OBESITY BEFORE BIRTH

ENDOCRINE UPDATES

Shlomo Melmed, M.D., Series Editor

For further volumes:
http://www.springer.com/series/5917

OBESITY BEFORE BIRTH

Maternal and Prenatal Influences on the Offspring

Edited by

Robert H. Lustig
Professor of Pediatrics
University of California
San Francisco, CA, USA

Springer

Editor
Robert H. Lustig, MD
Professor of Pediatrics
Division of Endocrinology
Director, Weight Assessment for Teen
and Child Health Program
University of California
San Francisco, CA 94143, USA

ISSN 1566-0729
ISBN 978-1-4419-7033-6 e-ISBN 978-1-4419-7034-3
DOI 10.1007/978-1-4419-7034-3
Springer New York Dordrecht Heidelberg London

Library of Congress Control Number: 2010935733

Printed on acid-free paper

Springer is part of Springer Science+Business Media (www.springer.com)

A gift for you

Enjoy your gift.

The editor would like to dedicate this volume to his family: his wife Julie and his two daughters, Miriam and Meredith. No academician could ask for more understanding, encouragement, sacrifice, and support – through service call, out-patient clinic, grant writing, mentoring others, and a busy lecture schedule. I am blessed beyond measure.

Preface

In my beginning is my end.
– T. S. Eliot, #2 of Four Quartets

Eliot had no idea that his observations on the life cycle would start even before birth. And indeed, one's earliest beginning predicts both the timing and means to that end. The concept that obesity was inherent, and not just the sum result of the behaviors of gluttony and sloth was surmised early in the twentieth century, but began in earnest with the postulation of a "thrifty genotype" by James Neel in 1962. However, the field lay dormant for another 30 years, awaiting biological and genetic confirmation. To compound the biological directive, the notion that prenatal biological influences could impact postnatal outcomes for obesity dates to 1989, when David Barker, an epidemiologist from Southampton, UK, first made the observation that now bears his name, the Barker hypothesis. He noted that maternal nutrition impacted on the fetus, such that small for gestational age infants were predicted to be at increased risk for obesity and metabolic syndrome in the future. Thus, the precept of developmental programming to amend one's genetic predisposition was advanced.

In the interval 21 years since Barker's discovery, numerous observations have slowly amended these two complementary hypotheses. Leptin, the first gene that of the energy balance pathway, was discovered in 1994. While already deemed essential for adult body weight regulation, Richard Simerly, then at Oregon Regional Primate Center, showed in animal models in 2004 that leptin likely was molding our hypothalami even before we took a swig of baby formula. Leptin opened up our understanding of the energy balance pathway, including genes such as MC4R, and their role in the genetics of obesity. Recent genome-wide association scans suggest that genetic linkages to obesity are primarily in the CNS. We learned in the late 1990s that large for gestational age and premature infants also became obese; and in the early 2000s that maternal obesity and weight gain during pregnancy are also risk factors. Furthermore epigenetics, which led credence to the ability of experiential phenomena in the mother to affect genetic expression in the newborn, was already a hot discipline when Randy Jirtle's group at Duke discovered in 2003 that they could alter offspring weight and color coat in genetically determined *Agouti* mice through altered maternal nutrition. This line of investigation has expanded exponentially ever since. The phenomenon of epigenetics has tied in very nicely with the above observations, explaining how vertical transmission of obesity can occur exclusive of DNA base changes. Lastly, data accrued by Retha Newbold at NIEHS and Bruce Blumberg at UC Irvine in 2005 found that environmental toxins not only contribute to obesity in adult animals but also program the liver and adipocyte during gestation. Moreover, each of these phenomena has been noted in human models. Lastly, we now recognize that developmental programming of obesity can be promulgated by actions in numerous target organs in the energy balance pathway. Actions on the hypothalamus can result in an altered energy setpoint; actions on the liver can result in an altered metabolic profile; and actions on the adipocyte can result in an altered storage capacity. These actions are not mutually exclusive, giving rise to phenotypes of hyperphagia (or not), insulin resistance (or not), and subcutaneous vs. visceral fat. Understanding these tissue-specific effects on these gestational perturbations will likely allow for understanding of the different obesity syndromes and their downstream co-morbidities.

Taken as a whole, these various phenomena clearly demonstrate that disruption of the normal energy balance paradigm during gestation has profound consequences for the offspring. These observations have led to a new branch of science and medicine: the Developmental Origins of Health and Disease (DOHaD). Given that (1) the obesity epidemic has gone global; (2) attempts at diet and exercise have failed to control the global obesity epidemic; and (3) we now have an epidemic of obese 6-month-olds, it is time to think “out of the box.” Is there an exposure that is causing this? Are pregnant women doing something to make their children fat? Are we promoting obesity before birth?

The purpose of this unique volume is to elucidate, in both animal and human models, the state-of-the-art evidence for each of these phenomena. The evidence, and indeed, our author roster, comes from around the world. Each of the sections of this volume (genetics, epigenetics, developmental programming, environmental obesogens) will start out with the role of pathogenetic mechanism in question in human obesity and will then follow up with the evidence in animal models. In this way, the strength and relevance of each of these pathogenetic mechanisms and their effects can be assessed.

It is hoped that by assembling each of these concepts in one volume, we will build a framework that will (1) inform physician and patient education into the causes of the obesity epidemic; (2) provide a nidus for further investigative efforts into the developmental nature of obesity and chronic disease; (3) provide a starting point for changes in policies to improve maternal–child health; and (4) provide data to assist public health officials to monitor and control environmental exposures, whether they be nutritional or toxicological.

San Francisco, CA
March 25, 2010

Robert H. Lustig

Contents

1 **Obesity: Nature or Nurture?** 1
Robert H. Lustig

Part I Genetic Disorders Leading to Obesity

2 **The Contribution of Heredity to Clinical Obesity** 25
Johanna C. Andersson and Andrew J. Walley

3 **Monogenic Disorders Within the Energy Balance Pathway** 53
Ivy R. Aslan, Sayali A. Ranadive, and Christian Vaisse

4 **Ciliary Syndromes and Obesity** 71
David S. Parker and Nicholas Katsanis

5 **Genome-Wide Association Studies and Human Population Obesity** 95
Ruth J.F. Loos and Tuomas O. Kilpeläinen

Part II Epigenetic Changes and the Development of Obesity

6 **Known Clinical Epigenetic Disorders with an Obesity Phenotype: Prader–Willi Syndrome and the *GNAS* Locus** 115
Merlin G. Butler

7 **Evidence for Epigenetic Changes as a Cause of Clinical Obesity** 147
Graham C. Burdge and Karen A. Lillycrop

8 **Epigenetic Changes Associated with Intrauterine Growth Retardation and Adipogenesis** 167
Sara E. Pinney and Rebecca A. Simmons

Part III Developmental Programming and the Development of Obesity

9 **Exposure to Diabetes In Utero, Offspring Growth, and Risk for Obesity** 193
Tessa Crume and Dana Dabelea

10 Maternal Weight Gain During Pregnancy and Obesity in the Offspring 205
Naomi E. Stotland and Janet C. King

11 Intrauterine Growth Restriction, Small for Gestational Age, and Experimental Obesity 215
Michael G. Ross, Ivan Huber, and Mina Desai

12 Experimental Models of Maternal Obesity and High-Fat Diet During Pregnancy and Programmed Obesity in the Offspring 241
Larissa Jane Prior, Geoffrey Albert Head, and James Andrew Armitage

13 High-Carbohydrate Intake Only During the Suckling Period Results in Adult-Onset Obesity in Mother as well as Offspring 261
Mulchand S. Patel and Malathi Srinivasan

14 Prenatal Stress, Glucocorticoids, and the Metabolic Syndrome . . 279
Amanda J. Drake and Jonathan R. Seckl

15 Hypothalamic Fetal Programming of Energy Homeostasis 301
Clement C. Cheung and Holly A. Ingraham

16 Adipocyte Development and Experimental Obesity 321
Elvira Isganaitis and Mary-Elizabeth Patti

Part IV Environmental Obesogens

17 The Obesogen Hypothesis of Obesity: Overview and Human Evidence 355
Jerrold J. Heindel

18 Perinatal Exposure to Endocrine Disrupting Chemicals with Estrogenic Activity and the Development of Obesity 367
Retha R. Newbold

19 The Role of Environmental Obesogens in the Obesity Epidemic . 383
Amanda Janesick and Bruce Blumberg

Index 401

Contributors

Johanna C. Andersson Department of Genomics of Common Disease, Faculty of Medicine, School of Public Health, Imperial College London, Hammersmith Hospital, London, UK, j.andersson@imperial.ac.uk

James Andrew Armitage Neuropharmacology Laboratory, Baker IDI Heart and Diabetes Institute, Melbourne, VIC, Australia; Department of Anatomy and Developmental Biology, Monash University, Clayton, VIC, Australia, james.armitage@med.monash.edu.au

Ivy R. Aslan Department of Endocrinology, Children's Hospital and Research Center, Oakland, 747 52nd Street, Oakland, CA 93609, USA, iaslan@mail.cho.org

Bruce Blumberg Department of Developmental and Cell Biology and Department of Pharmaceutical Sciences, University of California, Irvine, CA 92697-2300, USA, blumberg@uci.edu

Graham C. Burdge Institute of Human Nutrition, University of Southampton School of Medicine, Southampton SO16 6YD, UK, g.c.burdge@southampton.ac.uk

Merlin G. Butler Departments of Psychiatry and Behavioral Sciences and Pediatrics, Kansas University Medical Center, Kansas City, KS, USA, mbutler4@kumc.edu

Clement C. Cheung Departments of Pediatrics and Department of Cellular and Molecular Pharmacology, University of California, San Francisco, CA, USA, clement.cheung@ucsf.edu

Tessa Crume Department of Epidemiology, Colorado School of Public Health, University of Colorado, Denver, CO, USA, tessa.crume@ucdenver.edu

Dana Dabelea Department of Epidemiology, Colorado School of Public Health, University of Colorado, Denver, CO, USA, dana.dabelea@ucdenver.edu

Mina Desai Department of Obstetrics and Gynecology, David Geffen School of Medicine at Harbor-UCLA Medical School, Torrance, CA, USA, mdesai@obgyn.humc.edu

Amanda J. Drake Centre for Cardiovascular Science, The Queen's Medical Research Institute, University of Edinburgh, Edinburgh, UK, mandy.drake@ed.ac.uk

Geoffrey Albert Head Neuropharmacology Laboratory, Baker IDI Heart and Diabetes Institute, Melbourne, VIC, Australia, geoff.head@bakeridi.edu.au

Jerrold J. Heindel Division of Extramural Research and Training, National Institute of Environmental Health Sciences, Durham, NC, USA, heindelj@niehs.nih.gov

Ivan Huber Department of Obstetrics and Gynecology, Harbor-UCLA Medical Center, Torrance, CA, USA, ivan@randomtech.com

Holly A. Ingraham Department of Cellular and Molecular Pharmacology, University of California, San Francisco, CA, USA, holly.ingraham@ucsf.edu

Elvira Isganaitis Division of Cellular and Molecular Physiology, Joslin Diabetes Center, Harvard Medical School, Boston, MA, USA, elvira.isganaitis@joslin.harvard.edu

Amanda Janesick Department of Developmental and Cell Biology, University of California, Irvine, CA 92697-2300, USA, ajanesic@uci.edu

Nicholas Katsanis Department of Cell Biology, Center for Human Disease Modeling, Durham, NC 27710, USA, katsanis@cellbio.duke.edu

Tuomas O. Kilpeläinen MRC Epidemiology Unit, Institute of Metabolic Science, Addenbrooke's Hospital, Cambridge, UK, tuomas.kilpelainen@mrc-epid.cam.ac.uk

Janet C. King Children's Hospital Oakland Research Institute, Oakland, CA, USA, jking@chori.org

Karen A. Lillycrop School of Biological Sciences, University of Southampton, Southampton SO16 7PX, UK, k.a.lillycrop@soton.ac.uk

Ruth J.F. Loos MRC Epidemiology Unit, Institute of Metabolic Science, Addenbrooke's Hospital, Cambridge, UK, ruth.loos@mrc-epid.cam.ac.uk

Robert H. Lustig Division of Pediatric Endocrinology, Department of Pediatrics, University of California, San Francisco, CA 94143-0434, USA, rlustig@peds.ucsf.edu

Retha R. Newbold National Institute of Environmental Health Sciences (NIEHS), National Institutes of Health (NIH), Research Triangle Park, NC 27709, USA, newbold1@niehs.nih.gov; newboldretha@hotmail.com

David S. Parker Department of Cell Biology, Center for Human Disease Modeling, Durham, NC 27710, USA, dave.parker@duke.edu

Mulchand S. Patel Department of Biochemistry, School of Medicine and Biomedical Sciences, University at Buffalo, State University of New York, Buffalo, NY, USA, mspatel@buffalo.edu

Mary-Elizabeth Patti Division of Cellular and Molecular Physiology, Joslin Diabetes Center, Harvard Medical School, Boston, MA, USA, maryelizabeth.patti@joslin.harvard.edu

Sara E. Pinney Division of Endocrinology and Diabetes, Department of Pediatrics, The Children's Hospital of Philadelphia, University of Pennsylvania School of Medicine, Philadelphia, PA, USA, pinneys@email.chop.edu

Larissa Jane Prior Neuropharmacology Laboratory, Baker IDI Heart and Diabetes Institute, Melbourne, VIC, Australia, larissa.prior@bakeridi.edu.au

Sayali A. Ranadive Department of Endocrinology, Children's Hospital and Research Center Oakland, 747 52nd Street, Oakland, CA 93609, USA, sranadive@mail.cho.org

Michael G. Ross Department of Obstetrics and Gynecology, Harbor-UCLA Medical Center, Torrance, CA, USA, mikeross@ucla.edu

Jonathan R. Seckl Centre for Cardiovascular Science, The Queen's Medical Research Institute, University of Edinburgh, Edinburgh, UK, j.seckl@ed.ac.uk

Rebecca A. Simmons Division of Neonatology, Department of Pediatrics, The Children's Hospital of Philadelphia, University of Pennsylvania School of Medicine, Philadelphia, PA, USA, rsimmons@mail.med.upenn.edu

Malathi Srinivasan Department of Biochemistry, School of Medicine and Biomedical Sciences, University at Buffalo, State University of New York, Buffalo, NY, USA, malathi@acsu.buffalo.edu

Naomi E. Stotland Department of Obstetrics and Gynecology, University of California, San Francisco, CA, USA, stotlandn@obgyn.ucsf.edu

Christian Vaisse Department of Medicine, Diabetes Center, University of California, San Francisco, CA, USA, vaisse@diabetes.ucsf.edu

Andrew J. Walley Department of Genomics of Common Disease, Faculty of Medicine, School of Public Health, Imperial College London, Hammersmith Hospital, London, UK, a.walley@imperial.ac.uk

Chapter 1
Obesity: Nature or Nurture?

Robert H. Lustig

1.1 Introduction

The obesity epidemic shows no signs of relenting. There is now more obesity globally than malnutrition. Not only has obesity prevalence increased, but BMI distribution, the secular trend in increase in waist circumference, the increasing prevalence of comorbidities, and the incidence of obesity-related insulin resistance, and its spin-offs – the various components of the metabolic syndrome (type 2 diabetes, dyslipidemia, hypertension, cardiovascular disease) and the associated metabolic disturbances of nonalcoholic fatty liver disease and polycystic ovarian syndrome – continue to worsen. Furthermore, the increases in frequency of bariatric surgery around the world document that obesity and its comorbidities are increasing in frequency and severity globally. These increases have enormous negative connotations for both our health care dollars, as more people get sicker earlier and for longer, and for job productivity, as the obese have increased disability, time out of work, increased risk for dementia, and early death. Solving the obesity crisis is paramount; on this there is complete agreement. It has even been suggested in the USA that health care reform is nothing more or less than obesity reform. But how to solve it? A well-respected pediatrician and member of the antiobesity community once said to me, "I don't care what's causing the obesity epidemic. I just want to determine what to do about it." I respectfully disagree. "Eat less, exercise more" does not work. In order to solve this problem, we need to determine its cause(s). Thus, the need for this book. The chapters that follow denote specific biochemical and pathogenetic mechanisms by which obesity may occur.

One argument that continues to obstruct the discussion of what to do about the obesity epidemic is "Whose fault is it?" This argument can take many forms. Is it personal or societal? Is it biochemical or behavioral? Is it genetic or environmental? And for the purposes of this chapter, is it "nature" or "nurture"? This is not

R.H. Lustig (✉)
Division of Pediatric Endocrinology, Department of Pediatrics, University of California, San Francisco, CA 94143-0434, USA
e-mail: rlustig@peds.ucsf.edu

R.H. Lustig (ed.), *Obesity Before Birth*, Endocrine Updates 30,
DOI 10.1007/978-1-4419-7034-3_1,

just an academic argument, because such debates determine financial responsibility, allocations of care, access to programs, coverage by health insurance, and government payment. Here, I will attempt to demonstrate that each of these arguments is a "straw man" for the underlying pathophysiologic processes at work that foment this obesity epidemic.

1.2 Definitions

Although somewhat arbitrary, and with recognition of significant overlap, one set of theories for the development of obesity can be congregated into two paradigms: the "nature" camp and the "nurture" camp. For the purposes of this discussion and as an introduction to the rest of this volume, I will define "nurture" as a paradigm of empiricism or behaviorism. This is exemplified in the epistemological thesis of *tabula rasa* that individual human beings are born with no built-in content, in a word, "blank," and that their phenotype is built up from their cognitive experiences and sensory perceptions of the outside world. Such experiences are therefore imbued *after birth*. Conversely, I will define "nature" as a paradigm of nativism or innatism. Another way to express such a thesis is being *hardwired*, or possibly that their phenotype is built from sensory experiences from the inside world of the placenta. Thus, for purposes of this essay, nature can be equated with events *before birth*.

These paradigms extend themselves to discussions of the development of obesity. In its essence, energy balance obeys the first law of thermodynamics, which states that energy can neither be created nor destroyed; the total energy within a closed system remains constant. However, there are two disparate clinical interpretations of the first law, and the correct interpretation is open to question, dependent on which paradigm – "nature" or "nurture" – is favored.

1.3 The "Nurture" Interpretation

The "nurture" interpretation of the first law is thus stated: "If you eat it, you had better burn it, or you will store it." In this interpretation, the behaviors of increased energy intake and decreased energy expenditure are primary (and presumably learned) and the weight gain is a secondary result of these behaviors. Thus, many consider obesity to be a manifestation of these "aberrant behaviors" and therefore ascribe primacy to the behaviors associated with obesity. Included in this concept of "nurture" are individual phenomena such as food consumption, individual activity, and individual psychology; and societal and environmental phenomena such as food production, the activity environment, and societal influences [1]. The "nurture" interpretation also invokes the concept of "personal responsibility" for one's behavior, which serves society's current desire to place blame; which serves the obese individual as they would prefer to be portrayed as "perpetrator" rather than "victim;" and finally which serves as the cornerstone of both the government's and the insurance companies' restriction of obesity care delivery.

Numerous observations provide evidence for increased caloric intake fueling the obesity epidemic over the past 30 years, both in children [2] and in adults [3]. In a recent report evaluating data both from the US Department of Agriculture and from resting energy expenditure data from obese persons, Swinburn determined that increased caloric intake accounts for the entire US obesity epidemic [4]. In particular, calories from sugar-sweetened beverages have received the most attention [5] and has been the one food item that has been consistently linked with obesity [6, 7]. Fructose has been particularly scrutinized as a specific cause of obesity, insulin resistance, and metabolic syndrome [8–16].

Alternatively, decreased energy expenditure as a result of decreased physical activity has been implicated as a cause of obesity in some [17, 18], but not all [19], childhood studies. It is not clear when this decline started but there are age, sex, and racial covariates involved, which seem to correlate with the severity of obesity in children. In addition, screen time has been correlated directly with both obesity [20] and prevalence of metabolic syndrome in adolescents [21].

1.3.1 Risk Factors for Obesity Ascribable to "Nurture"

Aside from the obvious changes in the caloric and exercise milieu in which we find ourselves, numerous other processes associated with increased weight gain have been proffered as examples of environmental change. Many of these have a traditionally behavioral component. For example, sleep debt and decrease in smoking [22] are potentially malleable behaviors that might contribute to increased food intake. However, there are others that are not as clearly malleable but would nonetheless be classified within our environment. These include changes in ambient temperature and exposure to obesity-causing viruses such as adenovirus 36 [23]. Numerous behavioral changes occur in adolescence which might foster both increased caloric consumption and decreased activity [24]. Lastly, the concept of horizontal obesity transmission as a result of social networks was advanced by the Framingham study [25]. None of these exclude biochemical underpinnings to their efficacy, but each of them is felt to be specifically due to changes in exposure postnatally.

1.3.2 Problems with the "Nurture" Interpretation

The above associations with obesity suggest postnatal promotion of weight gain. However, they are just associations; none of these associations demonstrate clear directionality or mechanism. A second problem is that if childhood obesity were just about increased energy intake and decreased energy expenditure, then interventions focused on diet and exercise should be effective. Unfortunately, meta-analyses of the effects of dietary interventions to prevent [26] or treat [27] childhood obesity are salutary at best, as is true for exercise interventions [28]. Third, the concept of personal responsibility for obesity is not tenable in children. No child chooses to be obese. Children with childhood obesity experience a quality of life commensurate with children on cancer chemotherapy [29]. Obese children are ostracized by their peers [30]. Fourth and last, the greatest increase in prevalence is in the youngest members of society. The 2- to 5-year-old demographic is experiencing the most rapid rise in obesity and metabolic syndrome is even more frequent among obese children than it is for obese adults. Furthermore, young children are not responsible for food choices at home or at school and it can hardly be said that preschool children, in whom obesity is rampant [31], are in a position to accept personal responsibility. We even have an epidemic of obese 6-month-olds [32]. The obese 6-month-old is the "exception that proves the rule." While our society easily ascribes blame to our current dietary and exercise practices, how does this explain the obese 6-month-old?

To rationalize these arguments, we must understand what constitutes a behavior. *Stedman's Medical Dictionary* defines "behavior" as: "The stereotyped motor response to a physiological stimulus." This definition infers a physiological/biochemical basis underpinning behavior, which is evident in many medical disorders. For instance, if a child began to drink 10 gallons and urinate 10 gallons of water daily, the obvious diagnosis would be diabetes insipidus, a defect in vasopressin secretion or action. Although psychogenic water drinking could not be ruled out by history, it would be highly unlikely. Likewise, if a patient fell asleep at the wheel of a car or at the supper table, the initial diagnosis would be narcolepsy, which we now understand is a defect in stimulation by CNS orexins of the medullary reticular activating system [33, 34]. Even attention deficit disorder, obsessive compulsive disorder, and oppositional defiant disorder are thought to be biochemically based [35]. Thus, we routinely infer "biochemical" defects in many "behavioral" disturbances.

If obesity were merely the results of learned behaviors, then behavior/lifestyle interventions should be effective in reversing the process. Certainly, control of the environment by limiting access and insisting on physical activity results in weight loss [36]. And indeed, due to some notable, specific, and individual successes [37, 38], behavior/lifestyle modification in obese children has become the cornerstone of therapy. However, this is clearly not the case for the majority of obese children [39]. A review of the efficacy of lifestyle interventions in obese children stated: "... many interventions show success in knowledge and reported behaviors, but little effect on BMI or prevalence of overweight, most notably the large and expensive CATCH and Pathways trials" [40]. Indeed, recent meta-analyses of *treatment* of obese children demonstrate little response of BMI to dietary intervention [27] and even less response of BMI to exercise intervention [28]. However, because behavior/lifestyle modification is an "accepted" treatment, the general ethos is that any child who does not respond to lifestyle intervention must themselves, or their family, be noncompliant with the regimen. Indeed, the effects of altering lifestyle for obesity *prevention* are also underwhelming, showing minimal effects on behaviors and essentially no effect on BMI [26].

1.4 The "Nature" Interpretation

Conversely, the "nature" interpretation of the first law of thermodynamics is as follows: "If you are going to store it, and you expect to burn it, then you will have to eat it." Here, the weight gain is primary, presumably due to biochemical forces beyond one's control, and the witnessed behaviors of increased energy intake and decreased energy expenditure are secondary to the primary process of obligate weight gain.

This interpretation has become more approachable with the advent of the hormone leptin. The primacy of weight change in the first law is manifest during the starvation response. Everyone has a "personal leptin threshold," probably genetically set, above which the brain interprets a state of energy sufficiency [41]. The leptin-replete state is characterized by increased physical activity, decreased appetite, and increased feelings of well-being. However, in response to caloric restriction, leptin levels decline within 12 h, even before weight loss is manifest [42, 43], which is interpreted by the ventromedial hypothalamus (VMH) as starvation. Decline of leptin reduces α-melanocyte-stimulating hormone (α-MSH) release, which leads to reduced occupancy of the melanocortin-4 receptor (MC_4R). The resultant lack of anorexigenic pressure on the MC_4R results in changes in the efferent pathway of energy balance. Sympathetic nervous system (SNS) tone drops, resulting in a decline in resting energy expenditure (REE) and total energy expenditure in an attempt to conserve energy [44]. Uncoupling protein (UCP) levels decline with adipose tissue and skeletal muscle [45] as a result of decreased SNS activity in response to starvation [46]. Concomitantly, vagal tone is increased in order to slow the heart rate and myocardial oxygen consumption, increase β-cell insulin secretion in response to glucose, and increase adipose insulin sensitivity; all directed to increase energy storage [33, 46, 47]. These revert to baseline once caloric sufficiency is reestablished and leptin levels rise.

Examination of weight loss patterns in response to lifestyle and the obesity drugs dexfenfluramine, sibutramine, and orlistat demonstrates a rapid weight loss phase of 4 months, followed by a plateau [48]. Although reduced dietary intake and/or absorption continues, the plateau is inviolate. Although originally this plateau was viewed as a result of noncompliance or drug tachyphylaxis, it is actually due to a decline in resting energy expenditure, which occurs in response to the decline in serum leptin in order to offset the reduced caloric intake, termed the "starvation response" [49]. REE is dependent on nutritional status; in the energy-replete or over-replete state, REE is 50 kcal/kg fat-free mass, while in the weight-reduced state, REE is reduced to 40–42 kcal/kg fat-free mass [44, 50]. Thus, starvation results in a 20% increased efficiency of energy utilization [51]. Both obesity and starvation are states of free fatty acid mobilization and insulin resistance [52].

Obesity, with few exceptions, can be explained by either leptin deficiency or leptin resistance. The constitutional symptoms associated with obesity versus starvation are very similar: fatigue, malaise, lack of activity, inability to motivate, and depression. In each case, the VMH is unable to transduce the peripheral leptin signal, in starvation because of leptin inadequacy and in obesity because of leptin resistance [53, 54]. The difference is that giving leptin to obese leptin-sensitive individuals is extremely effective [55], while leptin administration to leptin-resistant individuals is not effective [56].

1.4.1 Risk Factors for Obesity Ascribable to "Nature"

The entirety of this book is dedicated to the various pathogenetic mechanisms associated with the "nature" camp. Numerous monogenic defects within the energy balance pathway have now been identified and characterized (Chapters 2–4). Each of these manifest normal birth weight but weight gain after birth is early, rapid, and unrelenting. In each of these, defects in leptin signaling, either due to leptin deficiency or due to downstream defects in leptin signal transduction, have been documented.

Genome-wide association scans (GWAS; see Chapter 5) have been extremely helpful in searching for other genetic loci associated with obesity. To date another 29 loci have been confirmed, many of which are in the CNS, giving rise to the concept that alterations in neural organization may underlie such propensity for obesity [57]. In particular, the associations with *FTO* and brain-derived neurotrophic factor (BDNF) are appealing, as these would tie genetic and neurodevelopmental phenomena together.

In addition, prenatal alteration of adipogenesis through epigenetic alterations leading to obesity has been documented in specific obesity syndromes, such as Prader–Willi syndrome (Chapter 6), and similar mechanisms are surmised in more general forms of obesity (Chapter 7). Alternatively, changes in fetal adaptation to a hostile environment, also known as "developmental programming," may be important. The hostile environment may include undernutrition, overnutrition, or maternal stress, transmitted through hormonal factors to the fetus. Such hormonal signals convey information about future threat, driving future energy storage even when there is no need to do so. This is certainly evidenced in the increased risk for future obesity that small-for-gestational age, large-for-gestational age, and premature babies manifest (Chapters 9, 10, 11, 12, 13, 14, 15, and 16). Clues to the possibility of prenatal overnutrition leading to future obesity include the increasing secular trend in birth weight found in many countries [57, 58]. A recent study [59] found that the rate of weight gain of mothers between their first and second child predicted increased birth weight in the second child, suggesting that maternal nutrition has long-lasting effects on the fetus.

Lastly, the possibility that toxins in our environment are programming surreptitious fetal adipose tissue development also has animal mechanistic support, and early human studies are at least suggestive, if not diagnostic of this mechanism of pathogenesis (Chapter 17). Numerous compounds in our environment act to induce adipocyte differentiation; fetal exposure may increase the "adipocyte load" fostering future obesity.

1.4.2 Problems with the "Nature" Interpretation

Although appealing mechanistically, the main knock against the "nature" interpretation is epidemiologic. Despite exhaustive searches, not that many people have the genetic mutations thus far elaborated. The only clinically meaningful mutation is MC4R deficiency, which accounts for somewhere between 2.5 and 5% of morbid obesity [60]. All the other mutations within the energy balance pathway are for the most part anecdotal and when combined do not account for even another 1%. Furthermore, GWAS studies (Chapter 5) suggest that a minority of weight gain is attributable to genetic loci. *FTO*, the most prevalent of the genetic association found thus far (found in 14% of children) [61], only accounts for 3.3 kg in extra weight in those homozygous for the "A" allele [62].

Lastly, if obesity is due to leptin resistance, then why has its prevalence only increased in the last 30 years? Certainly, genetics cannot explain this increase; the genetic pool does not change that fast. While epigenetic mechanisms are appealing, they also cannot explain the worldwide increase in prevalence of obesity, especially in such a short period of time. Presumably, some behavioral or environmental trigger is at work, something that is global and pervasive. The obvious answer is our food supply, with viruses, sleep deprivation, and changes in the built environment bringing up the rear. How to rationalize all these conflicts?

1.5 Toward a More Biochemical Understanding of the Nature Versus Nurture Argument

Instead of focusing on the timing (prenatal, postnatal) of the weight gain, perhaps we should focus on the pathophysiologic process itself. Could there be overarching phenomena, which are experienced at different times throughout the life cycle, which foment obesity, even prenatally? In the sections that follow, two specific biochemical phenomena associated with obesity are elaborated. Speculation is offered that their occurrence either in utero or postnatally sets up the adult, child, or baby for persistent weight gain and the metabolic syndrome.

1.6 Hyperinsulinemia and Leptin Resistance

Our clinical research program has been interested in the interplay between insulin and leptin in the VMH to affect leptin signal transduction. We believe that hyperinsulinemia acts as an "endogenous leptin antagonist" to promote leptin resistance. We postulate that this phenomenon can occur postnatally to promote weight gain, or possibly prenatally to reorganize the hypothalamus to foment risk for obesity in later life.

1.6.1 Postnatal Hyperinsulinemia, Leptin Resistance, and Obesity

Both insulin and leptin convey information to the CNS regarding long-term peripheral energy homeostasis. Insulin receptors colocalize to the same subpopulation of VMH neurons as do leptin receptors [63]. Both hormones have similarly anorexigenic effects when *acutely* administered into the CSF, as they decrease feeding behavior and induce satiety [64]. However, obesity is a state of *chronic* hyperinsulinemia and hyperleptinemia in the face of insulin and leptin resistance, and the negative feedback on food intake that should result from VMH exposure to both hormones is ineffective. Although insulin and leptin bind to separate receptors in the neurons of the VMH, they share the same signaling cascade, called insulin receptor substrate 2 (IRS2)/phosphatidyl inositol-3-kinase (PI3K) [65], and thus hyperinsulinemia may block leptin signaling. Numerous basic studies demonstrate that various knockouts within the CNS insulin signaling pathway can promote leptin sensitivity [66–73]. Transfection of the insulin receptor into HEK293 cells prevents leptin signaling upon insulin exposure [74]. Furthermore, insulin application blocks hypothalamic leptin-responsive neurons from firing [75]. Thus, hyperinsulinemia paradoxically turns the leptin negative feedback loop into a positive feedback loop or "vicious cycle" to foment obesity [76]. Appetite increases and weight accrues despite excess energy stores and hyperleptinemia, due to leptin resistance.

1.6.2 Two Clinical Paradigms Have Shown Improvement in Human Leptin Resistance

1.6.2.1 Forced Weight Loss

Rosenbaum et al. [77, 78] employed in-patient energy restriction to generate 10% weight loss to induce the starvation response. In these individuals, leptin declined, REE decreased, with commensurate decrease in serum triiodothyronine (T_3) levels. Exogenous administration of leptin in physiologic dosing to approximate the prestarvation leptin level resulted in further weight and fat decrease, along with return of REE and T_3 levels to the prestarvation state. Thus, in the prestarvation state, subjects were resistant to physiologic concentrations of endogenous leptin, while in the weight-reduced state, they were responsive to the same concentrations of exogenous leptin; thus, forced weight loss improved their inherent leptin sensitivity.

1.6.2.2 Insulin Suppression

This phenomenon of CNS leptin resistance is recapitulated in the syndrome of hypothalamic obesity. Hypothalamic damage can be a sequel of cranial insult due to head trauma, posterior fossa brain tumors, surgery, or radiation [79]. A direct relationship between hypothalamic damage and the rate of BMI increase and development of obesity has been noted in survivors of childhood brain tumors [80]. Death of VMH neurons prevents normal leptin signal transduction, resulting in "organic leptin resistance," which manifests as a chronic starvation response. Patients manifest an extremely poor quality of life with minimal physical activity despite adequate hormone replacement [79, 81]. Hypothalamic obesity is unresponsive to diet, exercise, and most pharmacologic manipulations. Bray and Gallagher [82] posited that the weight gain in hypothalamic obesity was a result of abnormal vagus nerve stimulation leading to increased β-cell insulin secretion. We hypothesized that suppression of β-cell insulin release should promote weight loss, despite the "organic leptin resistance." We examined the effects of the somatostatin analog octreotide (an agonist of the somatostatin-5 receptor on the β-cell, which is negatively coupled to the voltage-gated calcium channel) in children with hypothalamic obesity. In both a pilot, open-label trial [83] and a double-blind placebo-controlled trial [84], octreotide treatment resulted in insulin suppression and BMI stabilization, along with decreased caloric intake, increased spontaneous physical activity, and improvement in quality of life commensurates with the degree of insulin suppression, despite the organic leptin resistance.

We then postulated that a subset of obese adults without CNS insult also exhibit insulin hypersecretion, and might also respond to octreotide. In a pilot trial [85] and in a double-blind placebo-controlled trial [86], treatment with octreotide for 6 months resulted in significant weight and BMI loss (12.6 kg, BMI 4.3), but only in those (approximately 25%) who manifested insulin hypersecretion on their oral glucose tolerance tests. Despite the fact that leptin levels decreased by 50%, REE in these responders remained the same. We used the change in REE:leptin ratio as a surrogate index of change in leptin sensitivity within subjects. Indeed, the REE:leptin ratio increased in those who lost weight. Linear regression analysis between the change in REE:leptin and the change in insulin area under the curve demonstrated a significant negative correlation [87]. In other words, *insulin suppression improved leptin sensitivity*.

Both paradigms share at their core a reduction in systemic insulin concentrations. The similarity of outcome suggests that hyperinsulinemia may be a proximate cause of leptin resistance, promoting continued weight gain [76]. Teleologically, what could be the biological advantage of insulin–leptin hormonal antagonism? Leptin is a necessary signal to the VMH for the initiation of high-energy processes such as puberty and pregnancy [54]. Indeed, both puberty and pregnancy are insulin-resistant states [88]; leptin levels increase acutely; in adulthood or postpartum, insulin levels fall, weight stabilizes or is lost, and leptin levels return toward the baseline state [89, 90]. Insulin antagonism of leptin signal transduction is likely an integral control mechanism to insure reproductive competence. If leptin signaling were not modulable, the weight accrual required for reproductive competency during puberty and pregnancy would be compromised. The reversible antagonism of peripheral leptin action by insulin is advantageous for survival; since insulin causes energy deposition into fat, it makes sense that it should also be the central blocker of leptin.

1.6.3 Prenatal Hyperinsulinemia, Leptin Resistance, and Risk for Future Obesity

Follow-up studies of newborns born small-for-gestational age (SGA), large-for-gestational age (LGA), and premature have noted markedly increased risks for obesity, type 2 diabetes, and the metabolic syndrome in later life. The specific developmental aberration(s) that promote this phenomenon remain unknown. It is thought by some developmental biologists that SGA fetuses develop in a "mismatched" antenatal nutritional environment, which requires the organism to become energy efficient postnatally, leading to later obesity [91, 92]. However, this does not explain the same fate befalling LGA or premature offspring. An alternative thesis is that each of these three antenatal conditions is associated with insulin resistance at the level of the VMH, which could lead to attenuation of the leptin signal responsible for organizing the VMH to exert appropriate energy homeostasis.

1.6.4 Studies of SGA and Future Obesity

Documentation of the relationship of SGA with adult obesity and cardiovascular disease started with studies of the Dutch famine during World War II and its aftermath [93]. Several studies of newborns born SGA demonstrate that they are hyperinsulinemic and insulin resistant at birth, exhibit rapid catch-up growth in the early postnatal period, and develop obesity in childhood, with persistent insulin resistance and development of the metabolic syndrome. An analysis of Indian newborns born in India versus the UK [94] demonstrate that despite those born in India weighing 700 g less at birth, their glucose and insulin levels are markedly elevated. After adjustment for birth weight, the India-born babies demonstrate increased adiposity, four times higher insulin, and two times higher leptin levels than the UK-born babies. Thus, these babies are insulin resistant even at birth. Following such babies into childhood, there are numerous studies documenting insulin resistance during early childhood [95–97].

1.6.5 Studies of LGA and Future Obesity

Similarly, babies born LGA are hyperinsulinemic at birth [98]. Although most LGA babies are due to gestational diabetes mellitus (GDM) and exposure to hyperglycemia throughout the pregnancy, this is not always the cause. Follow-up of LGA babies without GDM demonstrates a doubling of prevalence of insulin resistance and metabolic syndrome, while LGA babies resulting from GDM manifest a threefold increase [99, 100]. Indeed, the "vertical" transmission of maternal diabetes to the offspring in the form of later obesity and diabetes has been documented in studies of Pima Indians [101, 102]. Conversely, obese women who underwent bariatric surgery reduced both the incidence of LGA offspring [103] and their future risk for obesity [104].

1.6.6 Studies of Prematurity and Future Obesity

Although there are no studies documenting hyperinsulinemia at birth in premature infants due to blood drawing issues, follow-up of these babies into early childhood also demonstrates increased weight gain and insulin resistance with compensatory insulin secretion that is inappropriately high for their degree of weight gain [105]. Thus, some aspect of prematurity leads to alteration in developmental programming and to the development of obesity and insulin resistance in later life.

1.6.7 Animal Models of Hypothalamic Maldevelopment: The Role of Neonatal Leptin

Animal models of gestational caloric restriction recapitulate the human condition and lead to SGA and insulin resistance at the birth of the offspring [106, 107], which manifests as later obesity with hypercaloric feeding [108]. Similarly, GDM in dams leads to future obesity and diabetes in offspring rats [109].

Several investigators have postulated that prenatal influences alter hypothalamic development and ultimately, postnatal regulation of energy balance in an adverse manner. For instance, gestationally diabetic dams give rise to offspring with decreases in the number and density of α-melanocyte stimulating hormone (α-MSH) and galanin (anorexigenic) neurons, and increases in the number and density of Neuropeptide Y (NPY) and Agouti-related protein (AGRP; orexigenic) neurons within the ventromedial hypothalamus (VMH); however, islet cell transplantation during the pregnancy restores both anorexigenic and orexigenic neurons to their baseline number and density [110]. This occurs as a consequence of improved glycemic control, and its attendant effects on neonatal fat metabolism [111].

Aside from its effects of signaling peripheral energy sufficiency to VMH neurons, it appears that leptin is also involved in the normal ontogeny and organization of the hypothalamus. Leptin-deficient mice (*ob/ob*) exhibit maldevelopment of hypothalamic architecture, with aberrant projections of neurons from the arcuate nucleus (the site of leptin receptors) to the paraventricular nucleus (the site of the melanocortin-4 receptors) [112]. This maldevelopment is notable as early as day 10 and worsens with age [112]. Defective neurotransmission of the anorexigenic signal within

VMH neurons is noted [113] and is thought to promote the hyperphagia that these animals experience. However, a single injection of leptin at birth can restore normal hypothalamic development and neurotransmission, even in the *ob/ob* mouse [113]. Histochemically, more synapses on α-MSH neurons and fewer synapses on NPY/AGRP neurons are evident even after one injection of leptin during the neonatal period.

This effect of neonatal leptin is also seen in the rat model of maternal undernutrition. Offspring of pregnant rats placed on food restriction during gestation are SGA and leptin deficient at birth. However, with adequate nutrition after the neonatal period, these animals become obese as adults, particularly when placed on high-fat chow after weaning [114]. These animals manifest insulin resistance at birth, with a steep weight trajectory thereafter, with insulin resistance and increased adiposity as adults. However, injection of leptin during the neonatal period restores normal weight gain and insulin levels in adulthood [114], suggesting that the leptin overrode an "organizational blueprint" for later obesity.

These data suggest that leptin exerts a trophic action on normal VMH ontogeny and development, which defends against obesity during the life of the animal [112]. However, either lack of leptin (as in the *ob/ob* mouse) or antagonism of leptin action in some fashion – for example, by the insulin resistance seen in the SGA, GDM-LGA, and premature models – may also prevent hypothalamic development and may also predispose the offspring to obesity in later life, especially in the setting of an overabundant food supply.

1.7 Stress, Glucocorticoids, and Visceral Adiposity

The amygdala is the neuroanatomic site of the stress-induced fear response [115, 116]. The amygdala synthesizes corticotropin-releasing hormone (CRH) and its neurotransmission is stimulatory to the HPA axis, with resultant cortisol secretion [117]. CRH-administered ICV evokes fear-like responses in animals [118], while inhibition of the CRH receptor prevents many manifestations of chronic stress [119, 120].

Stress and glucocorticoids are integral in promoting visceral adiposity and the metabolic syndrome. Adrenalectomized rats clamped with high levels of corticosterone (the rat glucocorticoid) demonstrate that exogenous fat intake is directly proportional to circulating glucocorticoid concentrations, although there is no effect on total chow intake [121], while amygdala activation by stress is dampened by the ingestion of energy-dense food [122], i.e., "comfort food" is "self-medication" for stress. In humans, glucocorticoid administration increases food intake directly [123]. Human research shows increased caloric intake of "comfort foods" (i.e., those with high energy density) after acute stress [124]. Chronic stress causes increased caloric intake of "comfort foods" (i.e., those with high energy density) but only among those with high cortisol reactivity [125–127]. People identifying themselves as "stress-eaters" exhibited significant increases in insulin, weight, and nocturnal cortisol during a stressful period compared to people who identified themselves as "stress noneaters" [128].

Thus, the high glucocorticoid levels associated with chronic stress may act as a feed-forward system, recruiting a central chronic stress response network [129] that alters the normal output of autonomic, neuroendocrine, and behavioral systems, biasing the usual responses toward increased HPA axis activity as well as accentuating fear-like behavior. Increased activity of this system increases ingestion of high energy density foods [122], with subsequent increased abdominal fat stores; possibly a marker of the metabolic syndrome in both rats and humans.

1.7.1 Postnatal Stress, Glucocorticoids, and Visceral Adiposity

Evidence of associations between elevated cortisol or markers of HPA axis dysregulation, psychological distress, and visceral adiposity in adults is compelling [130–137]. Job stress, depression, and cortisol are linked to the metabolic syndrome [137–140]. Psychosocial stresses correlate with risk of myocardial infarction in adults [141]; it is assumed that such patients exhibit increased HPA axis activation [142]. In the elderly, urinary glucocorticoid excretion is linked to various aspects of the metabolic syndrome, including blood pressure, fasting glucose and insulin, and waist circumference [143]. And of course, Cushing's syndrome, the prototypical disease of hypercortisolism, promotes visceral obesity and accelerated and severe CV mortality [144]. Even exogenous glucocorticoid administration is a risk factor for future CV events [145].

Stress and glucocorticoids have also been postulated to play a role in the metabolic syndrome in children [146], a time when eating patterns and adiposity levels are "programmed." Adverse childhood experiences predict both adult obesity [147] and metabolic dysfunction [148]. Several studies have shown relationships between stress and unhealthy dietary practices, including increased snacking in adolescents [149]. In a study of 9-year-olds, children who were both high on dietary restraint and felt more stressed by lab challenges tended to eat more comfort food [150]. Thus, childhood stress increases risk for obesity during adolescence and adulthood [151]. Lastly, glucocorticoid administration for acute lymphoblastic leukemia increases energy intake [152] and risk for future obesity [153].

1.7.2 Prenatal Stress, Glucocorticoid Exposure, and Risk for Future Visceral Adiposity

Maternal stress during pregnancy also appears to have long-lasting effects on the newborn. Numerous studies have demonstrated that increased maternal stress results in lower birth weight [154, 155], which, as we saw earlier, can predispose to obesity in later life. Offspring born of prenatal stress demonstrate altered glucose and insulin homeostasis upon reaching adulthood [156]. Prenatal stress, likely working through

CRH manufactured in the placenta, or possibly through maternal cortisol which overwhelms placental 11βHSD2 (which normally protects the fetus), may alter fetal metabolism in several ways. One correlate of prenatal stress and low birth weight is high umbilical cord cortisol levels [157]. Prenatal stress may also cause epigenetic changes in the methylation status of the CpG island in the NR3C1 gene, coding for the glucocorticoid receptor, which predicts altered neonatal stress reactivity [158].

Thus far, studies of prenatal glucocorticoid exposure in humans are sparse. The best studies are those conducted in offspring treated with dexamethasone in utero for congenital adrenal hyperplasia. Thus far, no effects on adiposity have been noted, although changes in cognition and behavior have been noted [159].

1.7.3 Prenatal Glucocorticoid Exposure in Animal Models

In animals, prenatal stress or glucocorticoid exposure appears to program risk for metabolic disorders. In rats, prenatal stress renders the offspring more vulnerable to a high-fat diet [160]. In rats, prenatal dexamethasone exposure increases ectopic fat distribution in response to a high-fat diet [161]. In nonhuman primates, prenatal dexamethasone exposure reduced birth weight and resulted in insulin resistance, glucose intolerance, and reduction in β-cell mass in the absence of changes in birth weight [162]. Lastly, prenatal dexamethasone administration to marmosets increased the placental expression of 11βHSD-1 in liver, pancreas, and fat post-natally, thus increasing the amplitude of glucocorticoid exposure within the fetus [163]. These data suggest that prenatal stress or glucocorticoid induction reduces birth weight (a risk factor for future adiposity) and has negative long-term effects on cardiometabolic fitness in the offspring.

1.8 Conclusions

Attempts at obesity prevention have recently gotten caught up in the question of "When is the best time to intervene?" Should we allocate resources to the adult, who is already obese and costing the medical system lots of money in comorbidities? Should we instead focus on the child, who is starting to demonstrate metabolic dysfunction, and will cost the system even more in the future? Should we focus on the infant to promote breastfeeding, one of the few interventions which work? Or should we focus on the pregnant woman, whose behaviors may set all of this in motion in the first place?

In this review, I hope I have shown that the argument of "nature" versus "nurture" in the development of obesity and metabolic syndrome is missing the point. Clearly, postnatal behaviors (such as altered nutrition and stress) have a biochemical underpinning, and those same behaviors when applied during pregnancy (in the form of antenatal nutrition and stress) drive the future biochemistry of the offspring. Thus, we humans are in a "vicious cycle" by which our biochemistry alters our behavior, which then alters the biochemistry of our next generation. Thus, the difference between "nature" and "nurture" is nothing more than when one chooses to examine the consequences of those biochemical effects. These effects can be pervasive, long-lasting, and vertically transmitted, expanding the affected population with each successive generation. And as a corollary, until we begin to understand the environmental forces that belie these changes and start to alter them, we can expect that the obesity epidemic will continue its parabolic curve of prevalence and comorbidity for generations to come.

Acknowledgments The author would like to thank Drs. Elissa Epel, Mary Dallman, Clement Cheung, Amanda Drake, Mark Tremblay, and Anastasia Hadjiyannakis for their collegiality and for their intellectual contributions to this treatise.

References

1. FORESIGHT. Tackling obesity: future choices – project report. 2nd ed. 2007. Government Office for Science http://www.foresight.gov.uk/Obesity/Obesity_final_part1.pdf.
2. Troiano RP, Briefel RR, Carroll MD, Bialostosky K. Energy and fat intakes of children and adolescents in the United States: data from the National Health and Nutrition Examination Surveys. Am J Clin Nutr. 2000;72:1343s–53s.
3. Centers for Disease Control. Trends in intake of energy and macronutrients – United States, 1971–2000. Morb Mortal Wkly Rep. 2004;53:80–2.
4. Swinburn B. Increased energy intake alone virtually explains all the increase in body weight in the United States from the 1970s to the 2000s. Eur Congr Obes (Amsterdam (Abstr.)). 2009;T1:RS3.3.
5. Duffey KJ, Popkin BM. Shifts in patterns and consumption of beverages between 1965 and 2002. Obesity. 2007;15:2739–47.
6. Malik VS, Schulze MB, Hu FB. Intake of sugar-sweetened beverages and weight gain: a systematic review. Am J Clin Nutr. 2006;84:274–88.
7. Vartanian LR, Schwartz MB, Brownell KD. Effects of soft drink consumption on nutrition and health: a systematic review and meta-analysis. Am J Public Health. 2007;97:667–75.
8. Le KA, Tappy L. Metabolic effects of fructose. Curr Opin Nutr Metab Care. 2006;9:469–75.
9. Rutledge AC, Adeli K. Fructose and the metabolic syndrome: pathophysiology and molecular mechanisms. Nutr Rev. 2007;65:S13–23.
10. Johnson RJ, Segal MS, Sautin Y, et al. Potential role of sugar (fructose) in the epidemic of hypertension, obesity and the metabolic syndrome, diabetes, kidney disease, and cardiovascular disease. Am J Clin Nutr. 2007;86:899–906.
11. Havel PJ. Dietary fructose: implications for dysregulation of energy homeostasis and lipid/carbohydrate metabolism. Nutr Rev. 2005;63:133–57.
12. Gross LS, Li S, Ford ES, Liu S. Increased consumption of refined carbohydrates and the epidemic of type 2 diabetes in the United States: an ecologic assessment. Am J Clin Nutr. 2004;79:774–9.
13. Elliott SS, Keim NL, Stern JS, Teff K, Havel PJ. Fructose, weight gain, and the insulin resistance syndrome. Am J Clin Nutr. 2002;76:911–22.
14. Dhingra R, Sullivan L, Jacques PF, et al. Soft drink consumption and risk of developing cardiometabolic risk factors and the metabolic syndrome in middle-aged adults in the community. Circulation. 2007;116:480–8.
15. Brown CM, Dulloo AG, Montani JP. Sugary drinks in the pathogenesis of obesity and cardiovascular diseases. Int J Obes. 2008;32:528–34.

16. Lim JS, Mietus-Snyder M, Valente A, Schwarz JM, Lustig RH. The role of fructose in the pathogenesis of NAFLD and the metabolic syndrome. Nat Rev Gastroenterol Hepatol. 2010;7:251–264.
17. Kimm SYS, Glynn NW, Kriska AM, et al. Decline in physical activity in black girls and white girls in adolescence. N Engl J Med. 2002;347:709–15.
18. Goran MI, Treuth MS. Energy expenditure, physical activity, and obesity in children. Pediatr Clin North Am. 2001;48:931–53.
19. Li S, Treuth MS, Wang Y. How active are American adolescents and have they become less active? Obes Rev. 2009; [epub Oct 27, 2009].
20. Marshall SJ, Biddle SJ, Gorely T, Cameron N, Murdey I. Relationships between media use, body fatness and physical activity in children and youth: a meta-analysis. Int J Obes Relat Metab Disord. 2004;28:1238–46.
21. Mark AE, Janssen I. Relationship between screen time and metabolic syndrome in adolescents. J Public Health. 2008;30:153–60.
22. Keith SW, Redden DT, Katzmaryk PT, et al. Putative contributors to the secular increase in obesity: exploring the roads less traveled. Int J Obes. 2006;30:1585–94.
23. Atkinson RL, Dhurandhar NV, Allison DB, et al. Human adenovirus-36 is associated with increased body weight and paradoxical reduction of serum lipids. Int J Obes. 2005;29: 281–6.
24. Jasik CB, Lustig RH. Adolescent obesity and puberty: the "perfect storm". Ann N Y Acad Sci. 2008;1135:265–79.
25. Christakis NA, Fowler JH. The spread of obesity in a large social network over 32 years. N Engl J Med. 2007;357:370–9.
26. Kamath CC, Vickers KS, Ehrlich A, et al. Clinical review: behavioral interventions to prevent childhood obesity: a systematic review and metaanalyses of randomized trials. J Clin Endocrinol Metab. 2008;93:4606–15.
27. McGovern L, Johnson JN, Paulo R, et al. Clinical review: treatment of pediatric obesity: a systematic review and meta-analysis of randomized trials. J Clin Endocrinol Metab. 2007;93:4600–5.
28. Shaw K, Gennat H, O'Rourke P, Del Mar C. Exercise for overweight or obesity. Cochrane Database Syst Rev. 2006;CD003817.
29. Schwimmer JB, Burwinkle TM, Varni JW. Health-related quality of life of severely obese children and adolescents. JAMA. 2003;289:1813–9.
30. Latner JD, Stunkard AJ. Getting worse: the stigmatization of obese children. Obes Res. 2003;11:452–6.
31. Ogden CL, Flegal KM, Carroll MD, Johnson CL. Prevalence and trends in overweight among US children and adolescents, 1999–2000. JAMA. 2002;288:1728–32.
32. Kim J, Peterson KE, Scanlon KS, et al. Trends in overweight from 1980 through 2001 among preschool-aged children enrolled in a health maintenance organization. Obesity. 2006;14:1164–71.
33. Hara J, Beuckmann CT, Nambu T, et al. Genetic ablation of orexin neurons in mice results in narcolepsy, hypophagia, and obesity. Neuron. 2001;30:345–54.
34. Mieda M, Yanigasawa M. Sleep feeding, and neuropeptides: roles of orexins and orexin receptors. Curr Opin Neurobiol. 2002;12:339–46.
35. Biederman J. Attention-deficit/hyperactivity disorder: a selective overview. Biol Psychiatry. 2005;57:1215–20.
36. Franco M, Orduñez P, Caballero B, et al. Impact of energy intake, physical activity, and population-wide weight loss on cardiovascular disease and diabetes mortality in Cuba, 1980–2005. Am J Epidemiol. 2007;166:1374–80.
37. Epstein LH, Roemmich JN, Raynor HA. Behavioral therapy in the treatment of pediatric obesity. Pediatr Clin North Am. 2001;48:981–93.
38. Mellin LM, Slinkard LA, Irwin CE. Adolescent obesity intervention: validation of the SHAPEDOWN program. J Am Diet Assoc. 1987;87:333–8.

39. Mun EC, Blackburn GL, Matthews JB. Current status of medical and surgical therapy for obesity. Gastroenterology. 2001;120:669–81.
40. Center for Weight and Health. Pediatric overweight: a review of the literature June 2001. http://www.cnr.berkeley.edu/cwh/news/announcements.shtml#lit_review (2001). Accessed Dec 1, 2009.
41. Leibel RL. The role of leptin in the control of body weight. Nutr Rev. 2002;60:S15–9.
42. Keim NL, Stern JS, Havel PJ. Relation between circulating leptin concentrations and appetite during a prolonged, moderate energy deficit in women. Am J Clin Nutr. 1998;68: 794–801.
43. Boden G, Chen X, Mozzoli M, Ryan I. Effect of fasting on serum leptin in normal human subjects. J Clin Endocrinol Metab. 1996;81:454–8.
44. Leibel RL, Rosenbaum M, Hirsch J. Changes in energy expenditure resulting from altered body weight. N Engl J Med. 1995;332:621–8.
45. Champigny O, Ricquier D. Effects of fasting and refeeding on the level of uncoupling protein mRNA in rat brown adipose tissue: evidence for diet-induced and cold-induced responses. J Nutr. 1990;120:1730–6.
46. Aronne LJ, Mackintosh R, Rosenbaum M, Leibel RL, Hirsch J. Autonomic nervous system activity in weight gain and weight loss. Am J Physiol. 1995;269:R222–5.
47. Lustig RH. The efferent arm of the energy balance regulatory pathway: neuroendocrinology and pathology. In: Donahoue PA, editor. Obesity and energy metabolism: research and clinical applications. Totowa, NJ: Humana; 2007. pp. 69–86.
48. Bray GA, Greenway FL. Current and potential drugs for treatment of obesity. Endocr Rev. 1999;20:805–75.
49. Elmquist JK, Maratos-Flier E, Saper CB, Flier JS. Unraveling the central nervous system pathways underlying responses to leptin. Nat Neurosci. 1998;1:445–50.
50. Rosenbaum M, Nicolson M, Hirsch J, Murphy E, Chu F, Leibel RL. Effects of weight change on plasma leptin concentrations and energy expenditure. J Clin Endocrinol Metab. 1997;82:3647–64.
51. Rosenbaum M, Vandenborne K, Goldsmith R, et al. Effects of experimental weight perturbation on skeletal muscle work efficiency in human subjects. Am J Physiol Regul Integr Comp Physiol. 2003;285:R183–92.
52. Boden G. Free fatty acids (FFA), a link between obesity and insulin resistance. Front Biosci. 1998;3:169–75.
53. Lustig RH. The "skinny" on childhood obesity: how our Western environment starves kids' brains. Pediatr Ann. 2006;35:898–907.
54. Flier JS. What's in a name? In search of leptin's physiologic role. J Clin Endocrinol Metab. 1998;83:1407–13.
55. Farooqi IS, Matarese G, Lord GM, et al. Beneficial effects of leptin on obesity, T-cell hyporesponsiveness, and neuroendocrine/metabolic dysfunction of human congenital leptin deficiency. J Clin Invest. 2002;110:1093–103.
56. Heymsfield SB, Greenberg AS, Fujioka K, et al. Recombinant leptin for weight loss in obese and lean adults: a randomized, controlled, dose-escalation trial. JAMA. 1999;282: 1568–75.
57. Ulijaszek SJ. Secular trend in birthweight among the Purari delta population, Papua New Guinea. Ann Hum Biol. 2001;28:246–55.
58. Davidson S, Litwin A, Peleg D, Erlich A. Are babies getting bigger? Secular trends in fetal growth in Israel – a retrospective hospital-based cohort study. Isr Med Assoc J. 2007;9: 649–51.
59. Ludwig DS, Currie J. The relationship between pregnancy weight gain and birth weight: a within family comparison. Lancet. 2010 Aug 4. [Epub ahead of print].
60. Vaisse C, Clement K, Durand E, Hercberg S, Guy-Grand B, Frougel P. Melanocortin-4 receptor mutations are a frequent and heterogeneous cause of morbid obesity. J Clin Invest. 2000;106:253–62.

61. Cecil JE, Tavendale R, Watt P, Hetherington MM, Palmer CN. An obesity-associated FTO gene variant and increased energy intake in children. N Engl J Med. 2008;359:2558–66.
62. Dina C, Meyre DGS, Durand E, Körner A, Jacobson P, Carlsson LM, et al. Variation in FTO contributes to childhood obesity and severe adult obesity. Nat Genet. 2007;39:724–6.
63. Baskin DG, Wilcox BJ, Figlewicz DP, Dorsa DM. Insulin and insulin-like growth factors in the CNS. Trends Neurosci. 1988;11:107–11.
64. Muntzel M, Morgan DA, Mark AL, Johnson AK. Intracerebroventricular insulin produces non-uniform regional increases in sympathetic nerve activity. Am J Physiol. 1994;267:R1350–5.
65. Niswender KD, Schwartz MW. Insulin and leptin revisited: adiposity signals with overlapping physiological and intracellular signaling capabilities. Front Neuroendocrinol. 2003;24:1–10.
66. Bence KK, Delibegovic M, Xue B, et al. Neuronal PTP1B regulates body weight, adiposity, and leptin action. Nat Med. 2006;12:917–24.
67. Mori H, Hanada R, Hanada T, et al. Socs3 deficiency in the brain elevates leptin sensitivity and confers resistance to diet-induced obesity. Nat Med. 2004;10:739–43.
68. Howard JK, Cave BJ, Oksanen LJ, Tzameli I, Bjorbaek C, Flier JS. Enhanced leptin sensitivity and attenuation of diet-induced obesity in mice with haploinsufficiency of SOCS3. Nat Med. 2004;10:734–8.
69. Kubota N, Terauchi Y, Tobe K, et al. Insulin receptor substrate 2 plays a crucial role in beta cells and the hypothalamus. J Clin Invest. 2004;114:917–27.
70. Choudhury AI, Heffron H, Smith MA, et al. The role of insulin receptor substrate 2 in hypothalamic and beta cell function. J Clin Invest. 2005;115:940–50.
71. Lin X, Taguchi A, Park S, et al. Dysregulation of insulin receptor substrate 2 in β-cells and brain causes obesity and diabetes. J Clin Invest. 2004;114:908–16.
72. Plum L, Ma X, Hampel B, et al. Enhanced PIP(3) signaling in POMC neurons causes K(ATP) channel activation and leads to diet-sensitive obesity. J Clin Invest. 2006;116:1886–901.
73. Munzberg H, Myers MG. Molecular and anatomical determinants of central leptin resistance. Nat Neurosci. 2005;8:566–70.
74. Kellerer M, Lammers R, Fritsche A, et al. Insulin inhibits leptin receptor signalling in HEK293 cells at the level of janus kinase-2: a potential mechanism for hyperinsulinaemia-associated leptin resistance. Diabetologia. 2001;44:1125–32.
75. Hill JW, Williams KW, Ye C, et al. Acute effects of leptin require PI3K signaling in hypothalamic proopiomelanocortin neurons in mice. J Clin Invest. 2008;118:1796–805.
76. Lustig RH. Childhood obesity: behavioral aberration or biochemical drive? Reinterpreting the first law of thermodynamics. Nat Clin Pract Endocrinol Metab. 2006;2:447–58.
77. Rosenbaum M, Murphy EM, Heymsfield SB, Matthews DE, Leibel RL. Low dose leptin administration reverses effects of sustained weight reduction on energy expenditure and circulating concentrations of thyroid hormones. J Clin Endocrinol Metab. 2002;87:2391–4.
78. Rosenbaum M, Goldsmith R, Bloomfield D, et al. Low-dose leptin reverses skeletal muscle, autonomic, and neuroendocrine adaptations to maintenance of reduced weight. J Clin Invest 2005;115:3579–86.
79. Poretti A, Grotzer MA, Ribi K, Schonle E, Boltshauser E. Outcome of craniopharyngioma in children: long-term complications and quality of life. Dev Med Child Neurol. 2004;46:220–9.
80. Lustig RH, Post SM, Srivannaboon K, et al. Risk factors for the development of obesity in children surviving brain tumors. J Clin Endocrinol Metab. 2003;88:611–6.
81. Harz KJ, Muller HL, Waldeck E, Pudel V, Roth C. Obesity in patients with craniopharyngioma: assessment of food intake and movement counts indicating physical activity. J Clin Endocrinol Metab. 2003;88:5227–31.
82. Bray GA, Gallagher TF. Manifestations of hypothalamic obesity in man: a comprehensive investigation of eight patients and a review of the literature. Medicine. 1975;54:301–33.

83. Lustig RH, Rose SR, Burghen GA, et al. Hypothalamic obesity in children caused by cranial insult: altered glucose and insulin dynamics, and reversal by a somatostatin agonist. J Pediatr. 1999;135:162–8.
84. Lustig RH, Hinds PS, Ringwald-Smith K, et al. Octreotide therapy of pediatric hypothalamic obesity: a double-blind, placebo-controlled trial. J Clin Endocrinol Metab. 2003;88: 2586–92.
85. Velasquez-Mieyer PA, Cowan PA, Arheart KL, et al. Suppression of insulin secretion promotes weight loss and alters macronutrient preference in a subset of obese adults. Int J Obes. 2003;27:219–26.
86. Lustig RH, Greenway F, Velasquez-Mieyer P, et al. A multicenter, randomized, double-blind, placebo-controlled, dose-finding trial of a long-acting formulation of octreotide in promoting weight loss in obese adults with insulin hypersecretion. Int J Obes. 2006;30(2):331–41.
87. Lustig RH, Sen S, Soberman JE, Velasquez-Mieyer PA. Obesity, leptin resistance, and the effects of insulin suppression. Int J Obes. 2004;28:1344–8.
88. Li HJ, Ji CY, Wang W, Hu YH. A twin study for serum leptin, soluble leptin receptor, and free insulin-like growth factor-1 in pubertal females. J Clin Endocrinol Metab. 2005;90: 3659–64.
89. Castracane VD, Hendrickx AG, Henson MC. Serum leptin in nonpregnant and pregnant women and in old and new world nonhuman primates. Exp Biol Med. 2005;230:251–4.
90. McLachlan KA, O'Neal D, Jenkins A, Alford FP. Do adiponectin, TNFα, leptin, and CRP relate to insulin resistance in pregnancy? Studies in women with and without gestational diabetes, during and after pregnancy. Diab Metab Res Rev. 2006;22:131–8.
91. Godfrey KM, Lillycrop KA, Burdge GC, Gluckman PD, Hanson MA. Epigenetic mechanisms and the mismatch concept of the developmental origins of health and disease. Pediatr Res. 2007;61:5R–10R.
92. Gluckman PD, Hanson MA, Cooper C, Thornburg KL. Effect of in utero and early-life conditions on adult health and disease. N Engl J Med. 2008;359:61–73.
93. Roseboom TJ, van der Meulen JH, Ravelli AC, Osmond C, Barker DJ, Bleker OP. Effects of prenatal exposure to the Dutch famine on adult disease in later life: an overview. Mol Cell Endocrinol. 2001;185:93–8.
94. Yajnik CS, Lubree HG, Rege SS, et al. Adiposity and hyperinsulnemia in Indians are present at birth. J Clin Endocrinol Metab. 2002;87:5575–80.
95. Arends NJ, Boonstra VH, Duivenvoorden HJ, Hofman PL, Cutfield WS, Hokken-Koelega AC. Reduced insulin sensitivity and the presence of cardiovascular risk factors in short prepubertal children born small for gestational age (SGA). Clin Endocrinol. 2005;62: 44–50.
96. Potau N, Gussinye M, Sanchez Ufarte C, Rique S, Vicens-Calvet E, Carrascosa A. Hyperinsulinemia in pre- and post-pubertal children born small for gestational age. Horm Res. 2001;56:146–50.
97. Yajnik CS, Fall CH, Vaidya U, et al. Fetal growth and glucose and insulin metabolism in four-year-old Indian children. Diabet Med. 1995;12:330–6.
98. Silverman BL, Landsberg L, Metzger BE. Fetal hyperinsulinism in offspring of diabetic mothers: association with the subsequent development of childhood obesity. Ann N Y Acad Sci. 1993;699:36–45.
99. Silverman BL, Rizzo TA, Cho NH, Metzger BE. Long-term effects of the intrauterine environment. The Northwestern University Diabetes in Pregnancy Center. Diab Care. 1998;21 Suppl 2:B142–9.
100. Boney CM, Verma A, Tucker R, Vohr BR. Metabolic syndrome in childhood: association with birth weight, maternal obesity, and gestational diabetes. Pediatrics. 2005;115:e290–6.
101. Knowler WC, Pettitt DJ, Savage PJ, Bennett PH. Diabetes incidence in Pima Indians: contributions of obesity and parental diabetes. Am J Epidemiol. 1981;113:144–56.
102. Dabelea D, Hanson RL, Lindsay RS, et al. Intrauterine exposure to diabetes conveys risk for type 2 diabetes and obesity: a study of discordant sibships. Diabetes. 2000;42:2208–11.

103. Marceau P, Biron S, Hould FS, et al. Outcome of pregnancies after obesity surgery. In: Guy-Grand B, Ailhaud G, editors. Progress in obesity research. John Libbey Eurotext, Montrouge, France 8th ed. 1999. pp. 795–802.
104. Kral JG, Biron S, Simard S, et al. Large maternal weight loss from obesity surgery prevents transmission of obesity to children who were followed for 2 to 18 years. Pediatrics. 2006;118:e1664–9.
105. Hofman PL, Regan F, Jackson WE, et al. Premature birth and later insulin resistance. N Engl J Med. 2004;351:2179–86.
106. Petry CJ, Ozanne SE, Wang CL, Hales CN. Effects of early protein restriction and adult obesity on rat pancreatic hormone content and glucose tolerance. Horm Metab Res. 2000;32:233–9.
107. Simmons RA, Templeton LJ, Gertz SJ. Intrauterine growth retardation leads to the development of type 2 diabetes in the rat. Diabetes. 2001;50:2279–86.
108. Vickers MH, Breier BH, Cutfield WS, Hofman PL, Gluckman PD. Fetal origins of hyperphagia, obesity, and hypertension and postnatal amplification by hypercaloric nutrition. Am J Physiol Endocrinol Metab. 2000;279:E83–7.
109. Boloker J, Gertz SJ, Simmons RA. Gestational diabetes leads to the development of diabetes in adulthood in the rat. Diabetes. 2002;51:1499–506.
110. Franke K, Harder T, Aerts L, et al. 'Programming' of orexigenic and anorexigenic hypothalamic neurons in offspring of treated and untreated diabetic mother rats. Brain Res. 2005;1031:276–83.
111. Harder T, Franke K, Fahrenkrog S, et al. Prevention by maternal pancreatic islet transplantation of hypothalamic malformation in offspring of diabetic mother rats is already detectable at weaning. Neurosci Lett. 2003;352(3):163–6.
112. Bouret SG, Draper SJ, Simerly RB. Trophic action of leptin on hypothalamic neurons that regulate feeding. Science. 2004;304:108–10.
113. Pinto S, Roseberry AG, Liu H, et al. Rapid rewiring of arcuate nucleus feeding circuits by leptin. Science. 2004;304:110–5.
114. Vickers MH, Gluckman PD, Coveny AH, et al. Neonatal leptin treatment reverses developmental programming. Endocrinology. 2005;146:4211–6.
115. Davis M, Whelan PJ. The amygdala: vigilance and emotion. Mol Psychiatry. 2001;6:13–34.
116. LeDoux J. Emotion circuits in the brain. Ann Rev Neurosci. 2000;23:155–84.
117. Sapolsky R, Krey L, McEwen B. The neuroendocrinology of stress and aging: the glucocorticoid cascade hypothesis. Endocrinol Rev. 1986;7:284–301.
118. Brown MR, Fisher LA. Corticotropin-releasing factor: effects on the autonomic nervous system and visceral systems. Fed Proc. 1985;44:243–8.
119. Smagin GN, Dunn AJ. The role of CRF receptor subtypes in stress-induced behavioural responses. Eur J Pharmacol. 2000;405:199–206.
120. Bakshi VP, Smith-Roe S, Newman SM, Grigoriadis DE, Kalin NH. Reduction of stress-induced behavior by antagonism of corticotropin-releasing hormone 2 (CRH2) receptors in lateral septum, or CRH1 receptors in amygdala. J Neurosci. 2002;22:7926–35.
121. La Fleur SE, Akana SF, Manalo SL, Dallman MF. Interaction between corticosterone and insulin in obesity: regulation of lard intake and fat stores. Endocrinology. 2004;145: 2174–85.
122. Dallman MF, Pecoraro N, Akana SF, et al. Chronic stress and obesity: a new view of "comfort food". Proc Natl Acad Sci. 2003;100:11696–701.
123. Tataranni PA, Larson DE, Snitker S, Young JB, Flatt JP, Ravussin E. Effects of glucocorticoids on energy metabolism and food intake in humans. Am J Physiol. 1996;271: E317–25.
124. Adam TC, Epel ES. Stress, eating, and the reward system. Physiol Behav. 2007;91:449–58.
125. Epel ES, McEwen BS, Seeman T, et al. Stress and body shape: stress-induced cortisol secretion is consistently greater among women with central fat. Psychosom Med. 2000;62:623–32.

126. Appelhans BM, Pagoto SL, Peters EN, Spring BJ. HPA axis response to stress predicts short-term snack intake in obese women. Appetite. 2010 Feb;54(1):217–20.
127. Epel ES, Lapidus R, McEwen BS, Brownell KD. Stress may add bite to appetite in women: a laboratory study of stress-induced cortisol and eating behavior. Psychoneuroendocrinology. 2001;26:37–49.
128. Adam TC, Epel ES. Stress, eating and the reward system. Physiol Behav. 2007 Jul 24;91:449–58.
129. Dallman MF, Pecoraro NC, La Fleur SE. Chronic stress and comfort foods: self-medication and abdominal obesity. Brain, Behav Immun. 2005;19:275–80.
130. Bjorntorp P, Rosmond R. Hypothalamic origin of the metabolic syndrome. Ann. N Y Acad Sci. 1999;892:297–307.
131. Epel E, McEwen B, Seeman T, et al. Can stress shape your body? Consistently greater stress-induced cortisol secretion among women with abdominal fat. Psychosom Med. 2000;62:623–32.
132. Thakore J, Richards P, Reznek R, Martin A, Dinan T. Increased intraabdominal fat in major depression. Biol Psychiatry 1997;41:1140–2.
133. Weber-Hamann B, Hentschel F, Kneist A, et al. Hypercortisolemic depression is associated with increased intra-abdominal fat. Psychosom Med. 2002;64:274–7.
134. Rosmond R, Dallman M, Bjorntorp P. Stress related cortisol secretion in men: relationships with abdominal obesity and endocrine, metabolic, and hemodynamic abnormalities. J Clin Endocrinol Metab. 1998;83:1853–9.
135. Rosmond R, Lapidus L, Marin P, Bjorntorp P. Mental distress, obesity, and body fat distribution in middle-aged men. Obes Res. 1996;4:245–52.
136. Ahlberg AC, Ljung T, Rosmond R, et al. Depression and anxiety symptoms in relation to anthropometry and metabolism in men. Psychiatry Res. 2002;112:101–10.
137. Wallerius S, Rosmond R, Ljung T, Holm G, Bjorntorp P. Rise in morning saliva cortisol is associated with abdominal obesity in men: a preliminary report. J Endocrinol Invest. 2003;26:616–9.
138. Vitaliano P, Scanlan J, Zhang J, Savage M, Hirsch I, Siegler I. A path model of chronic stress, the metabolic syndrome, and coronary heart disease. Psychosom Med. 2002;64:418–35.
139. Raikkonen K, Matthews KA, Kuller LH. The relationship between psychological risk attributes and the metabolic syndrome in healthy women: antecedent or consequence? Metabolism. 2002;51:1573–7.
140. Chandola T, Brunner E, Marmot M. Chronic stress at work and the metabolic syndrome: prospective study. BMJ. 2006;332:521–5.
141. Rosengren A, Hawken S, Ounpuu S, et al. Association of psychosocial risk factors with risk of acute myocardial infarction in 11,119 cases and 13,648 controls from 52 countries (the INTERHEART study): case-control study. Lancet. 2004;364:953–62.
142. Brunner EJ, Hemingway H, Walker BR, et al. Adrenocortical, autonomic, and inflammatory causes of the metabolic syndrome: nested case-control study. Circulation. 2002;106: 2659–65.
143. Andrew R, Gale CR, Walker BR, Seckl JR, Martyn CN. Glucocorticoid metabolism and the metabolic syndrome: associations in an elderly cohort. Exp Clin Endocrinol Diab. 2002;110:284–90.
144. Faggiano A, Pivonello R, Spiezia S, et al. Cardiovascular risk factors and common carotid artery caliber and stiffness in patients with Cushing's disease during active disease and 1 year after disease remission. J Clin Endocrinol Metab. 2003;88:2527–33.
145. Reynolds RM, Walker BR. Human insulin resistance: the role of glucocorticoids. Diab Obes Metab. 2003;5:5–12.
146. Charmandari E, Kino T, Souvatzoglou E, Chrousos GP. Pediatric stress: hormonal mediators and human development. Horm Res. 2003;59:161–79.
147. Greenfield EA, Marks NF. Violence from parents in childhood and obesity in adulthood: using food in response to stress as a mediator of risk. Soc Sci Med. 2009;68:791–8.

148. Danese A, Moffitt TE, Harrington H, et al. Adverse childhood experiences and adult risk factors for age-related disease: depression, inflammation, and clustering of metabolic risk markers. Arch Pediatr Adolesc Med. 2009;163:1135–43.
149. Oliver G, Wardle J. Perceived effects of stress on food choice. Physiol. Behav. 1999;66: 511–5.
150. Roemmich JN, Wright SM, Epstein LH. Dietary restraint and stress-induced snacking in youth. Obes Res. 2002;10:1120–6.
151. Johnson JG, Cohen P, Kasen S, Brook JS. Childhood adversities associated with risk for eating disorders or weight problems during adolescence or early adulthood. Am J Psychiatry. 2002;159:394–400.
152. Reilly JJ, Brougham M, Montgomery C, Richardson F, Kelly A, Gibson BE. Effect of glucocorticoid therapy on energy intake in children treated for acute lymphoblastic leukemia. J Clin Endocrinol Metab. 2001;86:3742–5.
153. Reilly JJ, Ventham JC, Newell J, Aitchison T, Wallace WH, Gibson BE. Risk factors for excess weight gain in children treated for acute lymphoblastic leukaemia. Int J Obes Relat Metab Disord. 2000;24:1537–41.
154. French NP, Hagan R, Evans SF, Godfrey M, Newnham JP. Repeated antenatal corticosteroids: size at birth and subsequent development. Am J Obstet Gynecol. 1999;180:114–21.
155. Bloom SL, Sheffield JS, McIntire DD, Leveno KJ. Antenatal dexamethasone and decreased birth weight. Obstet Gynecol. 2001;97:485–90.
156. Entringer S, Wüst S, Kumsta R, et al. Prenatal psychosocial stress exposure is associated with insulin resistance in young adults. Am J Obstet Gynecol. 2008;199:e1–7.
157. Phillips DI, Barker DJ, Fall CH, et al. Elevated plasma cortisol concentrations: a link between low birth weight and the insulin resistance syndrome? J Clin Endocrinol Metab. 1998;83:757–60.
158. Oberlander TF, Weinberg J, Papsdorf M, Grunau R, Misri S, Devlin AM. Prenatal exposure to maternal depression, neonatal methylation of human glucocorticoid receptor gene (NR3C1) and infant cortisol stress responses. Epigenetics. 2008;3:97–106.
159. Lajic S, Nordenström A, Hirvikoski T. Long-term outcome of prenatal treatment of congenital adrenal hyperplasia. Endocrinol Dev. 2008;13:82–98.
160. Tamashiro KL, Terrillion CE, Hyun J, Koenig JI, Moran TH. Prenatal stress or high-fat diet increases susceptibility to diet-induced obesity in rat offspring. Diabetes. 2009;58:1116–25.
161. Drake AJ, Raubenheimer PJ, Kerrigan D, McInnes KJ, Seckl JR, Walker BR. Prenatal dexamethasone programs expression of genes in liver and adipose tissue and increased hepatic lipid accumulation but not obesity on a high-fat diet. Endocrinology. 2010;151:1581–7.
162. De Vries A, Holmes MC, Heijnis A, et al. Prenatal dexamethasone exposure induces changes in nonhuman primate offspring cardiometabolic and hypothalamic-pituitary-adrenal axis function. J Clin Invest. 2007;117:1058–67.
163. Nyirenda MJ, Carter R, Tang JI, et al. Prenatal programming of metabolic syndrome in the common marmoset is associated with increased expression of 11beta-hydroxysteroid dehydrogenase type 1. Diabetes. 2009;58:2873–9.

Part I
Genetic Disorders Leading to Obesity

Chapter 2
The Contribution of Heredity to Clinical Obesity

Johanna C. Andersson and Andrew J. Walley

2.1 Introduction

In order to discuss the contribution of heredity to clinical obesity, we first need to define our terms of reference to give us the common ground that is needed to explore the relationship between heredity, the environment, and clinical obesity. This will also serve to introduce these subjects for later chapters of this volume covering other aspects of the relative contributions of heredity and environment to the final clinical outcome of obesity. The importance of understanding the mechanisms underlying obesity cannot be overstated. Global rates of obesity are rising fast in most countries and the economic implications for maintaining the health care systems of those countries under the increasing burden of comorbidities and ill health are enormous [1].

2.2 Defining Heredity

Heredity can simply be defined as the transmission of characteristic traits from parent to offspring. In the mid-nineteenth century, Mendel took this idea and by painstaking experimentation was able to formalize it as his two laws of heredity: the law of segregation and the law of independent assortment. The study of the science of heredity is genetics. In the twenty-first century, we now know the molecular basis of the principles of heredity and though our understanding of human genetics is by no means complete, the information that we have on DNA, the human genome sequence, epigenetics, and the environment all inform our understanding of heredity. We should be clear from the outset that using the term heredity does not imply that there is a purely genetic mechanism underlying the transmission of a trait. For many common traits, and for common obesity in particular, the influence of the environment is clearly strong.

A.J. Walley (✉)
Department of Genomics of Common Disease, Faculty of Medicine, School of Public Health, Imperial College London, Hammersmith Hospital, London, UK
e-mail: a.walley@imperial.ac.uk

R.H. Lustig (ed.), *Obesity Before Birth*, Endocrine Updates 30,
DOI 10.1007/978-1-4419-7034-3_2,

2.3 Clinical Obesity

As with heredity, a definition of clinical obesity is needed and for the purposes of this chapter, obesity is defined using the World Health Organization criteria (see http://www.who.int/mediacentre/factsheets/fs311/en/index.html). This defines adult obesity as a body mass index (BMI) greater than 30 kg/m^2, overweight as a BMI between 25 and 30 kg/m^2, and leanness as a BMI less than 25 kg/m^2. BMI has become widely accepted as a measure of obesity because of the simplicity and reproducibility of obtaining this measure in large numbers of people. It should not be used uncritically however, as BMI is affected by the proportion of heavier muscle tissue to lighter fat tissue, e.g., bodybuilders could be classed as clinically obese using the BMI definition alone. Equally, the specific presence of excess abdominal fat tissue, and not just excess fat tissue in general, is very important for determining health outcomes in obesity [2, 3] and the metabolic syndrome [4]. This has led to other simple measures such as waist–hip ratio (WHR) and skinfold thickness, and recently more sophisticated measures of body composition such as air displacement plethysmography and dual energy X-ray absorptiometry (DEXA) (see references [5, 6] for discussion of obesity-related phenotypes).

2.4 The Environment

The third basic term that we need to define is environment. In biological terms, the environment is the surroundings that an organism exists within and interacts with. Within this definition, and with respect to obesity, the environment can cover anything from food availability to infectious disease prevalence to provision of treatment. It is clear that the rapid rise in obesity seen over the last few decades cannot be due to genetic changes; therefore, environmental effects are extremely important to delineate. However, this does not rule out the possibility that the changing environment has revealed in our genome the presence of variants that are very predisposing factors for obesity.

2.5 The Obesogenic Environment and the Rise in Obesity

The rapid rise in obesity cannot be due to the slow changes in the human genome that occur over thousands of years in response to strong evolutionary pressures. This leaves us with two possibilities: either the rise in obesity is purely due to nongenetic changes or the environment has changed enough that positive genetic adaptations to the old environment are now having a negative effect in the new environment, resulting in obesity. This is why the phrase "obesogenic environment" was coined (first PubMed reference in 1999 [7]), as a way of referring to the current environment, which differs in many ways from the environment that existed prior to the mid-1950s, i.e., before the end of food rationing in the Allied countries after World

War II. Our current environment is considered obesogenic because of the ready availability of cheap, calorie-rich foods, the increasing trend toward office working due to automation and computerization of manual jobs, the rise of leisure pastimes such as video games that require little or no physical effort, and the ubiquity of the Internet allowing activities that previously required some physical effort, such as shopping or social interaction, to occur through a computer.

2.6 Why Aren't We All Obese?

It has been generally accepted, both within the medical profession and in the wider community, that obesity is simply the consequence of eating too much and exercising too little. However, despite many years of expensive public health campaigns and clear evidence that large numbers of people diet regularly, the rise in obesity continues. In a heavily regulated environment, anyone can be made to lose weight by forcing a reduction in their caloric intake. However, in the real world, exposed to the obesogenic environment every day, it is virtually impossible to sustain diet-induced weight loss over many years. While the environment is a fundamental factor in the rise of obesity, this raises the important question of why it is that not everyone is obese. Historically, obesity has always existed, though at much lower frequency, and there is no doubt that heredity has a role to play in the determination of our body size within a particular environment.

2.7 Is Obesity Heritable?

It is one thing to observe anecdotally that obesity seems to run in families and another to try and formally measure its heritability. Heritability is the proportion of the variation of a trait that is genetic in origin. As we have seen above, there are good reasons why we might think that obesity is wholly environmental. This probably explains why even though the evidence has been there since the 1960s [8], it has only been with the discovery of rare, monogenic, extreme obesity disorders (see Chapter 3) [9], syndromic forms of obesity (see Chapter 4) [10], and genome-wide association scans (see Chapter 5) that the academic community became open to the idea that common obesity could have a strong genetic basis. Many study designs exist that can give information on the heritability of a trait, and the ones used in the field of obesity research will be explored here, purely from the angle of what information they have provided about heredity and obesity. We will cover twin studies, adoption studies and studies of families. Case–control studies can provide additional information about the role of specific genes in heredity, and they will be discussed in this context. Finally, a short description of two specific confounding factors when investigating heredity and obesity will be mentioned. A detailed discussion of statistical approaches to calculating heritability statistics in these studies is beyond the scope of this chapter and the reader is referred to a recent review [11].

2.8 Twin Studies

Some of the first twin studies ever reported were conducted by Sir Francis Galton (1822–1911). In the 1870s he published a series of seminal articles arguing that heredity was a stronger factor than environment in determining the characteristics of twins [12]. The first systematic comparison of twins was reported by Siemens in 1924 [13]. He determined that any heritable disease will be more concordant in identical twins than in nonidentical twins, and concordance will be even lower in nonsiblings. In his experiments, he compared the numbers of pigmented skin lesions ("moles") in twins, and then correlated the mole counts between identical and nonidentical twins. The correlation was higher in identical twins (0.4) than in nonidentical twins (0.2), suggesting the importance of genetic factors in mole count.

Since then, twin studies have been widely used to help disentangle environmental and genetic effects. Several different study designs have been developed: the classical twin study, the extended twin study, which includes family members (parents, siblings, spouses) and in some cases virtual twins (same-age biological and nonbiological siblings reared together since birth), and studies of identical twins discordant for a trait of interest. Furthermore, obesity-related traits can be measured at a single time point (cross-sectional study) or multiple measurements can be taken at different time points (longitudinal study). An overview of twin study designs is given in Table 2.1.

Table 2.1 Overview of twin study designs

Twin study design	Key characteristics	Application
Classical	Comparison of phenotypes in MZ and DZ twins	Estimate the contribution of genetic and environmental effects
Extended	Family members (parents, siblings, spouses, offspring) included	Estimate G × E covariance, imprinting, parent-of-origin effects
Extended with virtual twins	Virtual twin, i.e., same-age nonbiological sibling (adoptee), included	Estimate common environmental effects that cannot be separated from nonadditive genetic effects using biological siblings only
Co-twin control	Twins answer questionnaires about themselves and their co-twin	Reduce the risk of misreporting often seen in self-reported data
Discordant MZ twins	Case–control study with perfectly matched control	Estimate environmental and epigenetic effects

Table of published twin study designs used in the investigation of heritability of obesity-related traits, including key characteristics and applications. Key: G × E = gene–environment interaction

2.8.1 Types of Twin Studies

2.8.1.1 The Classical Twin Study

The classical twin study compares the phenotypic resemblance of monozygotic (MZ; identical) and dizygotic (DZ; nonidentical) twin pairs. MZ twins are virtually 100% genetically identical whereas DZ twins share on average 50%. Comparison of MZ and DZ twins offers the first estimate of the extent to which genetic variation determines the phenotypic variation of the trait.

If MZ twins show a higher degree of similarity than DZ twins, this indicates that the trait is under some level of genetic control. The heritability (h^2) of a trait can be estimated from twice the difference between the correlation in MZ (r_{MZ}) and the correlation in DZ twins (r_{DZ}), i.e. ($h^2 = 2(r_{MZ}–r_{DZ})$. For example, a correlation of 0.4 in MZ twins and 0.2 in DZ twins gives a heritability estimate of 2(0.4–0.2), which equals 0.40 or 40%.

The proportion of the variance that is due to shared environment is the difference between the observed twin correlation and the heritability. In MZ twins, the proportion is $r_{MZ}–h^2$, and in DZ twins $r_{DZ}–h^2/2$, where r is the correlation between twins.

Traditionally, most twin studies have used analysis of variance (ANOVA) and intraclass correlations for analysis, but now most studies use structural equation modeling (SEM). In SEM, genotypic and environmental effects are modeled as the contribution of unmeasured variables to the potentially multivariate phenotypic differences between individuals. The contributions of the unmeasured variables are estimated as regression coefficients in the linear regression of the observed variables on the unmeasured variables. This means that SEM can accommodate the analysis of many covariates, including, e.g., gender differences in heritability.

2.8.1.2 The Extended Twin Study

The effects of cultural transmission, gene × environment covariance, and parent-of-origin can be determined by extending the classical twin study to include parents, siblings, spouses, and offspring. It can also be extended to include virtual twins. A virtual twin is a same-age nonbiological sibling, i.e., an adoptee who shares the same family environment but not the genetic background. Inclusion of virtual twins provides an opportunity to estimate common environmental effects on phenotypes that cannot be separated from the nonadditive genetic component using only biological siblings. In a relatively small study (929 individuals) using virtual twins [14], 64% of the variance in BMI was explained by nonadditive genetic effects with some contribution from common environmental factors. The study concluded that both genetic components and common environmental factors such as diet or exercise play an essential role in BMI.

2.8.1.3 The Co-twin Control Study

A study of 713 MZ and 698 same-sex DZ twin pairs aged 22–28 years were assessed for eating, dieting, and physical activity using structured questionnaires. Each twin was asked to describe their own eating and exercise habits as well as compare them to those of their co-twin. For all twin pairs, the co-twin for whom both twin pair members concordantly answered that this twin eats more, snacks more, eats more fatty foods, eats faster, and exercises less had significantly higher BMI and waist circumference. Multivariate regression analysis revealed co-twin differences in the amount of food consumed as the strongest independent predictor of intrapair differences in BMI and WC. This type of study design, while rarely used, improves the risk of misreporting that is often seen in subjective self-reports [15].

2.8.1.4 The Discordant MZ Twin Study

As might be expected in genetically identical individuals, phenotypic discordance is rare among MZ twins, but where these pairs can be identified, they can be viewed as perfectly genetically matched case–controls. This then allows the examination of either epigenetic or nongenetic environmental causes of obesity.

In a small study of seven MZ and nine DZ middle-aged twin pairs with long-term discordance for physical activity, but with very long follow-up, the effects of physically inactive versus active lifestyle were studied in relation to presence of fat tissue (visceral, liver, and intramuscular) assessed by magnetic resonance imaging [16]. The more active co-twin at the beginning of the study remained more active throughout the follow-up period of 32 years. Within-pair analyses carried out at the end of follow-up showed that the physically inactive twin had 50% greater visceral fat, 170% higher liver fat, and 54% higher intramuscular fat as compared with the active co-twin. All trends were similar for MZ and DZ twins. The use of discordant twins allowed the authors to conclude that regular physical activity is an important factor in preventing accumulation of high-risk fat over time, even after controlling for genetic liability and childhood environment.

Weight discordance is very rare among MZ twin pairs, but a study of 14 discordant MZ twin pairs from the FinnTwin16 study ($n = 658$ twin pairs) provides additional support for the utility of this approach. Discordance was defined as a difference in BMI equal to or greater than 4 kg/m^2. Ten concordant pairs were included as controls. The weight differences in the discordant pairs emerged at 18 years of age leading to an average discordance of 16.4 kg (5.6 kg/m^2) at 25.7 years of age. The heavier co-twin weighed more at birth (221 g, 1 kg/m^2), but the difference was gone by 6 months of age and only reappeared at 18 years of age. Although this twin sample was very small, it identified that young adulthood represents a critical period for weight gain irrespective of genetic background [17].

2.8.1.5 Twins Reared Apart

In rare cases, twins are reared apart and this offers the possibility of examining the correlation of traits between genetically identical sibling pairs that have been exposed to different environments. In a relatively small study of 53 MZ twin pairs from Finland, Japan, and America, estimates of heritability of BMI ranged between 0.5 and 0.7, consistent with other twin studies [18].

2.8.1.6 Twin Studies to Distinguish Between Genetic and Environmental Effects

Genetic effects can be divided into additive (A) and dominant (D) genetic effects. Environmental effects are typically divided into the common or shared environment (C) and the unique or nonshared environment (E).

Numerous twin studies in adults have demonstrated that BMI is influenced by additive genetic and unique environmental effects only [19]. On the other hand, most studies of children and young adolescents show a significant effect of common environment on children younger than 12 years [20–23]. The effect of the common environment then disappears during adolescence [24]. It is believed that this is due to greater parental influence over food choice and physical activity early in life as compared to adolescence.

2.8.2 Twin Studies and Obesity

Studies of MZ and DZ twins in the 1970s and 1980s resulted in identification of strong heritability for several obesity-related traits, such as skinfold thickness [25] and BMI [26]. Skinfold thickness was studied in children in 78 MZ and 144 DZ twin pairs. Significantly higher correlation coefficients were found in MZ twins compared to DZ twins. In the larger BMI study of 1,974 MZ and 2,097 DZ adolescent and adult twin pairs, the heritability estimate for BMI was reported to be between 0.77 and 0.84. The MZ twins also exhibited a markedly higher concordance rate for overweight than did DZ twins.

Further strong evidence of the heritability of BMI came from a study of identical twins separated at or near birth and brought up in different environments [27]. The study demonstrated that as adults, BMI was highly correlated between identical twins, but showed little correlation with that of their adoptive parents or siblings. Similar results have also been found in adoption studies not including identical twins (see below).

2.9 Genetic Linkage Studies Using DZ Twins

Variance due to early-life events is reduced in DZ twin pairs, making them highly valuable for linkage scans of complex traits, such as obesity. In one study, adult DZ female twin pairs from 1,094 pedigrees were studied for genome-wide linkage and positional candidate analysis, with the aim of identifying genes that play a role in regulating fat mass and distribution in women. Nonparametric multipoint linkage analyses showed linkage of the trait of central fat mass to 12q24 with LOD = 2.2, and for BMI to 8q11 with LOD = 1.3. These findings supported previously established linkage data [28–30]. Novel areas of suggestive linkage identified were for total fat percentage to 6q12 (LOD = 2.4) and for total lean mass to 2q37 (LOD = 2.4). Follow-up fine mapping in an extended cohort of 1,243 twin pairs reinforced the linkage for central fat mass to 12q24 (LOD = 2.6). Forty-five single nucleotide polymorphisms (SNPs) were chosen from twenty-six positional candidate genes in the area. Significant associations were found for SNPs in two genes: PLA2G1B ($p = 0.0067$) and P2RX4 ($p = 0.017$). These results suggested that genes involved in phospholipase and purinoreceptor pathways may regulate fat accumulation and distribution [31].

In a large meta-analysis [32], genome-wide linkage scans were performed using a 10 cM microsatellite marker map in 4,401 families (10,535 individuals) from six data sets of European origin from Australia, Denmark, Finland, The Netherlands, Sweden, and the UK from the GenomEUtwin cohort. This study found suggestive evidence for QTLs for BMI on 3q29 and 7q36 in the total sample set, with MLOD values of 2.6 and 2.4, respectively. Two individual cohorts showed strong evidence for three additional loci: 16q23 (MLOD = 3.7) and 2p24 (MLOD = 3.4) in the Dutch cohort, and 20q13 (MLOD = 3.2) in the Finnish cohort. In summary, this large twin cohort study provided evidence for suggestive linkage to BMI at two previously identified loci and strong evidence of linkage to three new loci. The results also suggested a smaller environmental variance between DZ twins than full siblings, with a corresponding increase in heritability for BMI as well as an increase in linkage signal in well-replicated regions.

2.10 Twin Studies of Obesity-Related Traits

Some of the historically important twin studies in obesity have already been mentioned. The following discussion of different obesity-related phenotypes provides a flavor of the most current research in these areas.

2.10.1 BMI in Children

As has already been mentioned, the use of BMI as a phenotype in obesity studies is widespread and it is no different when twin studies are considered. Rather than attempting to detail all studies in this area, the results of some notable studies examining obesity in childhood, adolescence, and adulthood are discussed. BMI is normally distributed in the general population and twin study designs have been utilized to understand the overlap between the etiology of obesity and normal variation in BMI in children. In a recent study [33], height and weight data were available from 2,342 same-sex twin pairs aged 7 and from 3,526 same-sex pairs aged 10 all from the UK. Twin method and model-fitting techniques were used to estimate genetic and environmental contributions to BMI. DeFries–Fulker (DF) extremes analysis was also used to investigate genetic and environmental influences on the mean difference between obese and normal-weight children. The results demonstrated a high heritability for BMI and obesity at both ages ($h^2 = 0.60$–0.74) and only a modest influence from shared environmental factors ($h^2 = 0.12$–0.22). The extremes analysis indicated that genetic and environmental influences on obesity are quantitatively and qualitatively similar across the whole range of BMI. The main conclusion was that obesity is simply one extreme result of the same genetic and environmental factors responsible for variation throughout the distribution of BMI.

A similar analysis [23] of more than 3,500 child twins with repeated assessments of BMI in a longitudinal sample indicated that the genetic influence on BMI becomes progressively stronger, with heritability increasing from 0.48 at age 4 to 0.78 at age 11. One suggested reason for the increasing heritability of the trait was the trend of children to increasingly select environments correlated with their genetic propensities.

While the heritability for height has been determined to be high [34], the other component of BMI, namely, weight has been less well explored. This was investigated using a longitudinal study of 231 MZ and 144 DZ male twin pairs born between 1973 and 1979 [35]. Anthropometric measurements of the subjects were obtained annually from birth to 18 years of age. The aim of the study was to determine the contribution of genetic and environmental factors to the development of relative weight during the growth period. The BMI at age 18 correlated with BMI at age 1 ($r = 0.32$) and this correlation increased steadily to age 17 ($r = 0.91$). The major part of these trait correlations (81–95%) was due to additive genetic factors, but unique environmental correlations were also present during the whole growth period. The results suggest persistent genetic regulation of BMI from age 1 to 18. In line with previous studies, this study showed a high heritability of obesity, as measured by BMI.

A very recent meta-analysis [36] of nine separate child twin studies identified a strong genetic effect on BMI variation at all ages. Heritability for BMI was moderate to high (0.55–0.93). Common environmental factors showed a strong effect in mid-childhood, but this effect disappeared in adolescence.

2.10.2 BMI in Adolescents

It is easy to see how the increasing independence that comes as children move into adolescence and young adulthood can result in reductions in shared environmental effects between twins. In order to investigate whether genetic effects are sex-limited, and whether nonadditive genetic effects contribute to BMI during these ages, a longitudinal study of BMI in 2,744 same-sex and 1,178 opposite-sex adolescents and young adult siblings was carried out [37]. Traits were measured at three separate time points: at baseline, after 1 year, and after 5 years. Models that included additive genetic, nonshared environment, and no sex-limited genetic effects gave the best fit with the data at all three measurement points. Heritable effects were large at all three measurements (0.75–0.86). The effects of nonshared environment were highly correlated between baseline and the first time point but less correlated between baseline and the last time point (at 5 years), indicating that the effects of environment change with maturity from adolescence into young adulthood. The results underscore the importance of understanding early genetic influences on BMI and highlight the role that novel environmental experiences have at later ages.

A study using two time points (average of 7 years apart) examined genetic and environmental effects over time on BMI in 1,306 European-American (EA) and 404 African-American (AA) adolescent and young adult female twin pairs [38]. For EA women, the majority of the variance (82% for each time point) in BMI was due to additive genetic effects, with the rest due to nonshared environment. For AA women, the nonadditive genetic effects accounted for the majority of the variance (68% at the first time point and 73% at the second) with some variance also due to nonshared environment and additive genetic effects.

A study of 4,884 twins and 2,509 singletons from Finland (aged 16–17 years) gave results similar to those above [39], in that genetic factors played a significant role in the variation of BMI. However, in this case, modeling suggested that the set of genes that explain variation in BMI may differ between males and females. It was noted that at this age, twin boys but not twin girls were leaner than singletons.

A longitudinal study of 4,368 individuals has been carried out [40] to examine the role of shared household environment, additive genetic, and shared genetic effects in BMI, and BMI change over time, in adolescents and young adults using two measurements taken 6 years apart. The study reported a heritability of 0.43 for BMI change. Significant household effects were modest and only found during young adulthood. They reported a moderate-to-strong genetic correlation (0.61) for shared genetic effects between BMI and BMI change during adolescence and a weak-to-moderate genetic correlation (0.23) during young adulthood.

2.10.3 BMI in Adults

Recently, a large longitudinal study of 5,278 adult twin pairs with three measurements over 15 years follow-up was reported [41], which was designed to analyze the genetic factors influencing changes in BMI over time. A substantial genetic influence on BMI (80% in males and 82% in females) was reported, with a moderate-to-high genetic influence on rate of change of BMI (58% in males and 64% in females). This study shows that the genetic effects influencing rate of change in BMI are likely to be different from those affecting BMI itself.

One recent result from adult twin-pair studies is that the effect of common environment appears to be inconsistent across different European countries [42]. A comparison of adult female twin pairs from the Netherlands (n = 222 MZ, 103 DZ) and Spain (n = 202 MZ, 235 DZ) was carried out. Age-related weight gain was significantly stronger in the Spanish sample. For BMI, both the genetic and the environmental variance components were larger in the Spanish arm of the study as compared to the Dutch arm.

2.10.4 Other Anthropometric Measures

In addition to BMI, a range of other anthropometric measures have been used to investigate obesity. Weight, waist circumference (WC), hip circumference, and waist–hip ratio (WHR) are just as useful in characterizing obesity in the population as is BMI [43, 44]. A more complex anthropometric measure is skinfold thickness, typically measured using calipers at multiple points on the body. While this is relatively simple and cost effective, it is significantly more time consuming and user dependent, and it is unclear what the exact relationship is between skinfold thickness at specific points on the body and obesity.

A study [45] using 4,020 twin pairs and SEM analysis demonstrated that an additive genetic effects, dominant/nonadditive genetic effects, and unique environmental effects model provided the best fit and allowing for sex-specific effects significantly improved the fit. The heritability of that proportion of weight unrelated to height was high: 0.61 in males and 0.73 in females.

To study the effect of the obesogenic environment on BMI and WC in children, a large study was carried out aiming to quantify genetic and environmental influences on BMI and central adiposity in children growing up during the time of dramatic rises in pediatric obesity. BMI and WC were analyzed in a UK sample of 5,092 twin pairs of ages 8–11 years using quantitative genetic model fitting for the univariate analyses and bivariate quantitative genetic model fitting for the analysis of covariance between BMI and WC [22]. Both BMI and WC showed high heritability (77% for both). About 60% of the genetic influence on WC was common to that of BMI and there was also a significant independent genetic effect on WC (40%). There was a very modest effect of shared environment on both BMI and WC, with the remaining environmental variance being nonshared. This demonstrated that the genetic influences on BMI and abdominal adiposity remain high in children born since the onset of the pediatric obesity epidemic. Even though most of the genetic effects on WC are common to BMI, 40% is attributable to independent genetic influences.

In a cross-sectional study of the genetic and environmental contribution to the variance of anthropometric traits in 259 twin pairs, triceps, subscapular, and suprailiac skinfold thickness, as well as waist circumference, height, and weight were measured using a standardized protocol [46]. A parsimonious model that included only additive genetic effects and nonshared environmental factors provided an adequate explanation for the variation in anthropometric traits. In this largely preadolescent population, different magnitudes of genetic effects were seen in males and females for waist circumference, biiliac diameter, and suprailiac skinfold.

2.10.5 Body Composition

Body composition is a broad term encompassing both categorical phenotypes such as somatotype (body type) and highly accurate phenotypes such as fat mass, which can be measured very accurately. Somatotype is a different approach to that of BMI as it is an attempt to categorize obesity based on relative fitness as well as adiposity. The three categories of somatotype are endomorph (substantial fat deposits, large waist), mesomorph (muscular, low adiposity, small waist, and large shoulders), and ectomorph (low adiposity, thin limbs, slim). The somatotype classification can be made more quantitative by using a sliding scale of all three features to classify a subject, e.g., individual scores for endomorphy, mesomorphy, and ectomorphy or a sum of all three.

In order to investigate the heritability of body fat distribution, a study of 108 MZ and 88 DZ Danish twins in two different age groups, 25–32 and 58–66, was carried out [47]. Body fat distribution was determined using DEXA. The intraclass correlations demonstrated higher correlations for MZ than DZ twins in both age groups. Modeling revealed a major genetic component of total and regional fat percentages in both age groups (h^2 estimates between 0.71 and 0.85). The study concluded that body fat distribution as determined by DEXA scans is under strong genetic control.

Genetic and environmental correlations between measures of obesity (BMI) and body fat distribution (WHR and subscapular/triceps skin thickness ratio (SSTR)) were examined in 133 MZ and 129 DZ adult elderly male twin pairs [48]. All measures were significantly correlated in twins, with BMI more closely related to WHR ($r = 0.52$) than SSTR ($r = 0.18$). Multivariate genetic analyses indicated a significant heritable component for each phenotype ($h^2 = 0.66$, 0.46, and 0.25 for BMI, WHR, and SSTR, respectively). The majority of the BMI–WHR correlation came from common genetic influences, suggesting that overall obesity and abdominal adiposity distribution are mediated, at least in part, by similar genetic influences. The results also indicated that the genetic influences on skinfold thickness distribution are independent of those on abdominal and overall body fat, supporting the hypothesis that WHR and SSTR indices do not assess the same aspects of body fat distribution.

Total body fat, central abdominal fat, and non-abdominal fat were measured using DEXA in 50 MZ and 36 DZ female adult twins [49]. A genetic influence was observed on total fat, central abdominal fat, and non-abdominal fat. The correlation among MZ twins for central abdominal fat was 0.66 compared to only 0.20 in DZ twins. After adjusting central abdominal fat for age and total body fat there was an independent genetic influence accounting for 70% of the population variance. This study concluded that the majority of interindividual variance in central abdominal fat in nonobese individuals is due to genetic factors. Since abdominal fat is associated with metabolic consequences, the inheritance of abdominal obesity may contribute to familial aggregation of insulin resistance, diabetes, and cardiovascular disease.

A more advanced look at the effects of genetics and environment on body composition was provided by a series of intervention studies in young adult male identical twins designed to determine if there was any evidence of interactions between genotype $\times$ overfeeding or genotype $\times$ negative energy balance, as measured by changes in body weight, body composition, fat distribution, and computerized tomography-assessed abdominal visceral fat [50]. Responses observed were more similar within twin pairs than between unrelated individuals. The intrapair resemblance in response was particularly strong for changes in body mass, body composition, subcutaneous fat distribution, and abdominal visceral fat. This study concluded that there are individuals at risk of gaining weight and body fat or who are resistant to weight loss and that this can be largely explained by genetic factors.

Correlation between body composition (using DEXA) as an adult and birth weight has been investigated using 2,228 DZ and 842 MZ female twins [51]. Multivariate regression models were used to identify both individual-specific associations and those mediated through shared environment. Significant associations were found between birth weight and DEXA measures for individuals; an increased birth weight of 1 kg corresponded to an increase of 1.72 kg in lean mass, 0.25 kg in fat mass, and a 0.05 unit increase in lean:fat mass ratio. Within pairs, the analysis showed that associations between birth weight and absolute levels of lean and fat mass were mediated through individual-specific effects, whereas the relation between birth weight and the proportion of lean to fat mass was mediated purely through factors common in twin pairs. This study concluded that higher birth weight is associated with a higher proportion of lean to fat mass as adults and that this effect is mediated through factors in the shared common environment rather than by individual-specific factors in utero.

A study of twin resemblance for somatotype was carried out in 62 MZ and 40 DZ twin pairs (males and females) aged 9–23 years [52]. The mean somatotype did not differ between the sexes but males were significantly more mesomorphic than female twins. Analysis was performed in two ways. First, each somatotype was treated as independent from the other two, and second, as a composite by statistically controlling for the other two. Intraclass variations were significantly higher among MZ than DZ twins of both sexes. Within-pair variation was lower in MZ than DZ twins of both sexes. These results suggested that genetic variation affects physique in adolescents and young adults.

In a very small study of somatotype, with only 28 female individuals (5 MZ and 9 DZ pairs) of ages 7–19, significant differences between MZ and DZ twins were found for height and somatotype [53]. The heritability for these measures was high (0.88–0.97). No significant differences were found between MZ and DZ twins for weight and BMI and the heritability was lower for these traits (0.42 and 0.52). This study indicated that somatotype may be more sensitive to genetic effects than BMI in females.

In a study of 105 same-sex twin pairs from Belgium followed between 10 and 18 years of age, multivariate path analysis was used to take into account the covariation between somatotype components, gender heterogeneity, and common environmental influences distinguished from genetic effects [54]. The heritability for all three somatotypes ranged from moderate to high. In boys the heritability was 0.21–0.88, 0.46–0.76, and 0.16–0.73 for endomorphy, mesomorphy, and ectomorphy, respectively, and in girls 0.76–0.89, 0.36–0.57, and 0.57–0.76, respectively. Sex differences were present from the age of 14 years onward. More than half of the variance in all somatotypes could be explained by common factors. This study provided evidence of a substantial genetic influence on the variability of somatotype and it emphasized the need for sex-specific analyses.

A study of genetic and environmental determination of variation of somatotype in 803 individuals from 424 Flemish adult twin pairs using multivariate path analysis was subsequently reported [55]. The study again found significant sex differences and significant covariation between the three somatotypes. The variance in somatotype could be explained by additive genetic effects, shared environment, and unique environment. In both males and females, more than 70% of the total variation could be explained by sources of variation shared by all three components of somatotype. This study indicated that the high heritability for mesomorphy and ectomorphy in adolescence was maintained in adulthood.

2.10.6 Eating Behavior

Eating behavior is clearly an important aspect in the development of obesity. Many believe that obesity originates in the brain as a neurobehavioral disorder, which is consistent with the current finding that most obesity-associated genes appear to be expressed in the brain rather than adipose tissue (see reference [56] for review). The difficulty with assessing eating behavior as a phenotype is that its measurement using questionnaires is notoriously unreliable, due to underreporting, particularly in obese subjects (see reference [57] for a review of measures of the food environment).

2.10.6.1 Restraint, Emotional Eating, and External Eating

One of the most extensive studies of the heritability of eating behavior and body weight-related traits was carried out in a Korean sample set [58]. The study group consisted of 2,144 subjects: 443 MZ and 124 DZ adult same-sex twins and 1,010 family members. The Dutch Eating Behavior Questionnaire (DEBQ) [59] was used to assess three eating behavior subscales measuring restraint, emotional eating, and external eating. Heritability was estimated using a variance components approach. After consideration of shared environmental effects and adjustment for age and sex, the heritability estimates among twins and their family members were 0.31 for restraint, 0.25 for emotional eating, and 0.25 for external eating. Heritability was high for measured current and self-reported body weight at 20 years old (0.77 and 0.70, respectively). All three subscales were associated with all weight-related traits after adjustment for age and sex. The results of this study suggest that eating behaviors and weight-related traits have a genetic influence and eating behaviors are associated with measures of obesity. These results are similar to results obtained in Western populations.

In a second study, the effects of genetic and environmental factors on cognitive and emotional aspects of dieting behavior, BMI, and responsiveness to fatty foods were investigated [60]. One thousand three hundred and twenty-six adult twin individuals, mostly females, from the UK and Finland completed the revised version of the Three-Factor Eating Questionnaire [61] and genetic modeling was carried out using linear structural equations. Heritability estimates were calculated separately for each country and sex and were 26–63% for cognitive restraint, 45–69%

for uncontrolled eating, and 9–45% for emotional eating. Interindividual genetic differences were responsible for 25–54% for the variation in liking and use frequency of fatty foods. No significant correlations were found between BMI and fatty food use or liking, but BMI was positively correlated with all of the dieting behaviors. This correlation was mostly genetic ($r = 0.16$–0.51). Uncontrolled eating was both genetically and environmentally associated with liking for salty and fatty foods ($r = 0.16$) and emotional eating was genetically associated with liking for salty and fatty foods ($r = 0.31$). In conclusion, the relation between BMI and diet appears to be mediated through dieting behaviors.

2.10.6.2 Satiety and Food Responsiveness

Aspects of appetite that have been implicated in obesity include responsiveness to satiety and responsiveness to food cues. A recent study assessed the relative contribution of genes and environment using 5,435 twins aged between 8 and 11 years [62]. Quantitative genetic model fitting gave heritability estimates of 63% for satiety responsiveness and 75% for food cue responsiveness. Shared and nonshared environmental influences were 21 and 16%, respectively, for satiety responsiveness, and 10 and 15%, respectively, for food cue responsiveness. The study concluded a high heritability of appetite traits and suggests that genetic vulnerability to weight gain could operate through behavioral and metabolic pathways. It was suggested that intervention strategies aimed at improving satiety responsiveness and reducing food cue responsiveness in high-risk individuals could help in preventing the development of obesity, but if there is a high genetic effect this approach would not likely be successful.

A second study of satiety responsiveness and food cue responsiveness in children used twins from two age groups: 3–5 years ($n = 572$) and 8–10 years ($n = 10364$) [63]. BMI was measured in both age groups and waist circumference in the older group. In both sets, higher BMI was associated with lower satiety responsiveness ($r = -0.19$ in 3–5 year olds and $r = -0.22$ in 8–11 year olds) and higher food cue responsiveness ($r = 0.18$ in both groups). Waist circumference was also associated with satiety responsiveness ($r = -0.23$) and higher food cue responsiveness ($r = 0.20$). By analyzing the data using weight categories, children in higher weight and WC categories had lower satiety responsiveness and higher food cue responsiveness. This was true for both age groups but more pronounced in 8–11 year olds. Association between appetite and adiposity supports a behavioral susceptibility model of obesity. Assessing appetite in childhood could help identify children at high risk of developing obesity while they are still normal weight, enabling targeted interventions to prevent obesity.

2.10.6.3 Eating Rate and Eating Styles

In order to investigate the hypothesis that speed of eating is related to greater adiposity and that eating rate is a heritable trait, a study of 254 10–12-year-old twin children was carried out [64]. There was significant linear association across three weight groups (obese/overweight, higher normal weight, and lower normal weight) for eating rate. Regression analysis demonstrated that eating rate correlated with BMI. In addition, the heritability of eating rate was high (0.62). This study showed that faster eating appears to be a heritable behavioral trait and is related to obesity.

In a prospective twin cohort study of 233 female and 2,060 male twins, the association of eating styles with overweight and obesity in young adults was investigated [65]. Twins were aged 16 at baseline (T1) and 22–27 at the time of nutritional assessment (T4). At T4, obesity was significantly cross-sectionally associated with restrictive eating, frequent snacks, eating in the evening, avoiding fatty foods, and failure to maintain healthy eating patterns ($p < 0.001$, 0.01, 0.01, and 0.05, respectively). These associations were independent of BMI at T1. After a multivariate analysis, only restrictive/overeating and health-conscious eating styles were significant correlates of obesity at T4, independent of gender and BMI at T1. The analysis was controlled for genetic background by restricting the analysis to MZ twin pairs discordant for obesity ($n = 39$ female pairs, 45 male pairs). Yet, restrictive/overeating eating style was still statistically significantly associated with excess weight. The study demonstrated that the eating styles of obese young adults differ from their normal-weight counterparts; and restrictive eating, overeating, and fewer healthy food choices are all associated with obesity.

2.10.7 Physical Activity

Physical activity is another aspect of behavior that is essential when considering the causes and treatment of obesity. Many studies support the role of physical activity in contributing to and especially maintaining weight loss [66]. One recent study has attempted to explore how physical activity and the proportion of energy as protein in the diet modify the genetic variation of BMI, WC, and percentage body fat (by bioelectrical impedance) in 756 Danish and 278 Finnish twin pairs aged 18–67 and 21–24, respectively [67]. High physical activity was associated with lower mean values for BMI, WC, and percentage body fat, and a high proportion of protein in the diet was associated with higher mean BMI, WC, and percentage body fat. This was statistically significant for WC in Danish men and Finnish women and for percentage body fat in Danish women. A meta-analysis of effects of physical activity on genetic variance of BMI, WC, and percentage body fat showed a significant modification by physical activity on BMI (–0.18; (95% CI –0.31 to 0.05) and WC (–0.14; 95% CI –0.22 to –0.05). The results suggest that in physically active individuals, the genetic variation in weight is reduced, possibly indicating that physical activity is able to modify the action of the genes responsible for predisposition to obesity.

Another recent study determined whether vigorous exercise shows evidence of a gene–environment correlation and gene × environment interaction with BMI among 2,710 MZ and 2,327 DZ male twin pairs [68]. The results show a significant modification of vigorous exercise on the additive genetic component of BMI, indicating a gene × environment interaction ($p < 0.001$). The genetic influence on BMI was highest among those that did not report vigorous exercise. The results are consistent with existing reports that vigorous exercise may mitigate some of the genetic influences on obesity.

A third large study also investigated whether physical activity modifies the degree of genetic influence on BMI and WC in 4,343 subjects from the FinnTwin16 Study [69]. Data were obtained using questionnaires and self-measurement of WC. The analysis was done using linear structural equations and gene × environment interaction models. Overall heritability estimates for BMI were 79% in males versus 78% in females, 56% versus 71% for WC, and 55% versus 54% for physical activity, respectively. They found an inverse relationship between physical activity and WC in males and females ($r = -0.12$ and $r = -0.18$, respectively) and between physical activity and BMI in females ($r = -0.12$). The heritability of both BMI and WC was significantly modified by physical activity. High physical activity specifically decreased the additive genetic component in BMI and WC. In summary, these results suggest that the individuals at greatest genetic risk of obesity would benefit the most from physical activity.

A longitudinal study of 146 twin pairs from the Finnish Twin Cohort over 30 years has allowed the follow-up necessary to determine the effect of physical activity on obesity and the role of environmental effects. All pairs were discordant for intensity and volume of leisure physical activity at baseline in 1975 and in 1981 [70]. Eighty-nine pairs were alive and participated in a follow-up interview in 2005 where self-measured weight and WC as well as physical activity during the whole follow-up were assessed. In the 42 twin pairs that were discordant throughout the follow-up period, the mean weight gain over 30 years was 5.4 kg less and the WC in the year 2005 was 8.4 cm smaller in the more active twin. These trends did not differ significantly between MZ and DZ twins. No significant differences were detected in weight and WC between the twins of 47 twin pairs that were not consistently discordant for physical activity. Persistent physical activity over 30 years was associated with a decreased rate of weight gain and with a smaller WC, even when partially controlling for genetic liability and childhood environment by studying twins.

Another study evaluated the relative contribution of genetic and environmental factors to the variation and covariation in activity-induced energy expenditure (AEE) and physical activity (PA) [71]. This was a small study, consisting of 12 MZ and 8 same-sex twin pairs of ages 18–39, because measurement of AEE is difficult and time consuming. AEE was measured in a respiration chamber for 24 h and with doubly labeled water in daily life for 2 weeks. PA was measured at the same time using a triaxial accelerometer. Analyses were performed using SEM to separate the observed variance into sex-adjusted additive genetic and common and unique environmental contributions. The results from the respiration chamber showed that common and unique environmental factors explained all of the variance in AEE and PA, with no genetic contribution. On the other hand, in daily life genetic factors explained 72 and 78% of the variance in AEE and PA, respectively, with unique environmental factors explaining the remaining variance. The same genetic factors explained 67% of the covariance between AEE and PA in daily life. In conclusion, this small study used gold standard measurements for AEE and PA and demonstrated that genetic factors explained a large part of the variation in AEE and PA in daily life, whereas environmental factors alone influenced variation in AEE and PA in the respiration chamber.

In summary, twin studies have provided good estimates of the heritability of obesity. Many different phenotypes can be used to assess obesity, each with different positive and negative aspects. Most studies have used BMI, with heritability estimates that are generally very high with a good concordance between studies, making it clear from twin studies that obesity has a genetic basis, whatever phenotype you consider.

2.11 Adoption Studies

The adoption study design is intended to clearly differentiate between the effects of genetics and environment. This is ideally achieved by contrasting the trait being measured between adoptive and biological siblings. If a trait is more similar between the adoptee and their biological rather than adoptive siblings then the trait is considered to have a stronger genetic basis and vice versa. However, this assumes that placement of the adopted child is random rather than selective, e.g., through an adoption agency rather than with other relatives, and it assumes that the prenatal environment, and any period of postnatal environment shared with biological parents, has no effect. Given that the average age at adoption from care in England for the year ending March 31, 2009 was 3 years and 9 months (figure from http://www.baaf.org.uk/info/stats/england.shtml), this is a significant length of time in the same environment as the biological parents. Given the inherent difficulties in recruiting and tracking both biological and adoptive families it is not surprising that few adoption studies have been carried out in obesity.

A recent systematic review [36] describes five adoption studies of childhood obesity [8, 72–75]. Of the four studies that included both natural and adopted families, the earliest, carried out in the UK, reported nonsignificant correlations between weight (adjusted for age and sex) of parents and adopted children and significant correlation between parents and biological children [8]. Two subsequent studies, one in the USA [72] and one in Canada [73], reported similar results. The US study also reported a correlation between mother and adoptive child (0.11, 95% CI 0.02–0.20) and the Canadian study reported that the correlation of weight/height in biological siblings was 0.37 ($p = 0.001$) compared to –0.03 ($p = 0.76$) for adopted siblings. A second US study, which utilized regular measures of BMI, was able to produce a heritability estimate of 0.09 at age 1, rising to 0.57 at age 9 [48]. The last report is a complete adoption study of 269 Danish adoptees involving both adoptive and biological families [75]. The average correlation between the adoptee and their biological siblings was 0.59 (95% CI 0.28–0.90) and with their adoptive siblings 0.14 (95% CI –0.13 to 0.41), demonstrating a strong influence of genetics on body mass index. A much lower correlation of 0.17 (0.03–0.31) with their biological mother and 0.17 (0.00–0.32) with their biological father was observed. No correlation was observed between the adoptee and their adoptive parents.

The contribution of the Danish group cannot be overstated as they are also responsible for the main adoption study of obesity in adults, initially reported in 1986 [76], and analyzed extensively in subsequent publications [77–79]. The initial study demonstrated that for a sample of 540 adult adoptees, there was a significant association between weight class (thin, median weight, overweight, or obese) of the adoptee and the BMI of their biological mother ($p < 0.0001$) and their biological father ($p < 0.02$). No significant association was observed with the adoptive parents [76]. Subsequent comparison of the adoptee weight class and full- and half-siblings' BMI demonstrated a highly significant trend of increasing BMI of full siblings with weight group for the adoptees ($p < 0.0001$) and a weaker trend for half-siblings ($p < 0.02$) [77]. Extension of the analysis to classify the adoptees using BMI and maximum BMI produced similar results, with correlation of BMI in the adoptee to biological mother, father, and full sibling being 0.15, 0.11, and 0.23, respectively ($p < 0.001$) [78]. Using a second measure of obesity, a silhouette score, similar correlations between adoptee obesity and their biological mother and full siblings were demonstrated. The correlation between adoptee and the biological father was nonsignificant [79]. Using a path analysis model, the heritability of obesity was subsequently estimated as 0.34 ($\pm$0.03), with no evidence for effects due to the shared family environment. All familial resemblance in adults was attributed to genetic effects [80]. However, this clearly meant that over 50% of the interindividual differences in BMI were due to individual environmental influences that were not shared.

2.12 Family-Based Studies

While twin and adoption studies are family based, the primary aspect of each is the sibling relationship. These are special cases of the wider family-based study design. Typically, family-based studies are based on the identification of one or more probands within a family, and then recruitment of the whole or part of the family. For genetic studies, families are useful as the siblings share a common environment; thus, this is assumed to be a good basis on which to explore the genetic basis of a phenotype as the environment can be controlled for. Family-based studies are typically used to investigate genetic linkage of a trait with markers on the human genome, so regions (and ideally genes) that are linked to the trait can be identified. Classically, nuclear families recruited on the basis of sibpairs discordant for the trait of interest have been used to maximize the potential to detect genetic influences on a trait in the presence of a shared environmental effect. However, concordant sibpairs can also be used, as well as recruiting large, multigenerational or consanguineous families, each of which has advantages. Discussion of the details and merits of family-based study designs is outside the remit of this chapter, so the reader is referred to two recent reviews of the subject [81, 82].

As heredity is the main concern of this chapter, what follows is not a comprehensive summary of the results of genetic linkage studies in obesity but an illustration of the evidence for heredity in obesity from family-based studies. Segregation analysis, the comparison of the observed proportion of affected subjects with the expected proportion given a specified mode of inheritance, has been the main method for trying to determine the genetic model that best fits the observed heredity patterns in obesity. In rare, monogenic forms of obesity, inheritance is autosomal recessive, though in the case of variants in the melanocortin-4 receptor gene, the frequency of mutation is sufficient that it is responsible for a small percentage of cases sampled from the general population [83], thus contributing to the more complex pattern of inheritance described for common obesity. Overall, the view of the field has been that the inheritance of common obesity is polygenic, with a possible role for one or two major genes [84–90]. Interestingly, analysis of the National Heart, Lung and Blood Institute Family Heart Study data gave a heritability value of 0.41–0.59, similar to the values obtained from twin studies [88]. Further complicating the picture of the heredity of common obesity, segregation analysis of the Swedish Obese Subjects study data suggested that below 20 years of age, a major gene effect was observed, while above the age of 20 a multifactorial mode of inheritance predominated [89].

In a genome-wide linkage study of BMI in the Amish [91], the heritability of obesity was estimated as 0.16–0.31 and for BMI percentile 0.40–0.52. Equally, in a genome-wide scan of Nigerian families for BMI, the heritability estimate was 0.46 ± 0.07. However, it should be noted that a study of intrafamilial correlation of BMI concluded that nonrandom mating and regional clustering may be inflating heritability estimates of BMI [92].

Analysis of the heritability of other obesity-related phenotypes has also demonstrated significant heritability values. For the trait of abdominal fatness (adjusted for total adiposity, age, and sex), a heritability of over 0.90 has been reported in a study of 300 South Indian families [93]. Eating behavior has a clear influence on obesity and in the Amish, heritabilities of 0.28 ± 0.09, 0.40 ± 0.10, and 0.23 ± 0.09 have been reported for the behavioral categories of restraint, disinhibition, and hunger, respectively [94]. Waist circumference is a commonly used obesity-related phenotype and in a recent study of the metabolic syndrome, waist circumference was reported to have a heritability of 0.38 ($p < 0.0001$) [95].

2.13 Case–Control Studies and the "Missing" Heritability Problem

As we have seen above, there have been many studies that have estimated heritability of common obesity and values obtained have been typically in the range of 0.5–0.7 for twin studies and 0.3–0.4 for adoption and family studies. Estimates of the contribution of individual genes to the total heritability of complex traits have emerged from genome-wide association (GWA) studies; see Chapter 5) [96] and this has revealed the so-called missing heritability problem [97]. For many complex traits, such as height or type 2 diabetes, large numbers of trait-associated loci have been identified (>20), but the proportion of the heritability that is explained by them is still low (<6%). The reasons for this are not clear at the moment, but there is little evidence that it is the overall heritability measure that is incorrect (see reference [97] for discussion). Although there are a few exceptions, such as age-related macular degeneration, where a few gene variants are responsible for most of the heritability, the current evidence suggests that common obesity has the same missing heritability problem as other common diseases.

There are two main issues with the design of the current generation of GWAS that could explain the failure to explain a substantial part of the heritability. The first is that the SNP markers that are used have a minor allele frequency of 5% or above. This was based on the original hypothesis of "common disease, common variant" [98], which suggested that any trait common in a population would most likely be associated with common variants. However, there is evidence that rare variants can have strong genetic effects in obesity [99] and the sum of the rare variants within a population could explain the missing heritability.

The second issue is that GWAS currently only addresses single nucleotide variation in the genome, while other types of variation may be associated with obesity. While GWAS arrays typically include markers that provide information on copy number variant (CNV) regions, the analysis of these data has proved problematic and initial conclusions have been that common CNVs cannot account for the missing heritability [100, 101]. However, by analogy to the situation with SNPs, the contribution of rare CNVs should not be underestimated, and in fact, there has been very recent evidence of the contribution of a rare CNV to obesity [102, 103]. Further sources of genomic variation include DNA methylation, telomere length, and histone modification, all of which could contribute to missing heritability in common obesity.

2.14 Heredity and Nongenetic Traits in Obesity

The problem with heredity is that it can sometimes be difficult to distinguish between genetic, environmental, or epigenetic mechanisms that may underlie the transmission of traits between parents and offspring. In obesity, at least two situations have been described where, for nongenetic reasons, traits predisposing offspring to obesity appear to be transmitted from the parents.

The first is the influence of the same-sex parent on body shape. Recently, it was reported that the body shape of a child was strongly correlated with that of its same-sex parent and not with the opposite-sex parent [104]. It is difficult to come up with a genetic explanation for this phenomenon and families share more or less the same environment for most of the time. The authors concluded that the best explanation was that the psychological predisposition of a child was to learn behaviors from its same-sex parent and this could include eating behavior. A child observing a parent eating large amounts of food quickly might be expected to follow their lead and overeat as well. Most published genetic studies of obesity successfully control for this effect by including sex as a covariate.

The second situation is the relationship between gut flora and obesity. Several publications examining the metagenome, the sum total of the bacterial and viral genomes that we are host to, have demonstrated that the gut flora is significantly different between obese and nonobese subjects (see reference [105] for review). As yet, there is insufficient evidence to decide whether this association is cause or effect. The heredity effect here is that the newborn continually shares the environment with its mother, and to a lesser extent its father, over the first few months of life as the child is slowly weaned onto solid food. This has the effect of the offspring "inheriting" a significantly biased proportion of its gut flora from its parents and a possible predisposition toward obesity as a consequence.

2.15 Conclusions

From all the evidence presented in this chapter, it should be clear to the reader that the majority of cases of obesity have a genetic basis. The contribution of the environment, both shared and individual, is variable, ranging from nothing for rare monogenic obesity to the majority of the effect in common obesity. Every case of obesity can be considered to be on a continuum, with a specific balance of genetic and environmental effects in each case (see Fig. 2.1). Monogenic obesity is almost purely genetic, with only drastic calorie restriction exerting an effect.

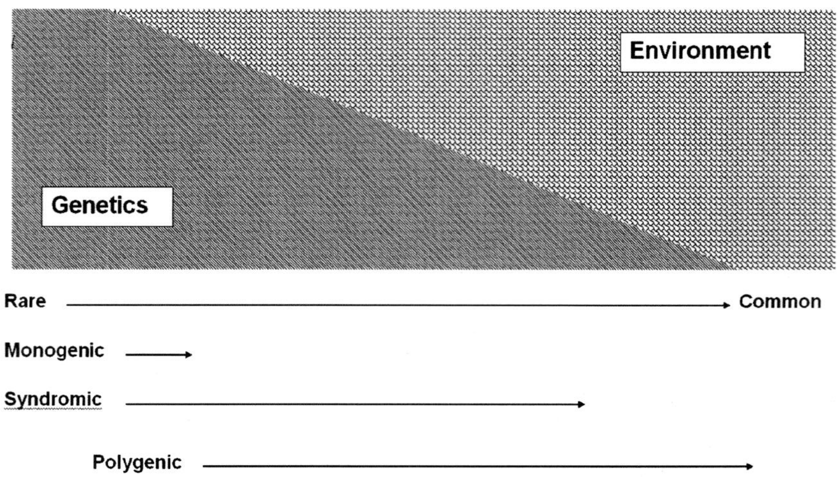

Fig. 2.1 The balance of genetic and environmental factors affecting obesity. Genetics and environment are shown as a balance of effects across the bulk of the spectrum, with regions of 100% genetics or environment at either end to emphasize the possibility of cases of clinical obesity being purely genetic (e.g., monogenic) or purely environmental (e.g., via learned behavior rather than genetics). The parts of the spectrum that the various forms of obesity occupy are shown below the figure, with monogenic disease being predominantly rare and genetic and common polygenic disease being caused by a balance of genes and environment

However, it should be remembered that even monogenic disease occurs in the context of a specific individual's genetic background, which may modify their outcome, e.g., BMI, in a specific environment. Syndromic obesity is more complex, as it may be monogenic or oligogenic, and obesity may not have to be present for diagnosis of the syndrome, e.g., in Bardet–Biedl syndrome. Both monogenic and syndromic subtypes of obesity are rare, presumably as a consequence of being severe disorders with consequent morbidity and mortality. Polygenic or complex obesity is common and had previously been suspected to be due to common variation in the genome. It is unlikely that common single nucleotide variations account for most of the heritability of obesity; whether it is rare variants of strong effect, other forms of genomic variation, or a combination of both remains an open question. It is already clear that copy number variation can contribute to obesity and there is every reason to believe that epigenetic mechanisms, such as DNA methylation or histone modification, could account for a significant part of the heritability of obesity.

References

1. James WP. WHO recognition of the global obesity epidemic. Int J Obes (Lond). Dec 2008;32 Suppl 7:S120–6.
2. Emery EM, Schmid TL, Kahn HS, Filozof PP. A review of the association between abdominal fat distribution, health outcome measures, and modifiable risk factors. Am J Health Promot. May–Jun 1993;7(5):342–53.
3. Pischon T, Boeing H, Hoffmann K, et al. General and abdominal adiposity and risk of death in Europe. N Engl J Med. Nov 13 2008;359(20):2105–20.
4. Fox CS, Massaro JM, Hoffmann U, et al. Abdominal visceral and subcutaneous adipose tissue compartments: association with metabolic risk factors in the Framingham Heart Study. Circulation. Jul 3 2007;116(1):39–48.
5. Bell CG, Walley AJ, Froguel P. The genetics of human obesity. Nat Rev Genet. Mar 2005;6(3):221–34.
6. Walley AJ, Asher JE, Froguel P. The genetic contribution to non-syndromic human obesity. Nat Rev Genet. Jul 2009;10(7):431–42.
7. Poston WS 2nd, Foreyt JP. Obesity is an environmental issue. Atherosclerosis. Oct 1999;146(2):201–9.
8. Withers RF. Problems in the genetics of human obesity. Eugen Rev. Jul 1964;56(2):81–90.
9. Montague CT, Farooqi IS, Whitehead JP, et al. Congenital leptin deficiency is associated with severe early-onset obesity in humans. Nature. Jun 26 1997;387(6636):903–8.
10. Goldstone AP, Beales PL. Genetic obesity syndromes. Front Horm Res. 2008;36:37–60.
11. Visscher PM, Hill WG, Wray NR. Heritability in the genomics era – concepts and misconceptions. Nat Rev Genet. Apr 2008;9(4):255–66.
12. Galton F. The history of twins, as a criterion of the relative powers of nature and nurture. Fraser's Mag. 1875;12:566–76.
13. Siemens HW. *Die Zwillingspathologie: Ihre Bedeutng, ihre Methodik, ihre biseherigen Ergebnisse (Twin Pathologies: Its Importance, Its Methodology, Its Previous Results)*. Berlin: Springer; 1924.
14. Segal NL, Feng R, McGuire SA, Allison DB, Miller S. Genetic and environmental contributions to body mass index: comparative analysis of monozygotic twins, dizygotic twins and same-age unrelated siblings. Int J Obes (Lond). Jan 2009;33(1):37–41.

15. Bogl LH, Pietilainen KH, Rissanen A, Kaprio J. Improving the accuracy of self-reports on diet and physical exercise: the co-twin control method. Twin Res Hum Genet. Dec 2009;12(6):531–40.
16. Leskinen T, Sipila S, Alen M, et al. Leisure-time physical activity and high-risk fat: a longitudinal population-based twin study. Int J Obes (Lond). Nov 2009;33(11):1211–8.
17. Pietilainen KH, Rissanen A, Laamanen M, et al. Growth patterns in young adult monozygotic twin pairs discordant and concordant for obesity. Twin Res. Oct 2004;7(5):421–9.
18. Allison DB, Kaprio J, Korkeila M, Koskenvuo M, Neale MC, Hayakawa K. The heritability of body mass index among an international sample of monozygotic twins reared apart. Int J Obes Relat Metab Disord. Jun 1996;20(6):501–6.
19. Maes HH, Neale MC, Eaves LJ. Genetic and environmental factors in relative body weight and human adiposity. Behav Genet. Jul 1997;27(4):325–51.
20. Koeppen-Schomerus G, Wardle J, Plomin R. A genetic analysis of weight and overweight in 4-year-old twin pairs. Int J Obes Relat Metab Disord. Jun 2001;25(6):838–44.
21. van Dommelen P, de Gunst MC, van der Vaart AW, Boomsma DI. Genetic study of the height and weight process during infancy. Twin Res. Dec 2004;7(6):607–16.
22. Wardle J, Carnell S, Haworth CM, Plomin R. Evidence for a strong genetic influence on childhood adiposity despite the force of the obesogenic environment. Am J Clin Nutr. Feb 2008;87(2):398–404.
23. Haworth CM, Carnell S, Meaburn EL, Davis OS, Plomin R, Wardle J. Increasing heritability of BMI and stronger associations with the FTO gene over childhood. Obesity (Silver Spring). Dec 2008;16(12):2663–8.
24. Lajunen HR, Kaprio J, Keski-Rahkonen A, et al. Genetic and environmental effects on body mass index during adolescence: a prospective study among Finnish twins. Int J Obes (Lond). May 2009;33(5):559–67.
25. Brook CG, Huntley RM, Slack J. Influence of heredity and environment in determination of skinfold thickness in children. Br Med J. Jun 28 1975;2(5973):719–21.
26. Stunkard AJ, Foch TT, Hrubec Z. A twin study of human obesity. JAMA. Jul 4 1986;256(1):51–4.
27. Stunkard AJ, Harris JR, Pedersen NL, McClearn GE. The body-mass index of twins who have been reared apart. N Engl J Med. May 24 1990;322(21):1483–7.
28. Gorlova OY, Amos CI, Wang NW, Shete S, Turner ST, Boerwinkle E. Genetic linkage and imprinting effects on body mass index in children and young adults. Eur J Hum Genet. Jun 2003;11(6):425–32.
29. Perusse L, Rice T, Chagnon YC, et al. A genome-wide scan for abdominal fat assessed by computed tomography in the Quebec Family Study. Diabetes. Mar 2001;50(3):614–21.
30. Mitchell BD, Cole SA, Comuzzie AG, et al. A quantitative trait locus influencing BMI maps to the region of the beta-3 adrenergic receptor. Diabetes. Sep 1999;48(9):1863–7.
31. Wilson SG, Adam G, Langdown M, et al. Linkage and potential association of obesity-related phenotypes with two genes on chromosome 12q24 in a female dizygous twin cohort. Eur J Hum Genet. Mar 2006;14(3):340–8.
32. Kettunen J, Perola M, Martin NG, et al. Multicenter dizygotic twin cohort study confirms two linkage susceptibility loci for body mass index at 3q29 and 7q36 and identifies three further potential novel loci. Int J Obes (Lond). Nov 2009;33(11):1235–42.
33. Haworth CM, Plomin R, Carnell S, Wardle J. Childhood obesity: genetic and environmental overlap with normal-range BMI. Obesity (Silver Spring). Jul 2008;16(7):1585–90.
34. Lettre G. Genetic regulation of adult stature. Curr Opin Pediatr. Aug 2009;21(4):515–22.
35. Silventoinen K, Pietilainen KH, Tynelius P, Sorensen TI, Kaprio J, Rasmussen F. Genetic and environmental factors in relative weight from birth to age 18: the Swedish young male twins study. Int J Obes (Lond). Apr 2007;31(4):615–21.
36. Silventoinen K, Rokholm B, Kaprio J, Sorensen TI. The genetic and environmental influences on childhood obesity: a systematic review of twin and adoption studies. Int J Obes (Lond). Jan 2010;34(1):29–40.

37. Haberstick BC, Lessem JM, McQueen MB, et al. Stable genes and changing environments: body mass index across adolescence and young adulthood. Behav Genet. Jan 20 2010 Jul; 40(4):495–504 (Epub Jan 20, 2010).
38. Duncan AE, Agrawal A, Grant JD, Bucholz KK, Madden PA, Heath AC. Genetic and environmental contributions to BMI in adolescent and young adult women. Obesity (Silver Spring). May 2009;17(5):1040–3.
39. Pietilainen KH, Kaprio J, Rissanen A, et al. Distribution and heritability of BMI in Finnish adolescents aged 16y and 17y: a study of 4884 twins and 2509 singletons. Int J Obes Relat Metab Disord. Feb 1999;23(2):107–15.
40. North KE, Graff M, Adair LS, et al. Genetic epidemiology of BMI and body mass change from adolescence to young adulthood. Obesity (Silver Spring). Oct 22 2010 Jul;18(7): 1474–6 (Epub Oct 22, 2009).
41. Hjelmborg JB, Fagnani C, Silventoinen K, et al. Genetic influences on growth traits of BMI: a longitudinal study of adult twins. Obesity (Silver Spring). Apr 2008;16(4):847–52.
42. Ordonana JR, Rebollo-Mesa I, Gonzalez-Javier F, et al. Heritability of body mass index: a comparison between the Netherlands and Spain. Twin Res Hum Genet. Oct 2007;10(5): 749–56.
43. McCarthy HD. Body fat measurements in children as predictors for the metabolic syndrome: focus on waist circumference. Proc Nutr Soc. Nov 2006;65(4):385–92.
44. McTigue KM, Hess R, Ziouras J. Obesity in older adults: a systematic review of the evidence for diagnosis and treatment. Obesity (Silver Spring). Sep 2006;14(9):1485–97.
45. Allison DB, Heshka S, Neale MC, Lykken DT, Heymsfield SB. A genetic analysis of relative weight among 4,020 twin pairs, with an emphasis on sex effects. Health Psychol. Jul 1994;13(4):362–5.
46. Bodurtha JN, Mosteller M, Hewitt JK, et al. Genetic analysis of anthropometric measures in 11-year-old twins: the Medical College of Virginia Twin Study. Pediatr Res. Jul 1990;28(1):1–4.
47. Malis C, Rasmussen EL, Poulsen P, et al. Total and regional fat distribution is strongly influenced by genetic factors in young and elderly twins. Obes Res. Dec 2005;13(12): 2139–45.
48. Cardon LR, Carmelli D, Fabsitz RR, Reed T. Genetic and environmental correlations between obesity and body fat distribution in adult male twins. Hum Biol. Jun 1994;66(3):465–79.
49. Carey DG, Nguyen TV, Campbell LV, Chisholm DJ, Kelly P. Genetic influences on central abdominal fat: a twin study. Int J Obes Relat Metab Disord. Aug 1996;20(8):722–6.
50. Bouchard C, Tremblay A. Genetic influences on the response of body fat and fat distribution to positive and negative energy balances in human identical twins. J Nutr. May 1997;127 5 Suppl:943S–7S.
51. Skidmore PM, Cassidy A, Swaminathan R, et al. An obesogenic postnatal environment is more important than the fetal environment for the development of adult adiposity: a study of female twins. Am J Clin Nutr. Aug 2009;90(2):401–6.
52. Song TM, Perusse L, Malina RM, Bouchard C. Twin resemblance in somatotype and comparisons with other twin studies. Hum Biol. Jun 1994;66(3):453–64.
53. Reis VM, Machado JV, Fortes MS, et al. Evidence for higher heritability of somatotype compared to body mass index in female twins. J Physiol Anthropol. Jan 2007;26(1):9–14.
54. Peeters MW, Thomis MA, Claessens AL, et al. Heritability of somatotype components from early adolescence into young adulthood: a multivariate analysis on a longitudinal twin study. Ann Hum Biol. Jul–Aug 2003;30(4):402–18.
55. Peeters MW, Thomis MA, Loos RJ, et al. Heritability of somatotype components: a multivariate analysis. Int J Obes (Lond). Aug 2007;31(8):1295–301.
56. O'Rahilly S, Farooqi IS. Human obesity: a heritable neurobehavioral disorder that is highly sensitive to environmental conditions. Diabetes. Nov 2008;57(11):2905–10.

57. McKinnon RA, Reedy J, Morrissette MA, Lytle LA, Yaroch AL. Measures of the food environment: a compilation of the literature, 1990–2007. Am J Prev Med. Apr 2009;36 4 Suppl: S124–33.
58. Sung J, Lee K, Song YM, Lee MK, Lee DH. Heritability of eating behavior assessed using the DEBQ (Dutch Eating Behavior Questionnaire) and weight-related traits: the healthy twin study. Obesity (Silver Spring). Oct 29 2010 May;18(5):1000–5 (Epub Oct 29, 2009).
59. van Strien T, Frijter JER, Bergers GPA, Defares PB. The Dutch Eating Behaviour Questionnaire (DEBQ) for assessment of restrained, emotional and external eating behaviour. Int J Eat Disord. 1986;5:295–315.
60. Keskitalo K, Tuorila H, Spector TD, et al. The three-factor eating questionnaire, body mass index, and responses to sweet and salty fatty foods: a twin study of genetic and environmental associations. Am J Clin Nutr. Aug 2008;88(2):263–71.
61. Stunkard AJ, Messick S. The three-factor eating questionnaire to measure dietary restraint, disinhibition and hunger. J Psychosom Res. 1985;29(1):71–83.
62. Carnell S, Haworth CM, Plomin R, Wardle J. Genetic influence on appetite in children. Int J Obes (Lond). Oct 2008;32(10):1468–73.
63. Carnell S, Wardle J. Appetite and adiposity in children: evidence for a behavioral susceptibility theory of obesity. Am J Clin Nutr. Jul 2008;88(1):22–9.
64. Llewellyn CH, van Jaarsveld CH, Boniface D, Carnell S, Wardle J. Eating rate is a heritable phenotype related to weight in children. Am J Clin Nutr. Dec 2008;88(6):1560–6.
65. Keski-Rahkonen A, Bulik CM, Pietilainen KH, Rose RJ, Kaprio J, Rissanen A. Eating styles, overweight and obesity in young adult twins. Eur J Clin Nutr. Jul 2007;61(7):822–9.
66. Jakicic JM. The effect of physical activity on body weight. Obesity (Silver Spring). Dec 2009;17 Suppl 3:S34–8.
67. Silventoinen K, Hasselbalch AL, Lallukka T, et al. Modification effects of physical activity and protein intake on heritability of body size and composition. Am J Clin Nutr. Oct 2009;90(4):1096–103.
68. McCaffery JM, Papandonatos GD, Bond DS, Lyons MJ, Wing RR. Gene × environment interaction of vigorous exercise and body mass index among male Vietnam-era twins. Am J Clin Nutr. Apr 2009;89(4):1011–8.
69. Mustelin L, Silventoinen K, Pietilainen K, Rissanen A, Kaprio J. Physical activity reduces the influence of genetic effects on BMI and waist circumference: a study in young adult twins. Int J Obes (Lond). Jan 2009;33(1):29–36.
70. Waller K, Kaprio J, Kujala UM. Associations between long-term physical activity, waist circumference and weight gain: a 30-year longitudinal twin study. Int J Obes (Lond). Feb 2008;32(2):353–61.
71. Joosen AM, Gielen M, Vlietinck R, Westerterp KR. Genetic analysis of physical activity in twins. Am J Clin Nutr. Dec 2005;82(6):1253–9.
72. Hartz A, Giefer E, Rimm AA. Relative importance of the effect of family environment and heredity on obesity. Ann Hum Genet. Oct 1977;41(2):185–93.
73. Biron P, Mongeau JG, Bertrand D. Familial resemblance of body weight and weight/height in 374 homes with adopted children. J Pediatr. Oct 1977;91(4):555–8.
74. Cardon LR. Genetic influence on body mass index in early childhood. In: Turner JR, Cardon, LR, Hewitt, JK, editors. Behavior genetic approaches in behavioral medicine. New York, NY: Plenum Press; 1995;3–13.
75. Sorensen TI, Holst C, Stunkard AJ. Childhood body mass index – genetic and familial environmental influences assessed in a longitudinal adoption study. Int J Obes Relat Metab Disord. Sep 1992;16(9):705–14.
76. Stunkard AJ, Sorensen TI, Hanis C, et al. An adoption study of human obesity. N Engl J Med. Jan 23 1986;314(4):193–8.
77. Sorensen TI, Price RA, Stunkard AJ, Schulsinger F. Genetics of obesity in adult adoptees and their biological siblings. BMJ. Jan 14 1989;298(6666):87–90.

78. Sorensen TI, Holst C, Stunkard AJ, Skovgaard LT. Correlations of body mass index of adult adoptees and their biological and adoptive relatives. Int J Obes Relat Metab Disord. Mar 1992;16(3):227–36.
79. Sorensen TI, Stunkard AJ. Does obesity run in families because of genes? An adoption study using silhouettes as a measure of obesity. Acta Psychiatr Scand Suppl. 1993;370: 67–72.
80. Vogler GP, Sorensen TI, Stunkard AJ, Srinivasan MR, Rao DC. Influences of genes and shared family environment on adult body mass index assessed in an adoption study by a comprehensive path model. Int J Obes Relat Metab Disord. Jan 1995;19(1):40–5.
81. Cupples LA. Family study designs in the age of genome-wide association studies: experience from the Framingham Heart Study. Curr Opin Lipidol. Apr 2008;19(2):144–50.
82. Laird NM, Lange C. Family-based methods for linkage and association analysis. Adv Genet. 2008;60:219–52.
83. Young EH, Wareham NJ, Farooqi S, et al. The V103I polymorphism of the MC4R gene and obesity: population based studies and meta-analysis of 29 563 individuals. Int J Obes (Lond). Sep 2007;31(9):1437–41.
84. Ness R, Laskarzewski P, Price RA. Inheritance of extreme overweight in black families. Hum Biol. Feb 1991;63(1):39–52.
85. Rice T, Borecki IB, Bouchard C, Rao DC. Segregation analysis of fat mass and other body composition measures derived from underwater weighing. Am J Hum Genet. May 1993;52(5):967–73.
86. Rice T, Borecki IB, Bouchard C, Rao DC. Segregation analysis of body mass index in an unselected French-Canadian sample: the Quebec Family Study. Obes Res. Jul 1993;1(4):288–94.
87. Lecomte E, Herbeth B, Nicaud V, Rakotovao R, Artur Y, Tiret L. Segregation analysis of fat mass and fat-free mass with age- and sex-dependent effects: the Stanislas Family Study. Genet Epidemiol. 1997;14(1):51–62.
88. Borecki IB, Higgins M, Schreiner PJ, et al. Evidence for multiple determinants of the body mass index: the National Heart, Lung, and Blood Institute Family Heart Study. Obes Res. Mar 1998;6(2):107–14.
89. Rice T, Sjostrom CD, Perusse L, Rao DC, Sjostrom L, Bouchard C. Segregation analysis of body mass index in a large sample selected for obesity: the Swedish Obese Subjects study. Obes Res. May 1999;7(3):246–55.
90. Feitosa MF, Borecki I, Hunt SC, Arnett DK, Rao DC, Province M. Inheritance of the waist-to-hip ratio in the National Heart, Lung, and Blood Institute Family Heart Study. Obes Res. Jul 2000;8(4):294–301.
91. Platte P, Papanicolaou GJ, Johnston J, et al. A study of linkage and association of body mass index in the Old Order Amish. Am J Med Genet C Semin Med Genet. Aug 15 2003;121C(1):71–80.
92. Magnusson PK, Rasmussen F. Familial resemblance of body mass index and familial risk of high and low body mass index. A study of young men in Sweden. Int J Obes Relat Metab Disord. Sep 2002;26(9):1225–31.
93. Davey G, Ramachandran A, Snehalatha C, Hitman GA, McKeigue PM. Familial aggregation of central obesity in Southern Indians. Int J Obes Relat Metab Disord. Nov 2000;24(11):1523–7.
94. Steinle NI, Hsueh WC, Snitker S, et al. Eating behavior in the Old Order Amish: heritability analysis and a genome-wide linkage analysis. Am J Clin Nutr. Jun 2002;75(6):1098–106.
95. Henneman P, Aulchenko YS, Frants RR, van Dijk KW, Oostra BA, van Duijn CM. Prevalence and heritability of the metabolic syndrome and its individual components in a Dutch isolate: the Erasmus Rucphen Family study. J Med Genet. Sep 2008;45(9):572–7.
96. Smith JG, Newton-Cheh C. Genome-wide association study in humans. Methods Mol Biol. 2009;573:231–58.

97. Manolio TA, Collins FS, Cox NJ, et al. Finding the missing heritability of complex diseases. Nature. Oct 8 2009;461(7265):747–53.
98. Reich DE, Lander ES. On the allelic spectrum of human disease. Trends Genet. Sep 2001;17(9):502–10.
99. Blakemore AI, Meyre D, Delplanque J, et al. A rare variant in the visfatin gene (NAMPT/PBEF1) is associated with protection from obesity. Obesity (Silver Spring). Aug 2009;17(8):1549–53.
100. Wellcome Trust Case Control Consortium, et al. Genome-wide association study of CNVs in 16,000 cases of eight common diseases and 3,000 shared controls. Nature. Apr 1 2010;464(7289):713–20.
101. Conrad DF, Pinto D, Redon R, et al. Origins and functional impact of copy number variation in the human genome. Nature. Apr 1 2010;464(7289):704–12.
102. Bochukova EG, Huang N, Keogh J, et al. Large, rare chromosomal deletions associated with severe early-onset obesity. Nature. Feb 4 2010;463(7281):666–70.
103. Walters RG, Jacquemont S, Valsesia A, et al. A new highly penetrant form of obesity due to deletions on chromosome 16p11.2. Nature. Feb 4 2010;463(7281):671–5.
104. Perez-Pastor EM, Metcalf BS, Hosking J, Jeffery AN, Voss LD, Wilkin TJ. Assortative weight gain in mother-daughter and father-son pairs: an emerging source of childhood obesity. Longitudinal study of trios (EarlyBird 43). Int J Obes (Lond). Jul 2009;33(7):727–35.
105. Ley RE. Obesity and the human microbiome. Curr Opin Gastroenterol. Jan 2010;26(1):5–11.

Chapter 3
Monogenic Disorders Within the Energy Balance Pathway

Ivy R. Aslan, Sayali A. Ranadive, and Christian Vaisse

3.1 Introduction

Obesity has become a significant public health concern due to its rising prevalence over the past 30 years [1]. Nationwide, nearly one in three adults is currently obese, compared to fewer than one in six 15 years ago [2]. Data from the Framingham study showed that in the United States, the lifetime risk of becoming overweight or obese is approximately 50 and 25%, respectively [3].

Childhood obesity has also reached epidemic proportions; in the United States today almost one-third of children and adolescents are overweight (BMI > 85%) [4]. Increased mortality in adults with obesity, hypertension, glucose intolerance, and hypercholesterolemia is well established. A recent report showed a similar association in children between obesity, hypertension, glucose intolerance, and premature death [5]. Specifically, 4,857 American Indian children without diabetes were followed. The rates of death from endogenous causes among children in the highest quartile of BMI were more than double those among children in the lowest BMI quartile, with glucose intolerance and hypertension as major risk factors.

Both environmental and genetic factors are involved in the onset and progression of weight gain [6]. Heritable factors contribute significantly to the development of obesity, since individuals exposed to the same environment have different degrees of vulnerability for obesity. The interaction between genetic predisposition and deleterious environmental factors plays a major role in the obese phenotype [7].

Epidemiologic studies have shown that genetic factors account for 40–70% of the population variation in BMI and that the heritability of obesity increases with its severity [8] (see Chapter 2). Both common variants with small effects [9, 10] (see Chapter 5) and rare variants with larger individual effects have been shown to contribute to the genetic predisposition to obesity [11]. The majority of genes that

C. Vaisse (✉)
Department of Medicine, Diabetes Center, University of California, San Francisco, CA, USA
e-mail: vaisse@diabetes.ucsf.edu

R.H. Lustig (ed.), *Obesity Before Birth*, Endocrine Updates 30,
DOI 10.1007/978-1-4419-7034-3_3, © Springer Science+Business Media, LLC 2011

contribute to this predisposition are still unknown, but the discovery and characterization of single gene defects have provided some insight into the hereditary nature of obesity.

3.2 Gene Mutations That Affect the Leptin–Melanocortin System

Several genes in which rare mutations cause severe monogenic or syndromic forms of obesity have been described and these have furthered our knowledge of the molecular pathways involved in food intake regulation and the control of body weight [12]. The genes implicated in these rare human monogenic forms of obesity encode proteins that have a role in the central regulation of energy homeostasis, in particular at the level of the hypothalamus.

This chapter focuses on obesity resulting from a mutation or deficiency of a single gene, defined as monogenic obesity. The majority of these monogenic obesity genes constitute regulatory step in the hypothalamic leptin–melanocortin system of energy homeostasis; e.g., melanocortin-4 receptor (MC4R), leptin, leptin receptor, proopiomelanocortin (POMC), and prohormone convertase 1/3 (PC1/3). In addition, other genes (*SIM1, BDNF,* and *NTRK2*) that are important for hypothalamic ontogeny and development are also associated with monogenic obesity.

The leptin–melanocortin system is a network of neurons centered in the hypothalamus, which regulates long-term maintenance of body weight in humans. This neuronal system integrates information about peripheral energy stores and affects changes in food intake behavior and basal energy expenditure. More specifically, leptin from adipocytes signals adequacy of the body's fat stores by binding to its receptors on two populations of neurons in the arcuate nucleus of the hypothalamus: orexigenic neurons that express AgRP (agouti-related peptide)/NPY (neuropeptide Y) and anorexigenic neurons that express POMC. These two groups of neurons have projections to the paraventricular nucleus (PVN) of the hypothalamus, as well as to other regions of the brain. When leptin binds to its receptor on POMC neurons, α-MSH is released, which activates the MC4R in the PVN to relay a satiety signal and cause a decrease in food intake. AgRP competes with α-MSH to bind MC4R; its binding to MC4R prevents anorexia and increases food intake. Leptin both activates POMC neurons and inhibits AgRP neurons, therefore acting in a concerted way to increase MC4R activation, and in so doing, decrease food intake and increase energy expenditure (Fig. 3.1).

3.2.1 Melanocortin-4 Receptor (MC4R)

The MC4R is a 332 amino acid protein encoded by a single exon gene localized on chromosome 18q22 [13, 14]. Disruption of this receptor leads to some of the most severe forms of human obesity [15]. MC4R is a G-protein-coupled

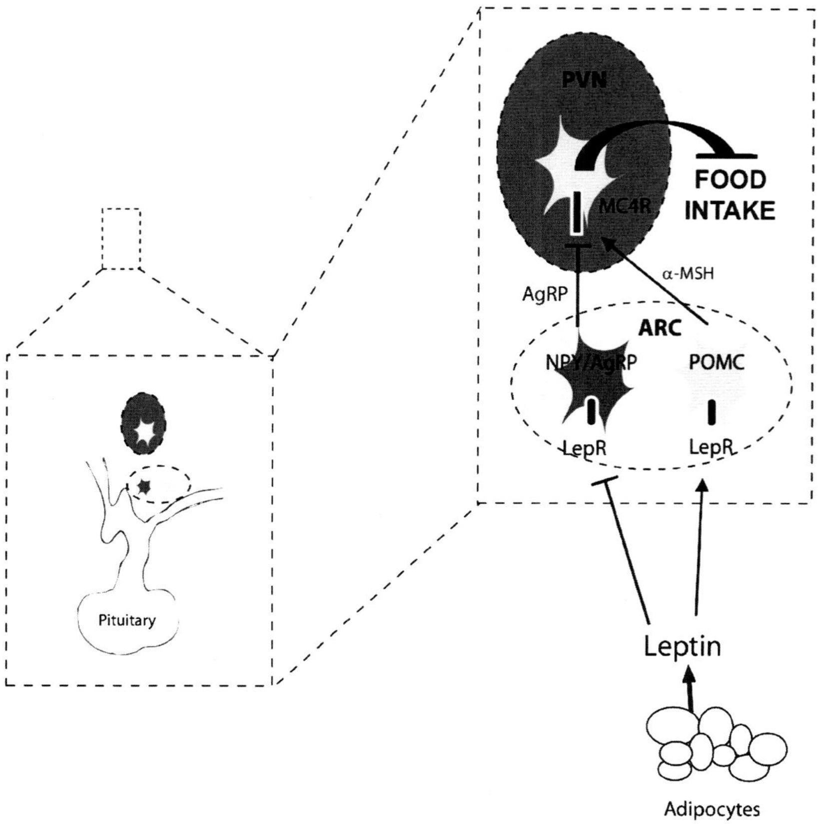

Fig. 3.1 The leptin–melanocortin system of energy balance. Hormones such as leptin convey information about the body's energy stores to the brain. Leptin is secreted by adipocytes in proportion to the body's fat mass. Leptin binds to its receptors on two populations of neurons in the arcuate nucleus (ARC) of the hypothalamus: the orexigenic agouti-related peptide (AgRP)/neuropeptide Y-expressing neurons and the anorexigenic POMC-expressing neurons. These groups of neurons have projections to the paraventricular nucleus of the hypothalamus and to other regions of the brain. The paraventricular nucleus of the hypothalamus (PVN) has a dense neuronal population that expresses MC4R. When leptin binds its receptor (LepR) on POMC neurons, α-melanocyte-stimulating hormone (α-MSH), a cleavage product of the POMC transcript, is released. Activation of MC4R in the PVN by α-MSH relays a satiety signal and causes a decrease in food intake. AgRP is an antagonist of MC4R and competes with α-MSH to bind MC4R. Binding of AgRP to MC4R leads to increased food intake. Leptin activates POMC neurons and inhibits AgRP neurons. Therefore, by activating its receptors on these two neuronal populations, leptin acts in a concerted way to increase MC4R activation by α-MSH and decrease its antagonism by AgRP, to cause a decrease in food intake. Mutations in genes with critical roles in the leptin–melanocortin system cause early-onset and severe obesity. Autosomal-recessive mutations in *leptin, LepR, POMC*, and *PC1/3*, and autosomal-dominant mutations in *MC4R* have been described

receptor (GPCR) that is expressed in hypothalamic nuclei involved in the regulation of food intake, particularly in neurons of the paraventricular nucleus (PVN) [16]. MC4R transduces its signal by coupling to the heterotrimeric $G_{s\alpha}$ protein and activating adenylate cyclase [13, 14]. MC4R regulates food intake and maintains long-term energy homeostasis by integrating signals provided by its agonist (α-MSH) and antagonist (AgRP) from neurons originating in the arcuate nucleus (ARC), which in turn are regulated by peripheral input mediated by leptin and insulin [17].

More than 100 mutations in the coding region of the *MC4R* gene have been described. Most of the detected rare *MC4R* mutations are missense mutations, which may or may not affect the function of the receptor. In order to show that non-synonymous mutations are responsible for disease, it is important to demonstrate the functional relevance of these mutations [18]. Functional studies of MC4R mutations associated with obesity indicate that multiple functional alterations contribute to their pathogenicity and that more severely impaired receptor function in vitro correlates clinically to earlier age of obesity onset and higher BMI. Each mutation impairs receptor function differently by affecting membrane expression or response to the agonist α-MSH to a variable degree [19].

MC4R mutations segregate with obesity in the families of the probands and are dominantly inherited with variable penetrance and expressivity. Patients with *MC4R* mutations have severe obesity and hyperphagia without other physical, hormonal, or developmental disorders, indicating that the function of MC4R is very specific for energy balance. Heterozygous MC4R mutations are the most common cause of monogenic obesity known, with a global prevalence of approximately 2.5% in severely obese individuals [17–20]. Homozygous MC4R mutations in humans are rare, with fewer than ten cases reported in the literature [17, 21–23]. These individuals, lacking both alleles of MC4R, are significantly more obese than heterozygotes.

Farooqi et al. have noted that MC4R deficiency is characterized by an increase in lean body mass, bone mineral density, increased linear growth, hyperphagia, and severe hyperinsulinemia. Furthermore, there was an age-related decrease in hyperinsulinemia and amelioration of hyperphagia with age in patients with MC4R heterozygous mutations [17]. However, in contrast to this reported "MC4R syndrome," we and others [20, 24–26] have not found a difference in insulin and glucose levels, blood pressure, and lipid profile between patients with MC4R mutations and obese volunteers without mutations [17].

A recent report showed that patients with heterozygous MC4R mutations have lower prevalence of hypertension compared with control subjects, suggesting that the melanocortin-4 signaling might control blood pressure through an insulin-independent mechanism [27]. Another recent study demonstrated that resting muscle sympathetic nerve activity, diastolic blood pressure, and heart rate were lower in MC4R mutations carriers as compared to control obese subjects, suggesting that central sympathetic outflow to the vasculature might depend on functional MC4R pathways [28].

3.2.2 Leptin

The hormone leptin was identified in 1994 by Fredman's group at Rockefeller University [29], who first showed that *ob/ob* mice are severely obese due to a mutation in the *leptin* gene. Others have since shown that peripheral administration of recombinant leptin reduced food intake, increased energy expenditure, and reduced body weight of leptin-deficient *ob/ob* mice [30–32]. Subsequently, leptin was shown to signal through the long isoform of the leptin receptor, a member of the interleukin-6 receptor family of class 1 cytokine receptors cloned in 1995 [33]. In humans, the first *leptin* gene mutation was described in 1997 in two severely obese cousins from a consanguineous Pakistani family, homozygous for a frameshift mutation (ΔG133) that leads to a truncated, unsecreted leptin molecule [34]. These patients had undetectable serum concentrations of leptin despite their obesity. Since then, few other patients have been described, including three Turkish patients homozygous for a missense mutation (R105Y) [35], six patients from four unrelated Pakistani families with the ΔG133 mutation [36, 37], a 3-year-old obese male Egyptian patient with a homozygous missense mutation (N103K) [38], and recently a 14-year-old Austrian girl with a new homozygous mutation (L72S) [39].

Congenital leptin deficiency is a rare autosomal-recessive disorder resulting from homozygous mutations in the *leptin* gene. Patients present with hyperphagia from birth and exhibit obesity as early as 6 months of age, lack of pubertal progression, and the majority of patients exhibit defective immunity [40]. Interestingly, a recent case had only mild obesity and normal T-cell responsiveness, despite the lowest recorded serum leptin levels [39]. Immeasurably low serum leptin levels make the diagnosis. Treatment with exogenous leptin is effective in restoring leptin signaling, with reduction in hyperphagia and body weight, induction of puberty, and improved immune regulation [37].

Heterozygous relatives of leptin-deficient subjects were studied to test the hypothesis that leptin has a dose–response effect on energy homeostasis [41]. Serum leptin levels in the heterozygous subjects were lower than expected per percent body fat and they had a higher prevalence of obesity than the control population, suggesting that the leptin-deficient haplotype can produce a graded response in terms of body composition across a broad range of plasma concentrations.

3.2.3 Leptin Receptor (LepR)

In contrast to leptin, a different strain of severely obese mice (*db/db*) was shown to be unresponsive to endogenous or exogenous leptin [42, 43] due to a deletion in the signaling form of the LepR. Defects in the *LepR* present either as homozygous or as compound heterozygous mutations. Three sisters from a consanguineous Algerian family were found to have a mutation truncating the LepR prior to its insertion in the membrane [44]. This family had symptoms and signs similar to those with leptin deficiency, including severe obesity early in life and hypogonadotropic hypogonadism; although they also had growth retardation, low thyroid levels, and low IGF-1 and IGFBP-3. Serum leptin in patients with LepR deficiency reflects BMI and fat mass, as it does in non-genetic obesity and other forms of monogenic obesity. It is important to note that the serum leptin levels in LepR deficiency are not any higher than would be predicted by the degree of obesity. Eight more individuals who had homozygous or compound heterozygous *LepR* mutations were identified in a highly consanguineous cohort of severely obese and hyperphagic patients [45]. Functional studies of these mutant receptors showed complete or partial loss of receptor signaling in response to leptin. Heterozygous carriers of *LepR* mutations are not severely obese, but do have increased fat mass [45].

3.2.4 Proopiomelanocortin (POMC)

POMC has a prominent role in the leptin–melanocortin system, as POMC-expressing neurons are the hypothalamic targets of leptin signaling, and α-MSH is the POMC cleavage product that activates MC4R. Therefore, lack of MC4R activation by α-MSH causes severe obesity in POMC deficiency.

The *POMC* gene is located on chromosome 2p22.3. It is approximately 8.6 kb and contains three exons [46]. The coding region of *POMC* is in exons 2 and 3 only. The *POMC* gene encodes the protein precursor POMC that is differentially cleaved into five biologically active peptides. Tissue-specific cleavage of POMC by pro-hormone convertases 1/3 and 2 leads to the production of ACTH in corticotropes of the anterior pituitary, and α-, β-, and δ-MSH and β-endorphin in the melanotropic cells of the hypothalamus and skin (Fig. 3.2). Loss-of-function mutations in *POMC* (homozygous or compound heterozygous) result in severe hyperphagia and obesity as a consequence of lack of MC4R activation by α-MSH; and adrenal insufficiency as a consequence of defective synthesis of ACTH. Obesity occurs

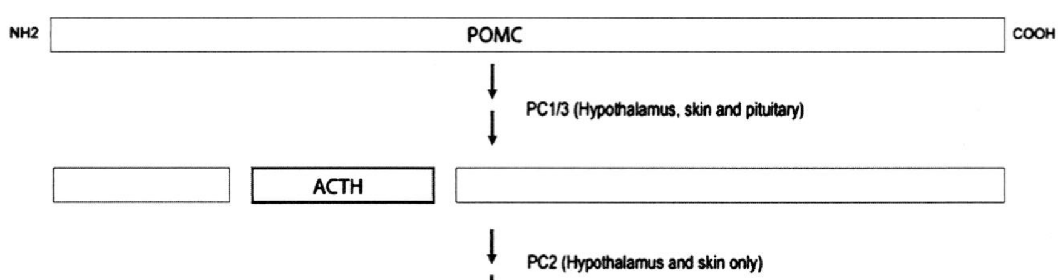

Fig. 3.2 Processing of POMC. POMC is processed by PC1/3 and PC2 into five biologically active proteins. In the corticotropes of the anterior pituitary, PC1/3 is expressed, but PC2 is not. Therefore, adrenocorticotropic hormone (ACTH) is the only biologically active POMC-derived peptide synthesized in the anterior pituitary. PC1/3 and PC2 are expressed in the melanotropes of the hypothalamus and skin. Thus, POMC is sequentially processed into α-, β-, and δ-MSH and β-endorphin in these tissues. The phenotype of POMC deficiency is explained by the tissue-specific lack of these cleavage products

despite profound glucocorticoid deficiency, a condition normally associated with weight loss [47]. Interestingly, *POMC*-null mice are hypersensitive to the adverse metabolic effects of glucocorticoids and develop diabetes mellitus 12 weeks after glucocorticoid replacement [48].

Only seven human cases of complete POMC deficiency have been reported. The first two patients with complete POMC deficiency were described in 1998. One patient was compound heterozygous for two mutations in exon 3 (G7013T and C7133D), and the other was homozygous for a base pair substitution in exon 2 (C3804A) that disrupted translation of the entire POMC protein [49]. Three more patients with homozygous or compound heterozygous *POMC* mutations causing congenital POMC deficiency were described in 2003 [50]. The sixth case was reported in a Turkish patient with a homozygous frameshift loss-of-function mutation (C6906D) with severe obesity and ACTH deficiency, but dark hair [51]. And most recently, the seventh case was described in a female patient of North African ancestry, homozygous for a frameshift mutation in the *POMC* gene (6922InsC) with severe obesity and multiple pituitary hormone deficiencies [52]. These patients presented in the newborn period with adrenal insufficiency and have required ongoing glucocorticoid replacement therapy to prevent adrenal crises. Hyperphagia leading to severe obesity usually begins in the first year of life. These patients have normal birth weight, the onset of rapid weight gain before 6 months of age, and weights exceeding 15 kg by 1 year, and 25 kg by 3 years. Red hair, due to lack of α-MSH activating MC1R in melanocytes, was initially reported as part of the clinical spectrum of congenital POMC deficiency. However, this finding is apparently variable, as the Turkish patient and the most recent patient from North Africa have black hair.

There is a significantly higher prevalence of overweight in heterozygous carriers of *POMC* mutations, supporting the idea that loss of one copy of *POMC* is sufficient to predispose to obesity [50, 51]. These patients with heterozygous *POMC* mutations have hyperphagia and obesity without other clinical manifestations [11].

3.2.5 Prohormone Convertase 1/3 (PC1/3)

PC1/3 and PC2 are serine endoproteases selectively expressed in neuroendocrine tissues and are essential in the cleavage of several proneuropeptides important for energy balance regulation. These neuropeptides include proTRH, proinsulin, proglucagon, proGHRH, POMC, pro-neuropeptide Y, and pro-cocaine–amphetamine-related transcript [53].

Defects in PC1/3 and PC2 lead to the inability to process various preprohormones to their active ligands, such as POMC to ACTH and α-MSH, proinsulin to insulin, and various gut propeptides to active hormones [54]. Three cases of PC1/3 mutations that cause severe obesity have been reported [54–57]. These patients also had mild hypocortisolism caused by partial ACTH deficiency, which was not as severe as in the patients with complete POMC deficiency. All three patients also had malabsorption caused by small bowel dysfunction. Improper processing of proglucagon in the intestinal cells to GLP-2, which has trophic effects on small bowel epithelium, may contribute to poor integrity of the small bowel mucosa in these patients. Two of the three patients had abnormalities of glucose homeostasis, such as postprandial hyperglycemia and reactive hypoglycemia, possibly due to abnormal processing of proinsulin to insulin in pancreatic β-cells [54, 55]. Other findings, such as hypogonadotropic hypogonadism in one patient and central hypothyroidism in another, may be attributed to impaired proTRH and proGnRH processing by PC1/3. Heterozygous *PC1/3* mutations are currently extremely rare in the differential diagnosis of monogenic obesity and the patients described above came to medical attention due to medical problems other than obesity. A high proinsulin-to-insulin ratio after a glucose load is the only laboratory evaluation available to determine PC1/3 deficiency. Carriers of *PC1/3* mutations do not have a clinically apparent obese phenotype.

3.3 Gene Mutations That Affect Neurodevelopment

3.3.1 SIM1

SIM1 is a transcription factor expressed in the PVN during development and after birth. In *SIM1* homozygous null mice, the PVN fails to develop, and these mice die perinatally. SIM1 heterozygous mice survive and develop early-onset obesity with increased linear growth, hyperinsulinemia, and hyperleptinemia. They are hyperphagic, but do not have decreased energy expenditure [58, 59].

The first human case of SIM1 deficiency was described in 2000. A 6-year-old girl had a balanced translocation interrupting one copy of *SIM1* on chromosome 6q [60]. Her obesity was not associated with any developmental abnormalities, syndromic features, or endocrine dysfunction. The description of obesity in children with chromosomal deletions in the 6q16 region (which contains *SIM1*), supports the role of SIM1 in the development of an obese phenotype [61–64]. A genome-wide search for childhood obesity-associated traits showed the strongest evidence of linkage on chromosome 6q22.31; of which *SIM1* was one of the likely candidate genes [64]. Eight patients with clinical features of Prader–Willi syndrome have been reported with interstitial deletions in chromosome 6q14–q21 [61–63, 65–69]. However, not all patients with deletion of *SIM1* exhibit a Prader–Willi like phenotype [68, 70].

More recently there is evidence that SIM1 may have an ongoing, post-developmental role in energy balance, and that it may function downstream of the MC4R to control food intake [60]. In mice, both SIM1 and MC4R are most abundantly expressed in the PVN [58] Additionally, MC4R knockout mice and SIM1 haploinsufficient mice have a remarkably similar phenotype of hyperphagia, obesity, increased linear growth, and increased sensitivity to a high-fat diet. Therefore, it is possible that SIM1 and MC4R are involved in the same hypothalamic pathway of control of food intake. However, the molecular pathways downstream of MC4R that regulate food intake are far from understood, and further studies are necessary to determine the exact role of SIM1.

3.3.2 Brain-Derived Neurotrophic Factor (BDNF)

BDNF acting through its receptor TRKB (tropomyosin-related kinase B) regulates proliferation, survival, and differentiation of many classes of neurons during development [71, 72]. In the adult nervous system, this ligand and its receptor regulate neuronal plasticity by controlling synaptic function and survival of neurons [72, 73].

BDNF has been shown to be important in the control of food intake [74, 75]. BDNF is an anorexigenic factor that is highly expressed in the mouse ventromedial hypothalamus (VMH) and is regulated by feeding status [71]. Postnatal deletion of BDNF in the mouse brain leads to hyperphagia, obesity, increased linear growth, hyperinsulinemia, and hyperleptinemia, similar to the MC4R knockout mouse; but BDNF deletion also leads to increased anxiety and hyperactivity [76]. Two lines of evidence support that MC4R signaling regulates BDNF expression in the VMH. First, deficiency in MC4R signaling reduces BDNF expression in the VMH, and second, the hyperphagia and rapid weight gain of MC4R-deficient mice on a high-fat diet are suppressed by administration of BDNF into the central nervous system. Together, these findings suggest that BDNF acts downstream of MC4R to modulate food intake [77].

The first human case of severe obesity due to haploinsufficiency of *BDNF* was reported in an 8-year-old girl [78]. The patient presented with hyperphagia, obesity, impaired cognition, impaired memory, nociception, and hyperactivity. She had a de novo paracentric inversion 46,XX,inv(11)p13p15.3 that contains the *BDNF* locus on chromosome 11. The authors show that the inversion does not disrupt the *BDNF* gene itself, but BDNF protein expression is compromised. Although it is possible that the inversion disrupts other unknown genes contributing to the patient's phenotype, the marked similarity of this patient's presentation to that of a patient with a *NTRK2* mutation (see below) supports the conclusion that her phenotype results from haploinsufficiency of *BDNF* [78]. As in *SIM1* haploinsufficiency, this patient's obesity may result from a lack of BDNF during hypothalamic development or from its impaired postnatal role in MC4R signaling and control of food intake.

BDNF haploinsufficiency and lower levels of BDNF were also found in patients with the WAGR syndrome (Wilms' tumor, aniridia, genitourinary anomalies, and mental retardation); these patients have contiguous gene deletions causing haploinsufficiency of the *WT-1* and *PAX6* genes on chromosome 11p13, approximately 4 Mb centromeric to *BDNF* (11p14.1). A subset of patients with this syndrome exhibit hyperphagia and obesity, depending on the extent of the contigious deletion. One study of 33 patients with WAGR syndrome and deletions on chromosome 11p showed a 58% prevalence of heterozygous *BDNF* deletions [79]. These patients had significant higher BMI and serum BDNF concentrations were approximately 50% lower among the patients with heterozygous BDNF deletions. They concluded that among patients with the WAGR syndrome, *BDNF* haploinsufficiency is associated with lower levels of serum BDNF and with childhood-onset obesity.

3.3.3 NTRK2

TRKB (tropomyosin-related kinase B), encoded by the *NTRK2* gene, is a neurotrophin receptor with high affinity for BDNF. As mentioned in the previous section, neurotrophins such as BDNF and their receptors regulate the development and maintenance of neurons, and specifically modulate the postnatal plasticity of hypothalamic neurons [72, 73, 80].

Homozygous null mutations of *NTRK2* and *BDNF* are postnatally lethal in mice [81] as these genes play a role in early brain development. The phenotype of partial deficiency of either of these genes includes hyperphagia and obesity [74, 77, 82].

One human case of a heterozygous de novo mutation in *NTRK2* has been reported [83]. This 8-year-old boy presented with hyperphagia, early-onset obesity; delayed development; stereotyped behaviors; and impaired memory, learning, and nociception. Functional studies of his missense mutation in *NTRK2* (Y722C) showed significantly impaired BDNF-induced receptor autophosphorylation as well as activation of signaling molecules downstream of the receptor [83, 84]. The authors also found decreased neurite outgrowth and cell survival in response to BDNF in cells transfected with the mutant receptor, suggesting that post-developmental neuronal plasticity is also affected by *NTRK2* mutations.

Screening a cohort of individuals with severe early-onset obesity and developmental delay revealed three other mutations in *NTRK2* (I98V, P660L, and T821A) that were not present in controls, but in vitro studies of these mutations did not reveal a significant difference in receptor function compared to wild type [84].

Although the exact role of these genes, *SIM1, BDNF*, and *NTRK2*, in the development of obesity has not yet clearly been delineated, their involvement in hypothalamic development and their postnatal function, possibly downstream of MC4R, seems likely based on data from mouse models.

3.4 Treatment

Of the monogenic forms of obesity described thus far, disease-specific clinical intervention is available only for congenital leptin deficiency. Treatment with daily subcutaneous injections of recombinant human leptin offers an excellent therapeutic outcome, for up to at least a 4-year treatment period. Previous reports showed that a decrease in therapeutic efficacy is seen due to the development of antibodies to the administered leptin, that has thus far been overcome by increases in leptin dosage [36, 37]. No subsequent follow-up data of ongoing leptin treatment has been published on these patients. Unfortunately, there is no beneficial effect of treatment with supraphysiologic doses of leptin in non-leptin-deficient individuals with non-genetic obesity [85].

Multiple other attempts have been made to treat patients with monogenic obesity, such as development of MC4R agonists to decrease hyperphagia, and treatment of POMC-deficient patients with thyroid hormone. Fan et al. tested the effect of an MC4R inverse agonist, ML0025376, in intracellular retained MC4R mutants and showed rescue of the mutant MC4R to the cell surface [86]. In addition, they showed that the rescued mutants are functional with increased cAMP production in response to the agonist. Further studies using this pharmacological chaperone in humans with MC4R mutations are needed to further evaluate its role as a therapeutic approach for this monogenic form of obesity. Another MC4R agonist, a synthetically produced cyclic peptide called LY2112688, was shown to cause yawning, stretching, penile erection, and higher blood pressure in obese volunteers without MC4R mutations [27]. Further studies of melanocortin agonists could be helpful in patients with *MC4R* haploinsufficiency. Krude et al. treated two patients with obesity due to POMC deficiency with $ACTH_{10}$ [50]. After 3 months of treatment, they showed no reduction in body weight or resting metabolic rate. Thyroid function test in those patients showed elevated TSH with borderline low total T4; thus they treated both patients in a prospective 1-year trial with increasing doses of levothyroxine. The treatment resulted in normal T4 values and low normal TSH; however, body weight was unaffected.

There is some evidence that the hyperphagia of patients with other forms of syndromic obesity responds to strict and intensive diet and lifestyle interventions. For instance, successful management of obesity in Prader–Willi syndrome patients can be accomplished with vigilant and vigorous control of food intake and adherence to a strict exercise program [87]. In contrast, Reinehr et al. showed that carriers of *MC4R* mutations could lose body weight with intense lifestyle intervention, but have difficulty maintaining the weight loss. Specifically, 514 obese children were followed during 1-year lifestyle intervention based on exercise, behavior, and nutrition therapy. They compared 16 children with missense *MC4R* mutations with 80 gender-matched children without *MC4R* mutations and 481 other children without *MC4R* mutations. Children with and without *MC4R* mutations reduced their body weight to a similar degree at the end of the 1-year intervention; however, the maintenance of weight loss among children with MC4R mutations failed in contrast to children without *MC4R* mutations [88].

Bariatric surgery is a promising weight-loss tool for selected severely obese patients for whom conventional medical and behavioral therapy has failed and this procedure has become a more common tool to achieve weight control and resolution of co-morbidities [89]. There are only limited available data on bariatric surgery outcome in patients with genetic disorders associated with obesity. Bariatric surgery has been shown to be anecdotally effective in some genetic syndromes associated with obesity and in patients with hypothalamic obesity. A report of an adolescent patient with Bardet–Biedl syndrome who underwent Roux-en-Y gastric bypass exhibited lower weight 3 years after surgery with a reduction in BMI from 52 to 34 kg/m^2 [90]. There are also several reports of bariatric surgery in patients with hypothalamic obesity following treatment of craniopharyngioma [91–93] as four patients achieved weight reduction, but post-operative complications developed in some. The underlying cause of the obesity in such patients is their inability to transduce the hypothalamic leptin signal, similar to patients with mutations in the leptin–melanocortin pathway but these patients also have hormone deficiencies and other associated neurological disorders which may interfere with the response to bariatric surgery.

One report suggested that carriers of genetic variations at the *MC4R* locus have poorer outcomes after gastric banding [94]. However, a majority of patients in this study carried *MC4R* polymorphisms that were not associated with obesity (i.e., found also in non-obese controls) and with no demonstrated functional effect on the MC4R protein. In addition, patients were included with binge eating disorder, who have been shown to exhibit poorer outcomes after bariatric surgery [95]. Further studies are therefore needed to evaluate the predictive role of *MC4R* mutations in outcome after bariatric surgery.

More generally, the observation that patients with hypothalamic obesity and other genetic syndromes may benefit from bariatric surgery supports further investigation of the role of this procedure in the treatment of these forms of obesity.

3.5 Conclusions

The hypothalamic leptin–melanocortin system is critical for the regulation of body weight in humans, since disruption of this signaling pathway leads to the most severe forms of human obesity known to date. Compromised hypothalamic energy regulation may also underlie the pathogenesis of less severe, later-onset obesity, and of obesity associated with other clinical and developmental defects. However, at this time, the known genetic causes of obesity only account for about 5% of all human obesity. The etiology of the remaining 95% of obesity is likely to be heterogeneous and polygenic and the identification of obesity-associated genes has been slow and challenging.

In general, the earlier the age of rapid weight gain and the more severe the body weight phenotype, the greater the likelihood of monogenic cause involving the leptin–melanocortin system will be found. However, even within the spectrum of genetic causes of obesity, a significant variability in severity of the phenotype exists. When evaluating an obese patient, the age at onset of weight gain, the phenotype of hyperphagia, a family history of consanguinity (for autosomal-recessive mutations), or a family history of obesity (for autosomal-dominant inheritance such as *MC4R* mutations) are important factors to elicit. Once the concern for a genetic cause for obesity is raised, the approach can be as follows. First, if the obesity is associated with any obvious clinical findings such as mental retardation, developmental delay, dysmorphic faces, or organ-specific defects of structure or function, then an evaluation for syndromic causes of the obesity should be pursued. Next, laboratory evaluation to look for subtle endocrine abnormalities such as hypothyroidism, hypocortisolism, hypogonadotropic hypogonadism, or for diagnostic clues such as extremely low fasting serum leptin, or abnormally high proinsulin to insulin ratio may be obtained. Finally, mutational analysis for the more common forms of monogenic obesity (*MC4R, leptin* and *LepR*) are now commercially available. However, in most cases, the management approach to severe obesity, even monogenetic disorders (with the exception of leptin deficiency), is currently the same regardless of the cause. Thus, further research to understand the pathogenic mechanisms underlying obesity is required for the development of similar rational and effective treatments. However, such research is challenging because of the great genetic heterogeneity of obesity versus the small number of patients with defined monogenic obesity. Although patients currently experience no direct benefit from the knowledge of the genetic basis of their disease, it is important from a research perspective to further explore the genetic cause of this phenotype. Only through elucidating the molecular mechanisms underlying obesity can this condition be rationally approached.

In summary, the study of patients with monogenic forms of obesity and gene discovery remains essential for insight into pathogenesis and therapy for obese patients.

References

1. Ogden CL, Flegal KM, Carroll MD, Johnson CL. Prevalence and trends in overweight among US children and adolescents, 1999–2000. JAMA. Oct 9 2002;288(14):1728–32.
2. Flegal KM, Carroll MD, Ogden CL, Curtin LR. Prevalence and trends in obesity among US adults, 1999–2008. JAMA. Jan 20 2010;303(3):235–41.
3. Vasan RS, Pencina MJ, Cobain M, Freiberg MS, D'Agostino RB. Estimated risks for developing obesity in the Framingham Heart Study. Ann Intern Med. Oct 4 2005;143(7):473–80.
4. Ogden CL, Carroll MD, Curtin LR, Lamb MM, Flegal KM. Prevalence of high body mass index in US children and adolescents, 2007–2008. JAMA. Jan 20 2010;303(3):242–9.
5. Franks PW, Hanson RL, Knowler WC, Sievers ML, Bennett PH, Looker HC. Childhood obesity, other cardiovascular risk factors, and premature death. N Engl J Med. Feb 11 2010;362(6):485–93.
6. Hill JO. Genetic and environmental contributions to obesity. Am J Clin Nutr. Nov 1998;68(5):991–2.
7. Swarbrick MM, Vaisse C. Emerging trends in the search for genetic variants predisposing to human obesity. Curr Opin Clin Nutr Metab Care. Jul 2003;6(4):369–75.
8. Maes HH, Neale MC, Eaves LJ. Genetic and environmental factors in relative body weight and human adiposity. Behav Genet. Jul 1997;27(4):325–51.
9. Frayling TM, Timpson NJ, Weedon MN, et al. A common variant in the FTO gene is associated with body mass index and predisposes to childhood and adult obesity. Science. May 11 2007;316(5826):889–94.
10. Loos RJ, Lindgren CM, Li S, et al. Common variants near MC4R are associated with fat mass, weight and risk of obesity. Nat Genet. Jun 2008;40(6):768–75.
11. Ranadive SA, Vaisse C. Lessons from extreme human obesity: monogenic disorders. Endocrinol Metab Clin North Am. Sep 2008;37(3):733–51.
12. Coll AP, Farooqi IS, O'Rahilly S. The hormonal control of food intake. Cell. Apr 20 2007;129(2):251–62.
13. Gantz I, Miwa H, Konda Y, et al. Molecular cloning, expression, and gene localization of a fourth melanocortin receptor. J Biol Chem. Jul 15 1993;268(20):15174–9.

14. Mountjoy KG, Robbins LS, Mortrud MT, Cone RD. The cloning of a family of genes that encode the melanocortin receptors. Science. Aug 28 1992;257(5074):1248–51.
15. Mountjoy KG, Mortrud MT, Low MJ, Simerly RB, Cone RD. Localization of the melanocortin-4 receptor (MC4-R) in neuroendocrine and autonomic control circuits in the brain. Mol Endocrinol. Oct 1994;8(10):1298–308.
16. Schwartz MW, Woods SC, Porte D Jr., Seeley RJ, Baskin DG. Central nervous system control of food intake. Nature. Apr 6 2000;404(6778):661–71.
17. Farooqi IS, Keogh JM, Yeo GS, Lank EJ, Cheetham T, O'Rahilly S. Clinical spectrum of obesity and mutations in the melanocortin 4 receptor gene. N Engl J Med. Mar 20 2003;348(12):1085–95.
18. Calton MA, Ersoy BA, Zhang S, et al. Association of functionally significant Melanocortin-4 but not Melanocortin-3 receptor mutations with severe adult obesity in a large North-American case control study. Hum Mol Genet. Dec 17 2008;18:1140–1147.
19. Lubrano-Berthelier C, Dubern B, Lacorte JM, et al. Melanocortin 4 receptor mutations in a large cohort of severely obese adults: prevalence, functional classification, genotype-phenotype relationship, and lack of association with binge eating. J Clin Endocrinol Metab. May 2006;91(5):1811–8.
20. Hainerova I, Larsen LH, Holst B, et al. Melanocortin 4 receptor mutations in obese Czech children: studies of prevalence, phenotype development, weight reduction response, and functional analysis. J Clin Endocrinol Metab. Sep 2007;92(9):3689–96.
21. Lubrano-Berthelier C, Le Stunff C, Bougneres P, Vaisse C. A homozygous null mutation delineates the role of the melanocortin-4 receptor in humans. J Clin Endocrinol Metab. May 2004;89(5):2028–32.
22. Dubern B, Bisbis S, Talbaoui H, et al. Homozygous null mutation of the melanocortin-4 receptor and severe early-onset obesity. J Pediatr. Jun 2007;150(6):613–7.
23. Kobayashi H, Ogawa Y, Shintani M, et al. A Novel homozygous missense mutation of melanocortin-4 receptor (MC4R) in a Japanese woman with severe obesity. Diabetes. Jan 2002;51(1):243–6.
24. Vaisse C, Clement K, Guy-Grand B, Froguel P. A frameshift mutation in human MC4R is associated with a dominant form of obesity. Nat Genet. Oct 1998;20(2):113–4.
25. Lubrano-Berthelier C, Cavazos M, Le Stunff C, et al. The human MC4R promoter: characterization and role in obesity. Diabetes. Dec 2003;52(12):2996–3000.
26. Mergen M, Mergen H, Ozata M, Oner R, Oner C. A novel melanocortin 4 receptor (MC4R) gene mutation associated with morbid obesity. J Clin Endocrinol Metab. Jul 2001;86(7):3448.
27. Greenfield JR, Miller JW, Keogh JM, et al. Modulation of blood pressure by central melanocortinergic pathways. N Engl J Med. Jan 1 2009;360(1):44–52.
28. Sayk F, Heutling D, Dodt C, et al. Sympathetic function in human carriers of Melanocortin-4 receptor gene mutations. J Clin Endocrinol Metab. Feb 10 2010;95(4):1998–2002.
29. Zhang Y, Proenca R, Maffei M, Barone M, Leopold L, Friedman JM. Positional cloning of the mouse obese gene and its human homologue. Nature. Dec 1 1994;372(6505):425–32.
30. Halaas JL, Gajiwala KS, Maffei M, et al. Weight-reducing effects of the plasma protein encoded by the obese gene. Science. Jul 28 1995;269(5223):543–6.
31. Pelleymounter MA, Cullen MJ, Baker MB, et al. Effects of the obese gene product on body weight regulation in ob/ob mice. Science. Jul 28 1995;269(5223):540–3.
32. Campfield LA, Smith FJ, Guisez Y, Devos R, Burn P. Recombinant mouse OB protein: evidence for a peripheral signal linking adiposity and central neural networks. Science. Jul 28 1995;269(5223):546–9.
33. Tartaglia LA, Dembski M, Weng X, et al. Identification and expression cloning of a leptin receptor. OB-R Cell. Dec 29 1995;83(7):1263–71.
34. Montague CT, Farooqi IS, Whitehead JP, et al. Congenital leptin deficiency is associated with severe early-onset obesity in humans. Nature. Jun 26 1997;387(6636):903–8.
35. Strobel A, Issad T, Camoin L, Ozata M, Strosberg AD. A leptin missense mutation associated with hypogonadism and morbid obesity. Nat Genet. Mar 1998;18(3):213–5.

36. Gibson WT, Farooqi IS, Moreau M, et al. Congenital leptin deficiency due to homozygosity for the Delta133G mutation: report of another case and evaluation of response to four years of leptin therapy. J Clin Endocrinol Metab. Oct 2004;89(10):4821–6.
37. Farooqi IS, Matarese G, Lord GM, et al. Beneficial effects of leptin on obesity, T cell hyporesponsiveness, and neuroendocrine/metabolic dysfunction of human congenital leptin deficiency. J Clin Invest. Oct 2002;110(8):1093–103.
38. Mazen I, El-Gammal M, Abdel-Hamid M, Amr K. A novel homozygous missense mutation of the leptin gene (N103K) in an obese Egyptian patient. Mol Genet Metab. Aug 2009;97(4):305–8.
39. Fischer-Posovszky P, von Schnurbein J, Moepps B, et al. A new missense mutation in the leptin gene causes mild obesity and hypogonadism without affecting T cell responsiveness. J Clin Endocrinol Metab. April 9 2010;95(6):2836–40.
40. Farooqi IS, O'Rahilly S. Monogenic human obesity syndromes. Recent Prog Horm Res. 2004;59:409–24.
41. Farooqi IS, Keogh JM, Kamath S, et al. Partial leptin deficiency and human adiposity. Nature. Nov 1 2001;414(6859):34–5.
42. Chua SC Jr., Chung WK, Wu-Peng XS, et al. Phenotypes of mouse diabetes and rat fatty due to mutations in the OB (leptin) receptor. Science. Feb 16 1996;271(5251):994–6.
43. Chen H, Charlat O, Tartaglia LA, et al. Evidence that the diabetes gene encodes the leptin receptor: identification of a mutation in the leptin receptor gene in db/db mice. Cell. Feb 9 1996;84(3):491–5.
44. Clement K, Vaisse C, Lahlou N, et al. A mutation in the human leptin receptor gene causes obesity and pituitary dysfunction. Nature. Mar 26 1998;392(6674):398–401.
45. Farooqi IS, Wangensteen T, Collins S, et al. Clinical and molecular genetic spectrum of congenital deficiency of the leptin receptor. N Engl J Med. Jan 18 2007;356(3): 237–47.
46. Owerbach D, Rutter WJ, Roberts JL, et al. The proopiocortin (adrenocorticotropin/beta-lipoprotein) gene is located on chromosome 2 in humans. Somatic Cell Genet. May 1981;7(3):359–69.
47. Farooqi S, O'Rahilly S. Genetics of obesity in humans. Endocr Rev. Dec 2006;27(7):710–8.
48. Coll AP, Challis BG, Lopez M, Piper S, Yeo GS, O'Rahilly S. Proopiomelanocortin-deficient mice are hypersensitive to the adverse metabolic effects of glucocorticoids. Diabetes. Aug 2005;54(8):2269–76.
49. Krude H, Biebermann H, Luck W, Horn R, Brabant G, Gruters A. Severe early-onset obesity, adrenal insufficiency and red hair pigmentation caused by POMC mutations in humans. Nat Genet. Jun 1998;19(2):155–7.
50. Krude H, Biebermann H, Schnabel D, et al. Obesity due to proopiomelanocortin deficiency: three new cases and treatment trials with thyroid hormone and ACTH4-10. J Clin Endocrinol Metab. Oct 2003;88(10):4633–40.
51. Farooqi IS, Drop S, Clements A, et al. Heterozygosity for a POMC-null mutation and increased obesity risk in humans. Diabetes. Sep 2006;55(9):2549–53.
52. Clement K, Dubern B, Mencarelli M, et al. Unexpected endocrine features and normal pigmentation in a young adult patient carrying a novel homozygous mutation in the POMC gene. J Clin Endocrinol Metab. Dec 2008;93(12):4955–62.
53. Nillni EA. Regulation of prohormone convertases in hypothalamic neurons: implications for prothyrotropin-releasing hormone and proopiomelanocortin. Endocrinology. Sep 2007;148(9):4191–200.
54. Jackson RS, Creemers JW, Ohagi S, et al. Obesity and impaired prohormone processing associated with mutations in the human prohormone convertase 1 gene. Nat Genet. Jul 1997;16(3):303–6.
55. O'Rahilly S, Gray H, Humphreys PJ, et al. Brief report: impaired processing of prohormones associated with abnormalities of glucose homeostasis and adrenal function. N Engl J Med. Nov 23 1995;333(21):1386–90.

56. Jackson RS, Creemers JW, Farooqi IS, et al. Small-intestinal dysfunction accompanies the complex endocrinopathy of human proprotein convertase 1 deficiency. J Clin Invest. Nov 2003;112(10):1550–60.
57. Farooqi IS, Volders K, Stanhope R, et al. Hyperphagia and early-onset obesity due to a novel homozygous missense mutation in prohormone convertase 1/3. J Clin Endocrinol Metab. Sep 2007;92(9):3369–73.
58. Michaud JL, Boucher F, Melnyk A, et al. Sim1 haploinsufficiency causes hyperphagia, obesity and reduction of the paraventricular nucleus of the hypothalamus. Hum Mol Genet. Jul 1 2001;10(14):1465–73.
59. Michaud JL, Rosenquist T, May NR, Fan CM. Development of neuroendocrine lineages requires the bHLH-PAS transcription factor SIM1. Genes Dev. Oct 15 1998;12(20):3264–75.
60. Holder JL Jr., Butte NF, Zinn AR. Profound obesity associated with a balanced translocation that disrupts the SIM1 gene. Hum Mol Genet. Jan 1 2000;9(1):101–8.
61. Villa A, Urioste M, Bofarull JM, Martinez-Frias ML. De novo interstitial deletion q16.2q21 on chromosome 6. Am J Med Genet. Jan 30 1995;55(3):379–83.
62. Gilhuis HJ, van Ravenswaaij CM, Hamel BJ, Gabreels FJ. Interstitial 6q deletion with a Prader-Willi-like phenotype: a new case and review of the literature. Eur J Paediatr Neurol. 2000;4(1):39–43.
63. Faivre L, Cormier-Daire V, Lapierre JM, et al. Deletion of the SIM1 gene (6q16.2) in a patient with a Prader-Willi-like phenotype. J Med Genet. Aug 2002;39(8):594–6.
64. Meyre D, Lecoeur C, Delplanque J, et al. A genome-wide scan for childhood obesity-associated traits in French families shows significant linkage on chromosome 6q22.31–q23.2. Diabetes. Mar 2004;53(3):803–11.
65. Wang JC, Turner L, Lomax B, Eydoux PA. 5-Mb microdeletion at 6q16.1–q16.3 with SIM gene deletion and obesity. Am J Med Genet A. Nov 15 2008;146A(22):2975–8.
66. Turleau C, Demay G, Cabanis MO, Lenoir G, de Grouchy J. 6q1 monosomy: a distinctive syndrome. Clin Genet. Jul 1988;34(1):38–42.
67. Varela MC, Simoes-Sato AY, Kim CA, Bertola DR, De Castro CI, Koiffmann CP. A new case of interstitial 6q16.2 deletion in a patient with Prader-Willi-like phenotype and investigation of SIM1 gene deletion in 87 patients with syndromic obesity. Eur J Med Genet. Jul–Aug 2006;49(4):298–305.
68. Klein OD, Cotter PD, Moore MW, et al. Interstitial deletions of chromosome 6q: genotype-phenotype correlation utilizing array CGH. Clin Genet. Mar 2007;71(3):260–6.
69. Stein CK, Stred SE, Thomson LL, Smith FC, Hoo JJ. Interstitial 6q deletion and Prader-Willi-like phenotype. Clin Genet. Jun 1996;49(6):306–10.
70. Le Caignec C, Swillen A, Van Asche E, Fryns JP, Vermeesch JR. Interstitial 6q deletion: clinical and array CGH characterisation of a new patient. Eur J Med Genet. Jul–Sep 2005;48(3):339–45.
71. Tapia-Arancibia L, Rage F, Givalois L, Arancibia S. Physiology of BDNF: focus on hypothalamic function. Front Neuroendocrinol. Jul 2004;25(2):77–107.
72. Huang EJ, Reichardt LF. Neurotrophins: roles in neuronal development and function. Annu Rev Neurosci. 2001;24:677–736.
73. Huang EJ, Reichardt LF. Trk receptors: roles in neuronal signal transduction. Annu Rev Biochem. 2003;72:609–42.
74. Kernie SG, Liebl DJ, Parada LF. BDNF regulates eating behavior and locomotor activity in mice. EMBO J. Mar 15 2000;19(6):1290–300.
75. Pelleymounter MA, Cullen MJ, Wellman CL. Characteristics of BDNF-induced weight loss. Exp Neurol. Feb 1995;131(2):229–38.
76. Rios M, Fan G, Fekete C, et al. Conditional deletion of brain-derived neurotrophic factor in the postnatal brain leads to obesity and hyperactivity. Mol Endocrinol. Oct 2001;15(10): 1748–57.
77. Xu B, Goulding EH, Zang K, et al. Brain-derived neurotrophic factor regulates energy balance downstream of melanocortin-4 receptor. Nat Neurosci. Jul 2003;6(7):736–42.

78. Gray J, Yeo GS, Cox JJ, et al. Hyperphagia, severe obesity, impaired cognitive function, and hyperactivity associated with functional loss of one copy of the brain-derived neurotrophic factor (BDNF) gene. Diabetes. Dec 2006;55(12):3366–71.
79. Han JC, Liu QR, Jones M, et al. Brain-derived neurotrophic factor and obesity in the WAGR syndrome. N Engl J Med. Aug 28 2008;359(9):918–27.
80. Biebermann H, Castaneda TR, van Landeghem F, et al. A role for beta-melanocyte-stimulating hormone in human body-weight regulation. Cell Metab. Feb 2006;3(2):141–6.
81. Klein R, Smeyne RJ, Wurst W, et al. Targeted disruption of the trkB neurotrophin receptor gene results in nervous system lesions and neonatal death. Cell. Oct 8 1993;75(1):113–22.
82. Lyons WE, Mamounas LA, Ricaurte GA, et al. Brain-derived neurotrophic factor-deficient mice develop aggressiveness and hyperphagia in conjunction with brain serotonergic abnormalities. Proc Natl Acad Sci USA. Dec 21 1999;96(26):15239–44.
83. Yeo GS, Connie Hung CC, Rochford J, et al. A de novo mutation affecting human TrkB associated with severe obesity and developmental delay. Nat Neurosci. Nov 2004;7(11): 1187–9.
84. Gray J, Yeo G, Hung C, et al. Functional characterization of human NTRK2 mutations identified in patients with severe early-onset obesity. Int J Obes (Lond). Feb 2007;31(2):359–64.
85. Heymsfield SB, Greenberg AS, Fujioka K, et al. Recombinant leptin for weight loss in obese and lean adults: a randomized, controlled, dose-escalation trial. JAMA. Oct 27 1999;282(16):1568–75.
86. Fan ZC, Tao YX. Functional characterization and pharmacological rescue of melanocortin-4 receptor mutations identified from obese patients. J Cell Mol Med. Sep 2009;13(9B):3268–82.
87. Schmidt H, Pozza SB, Bonfig W, Schwarz HP, Dokoupil K. Successful early dietary intervention avoids obesity in patients with Prader-Willi syndrome: a ten-year follow-up. J Pediatr Endocrinol Metab. Jul 2008;21(7):651–5.
88. Reinehr T, Hebebrand J, Friedel S, et al. Lifestyle intervention in obese children with variations in the melanocortin 4 receptor gene. Obesity (Silver Spring). Feb 2009;17(2):382–9.
89. Pories WJ. Bariatric surgery: risks and rewards. J Clin Endocrinol Metab. Nov 2008;93 11 Suppl 1:S89–96.
90. Daskalakis M, Till H, Kiess W, Weiner RA. Roux-en-Y gastric bypass in an adolescent patient with Bardet-Biedl syndrome, a monogenic obesity disorder. Obes Surg. Jan 2010;20(1): 121–5.
91. Rottembourg D, O'Gorman CS, Urbach S, et al. Outcome after bariatric surgery in two adolescents with hypothalamic obesity following treatment of craniopharyngioma. J Pediatr Endocrinol Metab. Sep 2009;22(9):867–72.
92. Inge TH, Pfluger P, Zeller M, et al. Gastric bypass surgery for treatment of hypothalamic obesity after craniopharyngioma therapy. Nat Clin Pract Endocrinol Metab. Aug 2007;3(8):606–9.
93. Muller HL, Gebhardt U, Wessel V, et al. First experiences with laparoscopic adjustable gastric banding (LAGB) in the treatment of patients with childhood craniopharyngioma and morbid obesity. Klin Padiatr. Nov–Dec 2007;219(6):323–5.
94. Potoczna N, Branson R, Kral JG, et al. Gene variants and binge eating as predictors of comorbidity and outcome of treatment in severe obesity. J Gastrointest Surg. Dec 2004;8(8):971–81, Discussion 981–972.
95. List JF, Habener JF. Defective melanocortin 4 receptors in hyperphagia and morbid obesity. N Engl J Med. Mar 20 2003;348(12):1160–3.

Chapter 4
Ciliary Syndromes and Obesity

David S. Parker and Nicholas Katsanis

4.1 Introduction

Recent advances in genomics, informatics, and population genetics have facilitated the identification of several regions in the human genome associated with obesity, metabolic syndrome, and other related traits, thus underscoring the promises that the genetic contribution of this common phenotype will be solved and that such discoveries can facilitate the understanding of the even more complex gene–environment interaction that is well documented in nonsyndromic forms of obesity.

However, with the exception of the association of variants near the *FTO* locus with obesity [1–3], our understanding of the genetic basis of this complex trait remains limited. Indeed, even the *FTO* locus, now reproduced in multiple studies and attaining significant association [4–11], accounts for only a modest fraction of genetic risk. The *FTO* risk allele is thought to contribute some 3 kg of excess body weight, and evidence pointing to the actual *FTO* message and protein in general obesity is circumstantial at best [12–18].

In contrast, the study of genetically simple forms of obesity, either as isolated phenotypes or in syndromic form, has provided the most valuable insights into the biology and biochemistry of energy homeostasis. Even though current evidence suggests that the loci for syndromic or Mendelian forms of obesity exert minimal contribution to the prevalence of common obesity, they have nonetheless provided us with a plethora of targets for pathways of metabolic relevance and therapeutic potential.

In this chapter, we will focus on the emerging link between ciliary dysfunction and energy dysregulation, which occurs both peripherally and at the level of CNS circuitry. The vertebrate cilium is an evolutionarily ancient subcellular organelle that has garnered much interest in recent years for its role in cell signaling and disease [19]. This organelle has been implicated in the processes of neuronal migration and specification, as well as a signal transducer/receiver in adipocytes, muscle, and

N. Katsanis (✉)
Department of Cell Biology, Center for Human Disease Modeling, Durham, 27710 NC, USA
e-mail: katsanis@cellbio.duke.edu

R.H. Lustig (ed.), *Obesity Before Birth*, Endocrine Updates 30,
DOI 10.1007/978-1-4419-7034-3_4,

numerous other tissues. Cilia have also been shown to play a role in body weight maintenance [20, 21]. Ciliary dysfunction underlies a family of human genetic disorders, a subset of which share obesity as a hallmark phenotype.

4.2 Ciliary Function, the Ciliopathies, and Clinical Phenotypes

The primary cilium projects apically from the surface of most vertebrate cells (Fig. 4.1). Historically, the major focus on cilia has been on their involvement in cell motility and/or fluid propulsion. However, the past decade has borne witness to rapid growth in the understanding of how cilia affect development and homeostasis. It is now known that cilia are complex sensory organelles that perform fundamental roles in cell communication, physiology, and development [19].

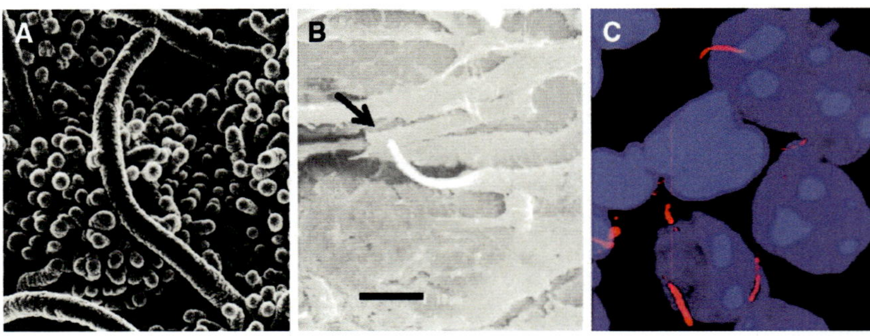

Fig. 4.1 Examples of cilia from different cell types. (**a**) Scanning electron micrograph of cilia on the node of the e8.0 mouse embryo [151]. (**b**) Scanning electron micrograph of cilia on a differentiating preadipocyte (*arrow*) [118]. (**c**) Confocal immunofluorescence image of promelanocortin-expressing cells of the hypothalamus. Cilia marked in red by antimonoacetylated tubulin; DAPI in blue [28]

The expanded appreciation for the roles of cilia in an increasing number of biological processes has coincided with the number of human clinical phenotypes linked to ciliary dysfunction. This collection of cilia-related pathologies, collectively referred to as ciliopathies [22], ranges in severity from embryonic lethal conditions, such as Jeune asphyxiating thoracic dystrophy (JATD) and Meckel–Gruber syndrome (MKS), to intermediate phenotypes, such as Bardet–Biedl syndrome (BBS) and Alström syndrome (ALMS), to isolated organ pathologies that include nephronophthisis (NPH) and some forms of Leber congenital amaurosis (LCA). At present, there exist over 30 known or predicted (based on phenotypes) ciliopathies [22]. Although individually rare, their combined frequency may exceed 1:1,000 live births [23].

Obesity is a hallmark of some, but not all, ciliopathies. Of the above list, only BBS and ALMS present with obesity as a predominant phenotype [20, 21], although this may be due to the fact that many ciliopathies, such as MKS, are lethal in the first year of life. In other cases, such as NPH, it is unclear whether obesity is absent or whether its penetrance is low and underappreciated. Importantly, genetic ablation of not only BBS proteins but also other ciliary and basal body proteins in the mouse has give rise to robust and tractable adipogenic phenotypes [24–30].

4.3 An Overview of the Primary Vertebrate Cilium

Cilia are microtubule-based organelles that nucleate at the basal body, a bundle of microtubules derived from, and associated with, the mother centrioles. Structurally, the cilium consists of a central microtubule scaffold (the axoneme) that is anchored at the basal body and projects apically from the cell, surrounded by a sheath of plasma membrane (Fig. 4.2). Typically, most vertebrate postmitotic cells possess a single cilium 2–5 μm in length [31].

At the basal body, microtubules are arranged in a characteristic pattern that consists of a radial array of nine microtubule triplets. Further along the axoneme in the transition zone, the nine microtubule bundles become doublets, and in the distal segment of the cilium the microtubule scaffold varies but usually consists of single microtubule fibers (Fig. 4.2a) [32, 33].

Historically, two classes of cilia have been described: motile cilia and nonmotile primary cilia, defined by the presence or absence of a central microtubule pair

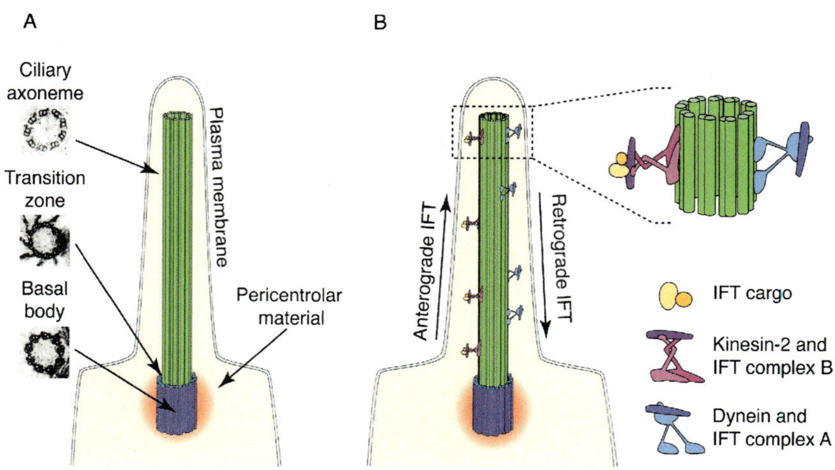

Fig. 4.2 The current model of primary cilia structure and IFT in vertebrates. (**a**) The vertebrate cilium consists of an apically oriented microtubule projection (the axoneme) ensheathed in the ciliary plasma membrane. The axoneme is tethered to the basal body, which is surrounded by pericentriolar material. Electron micrograph images for each portion of the cilium are shown on the left [34, 152]. (**b**) IFT is a bidirectional transport system [118]. Evidence supports a model whereby kinesin-2 and IFT complex B selectively transport cargo along the axoneme to the distal tip of the cilium (anterograde transport). Dynein and IFT complex A are then thought to transport proteins in the reverse (retrograde) direction back toward the cell body

("9+2" motile cilia or "9+0" nonmotile cilia). There are some notable exceptions to these classifications, such as the 9+0 motile nodal ependymal cilia in the central canal of the zebra fish spinal cord [34], the motile 9+0 nodal cilia that are essential for setting up left–right asymmetry in early mammalian development [35], and the immotile 9+2 cilia in the frog olfactory epithelium [36]. It should be noted, however, that both classes of cilia are able to perform sensory functions [37], suggesting that this ultrastructural dichotomization might be overly simplistic with respect to function.

4.4 Intraflagellar Transport (IFT)

Although the cilium is contiguous with the cytoplasm and plasma membrane and is not compartmentalized, it is a highly specialized subcellular environment due to the selective active transport of proteins along the axoneme through the process of IFT (Fig. 4.2b). The discovery and characterization of IFT owe much to the green algae *Chlamydomonas*, where IFT was first observed with light microscopy as the bidirectional movement of granular IFT particles along the cilium [38]. It is now known that IFT is the molecular-motor-mediated transport of cargo along the axoneme that allows specific proteins to be transported to the cilium and the ciliary membrane [39, 40].

IFT is a bidirectional transport system that employs two types of microtubule-based motors to shuttle cargo up and down the length of the cilium [40]. Anterograde IFT (toward the distal tip of the cilium and the plus end of the microtubule) is mediated by a heterotrimeric kinesin-2 motor, while retrograde IFT (toward the basal body and the minus end of the microtubule) is facilitated by cytoplasmic dynein 2. In addition, transport of ciliary proteins occurs in association with two protein raft complexes that bind to and accompany cargo: IFT complex B (anterograde transport) and IFT complex A (retrograde transport). IFT performs two broad functions in the cilium: first to deliver cargo required for cilium biogenesis and maintenance and second to transport cilium-based signaling molecules that regulate many cellular and developmental processes.

As protein synthesis is not thought to occur in cilia, the building and maintenance of cilia requires IFT to supply precursors and remove by-products. Using temperature-sensitive mutants of the protein *fla10* in *Chlamydomonas* (*Kif3a* in vertebrates, a component of the kinesin-2 complex), Kozminski et al. showed that *fla10* and anterograde IFT are both necessary and sufficient for ciliogenesis and maintenance [41]. When *fla10* is inactivated, cilia progressively become shorter, suggesting that IFT is necessary to maintain cilial length. In addition, cells at restrictive temperatures lose their ability to resynthesize cilia following deflagellation. A requirement for kinesin-2 for ciliogenesis has since been shown in several other organisms, including *Tetrahymena*, sea urchin, *Drosophila*, and mouse [35, 42–46].

Retrograde IFT is also required for the maintenance of cilial structure. Cytoplasmic dynein 2 (the retrograde motor) consists of at least four subunits [47, 48]. Mutation of the gene encoding DYNC2H1 (a subunit of the Dynein 2 motor) blocks retrograde IFT [49–51], resulting in the accumulation of material at the end of cilia, visualized as stunted cilia with bulbous distal tips [52, 53].

Aside from a general role in cilia formation and maintenance, IFT also transports specific proteins to the ciliary membrane [54, 55]. Several targeting motifs and post-translational modifications have been implicated in targeting proteins to cilia. For example, Smoothened (Smo), a seven-transmembrane serpentine protein integral to the Hedgehog (Hh) signaling pathway, localizes to cilia in vertebrates. The seventh transmembrane segment contains a hydrophobic and basic evolutionarily conserved motif that has been postulated to be necessary for ciliary localization and for Smo to transduce the Hh signal [56, 57]. A second example is an RVxP motif required for the ciliary localization of mammalian Polycystin-2, an integral membrane protein implicated in autosomal polycystic kidney disease.

Other proteins are targeted to cilia via posttranslational modifications. Amino-terminus myristoylation has been implicated in targeting several proteins to cilia in *Trypanosoma cruzi*, *Leishmania*, sea urchins, and cultured human cells [58–61]. In addition, there is at least one instance of casein kinase-2-dependent phosphorylation being required for the ciliary targeting of nephrocystin in human cells [62].

4.5 A Role for Cilia in Developmental Signaling

A major focus area of current ciliary biology centers on recent discoveries that have implicated ciliary function in paracrine signaling. The Hh and Wnt signal transduction pathways are highly conserved and play vital roles in the development of all metazoa [63, 64]. Their disruption causes a number of dramatic phenotypes in humans, and the connection of Hh and Wnt signaling to ciliary function has helped provide mechanistic explanations for some ciliopathy phenotypes.

4.5.1 Cilia and Hedgehog Signaling

The link between cilia and Hh signaling was initially made in an ethylnitrosourea screen in the mouse for mutants affecting embryonic development [65]. Loss-of-function phenotypes of two genes identified in this study suggested a block in Hh signaling, including neural tube defects and preaxial polydactyly. These genes were identified as Ift172 and Ift88, members of IFT complex B. Consistent with these data, mice mutant for *Kif3a*, a subunit of the IFT kinesin-2 motor used in IFT complex B, also exhibit phenotypes reminiscent of a loss of Hh signaling [65].

The Patched 1 (Ptc1) protein is both a negative regulator of the Hh pathway and the receptor for the Hh signal: in the absence of *ptc1* the Hh pathway is constitutively active. Double mutants of *ptc1* and *ift172*, *ift88*, or *kif3a* phenocopy the IFT single mutants (i.e., loss of Hh signaling), providing genetic evidence that IFT is required for the Hh pathway, either downstream or at the level of the Hh receptor [65]. Many proteins that function in the Hh pathway localize to cilia, including the transmembrane proteins Ptc1 and Smo, the cytoplasmic proteins SuFu and

Costal 2, and the downstream effectors of Hh signaling Gli2/Gli3. Upon activation of the Hh pathway, Ptc1 and Smo are recruited to cilia where Ptc1-dependent inhibition of Smo is relieved [66].

The Gli family of proteins (Gli1, Gli2, and Gli3 in vertebrates) are transcription factors capable of shuttling between the cytoplasm and the nucleus, where they direct the transcription of Hh target genes. Gli2 and Gli3 cease to function in primary limb bud cells lacking the IFT complex B component *ift88*, suggesting that IFT is required for their activity. Interestingly, Gli1 remains able to activate target gene expression under these conditions [67].

The connection between cilia, Hh signaling, and obesity is unclear. However, evidence does exist pointing to possible links. Exogenous Sonic hedgehog (one of three vertebrate hedgehog proteins) can inhibit adipogenesis and the expression of adipocyte markers, including leptin, C/EBPα, and PPARγ2, when applied to murine mesenchymal cells [68, 69]. In addition, the *FTM* gene (also called *RPGRIP1L*) encodes a protein that localizes to the basal body and contributes causal and modifying alleles to several ciliopathies [22, 70, 71]. Mice lacking *FTM* have Hh-like phenotypes such as left–right asymmetry defects, neural tube patterning defects, and preaxial polydactyly. Although mice lacking *FTM* have lower numbers of cilia in vivo compared to wild-type animals, cells isolated from $FTM^{-/-}$ mice can still form cilia but have a reduced response to Hh signaling [70]. These data suggest that *FTM* may be required for both Hh signaling via cilia and ciliogenesis or maintenance in vivo.

FTM is less than 1 kb from *FTO*. *FTM* and *FTO* are coregulated by the transcription factor CutL1 [72]. Several recent genome-wide association studies (GWAS) have associated multiple SNPs at this locus with obesity, including one that disrupts a putative CutL1 binding site [1–3]. Considering that functional evidence linking *FTO* to weight homeostasis is scarce [12–18] and that *FTM* and *FTO* are coregulated, it is possible that the obesity-associated SNPs at this locus also lead to misregulation of *FTM*. If so, it would provide a connection of *FTM* (and thus ciliary function and Hh signaling) to an inherited propensity toward obesity. Finally, Hh signaling can inhibit the differentiation of fat cells [68, 69], raising the possibility that aberrant Hh signaling due to ciliary dysfunction may be proadipogenic.

4.5.2 Cilia and Wnt Signaling

In contrast to Hh signaling, the role of cilia in Wnt signaling is not as clear. Initially, the connection between cilia and Wnt signaling was made through Inversin (Inv), a protein that localizes to cilia [73] and causes ciliopathy-like phenotypes in *inv* knockout mice [74–76]. Inv is capable of acting as a switch between the canonical and noncanonical (also called the planar cell polarity) Wnt pathways by regulating levels of the cytoplasmic Wnt signaling component Disheveled (Dvl) [77]. Subsequently, Inv was shown to have a negative effect on canonical Wnt signaling. In mice mutant for *kif3a* (which lack cilia as anterograde IFT is blocked), a Wnt pathway reporter gene is upregulated in embryos compared to littermate controls. Furthermore, MEFs from *kif3a*$^{-/-}$ animals are more sensitive to exogenously added Wnt protein than cells from control animals, consistent with cilia playing a negative role in canonical Wnt signaling [78]. Epistasis experiments suggest that this regulation occurs at or above the level of Dsh [78].

In zebra fish, knockdown of *BBS1* or *BBS4* causes convergent extension phenotypes consistent with a block in noncanonical Wnt signaling and a coincident expansion of the canonical Wnt target gene *axin2*, consistent with an upregulation of canonical Wnt signaling [79]. Furthermore, in ciliated human cells, knockdown of *BBS1*, *BBS4*, or *KIF3A* caused a marked increase in the response of a canonical Wnt reporter gene to exogenously added Wnt3a than in control cells.

However, two recent studies cast some doubt upon the role of cilia in canonical Wnt signaling. First, mouse embryos mutant for *kif3a*, *ift172*, or *ift88* have normal expression of the endogenous Wnt target *axin2* and the synthetic Wnt target BAT-gal, and MEFs isolated from these animals respond to exogenous Wnt3a in an identical manner to control cells [80]. Importantly, as a control the same MEFs were shown to lose their responsiveness to Shh, consistent with the notion that blocking IFT results in a block of Hh signaling. Second, zebra fish mutant for *oval* (*ift88* in mice and humans) lack cilia and have phenotypes consistent with deregulation of the Hh pathway, but no canonical or noncanonical Wnt phenotypes [81].

Despite first impressions, these studies are not irreconcilable. Experiments that show cilia as having a role in Wnt signaling concern proteins thought to reside at the basal body (i.e., Inv and the BBS proteins), while studies finding no connection between Wnt and cilia concern proteins important for IFT (Kif3a, Ift172, or Ift88). Consistent with a functional connection between Wnt signaling and basal bodies, knocking down all three *Xenopus dvl* genes disrupts ciliogenesis and the apical positioning of basal bodies [82]. This suggests the possibility that it is the basal body, not the cilia per se, that plays a role in Wnt signaling.

There are several connections between Wnt signaling and adiposity. Overexpression of Wnt10b in vitro inhibits the differentiation of preadipocytes into adipocytes, while blocking of Wnt signaling results in spontaneous adipogenesis [83]. Overexpression of Wnt10b in vivo under the control of the FAB4P enhancer reduces total body fat by approximately 50% [84]. Consistent with this, missense mutations in *Wnt10b* were associated with obesity in a human study [85] and myoblasts isolated from mice mutant for *Wnt10b* show increased adipogenic potential [86].

4.6 A Role for Primary Cilia in Appetite Control

Mouse models, in addition to in vitro data, have highlighted two molecular mechanisms by which ciliopathies may contribute to obesity. The first provides a possible explanation for the lack of satiety observed in BBS and ALS patients; the second raises the possibility that the primary cilium play a role in adipogenesis.

4.6.1 Leptin Signaling in the Hypothalamus Regulates Body Weight

How can defective ciliary function lead to a behavioral change such as hyperphagia? At least part of the answer might lie in a requirement for primary cilia to promote leptin signaling in the hypothalamus. Leptin is a 16-kDa adipocyte-derived peptide hormone that suppresses appetite. Leptin is secreted by white adipocytes in direct proportion to body weight; hence the more fat mass an individual accumulates the more leptin is secreted and the less one feels inclined to eat large meals [87]. Circulating concentrations of leptin in the blood reflect whole-body adiposity levels, with little direct connection to acute food intake [88].

Leptin crosses the blood–brain barrier, allowing leptin-responsive neurons in the brain to constantly monitor total body adiposity levels (Fig. 4.3). For example, an increase in body adiposity levels is accompanied by an increase in leptin levels in the blood, leading to increased leptin signaling in the brain, decreased appetite, and consequent weight loss [88, 89]. The opposite effect occurs when leptin levels decrease; humans and mice that lack leptin are hyperphagic and morbidly obese [87, 90], a phenotype that can be rescued by exogenous leptin administration [91, 92] (see Chapter 3).

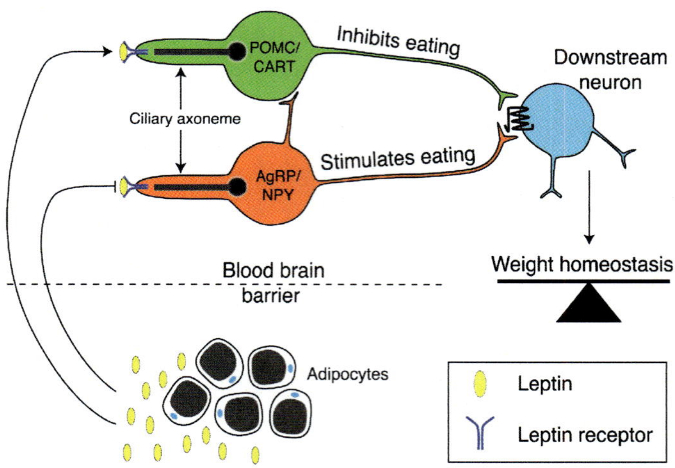

Fig. 4.3 Control of energy homeostasis by hypothalamic neurons. Adipocytes secrete the peptide hormone leptin into the circulation in direct proportion to body fat mass. Leptin crosses the blood–brain barrier and signals to two types of neurons in the arcuate nucleus of the hypothalamus, possibly via leptin receptors localized to cilia. Leptin signaling excites POMC/CART neurons and inhibits adjacent AgRP/NPY neurons, leading to downstream events that decrease appetite [153]

4.6.2 A Requirement for IFT in Leptin Signaling

It has been known for nearly half a century that neurons in the brain are ciliated [93]. Functional evidence that primary cilia play a role in leptin signaling comes from conditional knockouts of genes encoding IFT proteins Tg737/Ift88 and Kif3a, both of which are necessary for anterograde transport. As functional primary cilia are required for development in many cellular contexts, *tg737* and *kif3a* null mutants are lethal midgestation, with severe systematic defects [46, 94]. However, performing conditional knockouts with null alleles of these genes postnatally has uncovered essential roles for Tg737 and Kif3a later in development [28].

Consistent with a role for cilia in energy homeostasis, systemic conditional knockout of *tg737* or *kif3a* at 8–12 weeks of age under the control of the actin enhancer results in an almost immediate rapid and chronic weight gain [28]. These phenotypes are due to overeating, as conditional *kif3a*$^{-/-}$ mutant mice do not gain weight when diet restricted and become hyperphagic and gain fat mass rapidly when this restriction is lifted. About 14–16 weeks following *kif3a* ablation, *kif3a*$^{-/-}$ mice exhibit increased fat mass and increased serum levels of leptin and insulin, in addition to increased serum glucose following starvation [28].

To test if the hyperphagic behavior of conditional *kif3a*$^{-/-}$ animals is dependent upon a requirement for functional cilia in neurons, *synapsin1-cre* was used to create neuron-specific *kif3a* knockout mice [28]. These animals gained a significant amount of weight compared to age- and sex-matched control animals, indicating neuronal cilia are important to control body weight. Furthermore, knockout of *kif3a* in POMC/CART neurons also resulted in hyperphagia, obesity, and increased serum leptin. Immunostaining with antimonoglycylated tubulin to mark cilia shows a significant reduction of cilia in the hypothalamus of these mice, showing that loss of *kif3a* disrupts cilia formation in POMC-expressing cells [28].

It should be noted that the levels of obesity in the POMC neuronal *kif43a* knockout animal models is lower than in the system-wide *kif3a*$^{-/-}$ mice [28]. While this could be due to technical reasons, such as differing strengths of the actin and POMC enhancer constructs, it also suggests a possible role for IFT in weight homeostasis in other cell types.

Although it is currently unknown if cilia play a role in leptin signaling outside the accurate nucleus of the hypothalamus, there are data supporting a role for the leptin pathway influencing weight homeostasis from other areas of the brain. Interestingly, selective ablation of the leptin receptor (LepR) in POMC neurons results in less obesity than whole-animal LepR mutants [95]. Furthermore, LepR expressed in the ventromedial hypothalamus is required for normal body weight in a way unrelated to food intake [96]. Neurons of the caudal brainstem also express LepR, although in the brainstem activation of leptin signaling does not upregulate POMC expression, despite POMC being expressed in these cells [97, 98]. Finally, leptin acts on dopaminergic neurons of the ventral tegmental area to control appetite [99, 100].

4.6.3 BBS Proteins and the Control of Leptin Signaling

Like IFT, genetic experiments in mice clearly indicate a role for BBS genes in the regulation of appetite, specifically at the level of leptin signaling. The most common allele observed in BBS patients is a missense mutation in *BBS1* (*BBS1*^{M390R}) [101], and patients harboring this allele are obese and hyperphagic. *BBS1*$^{M390R/M390R}$ mice are also hyperphagic and do not respond to abnormally elevated blood leptin levels, suggesting that leptin signaling is attenuated in these animals [29].

BBS1 can interact with LepR in an in vitro pull-down assay, providing a potential biochemical link between leptin signaling and a BBS protein (Fig. 4.4a). Furthermore, the *BBS1*^{M390R} allele (which is sufficient to cause obesity in a mouse knock-in model of BBS) does not interact with LepR with the same affinity as the wild-type BBS1 protein, raising the possibility that the association of the BBSome with LepR may be necessary for leptin signaling to occur efficiently [30].

Other BBS proteins have also been linked with aberrant leptin signaling. Mice lacking *Bbs2*, *Bbs4*, and *Bbs6* are hyperphagic and obese with high levels of circulating leptin [27]. These mice also appear to have a perturbation of leptin signaling as they fail to upregulate POMC transcription in hypothalamic neurons in response to exogenously administered leptin, despite having normal expression levels of the LepR [30]. Further, leptin administration does not induce STAT3 phosphorylation in the hypothalamus, suggesting that leptin signaling is blocked prior to the activation of STAT3 in these animals. Notably, *Bbs2*$^{-/-}$ and *Bbs6*$^{-/-}$ mice have functional melanocortin receptors [30], further supporting the notion of a defunct leptin signaling pathway upstream of the melanocortin system.

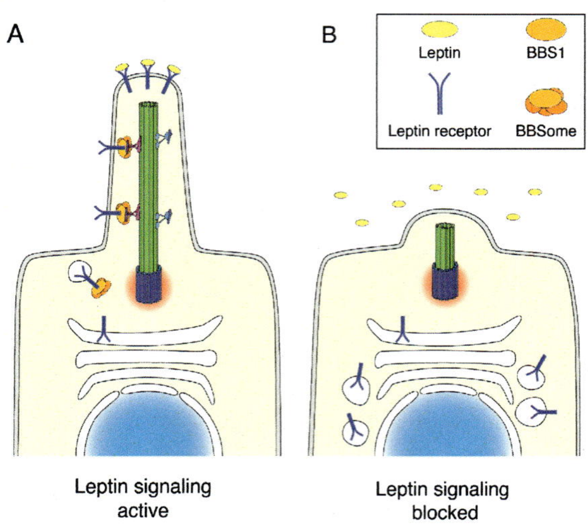

Fig. 4.4 A model describing the possible role for BBS proteins in leptin signaling. (**a**) In a wild-type hypothalamic neuron, BBS1 (a component of the BBSome) binds to the leptin receptor and guides it from the Golgi apparatus to the cilia where it functions to transduce the leptin signal. (**b**) In the absence of a functioning BBSome, cilia growth is inhibited and the leptin receptor remains in the vesicular transport machinery. Consequently, the leptin signal is not received by the neuron and appetite suppression is lost, resulting in hyperphagy and obesity

The mechanism by which BBS proteins facilitate leptin signaling is currently unclear, although some clues do exist. As discussed later, a subset of BBS proteins that form a multiprotein complex termed the BBSome may play a role in the transport of specific signaling molecules into the cilia. Consistent with this model, knockdown of *BBS1* or *BBS2* in a human cell line restricts the localization of a transfected leptin receptor to large perinuclear vesicles [30]. Thus, it is possible that in the absence of the BBSome, LepR is mislocalized and leptin signaling is blocked (Fig. 4.4b). Although there is no evidence that LepR is present in cilia, it is possible that (as in Hh signaling) there is a requirement for ciliary localization of LepR for proper signaling to occur. Although more studies are clearly required to elucidate the molecular and biochemical mechanisms, it is clear from genetic data that BBS proteins play a role in the leptin-dependent maintenance of a healthy body weight.

4.6.4 Other Roles for BBS Proteins in Neuronal Signaling and Obesity

Evidence suggests that BBS proteins play roles in CNS signaling events other than leptin signaling. The G protein-coupled receptors (GPCRs) somatostatin 3 (Sstr3) [102], serotonin receptor 6 [103, 104], melanin-concentrating hormone receptor 1 (Mchr1) [105, 106], and the downstream signaling effector type III adenylyl cyclase (ACIII) [107] all localize to neuronal cilia. Furthermore, BBS proteins are necessary and sufficient for the localization of the GPCRs to cilia. *Bbs2*$^{-/-}$ and *Bbs4*$^{-/-}$ animals have normal neuronal cilia that lack Sstr3 and Mchr1, and in cell culture, heterologous expression of Bbs2 or Bbs4 is sufficient to restore neuronal ciliary localization of both receptors [106].

Of these signaling molecules, Mchr1 and ACIII are known to play roles in energy homeostasis [108, 109]. Mice mutant for Mchr1 are lean [110], suggesting that Bbs-induced aberrant Mchr1 signaling does not explain the Bbs obesity phenotype. However, another study shows that *Mchr1*$^{-/-}$ mice are hyperphagic, with their leanness due to increased energy expenditure [111]. As hyperphagia is prevalent in BBS, it is possible that dysregulation of Mhcr1 signaling may play a role in BBS phenotypes. Polymorphisms at the ACIII locus have been correlated with obesity [108], and consistent with this, *AcIII* $^{-/-}$ mice are obese with larger adipocytes and higher circulating levels of leptin than littermate controls [112]. *AcIII* $^{-/-}$ mice are also hyperphagic and have decreased ACIII activity in the hypothalamus.

There is also evidence from *C. elegans* that BBS proteins may play a role in lipid metabolism. *tub-1* is the worm ortholog of the mouse *Tubby* gene; loss-of-function alleles of *Tubby* cause obesity in mice [113]. In worms, *tub-1* is expressed in ciliated neurons and *tub-1* mutants exhibit increased fat accumulation [114]. A screen for genetic modifiers of the *tub-1* phenotype identified 3-ketoacyl-CoA (*kat-1*). The human ortholog of *kat-1*, acetyl-CoA acetyltransferase (*ACAT1*), is elevated following lipid intake and plays a role in fatty acid β-oxidation in mitochondria. Furthermore, *Bbs-1* was identified in a screen for modifiers of the *kat-1* phenotype, suggesting a relationship between neuronal cilia, BBS proteins, and lipid metabolism [114].

4.7 Cilia and Adipogenesis

Aside from altering appetite, there is evidence to suggest that cilia play a more direct role in controlling body weight by regulating adipogenesis. Fat storage cells, or adipocytes, are derived from mesenchymal stem cells through a well-studied differentiation process termed adipogenesis [115, 116].

In vitro studies of preadipocyte cell lines show that adipogenesis proceeds via a temporally regulated transcriptional cascade. First, proadipogenic signals cause upregulation of the CCAAT-enhancer binding protein (C/EBP) family members C/EBPβ and C/EBPδ. These transcription factors subsequently induce the master adipogenic genes C/EBPα and peroxisome proliferator-activated receptor-γ (PPARγ), resulting in terminal adipocyte differentiation.

Several studies raise the possibility that ciliary genes could play a role in adipocyte differentiation. *BBS5*, *BBS6*, *BBS7*, *BBS8*, *BBS9*, and *BBS11* are expressed in adipose tissue isolated from mice, and all of these genes (with the exception of *BBS5*) are transcriptionally upregulated in a mouse preadipocyte cell line induced to undergo adipogenesis [117]. Induction of *BBS* genes occurs early in the adipogenic process, temporally coincident with the upregulation of C/EBPβ and C/EBPδ (approximately 2 days following induction). Expression of the *BBS* genes declined approximately 7 days following induction of differentiation, shortly before the upregulation of C/EBPα and PPARγ has been observed in cell culture models [117]. In a separate study in a human preadipocyte cell line undergoing adipogenesis, *BBS10* and *BBS12* have a temporally similar mRNA expression profile to the other *BBS* genes: high expression at early stages of adipocyte differentiation that decreases in subsequent days [118].

Consistent with the expression profile of *BBS* genes peaking early in adipogenesis, cilia have been observed in differentiating preadipocytes in vitro, but are absent from preadipocytes and mature adipocytes in human cells [118]. Interestingly, cilia that are present transiently during early adipogenesis harbor Wnt and Hh receptors; as mentioned previously there is evidence suggesting that both of these pathways are antiadipogenic.

Ciliogenesis in differentiating adipocytes is inhibited by RNAi-induced knockdown of *BBS10* and *BBS12*, and this treatment resulted in a modest activation of PPARγ and a modest inhibition of Wnt signaling, providing a possible mechanistic link between the antiadipogenic properties of cilia and the Wnt and Hh signaling pathways [118].

An alternative line of evidence supporting an antiadipogenic role for cilia comes from cultured dermal fibroblasts of *BBS10* and *BBS12* patients. When these cells are differentiated into fat-accumulating cells in vitro, they have higher triglyceride levels than control cells and also secrete increased leptin compared to control cells treated in the same manner [118].

4.8 The Human Ciliopathies and Obesity

The connection between cilia and the body weight homeostasis comes primarily from the observation that two ciliopathies, BBS and AS, share hyperphagia-induced obesity as a defining feature [22, 119]: nine out of every ten individuals with BBS or AS are severely overweight or obese [120–124].

Germane to any discussion of ciliopathies is the concept of allelic and phenotypic heterogeneity. Human phenotypes attributed to ciliary dysfunction exhibit significant inter- and intrafamilial variability; such phenotypes range along a continuum of prenatal lethality at one extreme to minimal weight gain on the other. The basis of this phenomenon is poorly understood and stems in part to the contribution of numerous modifying alleles on genes encoding ciliary proteins, in addition to primary causal mutations [23]. Underscoring such complexity is the sophisticated composition of cilia themselves.

As previously noted, the number of proteins that a cilium requires to function correctly is estimated to be as many as 1,000 [19, 125]. A mutation in any gene required for any aspect of ciliary function has the potential to result in any one of many phenotypes. Furthermore, many human ciliopathies arise when the mutational load of several genes involved in a specific ciliary process exceeds a certain functional threshold, resulting in cilia that are present (permitting viability), but function suboptimally (resulting in a phenotype). Practically, this means that multiple loci are likely affected for any given ciliopathy, with the number and location of mutations differing from patient to patient. This has been illustrated extensively in BBS, but is beginning to be documented in other ciliopathies as well [71, 126, 127].

4.9 Bardet–Biedl Syndrome

BBS (MIM 209900) is primarily an autosomal recessive disorder, with incidence varying from 1:160,000 in northern Europe [122, 128] to 1:13,500 in Kuwait and Newfoundland [129, 130]. While obesity is a hallmark of the syndrome, BBS is pleiotropic in its presentation. In 1866, Lawrence and Moon described the first BBS patient, an obese child with visual impairments and mental disabilities. In the 1920s, the addition of polydactyly and hypogenitalism by Bardet and Biedl characterized the syndrome further. BBS major phenotypes now include retinal degeneration, obesity, hypogonadism, polydactyly, renal dysfunction, and cognitive impairment, with phenotypic profile and severity varying between patients [119]. Obesity and retinal degeneration are the most common BBS symptoms (present in approximately 87 and 95% of cases, respectively). Polydactyly is also common (in 67% of cases), as is hypogenitalism in males (in 86% of male BBS patients [120–123]). BBS is complex genetically, as well as phenotypically: 14 different loci have been implicated in the disease to date (*BBS1-12*, *MKS1*, and *CEP290/NPHP6*), accounting for some 70% of the primary genetic lesions, and heterogeneity within individual loci is the rule rather than the exception [23].

All BBS-associated proteins studied to date localize to centrosomes, basal bodies, or cilia [131–136]. Sequence homology provides little insight as to the function of BBS proteins, and precisely how they function on a biochemical level is only recently coming to light.

Seven of the 14 BBS proteins are present in stoichiometric amounts in a stable complex, termed the BBSome [136, 137]. This 438-kDa complex consists of BBS1, BBS2, BBS4, BBS5, BBS7, BBS8, and BBS9, seven BBS proteins that are highly conserved among ciliated organisms [136, 138]. Cofractionation and pull-down experiments suggest that the BBSome transiently interacts with the core component of the centriolar satellites (PCM1) and the ciliary membrane [134, 136]. Furthermore, the BBSome interacts with Rabin8, a guanosyl exchange factor (GEF) for the small GTPase Rab8, through an interaction with BBS1 [136].

The Rab family of GTPases is the largest family of GTPases, with more than 60 known members in humans. Rab proteins act as organizers of vesicle transport, using GTP-dependent interactions with the core vesicular transport machinery to ensure vesicular cargo is delivered to the correct subcellular compartment [139]. GFP-Rabin8 can be seen at the centrosome and GFP-Rab8 localizes to the primary cilium in RPE cells. Interestingly, a mutant form of Rab8 that is GDP locked does not enter the cilium (and inhibits ciliogenesis), whereas a form of Rab8 that cannot hydrolyze GTP localizes to the cilium (and promotes ciliogenesis). This suggests that the GTP-bound form of Rab8 enters the primary cilium and might play a role in ciliary growth [136]. Furthermore, RNAi-mediated knockdown of Rabin8 inhibits cilial localization of Rab8. These data invoke a model in which the BBSome is transported by centriolar satellites to the basal body where, via the action of Rabin8, it becomes associated with $Rab8^{GTP}$ and enters the cilia [136].

The biochemical role(s) that the BBSome might play inside cilia has recently been investigated in *Chlamydomonas*. All eight subunits of the human BBSome are conserved in *Chlamydomonas*, which also contains a BBSome-like complex [140]. *BBS4* or *BBS7* mutants do not affect cilia assembly in this system (in contrast with other studies), but ciliary function is affected, as assayed by the lack of a phototactic response in mutant cells. The BBSome does not appear to be a core component of the IFT machinery in this system, as trafficking of IFT or cilia membrane proteins is not affected in a *BBS4* mutant. Consistent with this, the vast majority of BBS4 associates with a subset of IFT particles that cotransport BBS4 up and down cilia [140].

Intriguingly, *BBS1*, *BBS4*, and *BBS7* are required to export a specific set of proteins, including putative signaling molecules, from cilia in *Chlamydomonas* [140]. These data are consistent with data from *BBS1*, *BBS2*, *BBS4*, and *BBS6* knockout mice that show accumulation of membrane vesicles at the distal tip of cilia [141] and zebra fish *BBS* morphants that exhibit inhibited retrograde transport [142].

Taken together, these data point toward a model where the BBSome may selectively transport signaling molecules (such as transmembrane receptors) to cilia; such a model is consistent with the localization of Hh pathway components to cilia. It is possible that the transport of cell surface receptors to cilia may explain how cilia regulate appetite, as the leptin signaling pathway is disrupted in BBS and IFT mouse mutants, possibly due to the mislocalization of the leptin receptor [30]. Consistent with this hypothesis, mouse models ablated for *Bbs1* [29], *Bbs2*, and *Bbs4* [27] are hyperphagic and obese.

Another possible link between BBS and obesity is provided by the interaction between BBS4 and Necdin [143]. Necdin is one of four genes inactivated in Prader–Willi syndrome (PWS; see Chapter 6), a neurodevelopmental disorder resulting from a microdeletion on chromosome 15 [144]. Some of the hallmark phenotypes of PWS and BBS overlap, including hyperphagia with consequent obesity. In cotransfected cells, Necdin resides near the centrosome and can bind to BBS4, raising the possibility that these shared phenotypes could arise from dysfunctional cilia [143].

4.10 Alström Syndrome

Alström syndrome (MIM 203800), first described in 1959, is a monogenic autosomal recessive disorder caused by mutations in *ALMS1* [145–147]. Since the initial identification of AS, approximately 450 cases have been reported, suggesting AS is relatively rare [124]. Similar to BBS individuals, AS patients exhibit multiple complex phenotypes including early childhood obesity, blindness, neurosensory hearing loss, insulin resistance, type 2 diabetes, progressive hepatic and renal dysfunction, and hypogonadism [124]. Also reminiscent of BBS is the phenotypic variability of AS, even within families.

AS presents as a progressive disease, making diagnosis difficult at early stages [124]. Neurosensory problems develop early, with the onset of retinal dystrophy occurring weeks after birth and progressing throughout childhood such that most AS patients are legally blind by age 15 and are hearing impaired by age 21. Despite a normal birth weight, almost all AS patients become obese within 2–36 months [148] and develop hyperinsulinemia by age 4 and diabetes by age 16. Renal function also decreases with age, with renal failure being a common cause of death [148].

The functions of the ALMS1 protein are not clear. ALMS1 is a large protein, with a predicted ORF of 4169aa. However, like many of the genes responsible for BBS, ALMS1 has no sequence homology that is predictive of function [149], and no correlations have been made between mutations and specific phenotypes [146, 147]. Immunohistochemistry indicates that ALMS1 is expressed widely and localizes to the centrosome and basal body [149]. Furthermore, mass spectrometry showed that ALMS1 is a component of the centrosome [150].

There are several mouse models of Alström syndrome, and all suggest that Alms1 plays a role in maintaining weight balance [24–26]. *Alms1*$^{-/-}$ mutant mice are hyperphagic, rapidly gain weight, and exhibit greatly increased adiposity 8–12 weeks after birth when compared to littermates. They also become hyperinsulinemic, hyperglycemic, and develop type 2 diabetes over time (16–20 weeks after birth) [24–26]. In addition, *Alms1*$^{-/-}$ mice have high leptin and cholesterol levels and develop hepatic steatosis.

Cilia are present in *Alms1*$^{-/-}$ mice [24], and dermal fibroblast cells from a single AS patient had normal cilia as judged by acetylated α-tubulin staining. In contrast to these data, siRNA-mediated knockdown of *Alms1* in mouse kidney epithelial cells suggests that Alms1 is required for ciliogenesis [26]. This discrepancy is resolved by the observation that alleles of *Alms1* present in human ALMS patients (and mouse models) contain premature termination codons that truncate the *Alms1* protein and as such may represent hypomorphic *Alms1* alleles [24–26, 146, 147]. Indeed, a truncated version of the *Alms1* gene that resembles human disease alleles is sufficient to rescue the siRNA-induced loss-of-cilia phenotype in cells [26].

When ALMS1 is depleted from mouse kidney cells via siRNA, ciliogenesis and cilia function are affected. However, dermal fibroblast cells from a single AS patient had normal cilia as judged by acetylated α-tubulin staining [149]. This apparent contradiction is potentially explained by the fact that most AS patients have premature stop codons in ALMS1 that lead to a truncated protein, which presumably does not completely abrogate ALMS1 activity [24, 25, 146, 147].

4.11 Concluding Remarks

As discussed in this chapter, there are strong genetic links between the ciliopathies and obesity. Evidence from BBS and AS patients supported by mouse models of these disease states clearly shows that ciliary dysfunction can lead to rapid weight gain through hyperphagia and that at least part of this behavior is due to the inhibition of leptin signaling in the arcuate nucleus of the hypothalamus. In peripheral tissues, cilia may play a more direct role in the differentiation of adipocytes by modulating Hh and Wnt signaling.

But the molecular mechanisms by which these syndromes might cause obesity are not well understood. For example, the role of cilia in leptin signaling is the best characterized link between ciliary function and obesity, yet the cell-specific abolition of IFT within hypothalamic neurons does not recapitulate the weight gain induced by its systemic loss, and it is not known if LepR is present in cilia. However, despite difficulties in understanding the specific biochemical processes that control weight homeostasis, the strong genetic case for the role of cilia in body weight regulation and the mechanistic insights that have already been uncovered certainly support further investigation.

References

1. Frayling TM, Timpson NJ, Weedon MN, et al. A common variant in the FTO gene is associated with body mass index and predisposes to childhood and adult obesity. Science. May 11 2007;316(5826):889–94.

2. Dina C, Meyre D, Gallina S, et al. Variation in FTO contributes to childhood obesity and severe adult obesity. Nat Genet. Jun 2007;39(6):724–6.
3. Scuteri A, Sanna S, Chen WM, et al. Genome-wide association scan shows genetic variants in the FTO gene are associated with obesity-related traits. PLoS Genet. Jul 2007;3(7): e115.
4. Hinney A, Nguyen TT, Scherag A, et al. Genome wide association (GWA) study for early onset extreme obesity supports the role of fat mass and obesity associated gene (FTO) variants. PLoS One. 2007;2(12):e1361.
5. Liu Y, Liu Z, Song Y, et al. Meta-analysis added power to identify variants in FTO associated with type 2 diabetes and obesity in the Asian population. Obesity (Silver Spring). Endocr J. 2010;57(4):293–301.
6. Karasawa S, Daimon M, Sasaki S, et al. Association of the common fat mass and obesity associated (FTO) gene polymorphism with obesity in a Japanese population. Endocrinol J. Jan 6 2010. Vol 57(4):293–301.
7. Pausova Z, Syme C, Abrahamowicz M, et al. A common variant of the FTO gene is associated with not only increased adiposity but also elevated blood pressure in French Canadians. Circ Cardiovasc Genet. Jun 2009;2(3):260–9.
8. Hunt SC, Stone S, Xin Y, et al. Association of the FTO gene with BMI. Obesity (Silver Spring). Apr 2008;16(4):902–4.
9. Peeters A, Beckers S, Verrijken A, et al. Variants in the FTO gene are associated with common obesity in the Belgian population. Mol Genet Metab. Apr 2008;93(4):481–4.
10. Jacobsson JA, Danielsson P, Svensson V, et al. Major gender difference in association of FTO gene variant among severely obese children with obesity and obesity related phenotypes. Biochem Biophys Res Commun. Apr 11 2008;368(3):476–82.
11. Cha SW, Choi SM, Kim KS, et al. Replication of genetic effects of FTO polymorphisms on BMI in a Korean population. Obesity (Silver Spring). Sep 2008;16(9):2187–9.
12. Olszewski PK, Fredriksson R, Olszewska AM, et al. Hypothalamic FTO is associated with the regulation of energy intake not feeding reward. BMC Neurosci. 2009;10:129.
13. Jacobsson JA, Klovins J, Kapa I, et al. Novel genetic variant in FTO influences insulin levels and insulin resistance in severely obese children and adolescents. Int J Obes (Lond). Nov 2008;32(11):1730–5.
14. Tanofsky-Kraff M, Han JC, Anandalingam K, et al. The FTO gene rs9939609 obesity-risk allele and loss of control over eating. Am J Clin Nutr. Dec 2009;90(6):1483–8.
15. den Hoed M, Westerterp-Plantenga MS, Bouwman FG, Mariman EC, Westerterp KR. Postprandial responses in hunger and satiety are associated with the rs9939609 single nucleotide polymorphism in FTO. Am J Clin Nutr. Nov 2009;90(5):1426–32.
16. Sebert SP, Hyatt MA, Chan LL, et al. Influence of prenatal nutrition and obesity on tissue specific fat mass and obesity-associated (FTO) gene expression. Reproduction. Jan 2010;139(1):265–74.
17. Church C, Lee S, Bagg EA, et al. A mouse model for the metabolic effects of the human fat mass and obesity associated FTO gene. PLoS Genet. Aug 2009;5(8):e1000599.
18. Fischer J, Koch L, Emmerling C, et al. Inactivation of the Fto gene protects from obesity. Nature. Apr 16 2009;458(7240):894–8.
19. Gerdes JM, Davis EE, Katsanis N. The vertebrate primary cilium in development, homeostasis, and disease. Cell. Apr 3 2009;137(1):32–45.
20. Sen Gupta P, Prodromou NV, Chapple JP. Can faulty antennae increase adiposity? The link between cilia proteins and obesity. J Endocrinol. Dec 2009;203(3):327–36.
21. Mok C, HÈon E, Zhen M. Ciliary dysfunction and obesity. Clin Genet. 2010;77(1):18–27.
22. Badano JL, Mitsuma N, Beales PL, Katsanis N. The ciliopathies: an emerging class of human genetic disorders. Annu Rev Genomics Hum Genet. 2006;7:125–48.
23. Zaghloul NA, Katsanis N. Mechanistic insights into Bardet-Biedl syndrome, a model ciliopathy. J Clin Invest. Mar 2009;119(3):428–37.
24. Collin GB, Cyr E, Bronson R, et al. Alms1-disrupted mice recapitulate human Alstrom syndrome. Hum Mol Genet. Aug 15 2005;14(16):2323–33.

25. Arsov T, Silva DG, O'Bryan MK, et al. Fat aussie – a new Alstrom syndrome mouse showing a critical role for ALMS1 in obesity, diabetes, and spermatogenesis. Mol Endocrinol. Jul 2006;20(7):1610–22.
26. Li G, Vega R, Nelms K, et al. A role for Alstrom syndrome protein, alms1, in kidney ciliogenesis and cellular quiescence. PLoS Genet. Jan 5 2007;3(1):e8.
27. Rahmouni K, Fath MA, Seo S, et al. Leptin resistance contributes to obesity and hypertension in mouse models of Bardet-Biedl syndrome. J Clin Invest. Apr 2008;118(4):1458–67.
28. Davenport JR, Watts AJ, Roper VC, et al. Disruption of intraflagellar transport in adult mice leads to obesity and slow-onset cystic kidney disease. Curr Biol. Sep 18 2007;17(18): 1586–94.
29. Davis RE, Swiderski RE, Rahmouni K, et al. A knockin mouse model of the Bardet-Biedl syndrome 1 M390R mutation has cilia defects, ventriculomegaly, retinopathy, and obesity. Proc Natl Acad Sci USA. Dec 4 2007;104(49):19422–7.
30. Seo S, Guo DF, Bugge K, Morgan DA, Rahmouni K, Sheffield VC. Requirement of Bardet-Biedl syndrome proteins for leptin receptor signaling. Hum Mol Genet. Apr 1 2009;18(7):1323–31.
31. Praetorius HA, Spring KR. A physiological view of the primary cilium. Annu Rev Physiol. 2005;67:515–29.
32. Dutcher SK. Flagellar assembly in two hundred and fifty easy-to-follow steps. Trends Genet. Oct 1995;11(10):398–404.
33. Dutcher SK. Elucidation of basal body and centriole functions in *Chlamydomonas reinhardtii*. Traffic. Jul 2003;4(7):443–51.
34. Kramer-Zucker AG, Olale F, Haycraft CJ, Yoder BK, Schier AF, Drummond IA. Cilia-driven fluid flow in the zebrafish pronephros, brain and Kupffer's vesicle is required for normal organogenesis. Development. Apr 2005;132(8):1907–21.
35. Nonaka S, Tanaka Y, Okada Y, et al. Randomization of left-right asymmetry due to loss of nodal cilia generating leftward flow of extraembryonic fluid in mice lacking KIF3B motor protein. Cell. Dec 11 1998;95(6):829–37.
36. Reese TS. Olfactory cilia in the frog. J Cell Biol. May 1 1965;25(2):209–30.
37. Baldari CT, Rosenbaum J. Intraflagellar transport: it's not just for cilia anymore. Curr Opin Cell Biol. 2010 Feb;22(1):75–80.
38. Kozminski KG, Johnson KA, Forscher P, Rosenbaum JL. A motility in the eukaryotic flagellum unrelated to flagellar beating. Proc Natl Acad Sci USA. Jun 15 1993;90(12):5519–23.
39. Pedersen LB, Rosenbaum JL. Intraflagellar transport (IFT) role in ciliary assembly, resorption and signalling. Curr Top Dev Biol. 2008;85:23–61.
40. Scholey JM. Intraflagellar transport motors in cilia: moving along the cell's antenna. J Cell Biol. Jan 14 2008;180(1):23–9.
41. Kozminski KG, Beech PL, Rosenbaum JL. The Chlamydomonas kinesin-like protein FLA10 is involved in motility associated with the flagellar membrane. J Cell Biol. Dec 1995;131(6 Pt 1):1517–27.
42. Brown JM, Marsala C, Kosoy R, Gaertig J. Kinesin-II is preferentially targeted to assembling cilia and is required for ciliogenesis and normal cytokinesis in Tetrahymena. Mol Biol Cell. Oct 1999;10(10):3081–96.
43. Marszalek JR, Ruiz-Lozano P, Roberts E, Chien KR, Goldstein LS. Situs inversus and embryonic ciliary morphogenesis defects in mouse mutants lacking the KIF3A subunit of kinesin-II. Proc Natl Acad Sci USA. Apr 27 1999;96(9):5043–8.
44. Morris RL, Scholey JM. Heterotrimeric kinesin-II is required for the assembly of motile 9+2 ciliary axonemes on sea urchin embryos. J Cell Biol. Sep 8 1997;138(5):1009–22.
45. Sarpal R, Todi SV, Sivan-Loukianova E, et al. Drosophila KAP interacts with the kinesin II motor subunit KLP64D to assemble chordotonal sensory cilia, but not sperm tails. Curr Biol. Sep 30 2003;13(19):1687–96.
46. Takeda S, Yonekawa Y, Tanaka Y, Okada Y, Nonaka S, Hirokawa N. Left-right asymmetry and kinesin superfamily protein KIF3A: new insights in determination of laterality

and mesoderm induction by kif3A-/- mice analysis. J Cell Biol. May 17 1999;145(4): 825–36.
47. Pfister KK, Fisher EM, Gibbons IR, et al. Cytoplasmic dynein nomenclature. J Cell Biol. Nov 7 2005;171(3):411–3.
48. Rompolas P, Pedersen LB, Patel-King RS, King SM. Chlamydomonas FAP133 is a dynein intermediate chain associated with the retrograde intraflagellar transport motor. J Cell Sci. Oct 15 2007;120(Pt 20):3653–65.
49. Pazour GJ, Dickert BL, Witman GB. The DHC1b (DHC2) isoform of cytoplasmic dynein is required for flagellar assembly. J Cell Biol. Feb 8 1999;144(3):473–81.
50. Porter ME, Bower R, Knott JA, Byrd P, Dentler W. Cytoplasmic dynein heavy chain 1b is required for flagellar assembly in Chlamydomonas. Mol Biol Cell. Mar 1999;10(3): 693–712.
51. Signor D, Wedaman KP, Orozco JT, et al. Role of a class DHC1b dynein in retrograde transport of IFT motors and IFT raft particles along cilia, but not dendrites, in chemosensory neurons of living *Caenorhabditis elegans*. J Cell Biol. Nov 1 1999;147(3):519–30.
52. Huangfu D, Anderson KV. Cilia and Hedgehog responsiveness in the mouse. Proc Natl Acad Sci USA. Aug 9 2005;102(32):11325–30.
53. May SR, Ashique AM, Karlen M, et al. Loss of the retrograde motor for IFT disrupts localization of Smo to cilia and prevents the expression of both activator and repressor functions of Gli. Dev Biol. Nov 15 2005;287(2):378–89.
54. Rosenbaum JL, Witman GB. Intraflagellar transport. Nat Rev Mol Cell Biol. Nov 2002;3(11):813–25.
55. Christensen ST, Pedersen LB, Schneider L, Satir P. Sensory cilia and integration of signal transduction in human health and disease. Traffic. Feb 2007;8(2):97–109.
56. Corbit KC, Aanstad P, Singla V, Norman AR, Stainier DYR, Reiter JF. Vertebrate Smoothened functions at the primary cilium. Nature. 2005;437(7061):1018–21.
57. Dwyer ND, Adler CE, Crump JG, L'Etoile ND, Bargmann CI. Polarized dendritic transport and the AP-1 mu1 clathrin adaptor UNC-101 localize odorant receptors to olfactory cilia. Neuron. Aug 2 2001;31(2):277–87.
58. Godsel LM, Engman DM. Flagellar protein localization mediated by a calcium-myristoyl/palmitoyl switch mechanism. EMBO J. Apr 15 1999;18(8):2057–65.
59. Tull D, Vince JE, Callaghan JM, et al. SMP-1, a member of a new family of small myristoylated proteins in kinetoplastid parasites, is targeted to the flagellum membrane in Leishmania. Mol Biol Cell. Nov 2004;15(11):4775–86.
60. Quest AF, Harvey DJ, McIlhinney RA. Myristoylated and nonmyristoylated pools of sea urchin sperm flagellar creatine kinase exist side-by-side: myristoylation is necessary for efficient lipid association. Biochemistry. Jun 10 1997;36(23):6993–7002.
61. Ramulu P, Nathans J. Cellular and subcellular localization, N-terminal acylation, and calcium binding of Caenorhabditis elegans protein phosphatase with EF-hands. J Biol Chem. Jul 6 2001;276(27):25127–35.
62. Schermer B, Hopker K, Omran H, et al. Phosphorylation by casein kinase 2 induces PACS-1 binding of nephrocystin and targeting to cilia. EMBO J. Dec 21 2005;24(24):4415–24.
63. Croce JC, McClay DR. Evolution of the Wnt pathways. Methods Mol Biol. 2008;469:3–18.
64. Jiang J, Hui CC. Hedgehog signaling in development and cancer. Dev Cell. Dec 2008;15(6):801–12.
65. Huangfu D, Liu A, Rakeman AS, Murcia NS, Niswander L, Anderson KV. Hedgehog signalling in the mouse requires intraflagellar transport proteins. Nature. Nov 6 2003;426(6962):83–7.
66. Rohatgi R, Milenkovic L, Scott MP. Patched1 regulates hedgehog signaling at the primary cilium. Science. Jul 20 2007;317(5836):372–6.
67. Haycraft CJ, Banizs B, Aydin-Son Y, Zhang Q, Michaud EJ, Yoder BK. Gli2 and Gli3 localize to cilia and require the intraflagellar transport protein polaris for processing and function. PLoS Genet. Oct 2005;1(4):e53.

68. Spinella-Jaegle S, Rawadi G, Kawai S, et al. Sonic hedgehog increases the commitment of pluripotent mesenchymal cells into the osteoblastic lineage and abolishes adipocytic differentiation. J Cell Sci. Jun 2001;114(Pt 11):2085–94.
69. Zehentner BK, Leser U, Burtscher H. BMP-2 and sonic hedgehog have contrary effects on adipocyte-like differentiation of C3H10T1/2 cells. DNA Cell Biol. May 2000;19(5):275–81.
70. Vierkotten J, Dildrop R, Peters T, Wang B, Ruther U. Ftm is a novel basal body protein of cilia involved in Shh signalling. Development. Jul 2007;134(14):2569–77.
71. Khanna H, Davis EE, Murga-Zamalloa CA, et al. A common allele in RPGRIP1L is a modifier of retinal degeneration in ciliopathies. Nat Genet. Jun 2009;41(6):739–45.
72. Stratigopoulos G, Padilla SL, LeDuc CA, et al. Regulation of Fto/Ftm gene expression in mice and humans. Am J Physiol Regul Integr Comp Physiol. Apr 2008;294(4):R1185–R96.
73. Shiba D, Yamaoka Y, Hagiwara H, Takamatsu T, Hamada H, Yokoyama T. Localization of Inv in a distinctive intraciliary compartment requires the C-terminal ninein-homolog-containing region. J Cell Sci. Jan 1 2009;122(Pt 1):44–54.
74. Mochizuki T, Saijoh Y, Tsuchiya K, et al. Cloning of inv, a gene that controls left/right asymmetry and kidney development. Nature. Sep 10 1998;395(6698):177–81.
75. Morgan D, Turnpenny L, Goodship J, et al. Inversin, a novel gene in the vertebrate left-right axis pathway, is partially deleted in the inv mouse. Nat Genet. Oct 1998;20(2):149–56.
76. Phillips CL, Miller KJ, Filson AJ, et al. Renal cysts of inv/inv mice resemble early infantile nephronophthisis. J Am Soc Nephrol. Jul 2004;15(7):1744–55.
77. Simons M, Gloy J, Ganner A, et al. Inversin, the gene product mutated in nephronophthisis type II, functions as a molecular switch between Wnt signaling pathways. Nat Genet. May 2005;37(5):537–43.
78. Corbit KC, Shyer AE, Dowdle WE, et al. Kif3a constrains beta-catenin-dependent Wnt signalling through dual ciliary and non-ciliary mechanisms. Nat Cell Biol. Jan 2008;10(1): 70–6.
79. Gerdes JM, Liu Y, Zaghloul NA, et al. Disruption of the basal body compromises proteasomal function and perturbs intracellular Wnt response. Nat Genet. Nov 2007;39(11):1350–60.
80. Ocbina PJ, Tuson M, Anderson KV. Primary cilia are not required for normal canonical Wnt signaling in the mouse embryo. PLoS One. 2009;4(8):e6839.
81. Huang P, Schier AF. Dampened Hedgehog signaling but normal Wnt signaling in zebrafish without cilia. Development. Sep 2009;136(18):3089–98.
82. Park TJ, Mitchell BJ, Abitua PB, Kintner C, Wallingford JB. Dishevelled controls apical docking and planar polarization of basal bodies in ciliated epithelial cells. Nat Genet. Jul 2008;40(7):871–9.
83. Ross SE, Hemati N, Longo KA, et al. Inhibition of adipogenesis by Wnt signaling. Science. Aug 11 2000;289(5481):950–3.
84. Longo KA, Wright WS, Kang S, et al. Wnt10b inhibits development of white and brown adipose tissues. J Biol Chem. Aug 20 2004;279(34):35503–9.
85. Christodoulides C, Scarda A, Granzotto M, et al. WNT10B mutations in human obesity. Diabetologia. Apr 2006;49(4):678–84.
86. Vertino AM, Taylor-Jones JM, Longo KA, et al. Wnt10b deficiency promotes coexpression of myogenic and adipogenic programs in myoblasts. Mol Biol Cell. Apr 2005;16(4): 2039–48.
87. Zhang Y, Proenca R, Maffei M, Barone M, Leopold L, Friedman JM. Positional cloning of the mouse obese gene and its human homologue. Nature. Dec 1 1994;372(6505):425–32.
88. Woods SC, D'Alessio DA. Central control of body weight and appetite. J Clin Endocrinol Metab. Nov 2008;93 11 Suppl 1:S37–S50.
89. Coll AP, Farooqi IS, O'Rahilly S. The hormonal control of food intake. Cell. Apr 20 2007;129(2):251–62.
90. Montague CT, Farooqi IS, Whitehead JP, et al. Congenital leptin deficiency is associated with severe early-onset obesity in humans. Nature. Jun 26 1997;387(6636):903–8.
91. Friedman JM, Halaas JL. Leptin and the regulation of body weight in mammals. Nature. Oct 22 1998;395(6704):763–70.

92. Farooqi IS, Matarese G, Lord GM, et al. Beneficial effects of leptin on obesity, T cell hyporesponsiveness, and neuroendocrine/metabolic dysfunction of human congenital leptin deficiency. J Clin Invest. Oct 2002;110(8):1093–103.
93. Dahl HA. Fine structure of cilia in rat cerebral cortex. Z Zellforsch Mikrosk Anat. 1963;60:369–86.
94. Murcia NS, Richards WG, Yoder BK, Mucenski ML, Dunlap JR, Woychik RP. The Oak Ridge Polycystic Kidney (orpk) disease gene is required for left-right axis determination. Development. Jun 2000;127(11):2347–55.
95. Balthasar N, Coppari R, McMinn J, et al. Leptin receptor signaling in POMC neurons is required for normal body weight homeostasis. Neuron. Jun 24 2004;42(6):983–91.
96. Dhillon H, Zigman JM, Ye C, et al. Leptin directly activates SF1 neurons in the VMH, and this action by leptin is required for normal body-weight homeostasis. Neuron. Jan 19 2006;49(2):191–203.
97. Huo L, Grill HJ, Bjorbaek C. Divergent regulation of proopiomelanocortin neurons by leptin in the nucleus of the solitary tract and in the arcuate hypothalamic nucleus. Diabetes. Mar 2006;55(3):567–73.
98. Grill HJ, Schwartz MW, Kaplan JM, Foxhall JS, Breininger J, Baskin DG. Evidence that the caudal brainstem is a target for the inhibitory effect of leptin on food intake. Endocrinology. Jan 2002;143(1):239–46.
99. Hommel JD, Trinko R, Sears RM, et al. Leptin receptor signaling in midbrain dopamine neurons regulates feeding. Neuron. Sep 21 2006;51(6):801–10.
100. Fulton S, Pissios P, Manchon RP, et al. Leptin regulation of the mesoaccumbens dopamine pathway. Neuron. Sep 2006;51(6):811–22.
101. Mykytyn K, Nishimura DY, Searby CC, et al. Identification of the gene (BBS1) most commonly involved in Bardet-Biedl syndrome, a complex human obesity syndrome. Nat Genet. Aug 2002;31(4):435–8.
102. Handel M, Schulz S, Stanarius A, et al. Selective targeting of somatostatin receptor 3 to neuronal cilia. Neuroscience. Mar 1999;89(3):909–26.
103. Hamon M, Doucet E, Lefevre K, et al. Antibodies and antisense oligonucleotide for probing the distribution and putative functions of central 5-HT6 receptors. Neuropsychopharmacology. Aug 1999;21 2 Suppl:68S–76S.
104. Brailov I, Bancila M, Brisorgueil MJ, Miquel MC, Hamon M, Verge D. Localization of 5-HT(6) receptors at the plasma membrane of neuronal cilia in the rat brain. Brain Res. Jul 28 2000;872(1–2):271–5.
105. Berbari NF, Johnson AD, Lewis JS, Askwith CC, Mykytyn K. Identification of ciliary localization sequences within the third intracellular loop of G protein-coupled receptors. Mol Biol Cell. Apr 2008;19(4):1540–7.
106. Berbari NF, Lewis JS, Bishop GA, Askwith CC, Mykytyn K. Bardet-Biedl syndrome proteins are required for the localization of G protein-coupled receptors to primary cilia. Proc Natl Acad Sci USA. Mar 18 2008;105(11):4242–6.
107. Bishop GA, Berbari NF, Lewis J, Mykytyn K. Type III adenylyl cyclase localizes to primary cilia throughout the adult mouse brain. J Comp Neurol. Dec 10 2007;505(5):562–71.
108. Nordman S, Abulaiti A, Hilding A, et al. Genetic variation of the adenylyl cyclase 3 (AC3) locus and its influence on type 2 diabetes and obesity susceptibility in Swedish men. Int J Obes (Lond). Mar 2008;32(3):407–12.
109. Pissios P. Animals models of MCH function and what they can tell us about its role in energy balance. Peptides. Nov 2009;30(11):2040–4.
110. Shimada M, Tritos NA, Lowell BB, Flier JS, Maratos-Flier E. Mice lacking melanin-concentrating hormone are hypophagic and lean. Nature. Dec 17 1998;396(6712):670–4.
111. Kokkotou E, Jeon JY, Wang X, et al. Mice with MCH ablation resist diet-induced obesity through strain-specific mechanisms. Am J Physiol Regul Integr Comp Physiol. Jul 2005;289(1):R117–R24.
112. Wang Z, Li V, Chan GC, et al. Adult type 3 adenylyl cyclase-deficient mice are obese. PLoS One. 2009;4(9):e6979.

113. Coleman DL, Eicher EM. Fat (fat) and tubby (tub): two autosomal recessive mutations causing obesity syndromes in the mouse. J Hered. Nov–Dec 1990;81(6):424–7.
114. Mak HY, Nelson LS, Basson M, Johnson CD, Ruvkun G. Polygenic control of Caenorhabditis elegans fat storage. Nat Genet. Mar 2006;38(3):363–8.
115. Rosen ED, Walkey CJ, Puigserver P, Spiegelman BM. Transcriptional regulation of adipogenesis. Genes Dev. Jun 1 2000;14(11):1293–307.
116. MacDougald OA, Mandrup S. Adipogenesis: forces that tip the scales. Trends Endocrinol Metab. Jan–Feb 2002;13(1):5–11.
117. Forti E, Aksanov O, Birk RZ. Temporal expression pattern of Bardet-Biedl syndrome genes in adipogenesis. Int J Biochem Cell Biol. 2007;39(5):1055–62.
118. Marion V, Stoetzel C, Schlicht D, et al. Transient ciliogenesis involving Bardet-Biedl syndrome proteins is a fundamental characteristic of adipogenic differentiation. Proc Natl Acad Sci USA. Feb 10 2009;106(6):1820–5.
119. Quinlan RJ, Tobin JL, Beales PL. Modeling ciliopathies: primary cilia in development and disease. Curr Top Dev Biol. 2008;84:249–310.
120. Beales PL, Elcioglu N, Woolf AS, Parker D, Flinter FA. New criteria for improved diagnosis of Bardet-Biedl syndrome: results of a population survey. J Med Genet. Jun 1999;36(6): 437–46.
121. Green JS, Parfrey PS, Harnett JD, et al. The cardinal manifestations of Bardet-Biedl syndrome, a form of Laurence-Moon-Biedl syndrome. N Engl J Med. Oct 12 1989;321(15):1002–9.
122. Klein D, Ammann F. The syndrome of Laurence-Moon-Bardet-Biedl and allied diseases in Switzerland. Clinical, genetic and epidemiological studies. J Neurol Sci. Nov–Dec 1969;9(3):479–513.
123. Bell J. The Laurence-Moon syndrome. In: Penrose LS, editor. The treasury of human inheritance. London:Cambridge University Press; 1958. pp. 51–96.
124. Marshall JD, Beck S, Maffei P, Naggert JK. Alstrom syndrome. Eur J Hum Genet. Dec 2007;15(12):1193–202.
125. Gherman A, Davis EE, Katsanis N. The ciliary proteome database: an integrated community resource for the genetic and functional dissection of cilia. Nat Genet. Sep 2006;38(9):961–2.
126. Katsanis N. The oligogenic properties of Bardet-Biedl syndrome. Hum Mol Genet. Apr 1 2004;13 Spec No 1:R65–R71.
127. Kulaga HM, Leitch CC, Eichers ER, et al. Loss of BBS proteins causes anosmia in humans and defects in olfactory cilia structure and function in the mouse. Nat Genet. Sep 2004;36(9):994–8.
128. Beales PL, Warner AM, Hitman GA, Thakker R, Flinter FA. Bardet-Biedl syndrome: a molecular and phenotypic study of 18 families. J Med Genet. Feb 1997;34(2):92–8.
129. Farag TI, Teebi AS. Bardet-Biedl and Laurence-Moon syndromes in a mixed Arab population. Clin Genet. Feb 1988;33(2):78–82.
130. Farag TI, Teebi AS. High incidence of Bardet-Biedl syndrome amongst the Bedouin. Clin Genet. 1989;36:463–4.
131. Ansley SJ, Badano JL, Blacque OE, et al. Basal body dysfunction is a likely cause of pleiotropic Bardet-Biedl syndrome. Nature. Oct 9 2003;425(6958):628–33.
132. Li JB, Gerdes JM, Haycraft CJ, et al. Comparative genomics identifies a flagellar and basal body proteome that includes the BBS5 human disease gene. Cell. May 14 2004;117(4): 541–52.
133. Fan Y, Esmail MA, Ansley SJ, et al. Mutations in a member of the Ras superfamily of small GTP-binding proteins causes Bardet-Biedl syndrome. Nat Genet. Sep 2004;36(9):989–93.
134. Kim JC, Badano JL, Sibold S, et al. The Bardet-Biedl protein BBS4 targets cargo to the pericentriolar region and is required for microtubule anchoring and cell cycle progression. Nat Genet. May 2004;36(5):462–70.
135. Kim JC, Ou YY, Badano JL, et al. MKKS/BBS6, a divergent chaperonin-like protein linked to the obesity disorder Bardet-Biedl syndrome, is a novel centrosomal component required for cytokinesis. J Cell Sci. Mar 1 2005;118(Pt 5):1007–20.

136. Nachury MV, Loktev AV, Zhang Q, et al. A core complex of BBS proteins cooperates with the GTPase Rab8 to promote ciliary membrane biogenesis. Cell. Jun 15 2007;129(6): 1201–13.
137. Loktev AV, Zhang Q, Beck JS, et al. A BBSome subunit links ciliogenesis, microtubule stability, and acetylation. Dev Cell. Dec 2008;15(6):854–65.
138. Inglis PN, Boroevich KA, Leroux MR. Piecing together a ciliome. Trends Genet. Sep 2006;22(9):491–500.
139. Stenmark H. Rab GTPases as coordinators of vesicle traffic. Nat Rev Mol Cell Biol. Aug 2009;10(8):513–25.
140. Lechtreck KF, Johnson EC, Sakai T, et al. The *Chlamydomonas reinhardtii* BBSome is an IFT cargo required for export of specific signaling proteins from flagella. J Cell Biol. Dec 28 2009;187(7):1117–32.
141. Shah AS, Farmen SL, Moninger TO, et al. Loss of Bardet-Biedl syndrome proteins alters the morphology and function of motile cilia in airway epithelia. Proc Natl Acad Sci USA. Mar 4 2008;105(9):3380–5.
142. Yen HJ, Tayeh MK, Mullins RF, Stone EM, Sheffield VC, Slusarski DC. Bardet-Biedl syndrome genes are important in retrograde intracellular trafficking and Kupffer's vesicle cilia function. Hum Mol Genet. Mar 1 2006;15(5):667–77.
143. Lee S, Walker CL, Karten B, et al. Essential role for the Prader-Willi syndrome protein necdin in axonal outgrowth. Hum Mol Genet. Mar 1 2005;14(5):627–37.
144. Chen C, Visootsak J, Dills S, Graham JM Jr. Prader-Willi syndrome: an update and review for the primary pediatrician. Clin Pediatr (Phila). Sep 2007;46(7):580–91.
145. Alström CH, Hallgren B, Nilsson LB, Asander H. Retinal degeneration combined with obesity, diabetes mellitus and neurogeneous deafness: a specific syndrome (not hitherto described) distinct from the Laurence-Moon-Bardet-Biedl syndrome: a clinical, endocrinological and genetic examination based on a large pedigree. Acta Psychiatr Neurol Scand Suppl. 1959;129:1–35.
146. Hearn T, Renforth GL, Spalluto C, et al. Mutation of ALMS1, a large gene with a tandem repeat encoding 47 amino acids, causes Alstrom syndrome. Nat Genet. May 2002;31(1): 79–83.
147. Collin GB, Marshall JD, Ikeda A, et al. Mutations in ALMS1 cause obesity, type 2 diabetes and neurosensory degeneration in Alstrom syndrome. Nat Genet. May 2002;31(1):74–8.
148. Marshall JD, Bronson RT, Collin GB, et al. New Alstrom syndrome phenotypes based on the evaluation of 182 cases. Arch Intern Med. Mar 28 2005;165(6):675–83.
149. Hearn T, Spalluto C, Phillips VJ, et al. Subcellular localization of ALMS1 supports involvement of centrosome and basal body dysfunction in the pathogenesis of obesity, insulin resistance, and type 2 diabetes. Diabetes. May 2005;54(5):1581–7.
150. Andersen JS, Wilkinson CJ, Mayor T, Mortensen P, Nigg EA, Mann M. Proteomic characterization of the human centrosome by protein correlation profiling. Nature. Dec 4 2003;426(6966):570–4.
151. Eggenschwiler JT, Anderson KV. Cilia and developmental signaling. Annu Rev Cell Dev Biol. 2007;23:345–73.
152. Feistel K, Blum M. Three types of cilia including a novel 9+4 axoneme on the notochordal plate of the rabbit embryo. Dev Dyn. Dec 2006;235(12):3348–58.
153. Barsh GS, Schwartz MW. Genetic approaches to studying energy balance: perception and integration. Nat Rev Genet. Aug 2002;3(8):589–600.

Chapter 5
Genome-Wide Association Studies and Human Population Obesity

Ruth J.F. Loos and Tuomas O. Kilpeläinen

5.1 Introduction

Evidence from both family and twin studies suggest a strong heritability for obesity, ranging between 40 and 70% [1] (see Chapter 2). Despite the high heritability, the identification of genetic variants contributing to common obesity has long been unsuccessful. The complex etiology of obesity has been a challenge to geneticists. Common obesity is a multifactorial condition in which numerous genes, in interaction with each other and with the environment, may affect the risk of obesity [2]. Indeed, during the past 15 years, only a handful of obesity-susceptibility loci suggested by candidate gene or genome-wide linkage studies have been unequivocally established [3]. In light of the arduous past, the recent implementation of the genome-wide association (GWA) study approach represents a revolution in the search of susceptibility genes for obesity. Since the publication of the first wave of GWA studies for common obesity in 2007, least 15 susceptibility loci have been established, providing valuable insights into the genetic architecture of obesity.

GWA studies interrogate the whole genome by studying hundreds of thousands of single nucleotide polymorphisms (SNPs), the most common form of human genetic variation. The variation at such SNPs is determined using high-throughput genotyping chips that capture up to 80% of the common variation of the human genome, allowing the identification of obesity-susceptibility genes at the genome-wide level. Unlike candidate gene studies that rely on our current understanding of the biology of obesity, GWA studies are hypothesis-generating, aiming to identify new genes, previously unknown to play a role in a disease. By identifying new genes, GWA studies promise to provide new insights into the underlying mechanisms of obesity development.

R.J.F. Loos (✉)
MRC Epidemiology Unit, Institute of Metabolic Science, Addenbrooke's Hospital, Cambridge, UK
e-mail: ruth.loos@mrc-epid.cam.ac.uk

R.H. Lustig (ed.), *Obesity Before Birth*, Endocrine Updates 30,
DOI 10.1007/978-1-4419-7034-3_5, © Springer Science+Business Media, LLC 2011

During recent years, several large GWA studies for obesity-related traits have been carried out, leading to the succesful discovery of many new susceptibility loci. In this chapter, we describe the design, interpretation, discoveries, and future challenges of GWA studies in the field of obesity genetics.

5.2 Genome-Wide Association (GWA) Studies

5.2.1 The International HapMap Project and High-Throughput Genotyping – The Bedrocks of the Genome-Wide Association Approach

The aim of GWA studies is to capture the majority of common genetic variation in a population sample and to relate these variants (SNPs) to a trait or a disease [4]. The implementation of the genome-wide association approach would not have been possible without the growing knowledge of the human genome throughout the first decade of the 21st century. The completion of the Human Genome Project in 2003 provided the foundation for genome-wide studies by sequencing of all 3 billion base pairs of the human genome [5]. This project was followed by another large-scale collaboration, the International HapMap Project, launched in 2002, which built on the Human Genome Project. The International HapMap Project examined the common genetic variation across 3.1 million SNPs of 270 individuals from four ethnicities, providing insight into the genetic heterogeneity between individuals and ethnicities [6, 7]. The International HapMap Project later expanded to include 1,115 individuals from 11 populations. All the information is catalogued and made publicly available (http://hapmap.ncbi.nlm.nih.gov).

The HapMap not only catalogues the locations of SNPs and their frequencies in various populations, but also provides insight into how these SNPs are correlated (or in linkage disequilibrium) with each other [6]. These correlations exist because sets of nearby SNPs on the same chromosome are often inherited in blocks, called haplotypes. The great advantage of these correlations is that only a few SNPs are needed to uniquely identify all variants on a haplotype.

The documentation of these correlations between SNPs enabled geneticists to capture most of the common variation in human genome by genotyping only a subset of SNPs (known as tag SNPs or proxies) [7]. As such, by genotyping only a subset of roughly 500,000 SNPs, the genetic variation of 3.1 million SNPs can be studied in a more cost-efficient manner.

At the same time, vast advancements in technology have led to the development of high-throughput genotyping DNA microarrays or "chips" that enabled genotyping hundreds of thousands of SNPs in one single experiment [6]. The design of these SNP chips heavily relies on the SNP correlations reported by the HapMap as they aim to efficiently capture most of the common genetic variation by the careful selection of a few hundred thousands of tag SNPs. Since the first high-density SNP chips came on the market in 2005, the prices have dropped dramatically; for example, the company Affymetrix initially sold their 500 K SNP chip at ~$1,500 per chip, whereas 1 year later it was priced at less than $350. The relatively low cost of these SNP chips has allowed many research groups to genotype their population samples and to participate in international consortia.

5.2.2 Two-Stage Design of GWA Studies

A typical GWA study comprises of two stages: a discovery stage, followed by a replication stage (Fig. 5.1).

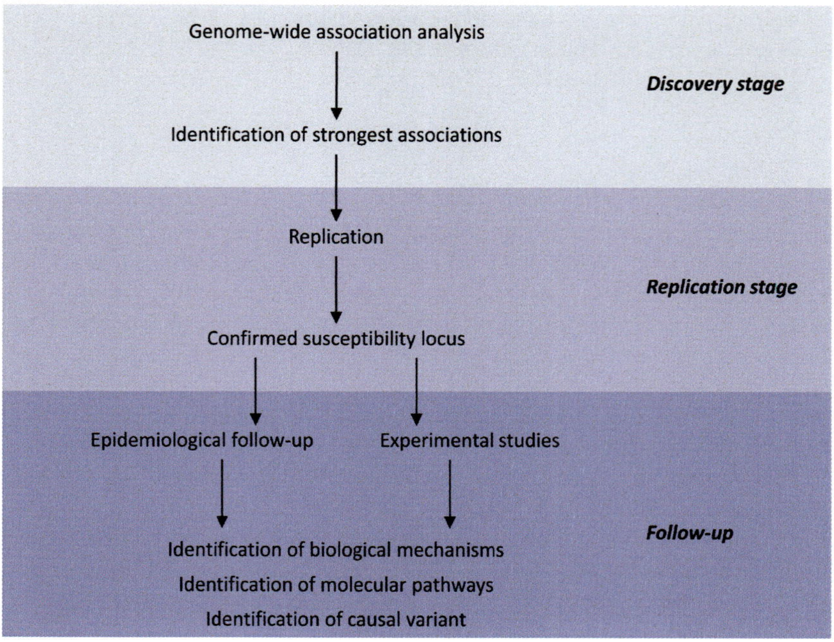

Fig. 5.1 Path from a genome-wide association study to the discovery and follow-up of a biologically relevant genetic locus

The *discovery stage* is the actual genome-wide analysis, in which each of the hundreds of thousands of SNPs is tested for association with a trait or a disease of interest. SNPs are coded as 0, 1, or 2, representing the number of "risk" alleles an individual carries. As such, the association tests the effect of each additional "risk" allele on a continuous trait or a binary outcome (e.g., a disease). Given the hundreds of thousands of association tests performed in a single study, the chance of false-positive findings is very high. To account for the multiple testing, the nominal P value to consider an association as significant must be very stringent; thus a $P < 5 \times 10^{-8}$ has been recommended as the minimum threshold to be reached after validation in the replication stage [8]. Typically, SNPs for which the association

P values reach $<10^{-7}$ or $<10^{-6}$ at the discovery stage are taken forward to the replication stage. Furthermore, only those associations that are validated in the replication stage are considered true findings.

The *replication stage* is performed in new series of samples that have the same study design as those used in the discovery stage and in which the total sample size is ideally at least as large as the sample size used at the discovery stage. The SNPs that were taken forward from the discovery stage are tested for association in the replication samples. Eventually the association results of the discovery and replication stage are combined. SNPs for which the P values reach the critical threshold of $< 5 \times 10^{-8}$ are considered confirmed loci ("hits"), whereas the other SNPs were likely false-positive findings.

The replication stage is often followed by a more in-depth investigation of the functional implications of the confirmed loci (Fig. 5.1).

5.2.3 Imputation

Over the past years, researchers have realized that collaboration is an important factor in the success of GWA studies. Through combining data from multiple groups, the sample size and thus also the statistical power of the study can be increased such that SNPs with even small effects can be identified with great confidence. However, when groups first started to collaborate they were faced with the fact that not all samples had been genotyped with the same SNP chip so that combining data was limited to SNPs common to the various chips. To make more efficient use of all available data, imputation software was developed that allowed imputing genotypes of SNPs that had not been genotyped, but for which information was available from the HapMap Project.

Imputation relies on the correlations between SNPs along the human genome documented by the HapMap Project. The strength of these correlations determine the accuracy with which untyped SNPs can be predicted on the basis of genotyped SNPs [7]. Before data from multiple studies are combined, each study imputes all SNPs from the HapMap and tests for association with the trait or disease of interest. Subsequently, summary statistics of all SNPs can be meta-analysed.

Imputation also increases the resolution of genome-wide scans as it provides data on all SNPs from the HapMap, rather than on a subset that is available on the SNP chip, which helps with the fine-mapping of the association signal.

5.2.4 Presentation of Genome-Wide Results

The results of the genome-wide scan are typically presented by plotting the association P values of the SNPs with the disease or trait of interest according to their physical location on the human genome. For ease of display, the statistics are

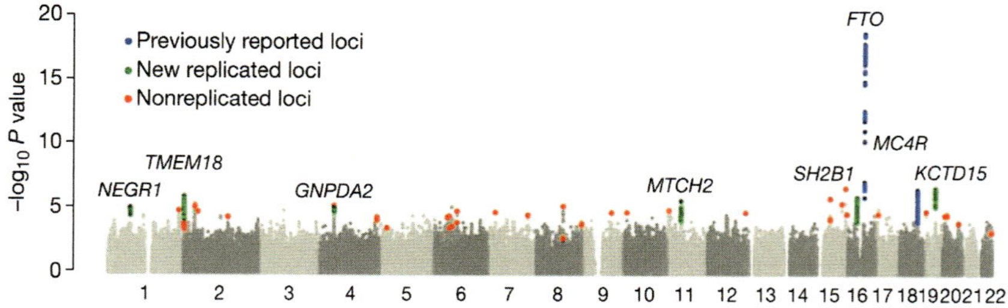

Fig. 5.2 Manhattan plot of the association between genome-wide data and BMI in the meta-analysis of the GIANT consortium. The $-\log_{10}P$ values for the association of each single nucleotide polymorphism with BMI are shown on the y-axis. The SNPs are plotted on the x-axis according to their chromosomal location. The SNPs that had previously been shown to associate with BMI are shown in *blue*. The SNPs that were taken forward from the discovery stage but did not replicate in the replication stage are shown in *red*. The six new loci that were replicated as new BMI hits are shown in *green*. Adapted from Ref. [16], with permission from Macmillan Publishers Ltd: Nature Genetics ©2009 (http://www.nature.com/ng/index.html)

typically shown as the $-\log_{10}$ of the P value, e.g., $P = 10^{-8}$ would be presented as "8" on the $-\log_{10}$ scale of the y-axis. The resulting plot is called a "Manhattan plot" (i.e., resembling the Manhattan skyline) (Fig. 5.2).

5.3 Three Waves of Discoveries

GWA studies have led to a rapid increase in the number of genetic loci implicated in predisposition to obesity. Three consecutive "waves" of discoveries can be distinguished, each characterized by a larger sample size and more confirmed loci compared to the preceding wave (Fig. 5.3).

The first wave in 2007 discovered the strongest known obesity risk locus so far, the fat mass and obesity-associated (*FTO*) gene [9–11]. Larger sample sizes were required in the identification of additional common variants with smaller effects, leading to extensive collaborative efforts and pooling of results from multiple genome-wide data sets. These genome-wide meta-analyses led to the identification of a locus near the melanocortin 4 receptor (*MC4R*) gene in the second wave of discoveries [12, 13] and to the detection of 17 more obesity loci in the third wave [14–18]. Altogether, these three waves of GWA studies have identified so far 19 new loci unequivocally associated with obesity-related traits.

5.3.1 First Wave – Discovery of FTO

The first wave of GWA studies was carried out in 2007 and consisted of three studies that each confirmed the *FTO* gene as the first gene unequivocally associated with common obesity. Although each of the three studies examined a different

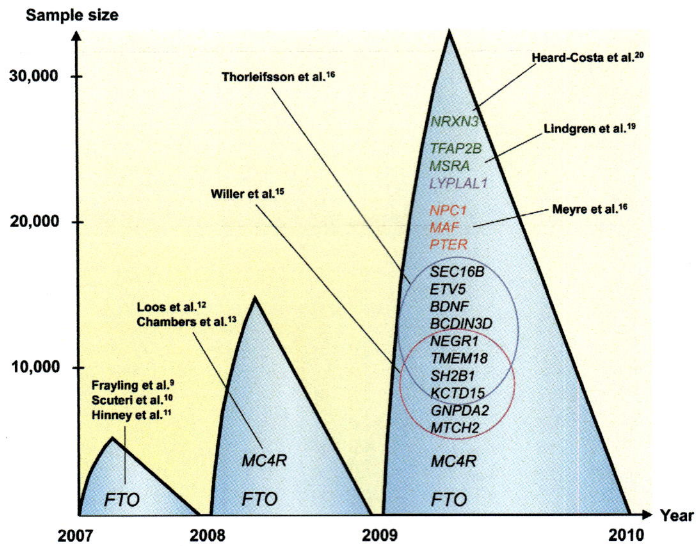

Fig. 5.3 Three waves of discoveries in genome-wide association studies on obesity-related traits. The loci discovered in genome-wide association studies for BMI, obesity risk, waist-to-hip ratio and waist circumference are shown in *black*, *red*, *purple*, and *green*, respectively

trait of interest, they all identified the same locus, reflecting the robustness of the observation.

Interestingly, the initial discovery was made with a GWA study for type 2 diabetes mellitus (T2DM), showing that SNPs in the first intron of *FTO* were highly significantly associated with T2DM [9]. Adjustment for BMI completely abolished the association between *FTO* and T2DM, indicating that the *FTO*–diabetes association was mediated through BMI. The association of *FTO* with BMI and obesity risk was subsequently confirmed in a meta-analysis of 13 cohorts, comprising 38,759 adults and children.

This initial report was soon followed by the publication of two other GWA studies, including a study on BMI among 4,741 Sardinians [10] and another on early-onset extreme obesity in 487 extremely obese young individuals and 442 healthy lean controls [11]. Both studies further confirmed *FTO* as the first robust obesity-susceptibility locus. Apart from *FTO*, several other variants that had been taken forward in these two GWA studies were not replicated in subsequent analyses [9–11].

5.3.2 Second Wave – Discovery of MC4R

The first wave of GWA studies was characterized by studies with relatively small sample sizes at the discovery stage that easily picked *FTO* as the low-hanging fruit. It was clear, however, that much larger sample sizes would be required to have sufficient statistical power for identifying additional common variants with smaller effects. As such, scientists from Europe and the USA combined forces and the GIANT (Genomic Investigation of Anthropometric Traits) consortium was launched [12]. The consortium combined data from seven studies to quadruple the sample size compared to the first wave of GWA studies. The resulting genome-wide meta-analysis, including 16,786 individuals of white European ancestry, confirmed *FTO* as the strongest signal and identified a new locus 188 kb downstream of the *MC4R* gene to be highly significantly associated with BMI and obesity risk. The *MC4R* gene (see Chapter 3) seemed an obvious candidate, as it is known to play a role in the hypothalamic regulation of food intake [19]. Furthermore, *MC4R* mutations are the commonest cause of monogenic obesity [20]. The same locus near *MC4R* was also identified in a relatively small GWA study of Indian-Asians ($n =$ 2,684) [13]. The higher frequency of the risk allele among Indian-Asians as compared to white Europeans (36% vs. 27%) may have provided the study sufficient statistical power to identify the association with a small sample at the discovery stage. The second wave of GWA studies thus confirmed a locus near the *MC4R* gene as the second locus robustly associated with obesity-related traits.

5.3.3 Third Wave – Discovery of Nine New Loci

For the third wave of discoveries, the discovery stage sample size of the GIANT consortium was doubled to 32,387 European adults [16]. Besides the confirmation of the *FTO* and near-*MC4R* loci as obesity-susceptibility loci, the meta-analysis additionally identified six new loci consistently associated with BMI. These include a locus near the neuronal growth regulator-1 (*NEGR1*), near the transmembrane protein 18 (*TMEM18*), in the SH2B adaptor protein-1 (*SH2B1*), near the potassium channel tetramerization domain containing-15 (*KCTD15*), near the glucosamine-6-phosphate deaminase-2 (*GNPDA2*), and in the mitochondrial carrier homologue-2 (*MTCH2*).

At the same time, the company deCODE genetics also performed a meta-analysis of four GWA studies for BMI, including 30,232 individuals of European descent and 1,160 African-Americans [15]. At the replication stage, eight new loci reached genome-wide significance, of which four (near *NEGR1*, near *TMEM18*, in *SH2B1*, near *KCTD15*) had also been identified by the GIANT consortium; while four others were new, including a locus in the SEC16 homologue-B (*SEC16B*), one between the ets variant-5 (*ETV5*) and diacylglycerol kinase (*DGKG*), one in brain-derived neurotrophic factor (*BDNF*), and one between the "BCDIN3 domain containing" (*BCDIN3D*) and the Fas apoptotic inhibitory molecule-2 (*FAIM2*).

While the GIANT consortium and deCODE genetics used BMI as the main outcome of their analyses, a third genome-wide association meta-analysis examined association with the risk of early-onset and morbid adult obesity in 1,380 cases and 1,416 controls [14]. Three new loci were identified, including in the

Niemann–Pick disease type C-1 (*NPC1*), near the v-maf musculoaponeurotic fibrosarcoma oncogene homologue (*MAF*), and near the phosphotriesterase related (*PTER*). In the replication stage it was shown that these loci also associate with BMI in population-based studies.

The GIANT consortium also performed a meta-analysis for measures of central obesity [17]. Two new loci were identified to be significantly associated with waist circumference: one locus near the transcription factor AP-2 beta (*TFAP2B*) and the second locus near the methionine sulfoxide reductase A (*MSRA*). A third locus near the lysophospholipase-like 1 (*LYPLAL1*) was associated with waist-to-hip ratio, but in women only. A second genome-wide association meta-analysis for waist circumference by the CHARGE (Cohorts for Heart and Aging Research in Genomic Epidemiology) consortium identified a fourth locus for central obesity in neurexin-3 (*NRXN3*) [18]. Of interest is that these four loci were also highly significantly associated with BMI [17, 18], suggesting that they not only affect central obesity but general obesity as well.

In summary, the three waves of genome-wide association studies for obesity-related traits have so far discovered 19 new susceptibility loci for common obesity in adults of white European descent.

5.4 Impact and Predictive Value of the Established Obesity Loci

The success of the three waves of GWA studies in 3 years has been tremendous, in particular when compared to the quantity of loci identified through 15 years of candidate gene and linkage studies. Obvious questions asked by the general public are whether the 19 established loci explain the heritability of BMI and whether they can predict a newborn's risk of obesity later in life.

Although the findings in GWA studies have been highly significant and reproducible in large population samples, the effect sizes of these new loci are rather small. The effect of genetic variation in intron 1 of the *FTO* gene is the strongest; each risk allele increases BMI by 0.26–0.66 kg/m^2 in individuals of European descent, equivalent to ~0.8–2.1 kg of body weight for a person 1.8 m tall (Table 5.1). The per-allele effect sizes for the other 18 established loci vary between 0.07 and 0.25 kg/m^2 for BMI (between ~230 and 810 g in body weight) in European populations (Table 5.1).

So far, only one large-scale study has been reported on the combined effect of 12 established obesity loci. In a population-based study of 20,000 adult men and women from the UK, a genetic predisposition risk score was calculated by summing the number of risk alleles carried by each individual [21]. Each additional risk allele increased the BMI by 0.15 kg/m^2 (or 444 g in body weight) and the risk of obesity by 10.8%. The average BMI of individuals with a high susceptibility (i.e., those carrying 17 or more risk alleles; 1.4% of the population) was 1.53 kg/m^2 (~5.7 kg of body weight) higher than of those with a low genetic susceptibility (those carrying six or fewer risk alleles; 1% of the population) [21]. This difference

Table 5.1 Genetic loci identified in large-scale high-density genome-wide association studies for BMI and extreme obesity

Nearest gene(s)	Chromosome	SNP[a]	BMI-Increasing allele	frequency (%)[b]	Effect size (kg/m^2)[c]	References
Near *NEGR1*	1p31	rs2815752	A	64	0.10–0.13	[15, 16]
SEC16B	1q25	rs10913469	C	25	0.11	[15]
Near *LYPLAL1*	1q41	rs2605100	G	69	0.06[d]	[17]
Near *TMEM18*	2p25	rs6548238	C	85	0.10–0.15	[15, 16]
Between *ETV5* and *DGKG*	3q27	rs7647305	C	80	0.19	[15]
Near *GNPDA2*	4p13	rs10938397	G	45	0.19	[16]
Near *TFAP2B*	6p12	rs987237	G	16	0.14[d]	[17]
Near *MSRA*	8p23	rs7826222	G	18	0.15[d]	[17]
Near *PTER*	10p12	rs10508503	C	91	0.07	[14]
MTCH2	11p11	rs10838738	G	36	0.07	[16]
BDNF	11p14	rs4923461	A	77	0.19	[15]
Between *BCDIN3D* and *FAIM2*	12q13	rs7138803	A	35	0.09	[15]
NRXN3	14q31	rs10146997	G	21	0.10	[18]
SH2B1	16p11	rs7498665	G	38	0.15	[15, 16]
FTO	16q12	rs9939609	A	46	0.26–0.66	[9, 10, 11]
Near *MAF*	16q23	rs1424233	A	56	0.13	[14]
NPC1	18q11	rs1805081	A	53	0.14	[14]
Near *MC4R*	18q21	rs17782313	C	27	0.22–0.25	[12, 13]
Near *KCTD15*	19q13	rs29941	C	68	0.06–0.17	[15, 16]

Effect sizes represent the increase in body mass index (BMI) for each additional risk allele. Effect sizes were derived from the replication stage of the genome-wide association studies, except for Frayling et al. [9], Scuteri et al. [10], Loos et al. [12], and Heard Costa et al. [18]

[a]Other SNPs in the same haplotype (correlating SNPs) show similar association

[b]Frequency of the BMI-increasing allele in the CEU Population (European ancestry) of the HapMap Phase III

[c]For loci for which the effect size was not reported in absolute BMI value, the effect size was estimated from z-scores, assuming a SD of 4.3 kg/m^2

[d]Effect size calculated from the effect size on waist circumference (*TFAP2B* and *MSRA*) or waist-to-hip ratio (*LYPLAL1*)

is substantial and solely due to difference in genetic background. However, it should be highlighted that it only compares the 1–2% extremes of the population. The 12 loci explained only 0.9% of the inter-individual variation in BMI in the total population [21]. This study also estimated the predictive value to obesity using these 12 loci by calculating the area under the receiver operating characteristic (ROC) curve (AUC). The ROC-AUC can vary between 0.50 (no predictive value) and 1 (perfect prediction). In this cross-sectional study, the AUC was estimated to be 0.574, suggesting that these 12 loci cannot be used to predict whether an individual will be obese or not.

5.5 Follow-Up and Functional Characterization of the Established Loci

While the effect sizes of the newly established obesity loci are small and the explained variance and predictive values are low, the primary value and implementation of this new knowledge lies in increasing our understanding of the physiological pathways through which they increase the risk of obesity.

A systematic follow-up of the associations of the newly identified loci with more refined obesity-related traits such as body fat percentage and fat distribution and with intermediary traits that are assumed to induce weight gain, such as physical activity behavior and dietary intake, may lead to new insights into the physiological mechanisms of these loci. Apart from follow-up through epidemiological studies, the functional characterization of the loci in molecular and physiological studies, such as transgenic animal models or cellular over-expression studies, may unlock doors to new, larger biological pathways that may even point to pharmaceutical targets.

As the flurry of discoveries is very recent, the physiological mechanisms that link the genetic loci to weight gain are not yet well understood. However, new insights into the functions of the *FTO* gene have started to accumulate. *FTO* encodes a 2-oxoglutarate-dependent nucleic acid demethylase that catalyses the demethylation of 3-methylthymine in single-stranded DNA [22, 23]. In rodents, *FTO* mRNA expression is particularly abundant in the hypothalamic nuclei that control energy balance in the brain and its expression is dependent on the energy state [22, 24, 25]. Studies in humans have supported this neuronal hypothesis as *FTO* SNPs were found to be associated with increased appetite, reduced satiety, and higher energy intake [26–30]. More recent data in mice, however, has challenged the earlier findings by providing strong evidence of a peripheral role of *FTO*. Loss of *FTO* in mice leads to a significant reduction in adipose tissue and lean body mass as a consequence of increased energy expenditure and systemic sympathetic activation [31]. *FTO* may thus affect adiposity through controlling energy expenditure. So far, most studies in humans have not been able to confirm association between *FTO* and resting energy expenditure [26, 27, 30, 32–34]. In healthy women, however, lipolytic activity was reported to be lower in carriers of the *FTO* risk allele, independent of BMI, which supports the hypothesis of a peripheral role of *FTO* [35].

The *MC4R* gene is an obvious candidate gene as *MC4R* mutations are the commonest cause of monogenic early-onset obesity [20] (see Chapter 3). However, the recently established locus is located as far as 188 kb downstream from the *MC4R* gene. Although it has not yet been confirmed whether the observed associations with obesity risk indeed reflect *MC4R* function, the association of this locus with increased height and childhood obesity is consistent with the phenotype seen in severe coding mutations in *MC4R* [12].

The physiological implications of most of the remaining 17 loci remain largely unexplored. Nevertheless, a few preliminary insights are available. For example, several of the established obesity loci locate in or near genes that are highly expressed or known to act in the brain and hypothalamus, emphasizing the role of the central nervous system in control of body weight. Also, the *SH2B1* and *BDNF* genes have a fairly strong biological candidacy. Sh2b-knockout mice develop obesity through an effect on leptin signaling [36], and genetic variation in *BDNF* has previously been associated with eating behavior and BMI in candidate gene studies [37].

For many of the established loci, the associated variants are located in noncoding regions, rather than in the amino acid coding part of the gene [12, 14–17]. This might indicate that these variants play a role in the up- or down-regulation of genes from a distance. Alternatively, it suggests that the identified variants are not causal but correlate with the causal variants that are located in genes nearby.

Indeed, pinpointing the causal variants of the established obesity loci is one of the major challenges for future research. Fine-mapping of a genetic signal to identify the causal variant is a laborious process, which requires deep sequencing of the surrounding region, followed by the genotyping of numerous variants of interest in a population sufficiently large to provide the statistical power for distinguishing between association signals. Some loci span very large regions in the genome, sometimes with a complex genetic architecture, making the task even more challenging. Furthermore, in some cases where SNPs are highly correlated, fine-mapping the causal variant may be impossible. The study of different ethnicities with a distinct pattern of SNP correlations [38] may help in such situations.

5.6 Clinical Applications

Despite the small effects of the 19 established obesity loci on BMI, their discovery promises to provide new insights into the complex physiology that governs the regulation of energy balance, and may provide new opportunities for the development of new therapies in the future. The discovery of *SUR1* and *PPARG* genes, the molecular targets of two commonly used glucose-lowering drugs, as susceptibility loci for type 2 diabetes, elegantly demonstrates that variants with very modest effects provide important clues to key drug targets [39].

As new GWA studies will identify more loci, the risk prediction of obesity may improve in the future. However, given that the genes and lifestyle both contribute equally to the risk of obesity, it remains to be seen whether genetic loci will ever be able to accurately predict obesity risk.

Therefore, the most important contribution of the newly identified loci is likely toward increasing our understanding of the physiological mechanisms that underlie the risk of developing obesity. The current state of knowledge is, however, many steps from clinical applications, and extensive efforts are still required to translate the new discoveries into mainstream health care.

5.7 Approaches for Identifying More Loci for Obesity Through GWA Studies

Despite the revolutionary success of GWA studies in discovering new susceptibility loci for obesity, the "missing heritability" suggests that many more loci are likely to be uncovered. Various approaches have been proposed for identifying these additional loci through GWA studies.

5.7.1 Increased Sample Size

The statistical power of GWA studies to identify new loci depends largely on the sample size at the discovery stage. Current GWA studies, with up to 35,000 samples, have been able to identify only genetic loci of which the smallest effect size was 0.06 kg/m^2 and lowest minor allele frequency was 9%. To identify variants that are less frequent and/or have smaller effects, GWA studies need to be scaled up. Therefore, in the upcoming fourth wave of GWA studies, the sample size of the discovery stage GIANT consortium will be increased to >120,000 individuals, i.e., fourfold compared to the studies in the third wave [16]. These extensive efforts are likely to lead to the discovery of multiple new obesity-susceptibility loci.

5.7.2 Studies in Populations of Different Ethnic Backgrounds

The vast majority of GWA studies for obesity-related traits have been performed in populations of white European ancestry. As the genetic architecture, including the frequency of genetic variants and the correlation between them, differs across ethnicities and also the genetic effects may vary, the statistical power to identify new loci may vary across populations of different ancestry. Therefore, the study of ethnicities other than white European may provide new opportunities to discover additional obesity-susceptibility loci. This is elegantly illustrated by the GWA studies in Indian-Asians, which needed only 2,684 individuals at the discovery stage to identify the near *MC4R* locus, whereas the GWA studies in white Europeans required 16,876 individuals to find the same locus [12]. The higher frequency of the risk allele in Indian-Asians (36%) compared to white Europeans (27%) likely provided the former more power to identify this locus with a smaller sample size.

5.7.3 Genome-Wide Association Studies in Children and Adolescents

So far, only one relatively small GWA studies on the risk of early obesity has been reported [11]. By comparing 487 extremely obese children and adolescents to 442 healthy lean controls, this genome-wide association study could only confirm the *FTO* locus.

As genetic effects vary over the life course and sometimes they may be larger during childhood because of limited environmental influence, performing GWA studies in children and adolescents might be another avenue to reveal new obesity-susceptibility loci.

A longitudinal study on the influence of the *FTO* and *MC4R* loci in a birth cohort born in 1946 showed that the effects of both loci increased during childhood and adolescence, reaching its largest impact at around the age of 20 years, followed by a subsequent weakening of the effect throughout adulthood [40]. These findings suggest that the genetic effects vary over the life course. Alternatively, they might reflect the effects of a time period.

5.7.4 Studies on Other Obesity-Related Traits than BMI

BMI is an inexpensive, non-invasive measure of obesity that is available in most cohorts [41]. Hence, it has been the most commonly studied outcome in recent GWA studies. However, BMI is also a heterogeneous phenotype that is affected by varying proportions of lean mass and is thus not a very accurate measure of adiposity at the individual level. By using more accurate measures of adiposity, such as body fat percentage, the power to detect new loci may be increased. However, such measures are often more expensive and harder to obtain and will be available in few cohorts. Whether the gain in power through improved measurement accuracy compensates for the loss in power due to smaller sample size remains to be determined in upcoming GWA studies for other traits, e.g., body fat percentage.

5.7.5 Studies on the Risk of Obesity

GWA studies on the risk of obesity may also identify loci that are different from those identified through analyses of BMI. The increase in the prevalence of obesity in Western populations seems mainly to be driven by individuals who were already above the median of the BMI distribution of the population, whereas the median BMI has increased less over time [42, 43]. Thus, the BMI distribution is becoming more and more right-skewed. This suggests that the genetic susceptibility to gain weight in an obesogenic environment lies particularly in those who are already at the extreme right of the BMI distribution. Therefore, case–control analyses that compare obese with non-obese individuals may identify loci that are different from those identified with BMI.

5.7.6 Studies on Intermediary Traits of Obesity

Obesity-susceptibility loci will lead to increased BMI through their effects on energy balance. GWA studies of physical activity (i.e., energy expenditure) and dietary factors (i.e., energy intake) could reveal new obesity-predisposing loci than that may not be identified by studying BMI.

The only GWA study for leisure-time exercise behavior that has been performed so far included 1,644 Dutch and 978 American individuals that were interchangeably used as a both discovery and a replication cohort [44]. Although the analyses suggested association with exercise behavior of SNPs in the 3′-phosphoadenosine 5′-phosphosulfate synthase-2 (*PAPSS2*), near spermatogenesis-associated serine-rich 2-like (*SPATS2L*), and near chromosome 18 open reading frame-2 (*C18orf2*) loci, none of the loci reached genome-wide significance.

The main challenge when studying intermediate traits such as physical activity and food intake is the measurement of these traits in an accurate and objective manner. Most often questionnaires are used that differ across studies. This inaccuracy and heterogeneity of measurements will lower the power and hamper pooling of data for meta-analyses. Therefore, harmonization of measures of lifestyle factors across studies will be essential to achieve a uniform phenotype that can be meta-analysed across cohorts.

5.7.7 Studies on Gene–Lifestyle Interaction

Obesity-susceptibility loci may interact with lifestyle factors such that genetically susceptible individuals gain more weight in an obesogenic environment than those who are genetically protected. GWA studies that take lifestyle factors into account may therefore identify obesity loci that have previously not been identified.

Genome-wide gene–lifestyle interaction studies will identify obesity-susceptibility loci that are environment-sensitive, e.g., the effect of these loci may be more pronounced in individuals who live an unhealthy lifestyle, while they may have no influence in individuals who live a healthy lifestyle.

So far, no genome-wide gene–lifestyle interaction studies for BMI or obesity risk have been reported. Similar to GWA studies of intermediate traits, described above, gene–environment interaction studies will require the harmonization of lifestyle measures before data can be combined in meta-analyses large enough to detect interaction effects, which typically require sample sizes larger than those needed for the study of main effects [45, 46].

Thus far, gene–lifestyle interaction studies have focused on *FTO*. Four studies have reported significant interaction between a *FTO* variant and physical activity on the level of BMI [34, 47–49]. In these studies, the BMI-increasing effect of *FTO* was more pronounced in sedentary individuals compared to physically active individuals, suggesting that the genetic susceptibility toward obesity induced by *FTO* can be overcome, at least in part, by adopting a physically active lifestyle.

5.7.8 Replication of Variants with Less Stringent Significance Thresholds

Typically stringent *P* value thresholds are used to decide which loci are taken forward from the discovery stage to the replication stage to avoid too many false-positive findings at replication [8]. However, true loci may well be hidden among the variants not reaching these stringent *P* value cut-offs. To validate such variants, several large-scale consortia that study metabolic traits, including anthropometric traits, lipids, glucose and insulin levels, cardiovascular disease, and T2DM, have developed a custom-made SNP chip of 200,000 SNPs, called the "MetaboChip". This chip contains SNPs of which significance just missed the threshold to be taken forward for replication in well-powered GWA studies for metabolic and cardiovascular disease and traits. Because of the less significant levels of association, replication of the MetaboChip SNPs will require even larger sample sizes than those needed in GWA studies. It is hoped that the low cost of this chip (~$40) will encourage many research groups to participate in this extensive collaborative effort to identify more susceptibility loci.

5.7.9 Genome-Wide Association of Copy Number Variants (CNVs)

Copy number variants are genomic sequences of roughly 1 kb to 3 Mb in size which are deleted or duplicated in varying numbers. Although not as frequent as SNPs, CNVs occur commonly in the human genome [50], and the extent to which CNVs might contribute to common disease is currently uncertain. Nevertheless, two genome-wide CNV association studies found convincing evidence of a rare, highly penetrant 593-kb deletion at chromosome 16p11.2 to be associated with morbid obesity (BMI $\geq$ 40 kg/m^2) [51, 52]. This deletion encompasses the *SH2B1* gene that was previously found to be associated with diet-induced obesity in sh2b-knockout mice. Common variants near this gene have also been identified in GWA studies for BMI of common obesity [16]. These findings highlight the value of using a variety of strategies to increase our insights into the genetic architecture of human obesity.

5.7.10 More Comprehensive Genotyping Chips

GWA studies have so far relied on the "common disease, common variant" hypothesis, i.e., genetic influences on common diseases and traits are attributable to "common" (present in >1% of the population) SNPs [53–55]. However, there may be disease-causing variants that are less frequent, as illustrated by the CNV analysis in morbidly obese patients [51, 52].

While the International HapMap catalogues most of the common genetic variations of the human genome, it does not capture rarer variants. To that extend, a new project called the 1,000 Genomes Project was started in January 2008 [56]. The project is another international collaboration that involves the sequencing of more than 1,000 genomes of people from around the world. This will allow identifying the less frequent variants that are currently not available in the HapMap [56]. The project is expected to reveal new loci by increasing the detection of rare genetic variants and by providing a new resource for the next generation of genome-wide chips.

5.8 Conclusions

With GWA studies, gene discovery for common obesity has entered a new era. Altogether 19 new susceptibility loci have been discovered during the past 3 years, and the findings promise to provide valuable new insights into the pathophysiological mechanisms and pathways that underlie obesity development. The currently identified loci explain only a fraction of the inter-individual variability in BMI, suggesting that many new loci remain to be found. Translating the accumulating genetic discoveries into mainstream health care remains a challenge ahead. First, we need to learn more about the causal variants and the physiological pathways through which they confer obesity.

References

1. Maes HH, Neale MC, Eaves LJ. Genetic and environmental factors in relative body weight and human adiposity. Behav Genet. Jul 1997;27(4):325–51.
2. Lander ES, Schork NJ. Genetic dissection of complex traits. Science. Sep 1994;265(5181):2037–48.
3. Loos RJ. Recent progress in the genetics of common obesity. Br J Clin Pharmacol. Dec 2009;68(6):811–29.
4. Pearson TA, Manolio TA. How to interpret a genome-wide association study. JAMA. Mar 2008;299(11):1335–44.
5. International human genome sequencing consortium. Finishing the euchromatic sequence of the human genome. Nature Oct 2004;431(7011):931–45.
6. A haplotype map of the human genome. Nature Oct 2005;437(7063):1299–320.
7. Frazer KA, Ballinger DG, Cox DR, et al. A second generation human haplotype map of over 3.1 million SNPs. Nature. Oct 2007;449(7164):851–61.
8. de Bakker PI, Ferreira MA, Jia X, Neale BM, Raychaudhuri S, Voight BF. Practical aspects of imputation-driven meta-analysis of genome-wide association studies. Hum Mol Genet. Oct 2008;17(R2):R122–8.
9. Frayling TM, Timpson NJ, Weedon MN, et al. A common variant in the FTO gene is associated with body mass index and predisposes to childhood and adult obesity. Science. May 2007;316(5826):889–94.
10. Scuteri A, Sanna S, Chen WM, et al. Genome-wide association scan shows genetic variants in the FTO gene are associated with obesity-related traits. PLoS Genet. Jul 2007;3(7):e115.
11. Hinney A, Nguyen TT, Scherag A, et al. Genome wide association (GWA) study for early onset extreme obesity supports the role of fat mass and obesity associated gene (FTO) variants. PLoS One. 2007;2(12):e1361.
12. Loos RJ, Lindgren CM, Li S, et al. Common variants near MC4R are associated with fat mass, weight and risk of obesity. Nat Genet. Jun 2008;40(6):768–75.
13. Chambers JC, Elliott P, Zabaneh D, et al. Common genetic variation near MC4R is associated with waist circumference and insulin resistance. Nat Genet. Jun 2008;40(6):716–8.
14. Meyre D, Delplanque J, Chevre JC, et al. Genome-wide association study for early-onset and morbid adult obesity identifies three new risk loci in European populations. Nat Genet. Feb 2009;41(2):157–9.
15. Thorleifsson G, Walters GB, Gudbjartsson DF, et al. Genome-wide association yields new sequence variants at seven loci that associate with measures of obesity. Nat Genet. Jan 2009;41(1):18–24.
16. Willer CJ, Speliotes EK, Loos RJ, et al. Six new loci associated with body mass index highlight a neuronal influence on body weight regulation. Nat Genet. Jan 2009;41(1):25–34.

17. Lindgren CM, Heid IM, Randall JC, et al. Genome-wide association scan meta-analysis identifies three Loci influencing adiposity and fat distribution. PLoS Genet. Jun 2009;5(6):e1000508.
18. Heard-Costa NL, Zillikens MC, Monda KL, et al. NRXN3 is a novel locus for waist circumference: a genome-wide association study from the CHARGE Consortium. PLoS Genet. Jun 2009;5(6):e1000539.
19. Huszar D, Lynch CA, Fairchild-Huntress V, et al. Targeted disruption of the melanocortin-4 receptor results in obesity in mice. Cell. Jan 1997;88(1):131–41.
20. Farooqi IS, Keogh JM, Yeo GS, Lank EJ, Cheetham T, O'Rahilly S. Clinical spectrum of obesity and mutations in the melanocortin 4 receptor gene. N Engl J Med. Mar 2003;348(12):1085–95.
21. Li S, Zhao JH, Luan J, et al. Cumulative effects and predictive value of common obesity-susceptibility variants identified by genome-wide association studies. Am J Clin Nutr. Jan 2010;91(1):184–90.
22. Gerken T, Girard CA, Tung YC, et al. The obesity-associated FTO gene encodes a 2-oxoglutarate-dependent nucleic acid demethylase. Science. Nov 2007;318(5855):1469–72.
23. Sanchez-Pulido L, Andrade-Navarro MA The FTO (fat mass and obesity associated) gene codes for a novel member of the non-heme dioxygenase superfamily. BMC Biochem. 2007;8:23.
24. Fredriksson R, Hagglund M, Olszewski PK, et al. The obesity gene, FTO, is of ancient origin, up-regulated during food deprivation and expressed in neurons of feeding-related nuclei of the brain. Endocrinology. May 2008;149(5):2062–71.
25. Stratigopoulos G, Padilla SL, LeDuc CA, et al. Regulation of Fto/Ftm gene expression in mice and humans. Am J Physiol Regul Integr Comp Physiol. Apr 2008;294(4):R1185–96.
26. Cecil JE, Tavendale R, Watt P, Hetherington MM, Palmer CN. An obesity-associated FTO gene variant and increased energy intake in children. N Engl J Med. Dec 2008;359(24): 2558–66.
27. Haupt A, Thamer C, Staiger H, et al. Variation in the FTO gene influences food intake but not energy expenditure. Exp Clin Endocrinol Diab. Apr 2009;117(4):194–7.
28. Timpson NJ, Emmett PM, Frayling TM, et al. The fat mass- and obesity-associated locus and dietary intake in children. Am J Clin Nutr. Oct 2008;88(4):971–8.
29. Wardle J, Carnell S, Haworth CM, Farooqi IS, O'Rahilly S, Plomin R. Obesity associated genetic variation in FTO is associated with diminished satiety. J Clin Endocrinol Metab. Sep 2008;93(9):3640–3.
30. Wardle J, Llewellyn C, Sanderson S, Plomin R. The FTO gene and measured food intake in children. Int J Obes (Lond). Jan 2009;33(1):42–5.
31. Fischer J, Koch L, Emmerling C, et al. Inactivation of the Fto gene protects from obesity. Nature. Apr 16 2009;458(7240):894–8.
32. Berentzen T, Kring SI, Holst C, et al. Lack of association of fatness-related FTO gene variants with energy expenditure or physical activity. J Clin Endocrinol Metab. Jul 2008;93(7):2904–8.
33. Hakanen M, Raitakari OT, Lehtimäki T, et al. FTO genotype is associated with body mass index after the age of 7 years but not with energy intake or leisure-time physical activity. J Clin Endocrinol Metab. Apr 2009;94(4):1281–7.
34. Rampersaud E, Mitchell BD, Pollin TI, et al. Physical activity and the association of common FTO gene variants with body mass index and obesity. Arch Intern Med. Sep 2008;168(16):1791–7.
35. Wahlen K, Sjolin E, Hoffstedt J. The common rs9939609 gene variant of the fat mass- and obesity-associated gene FTO is related to fat cell lipolysis. J Lipid Res. Mar 2008;49(3): 607–11.
36. Ren D, Zhou Y, Morris D, Li M, Li Z, Rui L. Neuronal SH2B1 is essential for controlling energy and glucose homeostasis. J Clin Invest. Feb 2007;117(2):397–406.
37. Shugart YY, Chen L, Day IN, et al. Two British women studies replicated the association between the Val66Met polymorphism in the brain-derived neurotrophic factor (BDNF) and BMI. Eur J Hum Genet. Aug 2009;17(8):1050–5.

38. Gabriel SB, Schaffner SF, Nguyen H, et al. The structure of haplotype blocks in the human genome. Science. Jun 2002;296(5576):2225–9.
39. Moore AF, Florez JC. Genetic susceptibility to type 2 diabetes and implications for antidiabetic therapy. Annu Rev Med. Feb 2008;59:95–111.
40. Hardy R, Wills AK, Wong A, et al. Life course variations in the associations between FTO and MC4R gene variants and body size. Hum Mol Genet. Feb 2010;19(3):545–52.
41. Bouchard C. BMI, fat mass, abdominal adiposity and visceral fat: where is the "beef"?. Int J Obes (Lond). Oct 2007;31(10):1552–3.
42. Flegal KM. Epidemiologic aspects of overweight and obesity in the United States. Physiol Behav. Dec 2005;86(5):599–602.
43. National Center for Health Statistics. 2008 – With Chartbook on Trends in the Health of Americans; Centers for Disease Control and Prevention, Health, United States, 2008.
44. DE Moor MH, Liu YJ, Boomsma DI, et al. Genome-wide association study of exercise behavior in dutch and American adults. Med Sci Sports Exerc. Oct 2009;41(10):1887–95.
45. Luan JA, Wong MY, Day NE, Wareham NJ. Sample size determination for studies of gene-environment interaction. Int J Epidemiol. Oct 2001;30(5):1035–40.
46. Wong MY, Day NE, Luan JA, Chan KP, Wareham NJ. The detection of gene-environment interaction for continuous traits: should we deal with measurement error by bigger studies or better measurement? Int J Epidemiol Feb 2003;32(1):51–7.
47. Andreasen CH, Stender-Petersen KL, Mogensen MS, et al. Low physical activity accentuates the effect of the FTO rs9939609 polymorphism on body fat accumulation. Diabetes. Jan 2008;57(1):95–101.
48. Cauchi S, Stutzmann F, Cavalcanti-Proenca C, et al. Combined effects of MC4R and FTO common genetic variants on obesity in European general populations. J Mol Med. May 2009;87(5):537–46.
49. Vimaleswaran KS, Li S, Zhao JH, et al. Physical activity attenuates the body mass index-increasing influence of genetic variation in the FTO gene. Am J Clin Nutr. Aug 2009;90(2):425–8.
50. Tuzun E, Sharp AJ, Bailey JA, et al. Fine-scale structural variation of the human genome. Nat Genet. Jul 2005;37(7):727–32.
51. Bochukova EG, Huang N, Keogh J, et al. Large, rare chromosomal deletions associated with severe early-onset obesity. Nature. Feb 2010;463(7281):666–70.
52. Walters RG, Jacquemont S, Valsesia A, et al. A new highly penetrant form of obesity due to deletions on chromosome 16p11.2. Nature. Feb 2010;463(7281):671–5.
53. Collins FS, Guyer MS, Charkravarti A. Variations on a theme: cataloging human DNA sequence variation. Science. Nov 1997;278(5343):1580–1.
54. Pritchard JK. Are rare variants responsible for susceptibility to complex diseases?. Am J Hum Genet Jul 2001;69(1):124–37.
55. Reich DE, Lander ES. On the allelic spectrum of human disease. Trends Genet. Sep 2001;17(9):502–10.
56. Via M, Gignoux C, Burchard EG. The 1,000 genomes project: new opportunities for research and social challenges. Genome Med. Jan 2010;2(1):3.

Part II
Epigenetic Changes and the Development of Obesity

Chapter 6
Known Clinical Epigenetic Disorders with an Obesity Phenotype: Prader–Willi Syndrome and the *GNAS* Locus

Merlin G. Butler

6.1 Introduction

Prader–Willi syndrome (PWS) is a neurodevelopmental disorder characterized by infantile hypotonia, feeding difficulties, hypogonadism and hypogenitalism, mental deficiency (average IQ of 65), behavioral problems (skin picking, stubbornness, temper tantrums), short stature with small hands and feet due to growth hormone deficiency, hypopigmentation, hyperphagia in early childhood with subsequent obesity, and a characteristic facial appearance (narrow bifrontal diameter, short upturned nose, downturned corners of the mouth, almond-shaped eyes, sticky saliva, and enamel hypoplasia). PWS arises from lack of expression of paternally inherited genes known to be imprinted in the chromosome 15q11–q13 region. This syndrome is considered the most common genetic condition leading to life-threatening obesity and estimated to occur at a frequency of 1 in 10,000–20,000 individuals. An estimated 350,000–400,000 people are affected worldwide. PWS has been observed in all races and ethnic groups, but reported disproportionately more in Caucasians [1–3].

A de novo paternally derived chromosome 15q11–q13 deletion is seen in about 70% of PWS subjects, while maternal disomy 15 (both 15 s from the mother) accounts for about 25% of cases, and the remaining individuals have imprinting defects (either microdeletions or epimutations) in the imprinting center located in the 15q11–q13 region or from chromosome 15 translocations. Most cases are sporadic with recurrence of less than 1%; however, the risk might be much higher (e.g., 50%) in those PWS families in which the father carries an imprinting center defect due to a microdeletion inherited from his mother. PWS and Angelman syndrome (an entirely different clinical syndrome generally due to a maternally derived deletion of the 15q11–q13 region) were the first examples in humans of genomic imprinting or the differential expression of genetic information depending on the parent of origin [4].

M.G. Butler (✉)
Departments of Psychiatry & Behavioral Sciences and Pediatrics, Kansas University Medical Center, Kansas City, KS, USA
e-mail: mbutler4@kumc.edu

R.H. Lustig (ed.), *Obesity Before Birth*, Endocrine Updates 30,
DOI 10.1007/978-1-4419-7034-3_6,

Adipogenesis and obesity are determined before birth by epigenetics in PWS and other obesity-related disorders. Epigenetics refers to the heritable but reversible regulation of various genetic functions including gene expression influenced by stochastic and environmental factors. The epigenetic status of a gene can be tissue specific and developmentally regulated but essential for normal cellular development and differentiation. The epigenetic process is mediated through modifications of DNA and histones through mechanisms usually involving methylation without altering the DNA sequence. Other clinical disorders in humans due to genomic imprinting exist besides PWS and Angelman syndrome, including Silver–Russell syndrome, Beckwith–Weidemann syndrome, Albright hereditary osteodystrophy, and uniparental disomy 14. Specific information regarding the known clinical epigenetic disorders with obesity will be discussed in this chapter. These include PWS and chromosome 15, along with epigenetic defects involving the complex *GNAS* gene locus on chromosome 20 causing Albright hereditary osteodystrophy (pseudohypoparathyroidism – PHP and pseudopseudohypoparathyroidism – PPHP) and McCune–Albright syndrome.

6.2 Genomic Imprinting

Genomic imprinting, a process first described in plant genetics and not recognized in humans until its discovery in PWS, is an epigenetic phenomenon whereby the phenotype is modified depending on the parental sex contributing the allele. It involves methylation of cytosine bases in the CpG dinucleotides of the DNA molecule and the regulatory elements of genes. Nearly all imprinted genes have a CpG-rich differentially methylated region (DMR) which usually relates to allele repression. Epigenetic changes (such as methylation) to genes arise during gametogenesis and result in altered gene expression, dependent on the parent of origin, producing monoallelic expression of either the maternal or paternal allele of a particular imprinted locus known to affect animal growth, development, and viability. This process is reversible in gametogenesis by marking a genomic sequence that is parent specific. Many imprinted genes are arranged in clusters (imprinted domains) on different chromosomes and are under the control of an imprinting center [5–7].

The expression of imprinted genes may be tissue- and stage specific with one of the parental alleles being differentially expressed only at a specific developmental stage or in certain cells. The transcription rate of genes that influence growth can be regulated by the imprinting process through a fine balance between the expression of the two parental alleles. However, genomic imprints are erased in both germlines and reset accordingly and are reversible depending on the parent of origin. This leads to differential expression in the course of development. DNA methylation patterns are established and maintained during development by three distinct DNA cytosine methyltransferases (Dnmt1, Dnmt3a, and Dnmt3b). In mammalian somatic cells, cytosine methylation occurs in 60–80% of all CpG dinucleotides that are not randomly distributed in the genome. Heavily methylated heterochromatin and repetitive sequences appear to contribute to gene silencing while most CpG islands located at the promoter regions of active genes are methylation free [6, 8, 9].

About 1% of all mammalian genes are thought to be imprinted while many imprinted genes are candidates for human diseases including cancer, obesity, and diabetes. A genome-wide search for imprinted genes in the human genome identified over 150 imprinted genes involving 115 chromosome bands for at least 100 conditions due to inappropriate genetic alterations, including deletions of genes or uniparental disomy of chromosome regions [8, 9].

Imprinted genes are targets for environmental factors, including nutrition influencing expression through epigenetics without changing the DNA nucleotide coding structure. When imprinted genes are clustered together and under the regulation of a single imprinting-controlling element, it suggests a possible involvement of higher order regulatory elements for allelic-specific DNA replication. In addition, genes contributed by the mother generally replicate or express at different rates than genes contributed by the father. Many imprinted genes are known to be growth factors, such as insulin-like growth factors (e.g., *IGF2* in Beckwith–Wiedemann syndrome), or as regulators of gene expression controlling growth (e.g., the *GRB10* gene in Silver–Russell syndrome). Paternally expressed genes generally enhance growth, whereas maternally expressed genes appear to suppress growth. Therefore, imprinting disorders are associated with both genetic (e.g., deletions) and epigenetic mutations or defects including disruption of DNA methylation within the imprinting controlling regions of these genes. The process of turning on and off genes, particularly developmental genes, is ongoing throughout the life cycle of mammals and is influenced by tissue specificity and timing. Understanding DNA methylation and gene regulation impacted by the environment and epigenetic mechanisms will be important to identify and treat human disorders due to errors in genomic imprinting.

6.3 Genetic Subtypes and Clinical Differences in PWS

6.3.1 Genetics

In 1956, Prader, Labhart, and Willi [10] were the first to report this syndrome, while Ledbetter and others [11] in 1981 were the first to report an interstitial deletion of the proximal long arm of chromosome 15 including the 15q11–q13 region. Butler and Palmer [12] in 1983 were the first to report that the origin of the chromosome 15 deletion was de novo in origin or due to a new event and found that the chromosome 15 leading to the deletion was donated only from the father. Later in 1989, Nicholls, Butler, and others [13] reported that PWS individuals with normal appearing chromosome 15s had both 15s inherited from the mother and coined the term *maternal disomy 15*. Maternal disomy 15 is the second most frequent genetic finding in PWS due to an error in meiosis with two maternal chromosome 15s in the oocyte and fertilized by a sperm with one chromosome 15. This leads to a zygote with trisomy 15, which is not compatible with development. Trisomy 15 is a relatively common cause of early miscarriages. Through a trisomy rescue event, one of the two maternal chromosome 15s will be lost from the trisomic cell in two-thirds of the trisomic 15 pregnancies. This results in a normal set of chromosomes. However, in the remaining one-third of trisomic 15 pregnancies through a trisomy rescue event, the paternal chromosome 15 is lost leaving the cell with two maternal chromosome 15s and a normal count of 46 chromosomes. Thus, the fetus is delivered with PWS and normal cytogenetic findings, but with maternal disomy 15.

Maternal disomy 15 causing PWS is of two types: heterodisomy and isodisomy. The disomic type may also impact on the pregnancy and clinical outcome. Most PWS subjects with maternal disomy 15 have the heterodisomic form. Maternal heterodisomy occurs when the baby inherits each of the mother's two chromosome 15s. Maternal isodisomy results when two identical chromosome 15s are inherited from the mother as a result of nondisjunction in meiosis II or from nondisjunction in meiosis I with a crossing over event or possibly a somatic recombination in early pregnancy producing a segmental or partial form of isodisomy for only a region of chromosome 15. Maternal isodisomy may also lead to other genetic disorders in the PWS individual. For example, if the mother is a carrier of an autosomal recessive gene mutation located on chromosome 15 and that chromosome region (e.g., due to segmental isodisomy) or the entire chromosome representing isodisomy (e.g., nondisjunction in meiosis II producing identical chromatids and therefore chromosomes), then the offspring would present with PWS and also the recessive genetic disorder by inheriting both of the mother's recessive alleles. As in other nondisjunction cases, the risk of maternal disomy 15 increases with maternal age [14, 15].

To determine if maternal disomy 15 in PWS contributes to disturbances in gestational age by impacting on placental structure or function secondary to the abnormal chromosomal number in the placental cells or in mechanisms leading to the maternal disomy status, Butler et al. [16] reported gestational age data in PWS pregnancies grouped by genetic subtypes and found that postterm deliveries (>42 weeks gestation) were more common in the maternal disomy group compared to the deletion group. Although there are no recognized growth factor genes in the proximal long arm of chromosome 15 that should affect placental growth or other imprinted genes in humans on chromosome 15, disturbances of growth factors influenced by maternal disomy 15 may contribute to abnormalities of placental growth or function in PWS and pregnancy outcome. However, the insulin-like growth factor receptor 1 (*IGF1R*) gene is located on the distal long arm of chromosome 15 and involved with growth and development. *IGF1R* is a member of a gene family of growth factors and receptors which is genetically imprinted in humans and transmits the effects of major growth factors (IGF1 and IGF2) during pre- and postnatal growth. Imprinting disturbances on chromosome 11 including the *IGF2* gene are known to cause Beckwith–Wiedemann syndrome, an overgrowth syndrome with abnormal placental growth and polyhydramnios [17, 18]. One could speculate that differences in gestational age in PWS subjects with maternal disomy 15 compared with those PWS subjects with the 15q11–q13 deletion could be triggered by maternal disomy 15 and/or trisomy 15 rescue events in early pregnancy on placenta and fetal growth. Imprinted gene products are critical regulators of growth and development. More research is needed to further address the observations of abnormal gestation in pregnancies with PWS and maternal disomy 15.

To further investigate the trisomy rescue event and timing in abnormal cells from the early pregnancy in PWS, the X chromosome inactivation ratio using the polymorphic androgen receptor (*AR*) gene located at Xq11.2 can be used to access X inactivation patterns in those females informative for the polymorphic CAG repeat site following DNA digestion with methyl-sensitive restriction enzymes (e.g., *HpaII*) and PCR amplification. X chromosome skewness (i.e., one X chromosome may be more or less active compared with the second X chromosome in somatic cells) is assigned at an arbitrary ratio of highly skewed (e.g., >80%:20%) and is considered to be an uncommon event [19, 20]. The inactivation of the X chromosome in females is generally considered random with regard to which X is inactivated to allow for equal gene dosage for X-linked genes in normal females and males. In certain cases, the X chromosome inactivation skewness is no longer random but is skewed. X chromosome skewness occurs in X-autosomal chromosome rearrangements, mutations of the gene controlling the X inactivation process (i.e., *XIST*), or in certain X-linked disorders (e.g., Rett syndrome) [21]. Since about 2% of pregnancies detected by chorionic villus sampling are associated with confined placental mosaicism, it may be a significant contributor to both skewed X inactivation observed in some newborns and expression of X-linked recessive diseases in females [22].

Butler et al. [20] reported results from a cohort of PWS females with either the 15q11–q13 deletion or maternal disomy 15 and compared with findings, female controls using the androgen receptor gene assay system in peripheral blood. A significantly larger number of PWS females with maternal disomy were found with extreme X chromosome skewness (95%:5%) compared with PWS deletion or control females. These results indicated that if a trisomy rescue event occurred in early embryo development and a small number of cells survived, then a selective advantage for cell proliferation occurs, leading to extreme X chromosome skewness in the PWS female with maternal disomy 15. Because of extreme X chromosome skewness, these PWS females could be at risk for X-linked recessive gene disorders if the X-linked gene mutation is present on the active skewed X chromosome.

6.3.2 Deletion Versus Maternal Disomy 15

Clinical differences have been reported over the past 30 years since the discovery of the two genetic subtypes (deletion and maternal disomy 15) in PWS. PWS individuals with the typical chromosome 15 deletion are more homogeneous in their clinical presentation with hypopigmentation due to the deletion of the *P* gene involved with pigment formation. PWS subjects with maternal disomy 15 have fewer typical facial features. Those with the typical deletion are also thought to have a lower birth weight, more skin picking, an unusual skill with jigsaw puzzles, a higher pain threshold, and more articulation problems than those with maternal disomy 15. The diagnosis of PWS is often delayed in those with maternal disomy 15 compared with the 15q deletion, reflecting a milder phenotype in the maternal disomy subjects [2].

Behavioral problems including obsessive–compulsive and self-injurious behavior are frequently reported in PWS. Self-injurious behavior in individuals with intellectual impairment, autism, and developmental disabilities without PWS ranges from 5 to 60%. However, self-injurious behavior is reported in about 70% of PWS adolescents. Self-injurious behavior, particularly skin picking, is commonly seen in PWS individuals with the typical 15q11–q13 deletion. Additionally, PWS individuals hoard and arrange items excessively. Compulsive symptoms have been found in about 60% of PWS patients with compulsions being more common in deletion subjects compared with those having maternal disomy 15. In addition, acute psychosis has been reported in PWS, particularly adults with maternal disomy 15 and possibly more seizures in the PWS deletion subjects. However, PWS children with the 15q11–q13 deletion show more relative strengths in standardized visual–spatial tasks such as object assembly compared with age- and IQ-matched controls with mixed mental retardation. Interestingly, PWS subjects outperform normal peers in proficiency at jigsaw puzzle placement [23].

Measures of intelligence and academic achievement in PWS have shown that those with maternal disomy 15 have significantly higher verbal IQ scores than those with the deletions. PWS deletion subjects also score higher on object-assembly subtests and discrimination of shape and kinetic motion measures than the maternal disomy 15 subjects, supporting specific visual perceptual skills as relative strengths in the PWS deletion group. However, PWS individuals with maternal disomy 15 perform better than either typical deletion or comparison subjects in visual recognition and memory tasks. Superior visual recognition memory in the maternal disomy 15 subjects further supports the possible role of two active alleles of maternally expressed genes from chromosome 15 [2, 24].

Although PWS individuals share common characteristics, deletion subjects have poorer outcomes in academic achievement and more obsessions compared with maternal disomy 15 individuals. Because paternally expressed genes are inactive in both subtypes, the increased severity associated with the deletion must be due to reduced expression of hemizygous genes and compensated when two maternal copies are present. In addition, disruption of interactive genes outside of chromosome 15 may be altered by the expression of chromosome 15 genes.

6.3.3 Molecular Genetics and Deletion Types in PWS

PWS is thought to be a contiguous gene syndrome with several imprinted (paternally expressed) genes in the 15q11–q13 region. This region contains between 7 and 8 million DNA base pairs including a large cluster of imprinted genes but also a nonimprinted domain [25] (Fig. 6.1). Novel DNA sequences have been identified with low copy repeats clustered at or near the two major proximal chromosome

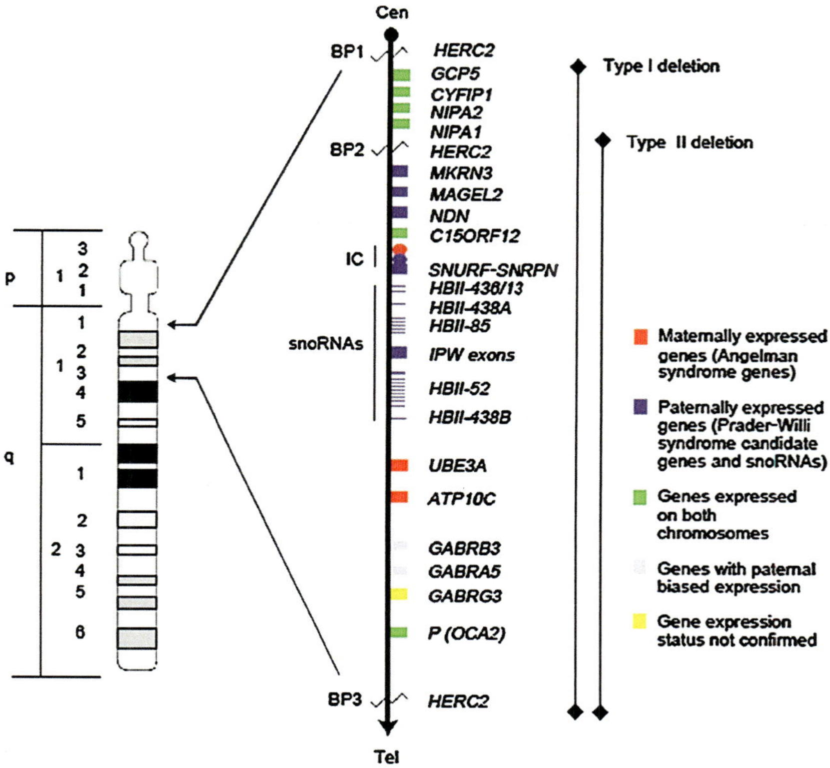

Fig. 6.1 High-resolution chromosome 15 ideogram, location, and order of genes in the 15q11–q13 region and patterns of expression. The gene order is based on the UCSC Genome Bioinformatics web site (http://genome.ucsc.edu). snoRNAs indicate small nucleolar RNAs. About 40% of subjects with the typical deletion have the Type I deletion and approximately 60% have the smaller Type II deletion. *Source*: Reproduced from reference [4] with permission

breakpoints (BP1 and BP2) and the distal breakpoint (BP3) in the 15q11–q13 region. The typical PWS deletion consists of two classes, Type I and Type II, depending on the size and chromosome breakpoint position. The larger Type I (TI) deletion involving breakpoint 1 (BP1) is nearer to the centromere and located proximal to the microsatellite marker D15S1035, while the smaller Type II (TII) deletion involves breakpoint 2 (BP2) and distal to D15S1035. Breakpoint 3 (BP3) is located distally and common to both typical deletion subgroups.

Butler et al. [25] used high-resolution array comparative genomic hybridization (aCGH) in PWS subjects and found that BP1 spanned a region from 18.68 to 20.22 Mb from the p-terminus of chromosome 15, BP2 from 20.81 to 21.36 Mb, and BP3 from 25.94 to 27.29 Mb. The Type I deletion ranged in size from 5.72 to 8.15 Mb (mean 6.583) and the Type II deletion from 4.77 to 6.44 Mb (mean 5.33). A subset of the Type I subjects showed larger deletions including the loss of at least three genes/transcripts (i.e., *LOC283755*, *POTE5*, and *OR4N4*) in addition to the four genes recognized between BP1 and BP2 (i.e., *GCP5*, *CYFIP1*, *NIPA1*, and *NIPA2*). Occasionally, PWS subjects will have duplications of the 15q11 region in addition to the typical deletion. PWS subjects with the larger typical Type I deletion (involving BP1 and BP3) have more clinical problems such as obsessive–compulsive disorders, self-injury, and poorer academic performance than those PWS subjects with the smaller Type II deletions (involving BP2 and BP3). Atypical deletions that are greater or smaller than the typical Type I or Type II deletion have been reported, but account for only a small percentage of those with deletions of chromosome 15q11–q13 region.

At least 70 nonredundant genes/transcripts are recognized in the 15q11–q13 region, and at least a dozen genes are imprinted and paternally expressed. Methylation DNA testing which measures the methylation status of genes in the region can be used for laboratory diagnosis and is considered to be 99% accurate in the diagnosis of PWS. However, it will not identify the specific genetic subtype (deletion, maternal disomy, or an imprinting defect). Additional testing besides FISH is required to identify maternal disomy 15 or imprinting defects such as genotyping of informative DNA markers from the 15q11–q13 region, DNA sequencing, or aCGH studies [4].

Several paternally expressed genes or transcripts are mapped to the 15q11–q13 region including *SNRPN* (small nuclear ribonucleoprotein N) and a second protein coding sequence (*SNURF* or *SNRPN* upstream reading frame) as well as multiple copies of C/D box small nucleolar RNAs (snoRNAs) or *SNORDs* thought to participate in RNA processing. Other protein coding genes located on the centromeric side of *SNRPN* include *MKRN3*, *MAGEL2*, *NDN*, and *C15orf2* and are involved directly or indirectly in brain development and function. The promoter and first exon of *SNURF–SNRPN* are integral components of the imprinting center that controls regulation of imprinting throughout the chromosome 15q11–q13 region. The imprinting center has a bipartite structure composed of five domains impacting maternal and paternal specific epigenetic patterns of gene expression. It spans 35 kilobases (kb) and contains a 4.3-kb sequence implicated in PWS including the *SNRPN* promoter/exon 1 and an 880-bp sequence located just upstream to the SNRPN transcription start site implicated in Angelman syndrome. Therefore, exons 4–10 of the bicistronic gene *SNURF–SNRPN* encode a core spliceosomal protein (SmN) involved in mRNA splicing in the brain, whereas exons 1–3 encode a 71-amino-acid protein enriched in arginine residues. A disruption of this complex locus will cause loss of function of paternally expressed genes in this region, leading to PWS [26].

Necdin (*NDN*), a member of the melanoma-associated antigen gene (MAGE) family of proteins, is expressed only from the paternal allele in the 15q11–q13 region. The MAGE family of proteins is implicated in cell-cycle proliferation, differentiation, and apoptosis. Necdin is detected in all developing neurons of the embryonic mouse, in both the central and peripheral nervous system, with the highest expression levels in the diencephalon and hindbrain. Necdin has been shown to be essential for axonal outgrowth and is expressed in specific brain structures (hypothalamus, thalamus, and pons) suggesting a developmental role. Mice deficient for necdin show delayed migration of the sympathetic neurons of the superior cervical ganglia, hypothalamic deficiency, neonatal lethality, and respiratory problems and abnormal behavior similar to that seen in PWS. Therefore, dysregulation of cytoskeletal rearrangements consequent to loss of necdin provides evidence for an intracellular signaling defect in murine and human cells [27].

The *MAGEL2* gene is paternally expressed in various brain regions (most notably the hypothalamus) and belongs to the MAGE family of proteins. Mice with a targeted deletion of *MAGEL2* display hypoactivity and disturbed metabolism, blunted circadian rhythm, decreased fertility, and increased adiposity, all features consistent with the PWS phenotype. Abnormal neurochemistry is detected in brain samples of *MAGEL2*-null mice including decreased serotonin levels although the mice display relatively normal learning abilities [28]. Therefore, *MAGEL2* may play an important role in circadian rhythm, brain structure, behavior, and maintenance of fertility in humans [29].

The *MKRN3* gene or *ZNF127* is a member of the makorin (MKRN) RING finger protein gene family encoding proteins (makorins) with a characteristic array of zinc-finger motifs and is present in a wide variety of eukaryotes. There are nine recognized MKRN gene family loci distributed in the human genome. The putative encoded ribonucleoproteins show a distinctive array of zinc-finger motifs including two to four C(3)H zinc fingers and a highly conserved RING zinc finger. The *MKRN3* is encoded in the complex imprinted area of chromosome 15q11–q13 region and is paternally expressed. The MKRN gene family is considered ancient with orthologs found in the fruitfly and nematode. There appears to be abundant expression in developing brain and nervous system [30].

Two additional novel genes have been reported by Buiting et al. [31] located between *NDN* and *C15orf2* in the 15q11–q13 region and called *PWRN1* and *PWRN2*. *PWRN1* is a novel alternative start site for *SNURF–SNRPN*. *PWRN2* is a male germ cell-specific gene expressed from the haploid genome. Other genes implicated in PWS include *IPW* (for "imprinted in Prader–Willi") and the series of highly repeated sequences encoding small nucleolar RNAs (snoRNAs) or *SNORDs*. *IPW* is a component of the large *SNURF–SNRPN* transcript and is spliced and polyadenylated but apparently does not encode a protein. However, it could represent functional RNA, similar to the *H19* and *XIST* genes. Also encoded within the *SNURF–SNRPN* transcript are multiple C/D box snoRNAs. The single-copy snoRNA genes are *SNORD64*, *SNORD107*, *SNORD108*, *SNORD109A*, and *SNORD109B* previously referred to as HBII-13, HBII-436, HBII-437, HBII-438A, and HBII-438B, respectively. Two snoRNA gene clusters in the region are *SNORD115* (previously HBII-52) and *SNORD116* (previously HBII-85) and are encoded in a tandemly repeated array of 47 or 24 units, respectively, and paternally expressed. Deletions of snoRNAs have also been implicated in causing a PWS phenotype [4, 32].

Two imprinted maternally expressed genes (*UBE3A* and *ATP10C*) that are paternally silenced are also present in this chromosome region. The *UBE3A* gene causes Angelman syndrome. Other genes located in the distal area of the 15q11–q13 region are several gamma aminobutyric acid (GABA) receptor subunits called *GABRB3*, *GABRA5*, and *GABRG3*. The receptor subunit genes for GABA, a major inhibitory neurotransmitter, are reported as paternally biased with loss of the paternal allele resulting in reduction in expression of greater than 50% [33, 34]. The paternal allele accounts for a larger percentage of gene expression than the maternal allele. GABA has also been implicated in a number of symptoms associated with PWS including hunger, obsessive–compulsive disorder, and altered visual perception and memory. GABA is widely distributed in the central nervous system and it is estimated that 40% of the brain and spinal cord neurons utilize GABA as their neurotransmitter, making it the most important inhibitory brain neurotransmitter in humans. Furthermore, plasma GABA levels were found to be increased by three- to fourfold in PWS individuals compared with control subjects [35]. Lastly, the distal area of 15q11–q13 codes for the *P* gene of pigment production. *P* gene mutations are known to cause oculocutaneous albinism II. These genes are not imprinted and expressed from both alleles.

The three breakpoint sites (BP1, BP2, and BP3) located at the ends of the 15q11–q13 region contain a large transcribed gene (*HERC2*) with many partially duplicated copies, some of which are transcribed. The functional *HERC2* gene located at breakpoint BP3 encodes a highly conserved protein distantly related to *HERC1*, a guanine nucleotide exchange factor (GEF) implicated in vesicular trafficking and degradation pathways in the cell [36, 37]. *HERC2* repeated sequences have also been implicated in unequal crossing over in meiosis and may participate in the development of the typical 15q11–q13 Type I and Type II deletions seen in PWS and AS subjects. In addition, the environment may influence recombination and the deletion process in this chromosome region with the involvement of the repeated sequences. However, no difference in the number of chromosome and chromatid aberrations was reported previously in cells grown in conditions to induce damage, and no clustering of chromosome/chromatid breaks or sister chromatid exchanges was seen in PWS subjects or their parents [38].

6.3.4 Clinical Findings Associated with Type I Versus Type II Deletions

Butler et al. [39] reported that different multiple psychological, cognitive, and behavioral test results were found in 12 young adults with PWS with the longer Type I deletion involving breakpoints BP1 and BP3 versus 14 young adults with PWS having the shorter Type II deletion involving BP1 and BP3. PWS individuals with the longer Type I deletions scored significantly worse in self-injurious and maladaptive behavior assessments as compared to PWS subjects with Type II deletions. Obsessive–compulsive behavior was also more evident in PWS subjects with Type I deletions.

Interestingly, individuals with shorter deletions exhibited significantly more self-injury than those with maternal disomy 15 but less than those with longer deletions.

Psychobehavioral characteristics of PWS individuals with Type I deletions involving BP1 were similar in several aspects to individuals with uncharacterized typical deletions, but differed from those with Type II deletions involving BP2. Those with Type II deletions resembled more closely those PWS individuals with maternal disomy 15.

Several academic achievement scores differed between those with shorter or longer typical deletions reflecting a difference in intellectual functioning and visual perceptional skills affecting reading, supporting that loss of genetic material between BP1 and BP2 increases the severity of behavioral and psychological problems in PWS. Adaptive behavior scores were generally worse in individuals with PWS and the Type I deletion, and specific obsessive–compulsive behaviors were more evident in the Type I individuals compared with those with maternal disomy 15. Individuals with PWS with Type I deletions also had poorer reading and math skills as well as visual–motor integration, poorer adaptive behavior, and more compulsions than subjects with Type II deletions. They have more severe compulsions related to grooming and bathing and compulsions are more disruptive to daily living. Intellectual ability and academic achievement were poorer in subjects with Type I deletions. Visual processing was also noted to be poor in subjects with Type I deletions compared with Type II. Figure 6.2 represents a typical adult male with PWS and the Type I deletion.

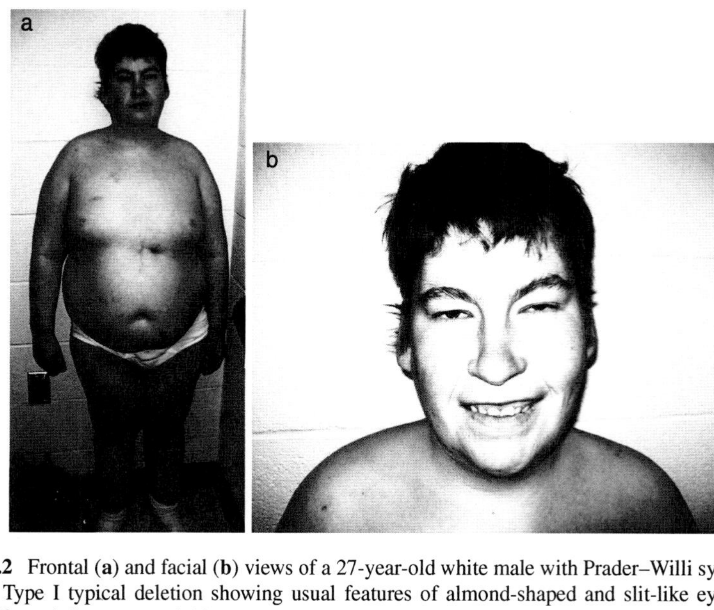

Fig. 6.2 Frontal (**a**) and facial (**b**) views of a 27-year-old white male with Prader–Willi syndrome and a Type I typical deletion showing usual features of almond-shaped and slit-like eyes, narrow bifrontal diameter, and thin upper lip along with central obesity. Small hands and a previous gastrostomy site in the upper abdomen can also be seen

6.3.5 Expression of Four Genes Between BP1 and BP2 in PWS

The behavioral, cognitive, and psychological differences seen in those PWS subjects with the Type I deletion compared with those with the Type II deletion led Bittel et al. [40] to investigate the expression of the four biallelically expressed genes between BP1 and BP2. As adaptive behavior, obsessive–compulsive behaviors, reading, math, and visual–motor integration assessments were generally poorer in individuals with PWS and the Type I deletion versus PWS with the Type II deletion or maternal disomy 15, the four genes (*NIPA1*, *NIPA2*, *CYFIP1*, and *GCP5*) localized between breakpoints BP1 and BP2 in the chromosome 15q11–q13 region are possible candidates for behavior and intellectual ability differences. Bittel et al. [40] quantified messenger RNA levels of these four genes in actively growing lymphoblastoid cells derived from eight young adults with PWS with the Type I deletion and from nine young adults with the Type II deletion. Messenger RNA levels were correlated with validated psychological and behavioral scales administered by trained psychologists blinded to genotype status. Messenger RNAs from *NIPA1*, *NIPA2*, *CYFIP1*, and *GCP5* were reduced but detectable in the subjects with PWS with the TI deletion, supporting biallelic expression (see Fig. 6.3).

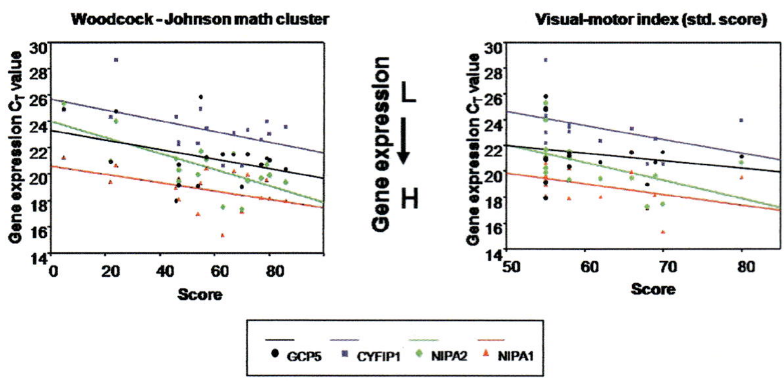

Fig. 6.3 Correlations of gene expression (based on a C_T value representing the PCR cycle threshold for gene expression detection) for *NIPA1*, *NIPA2*, *CYFIP1*, and *GCP5* and Woodcock–Johnson math cluster measures and visual–motor index scores. Significant negative correlations were observed for the *NIPA2* gene when comparing gene expression C_T values and test scores. Higher C_T values indicate lower gene expression in lymphoblastoid cells analyzed from the Prader–Willi syndrome subjects

Three of these genes have been implicated in central nervous system development and/or function. *NIPA1* has been associated with spastic paraplegia. *NIPA2* is conserved in vertebrates and widely expressed, including the central nervous system, and recently identified as a magnesium transporter. The *CYFIP1* gene codes for a protein that is present in synaptosomal extracts and interacts with FMRP, the protein product of the *FMR1* gene, which is responsible for fragile X syndrome. *GCP5* is a member of the cytoskeleton tubulin complex in cells. Although all four of the genes examined seemed to contribute to some degree to the parameters measured, *NIPA2* seemed to have the greatest impact because a larger number of phenotypic parameters were noted with significant correlations with *NIPA2* mRNA levels. The coefficient of determination indicated the quantity of messenger RNA of the four genes explained from 24 to 99% of the variation of the behavioral and academic parameters measured, particularly NIPA2 which accounted for as much as 75% of the variation seen in behavior scores and academic achievement. By comparison, the coefficient of determination for deletion type alone explained 5–50% of the variation in the assessed parameters. Understanding the influence of gene expression on behavioral and cognitive characteristics in humans is in the early stage of research development. These data suggest that *NIPA1*, *NIPA2*, and *CYFIP1* may have a greater influence on the studied behavioral and cognitive parameters than does *GCP5*. Additional research is needed to identify the function of these genes and their interaction with gene networks to clarify the potential role they play in central nervous system development and function. These data imply that genotype may influence medical care. For example, better educational programs and treatment plans can be tailored for each PWS patient depending on genetic subtype and associated phenotypic characteristics to improve the quality of life and clinical outcome (e.g., higher verbal IQ and visual memory in maternal disomy 15 PWS subjects and more compulsions and self-injury in Type I deletion PWS subjects) [2, 40–42].

6.4 PWS with Atypical 15q11–q13 Deletions or Translocations and Causative Genes

A female patient was recently reported with an atypical deletion involving the chromosome 15q11–q13 region due to an unbalanced translocation of chromosomes X and 15. This patient had a paternal deletion of the region including only the *MKRN3*, *MAGEL2*, and *NDN* genes. She presented with obesity, mental retardation, and a high pain threshold, but lacked other features of PWS [43]. Therefore, the authors concluded that a paternal deficiency of *MKRN3*, *MAGEL2*, and *NDN* in this rare patient was not sufficient to cause the complete phenotype of PWS.

Recently, Sahoo et al. [44] described a male child with several features of PWS, such as neonatal hypotonia, feeding problems, obesity, and hypogenitalism. Atypical features included high birth weight, macrosomia, macrocephaly, absence of mental retardation, and an atypical face. The patient was deleted for the paternal copies of *SNORD109A*, the *SNORD116* gene cluster, and half of the *SNORD115* gene cluster.

More recently, Smith et al. [45] reported a 19-year-old male with hyperphagia and severe obesity, mild learning difficulties, and hypogonadism, in whom diagnostic tests for PWS were negative. They identified a 187-kb microdeletion of chromosome 15q11–q13 encompassing the noncoding small nucleolar RNAs (including *SNORD116*) in this patient which were not expressed in peripheral lymphocytes. They concluded that there was evidence for the role of a particular family of noncoding RNAs in human energy homeostasis, growth, and reproduction, specifically the *SNORD116* cluster, in the expression of several abnormal clinical findings in PWS.

In addition, Kanber et al. [43] reviewed six patients with balanced translocations affecting the *SNURF–SNRPN* locus and described as having typical PWS or PWS-like phenotype. The snoRNA genes located in the large *SNURF–SNRPN* transcripts may be responsible for at least several features of PWS. These include several single-copy snoRNA genes (*SNORD64*, *SNORD107*, *SNORD108*, *SNORD109A*, and *SNORD109B* – earlier referred to as HBII-13, HBII-436, HBII-437, HBII-438A, and HBII-438B, respectively) and the two snoRNA gene clusters, *SNORD115* and *SNORD116*. Because the *SNORD116* gene cluster maps distal to the six balanced translocation breakpoints in these patients with features of PWS, it is not expressed further, supporting a role in PWS. Hence, recent clinical reports of small deletions involving the paternally expressed snoRNAs (e.g., *SNORD116* and partial deletion of *SNORD115*) in individuals with obesity, hypotonia, and other features of PWS have led investigators to speculate on PWS causative genes in the 15q11–q13 region.

The role of *SNORD116* in humans is not known although deletion in mice of this snoRNA causes hyperphagia and growth deficiency. Kishore and Stamm [46] also reported that the paternally expressed snoRNA *SNORD115* regulates alternative splicing of the serotonin 5-HT_{2C} receptor by binding to a silencing element in exon Vb of this receptor gene. If *SNORD115* is not present or functional on chromosome 15, then an alternative form of the serotonin receptor is produced with altered reduced function. This serotonin receptor is involved with behavior influencing eating patterns. Therefore, a defect in pre-mRNA processing by snoRNAs may contribute to hyperphagia and other features recognized in PWS.

Additional patients with a *SNORD116* deletion are needed to define the role of *SNORD116* and other genes involved in PWS. Therefore, PWS is not caused by a single locus defect, but by a deficiency of several genes in the region that includes *SNURF–SNRPN* and the *SNORD* genes. Furthermore, it is possible that deficiencies of *MKRN3*, *MAGEL2*, and/or *NDN* are necessary, although not sufficient, to generate the full PWS phenotype. To further understand the role of the 15q11–q13 genes in PWS, more patients need to be reported and genetically evaluated.

6.5 Gene Expression in PWS

PWS is caused by loss of function of paternally expressed genes in the 15q11–q13 region; however, there is a paucity of data on transcriptome variation. Genes in *Cis* (located on chromosome 15 in PWS) are affected by disturbances of chromosome 15, while *Trans* affects those genes disturbed on other chromosomes but impact on the PWS phenotype. Therefore, the interaction of genes located throughout the genome and disturbed gene networks needs further clarification in PWS.

To further characterize these genetic alterations, Bittel et al. [33] used custom-made microarrays to examine expression of genes/transcripts from 15q11–q13 and found a higher level of regulatory mechanisms were perturbed in PWS. For example, several genes/transcripts acting in *Cis* (e.g., *GABRA5* and *GABRB3*) showed increased expression in PWS lymphoblastoid cell lines established from individuals with maternal disomy 15 compared with those having typical deletions. However, the genes in *Cis* produced less total RNA represented by lower expression in PWS individuals with maternal disomy 15 than controls having one maternal and one paternal copy of the same gene, supporting paternal bias of expression. Several transcripts outside of the deleted 15q11–q13 region showed increased expression in PWS individuals with typical deletions relative to controls or PWS individuals with maternal disomy. These observations were confirmed in cells in Angelman syndrome, using similar methods [34]. Presumably, this expression pattern is a consequence of repositioning of genes in the proximal long arm region outside of the deleted segment and with altered chromatin structure from the deletion process in the deleted chromosome 15.

Bittel et al. [47] used whole-genome microarrays to analyze gene expression, microarray, and quantitative RT-PCR analysis with RNA isolated from lymphoblastoid cells from PWS male subjects (four with 15q11–q13 deletion and three with UPD) and three age- and cognition-matched nonsyndromic comparison males. More than 47,000 probes were examined in the microarrays and 23,383 were detectable. Of these detectable probes, 323 had significantly different expression levels with at least 1.5-fold difference in detection in the PWS lymphoblastoid cells relative to comparison cells. Fourteen genes detected were related to neurodevelopment and function. As expected, there was no evidence of expression of paternally expressed genes from the 15q11–q13 region (e.g., *SNRPN*) in the PWS cells. Alterations in expression of the neurotransmitter serotonin receptor genes (e.g., *HTR2B*) and genes involved in eating behavior and adiposity involving melanocortin receptors, orexin, and oxytocin receptors (*ADIPOR2*, *MC2R*, *HCRT*, *OXTR*) were also identified with increased or decreased levels. Other genes of interest with reduced expression in PWS subjects included *STAR* (a key regulator of steroid synthesis) and *SAG* (an arrestin family member which desensitizes G protein-coupled receptors). Quantitative RT-PCR studies for *SAG*, *OXTR*, *STAR*, *HCRT*, and *HTR2B* were undertaken using RNA isolated from their lymphoblastoid cells and available brain tissue (frontal cortex) from separate individuals with PWS and control subjects. Modest changes were found in expression of several genes involved in energy metabolism.

6.6 Clinical Stages and Natural History of PWS

PWS can be divided into two major clinical stages of development (see Table 6.1 for list of common features in PWS). The first stage is characterized by infantile hypotonia, temperature instability, a weak cry, a poor suck with feeding difficulties often requiring tube feedings, delayed developmental milestones, and underdevelopment of the sex organs. The second stage occurs in early childhood beginning

Table 6.1 Natural history and clinical course development in Prader–Willi syndrome

Stage 1		Stage 2	
Pregnancy and delivery	Neonatal and infancy	Childhood	Adolescence and adulthood
Reduced fetal activity	Narrow forehead	Short stature	Short stature
Breech presentation	Undescended small testicles	Small hands and feet	Small hands and feet
Pre- or postterm delivery	Small genitals	Light skin and eye color	Scoliosis
	Hypotonia and decreased muscle mass	Almond-shaped or slit-like eyes	Osteoporosis
	Poor suck and feeding problems	Strabismus	Delayed puberty
	Sticky dry saliva	Vision changes (myopia)	Diabetes mellitus
	Weak cry	Self-injury (skin or rectal picking)	Depression
	Temperature instability	Enamel defects and dental caries	Excessive sleepiness
	Developmental delay	Excessive appetite/food foraging	
		Obesity (central)	
		Intellectual disability	
		Behavioral problems	
		Temper tantrums	
		Stubbornness	
		Obsessive–compulsive behavior	

around 2 years of age and is characterized by an insatiable appetite with rapid weight gain and obesity if caloric restriction is not in place. Continued developmental delay is noted with an average IQ of 65. Other features seen during this stage include speech problems, food foraging and rumination, daytime sleepiness, physical inactivity, decreased pain sensitivity and self-injurious behavior, strabismus, scoliosis, obstructive sleep apnea, and abnormal oral pathology [1, 2, 48–51]. In addition, those with the 15q11–q13 deletion are prone to hypopigmentation and self-injurious behavior (skin picking) at a greater rate while those with maternal disomy 15 may have higher verbal IQ scores and better memory retention. The typical 15q11–q13 deletion seen in either PWS or AS is classified into two types, Type I and Type II, depending on the size and chromosome 15 breakpoint position [39, 52] (see Fig. 6.1).

Approximately 50% of children with PWS develop temper tantrums and stubbornness between 3 and 5 years of age and may also display depression during adolescence and adulthood. Behavioral problems may sometimes be precipitated by withholding food. About one-half of children with PWS function in the low to normal intelligence range (70–100 IQ) and the remaining PWS children (and adults) function in the mild to moderate range (50–70 IQ). Children with PWS tend to be affectionate and caring. However, changes in routine can be disruptive for many adolescents and adults with PWS. Poor peer interaction, immaturity, and inappropriate social behavior are often present. Many children with PWS begin school in mainstream settings, but due to behavioral problems and learning deficiency, children with PWS often require special education services. By elementary school age, children with PWS may steal or hide food at home or at school to be eaten later. Many children with PWS have reading and math difficulties. Recent evidence indicates that behavior and academic achievement skills may vary depending on the genetic subtype [40].

Other endocrine disturbances including diabetes mellitus, central adrenal insufficiency, and hypothyroidism are also noted in PWS. Adolescents with PWS do not mature sexually as rapidly as their peers, although this may be due to low gonadotropin production or the excessive estrogen milieu due to their adiposity [2]. Recent data suggest that delayed puberty in PWS may be due to primary testicular and ovarian dysfunction [53, 54].

Adolescents and young adults with PWS look younger than their chronological age. About one-third of appropriately aged females have menstrual periods although not regular. Adolescent girls are unlikely to become pregnant and males with PWS are thought to be sterile [53]; however, there are at least three adult females with PWS confirmed by molecular genetic studies reported to have given birth. One adult female with PWS having the 15q11–q13 deletion gave birth to an infant with Angelman syndrome [2, 24].

Typical adolescent rebelliousness can often be exaggerated in PWS by the constant struggle with parents and teachers over access to food. By late adolescence, some PWS individuals begin stealing food from stores and rummaging through discarded lunch bags or trash cans. Parents may find it necessary to lock the refrigerator and cabinets containing food to prevent excessive eating. Despite these precautions, PWS subjects often pry open locked cabinets to gain access to food. Because of hyperphagia, lack of satiety, and an inability to vomit, stomach rupturing is a reported cause of death in PWS [55]. Thus, this remarkable eating disorder and complications of obesity can reduce the life expectancy of a PWS person. Adolescents with PWS may weigh 250–300 pounds by their late teens. Adults with PWS are short if not treated with growth hormone. The average adult male with PWS without growth hormone therapy is 155 cm and the adult female is 147 cm. Small hands and feet are particularly evident during adolescence and adulthood in PWS [24].

As a result of better awareness and recent advances in genetic testing, the diagnosis of PWS is made at an earlier age than in the past. Early diagnosis is important since nutritional intervention is required to maintain a healthy weight status. Caloric restriction (e.g., approximately 60% of normal) throughout life is important to control the obesity and comorbidities. As noted, therapy with GH is frequently prescribed during infancy or early childhood to improve stature, body composition, muscle mass, energy level, and metabolism, but no specific medication has universally benefited the behavioral problems commonly seen in PWS. Specific serotonin reuptake inhibitors have helped control skin picking and depression in affected individuals. However, obesity continues to be a lifelong concern. If weight is adequately controlled, life expectancy should be similar to that of other mildly intellectually impaired individuals, which approximates a death rate of 3% per year [2, 56].

6.7 Fatness Patterns and Body Composition Measures in PWS

Early research focused on the characterization of obesity in PWS with attempts to describe the patterning of fatness through a comprehensive assessment of skinfold measurement at several standard body sites. Meaney and Butler [57, 58] evaluated repeated measurements of 26 anthropometric variables, including skinfold thicknesses at seven body sites: triceps, forearm, subscapular, abdomen, suprailiac, thigh, and medial calf; weight; height; sitting height; four circumferences; four head dimensions; and eight hand and food measurements in a group of 40 non-growth hormone-treated PWS individuals ranging in age from 0.1 to 39 years. Anthropometric data grouped by age, sex, and chromosome type were compared with normative data for skinfolds. The results suggested that males with PWS had three times the fatness scores of other males their age, while scores for PWS females averaged only twice those of normal. The highest measurement in PWS subjects was for medial calf skinfold, while the triceps skinfold had the lowest average value.

Height, weight, and triceps and subscapular skinfold measurements revealed negative correlations with age for height, suggesting a relative slowing down of linear growth compared with normal individuals. The overall body fat estimate was 42% in PWS based on triceps alone, or triceps and medial calf skinfolds using standardized formulas for calculations of body fat estimates. More females than males were below the 5th percentile for height, particularly from 2 to 16 years of age. Most females and males were in the normal range for sitting height, indicating that the short stature which is common in this syndrome due to growth hormone deficiency may be related to a shorter lower body segment compared with upper body in both sexes.

Talebizadeh and Butler [59] further reported on fatness patterns and lipid, leptin, glucose, and insulin levels in subjects with simple obesity or non-growth hormone-treated PWS. They analyzed fasting peripheral blood samples and cross-sectional magnetic resonance image (MRI) scans at the level of the umbilicus for fatness measures in 55 obese (average age = 26 years) and non-growth hormone-treated PWS (average age = 22 years) subjects ranging in age from 10 to 49 years. PWS subjects were shorter and weighed less than the obese controls. Twenty-three of the 37 PWS subjects met the criteria for obesity (BMI > 95th percentile). Subcutaneous fat area (SFA) and intra-abdominal visceral fat area (VFA) were calculated, but no significant differences were observed for SFA and VFA between the PWS subjects judged to be obese versus control subjects with simple obesity. Fasting insulin levels were significantly lower in the obese PWS subjects compared with subjects with simple obesity. Insulin resistance was lower and insulin sensitivity higher in PWS subjects compared with obese controls. Adiponectin levels were also studied and found to be higher in PWS subjects compared with matched obese controls. As with other forms of obesity, PWS subjects with higher VFA may also be at a higher risk of obesity-related complications compared to PWS subjects with less lower VFA.

The development of obesity requires an energy imbalance with the rate of triglyceride synthesis and fat storage exceeding that of fat mobilization and utilization. The massive accumulation of adipose tissue observed in PWS and the unusual fat patterning further suggests abnormalities in fat mobilization and oxidation or triglyceride synthesis and storage related to genetic changes in the syndrome [58]. Specifically, individuals with a significant accumulation of intra-abdominal visceral fat are particularly at risk for obesity-related complications. Furthermore, increased visceral fat plays an integral role in the development of insulin resistance, glucose intolerance, and hyperlipidemia in obese subjects without PWS. Other studies have shown visceral adipose tissue and metabolic complications are reduced in adult females with PWS which is in contrast to that expected by their physical inactivity, hypogonadism, and growth hormone deficiency [60]. Furthermore, an unusual and excessive distribution of body fat is observed in non-growth hormone-treated PWS subjects with marked obesity following weight loss. However, a sex reversal fat pattern is seen in PWS with males having greater subcutaneous fat compared with females even at an early age [58].

To further characterize the body composition of PWS subjects compared with simple obesity, Theodoro, Talebizadeh, and Butler [61] used DEXA to study 48 non-growth hormone-treated PWS individuals and 24 obese controls from 10 to 49 years of age. Body composition measures were calculated from the DEXA results and regional fat and lean mass patterns characterized. Significant differences were found between the PWS and obese groups for lean measures involving the arms, legs, and trunk with total lean mass being significantly lower in PWS than in obese subjects for arms, trunk, and especially legs. Furthermore, two body regions (legs and trunk) showed significant differences for fat and lean measures between PWS and obese males. However, significant differences between PWS and obese females for these measures were found only for legs. Obese females had significantly greater arm fat, arm lean, leg lean, trunk fat, trunk lean, total body fat, total body lean, and BMI compared with age-matched female PWS subjects. Although individuals with simple obesity have more overall fat and lean mass by weight compared with PWS subjects, PWS subjects had increased adiposity or percentage of fat with significantly less lean mass in all body regions studied than individuals with simple obesity. Therefore, PWS subjects have more fat and less lean tissue relative to individuals with simple obesity, with males contributing more to these discrepancies than females. Furthermore, PWS males presented with a more feminine fat pattern. This may relate to the delayed sexual development and small gonads seen in PWS subjects, which contributes to decreased testosterone levels in males and thus interferes with muscle growth and with the subsequent loss of subcutaneous fat that normally occurs after puberty.

6.8 Obesity and Nutritional Management in PWS

Ghrelin and peptide YY (PYY) are small peptides produced by the gastrointestinal organs and are only a few of the several neuroendocrine peptides involved in appetite regulation (ghrelin stimulates eating whereas PYY inhibits eating) [62–65]. Elevated fasting plasma ghrelin levels have been reported in infants, children, and adults with PWS; therefore, potentially new classes of antiobesity drugs (e.g., ghrelin antagonists) that impact on ghrelin levels and eating behavior may have a role in the treatment of PWS. In addition, functional brain imaging (fMRI) studies in PWS and normally developing subjects using food and nonfood stimulation pictures at the time of fasting (premeal) and after food consumption (postmeal) showed significant differences between the two groups. Premeal fMRI studies showed neutral responses in the PWS subjects compared with controls; however, postmeal fMRI results showed increased activation in the limbic and paralimbic areas (orbital frontal cortex, prefrontal cortex, and amygdala) in PWS subjects compared with controls, indicating a lack of satiation in PWS subjects [66].

Energy expenditure components are estimated by a variety of methods but comprised of resting metabolism, thermic effects of food (energy required to consume and digest food), and physical activity (leisure or planned exercise). Resting metabolic rate and thermal effects of food generally represent stable components of total energy expenditure with resting metabolism accounting for approximately 60% of energy expenditure, thermic effects of food accounting for about 10%, and the remaining due to physical activity [67]. Pharmacological agents for weight management PWS have been met with limited success including appetite suppressant and antiabsorptive agents marketed for obesity treatment. However, these agents have not been systematically studied in PWS. Because of hyperphagia and concern for gastric rupturing in PWS [55], surgically decreasing stomach volume could pose unwanted and life-threatening risks. Therefore, bariatric surgical procedures which limit stomach size in PWS subjects are discouraged [2, 68].

Obesity can be a major health problem in PWS and life-threatening if not controlled. Obesity in PWS results from hyperphagia and persistent hunger, decreased perception of satiety, decreased physical activity and metabolic rate, and impaired emesis. Weight control and dietary restrictions are key management issues with caloric intake restricted to 6–8 kcal/cm of height for weight loss beginning in early childhood for non-growth hormone-treated PWS children and to 10–12 kcal/cm of height to maintain weight. For adolescents and adults with PWS, a general recommendation of 800/1,000 kcal/day is advised to achieve weight loss [69, 70]. An acceptable caloric reduction plan in use in the general population includes 60% carbohydrate, 15% protein, and 25% fat, while an approach for PWS may include one-third of calories from protein, two-fifths from carbohydrate, and the remainder from fat. Adequate protein during times of caloric restriction is needed to conserve lean body mass. Food exchange programs (e.g., American Dietetic Association) for starch/bread, vegetables, fruit, meat, dairy products, and fat can be utilized to assist in the nutritional needs of the PWS child during periods of growth. Restricted caloric intake requires vitamin and mineral (calcium) supplementation under close supervision of an experienced dietitian during the toddler years and beyond to minimize excessive weight gain and osteoporosis. The regime requires regular dietary counseling of care providers and analysis of food records to identify individual nutritional deficiencies. It is equally important to relate weight loss with body composition changes using DEXA (dual-energy x-ray absorptiometry) scans [71].

A careful and vigilant food monitoring program is essential for the child or adult with PWS to address their obesity issues. This includes close supervision at all times at school, on the school bus, visits to the grandparents, or in the work setting. Nutritional management in PWS can be separated into four major categories: (1) control of underweight during infancy and overweight during early childhood and beyond, (2) optimization and conservation of lean body mass, (3) special nutritional considerations, and (4) treatment of obesity related comorbidities.

The typical PWS body composition includes increased fat mass and decreased muscle mass and bone density compared to the general population. The goal of nutritional management of PWS is to provide optimal nutrition for health and growth, achieve weight control, and preserve (or increase) lean body mass. Oral intake during the first 2 years of life requires adjustment to maintain weight for length measures between the 25th and 80th percentile. Published growth standards for PWS are available to aide in monitoring their growth parameters [2, 72]. Effective strategies for nutritional management should include involvement of the patient, family members, and care providers to cope with weight and behavior control issues seen in PWS. Some of these strategies include locking away food; keeping limited amounts of food in the home; continual close supervision particularly around food or food-related events; providing non-food-related rewards; supplying smaller proportions of food servings by using smaller plates and bowls at mealtime; allowing the child to participate in menu planning, preparation, and posting; counting calories; and having less high-dense food available. Keeping strict mealtime regimes and unwavering consistency by both parents and care providers in and outside of the residence are important. Exercise programs that are tailored for each PWS person are encouraged with 30 min of sustained activity for three to five times per week. Obesity can be controlled in PWS subjects, but a lifetime commitment and close observation are required by all involved in their care [2, 71].

Growth hormone treatment will also impact these areas of nutritional management. The use of human recombinant growth hormone (GH) to treat GH deficiency common in PWS has improved the quality of life in PWS individuals with beneficial effects on height and body composition by expanding lean mass. The increase of lean mass (muscle) raises the metabolic rate and increases physical activity and energy expenditure which lead to a decreased fat mass. Individuals with PWS have lower lean body mass (LBM) compared with controls, which should contribute to a reduced basal energy expenditure level. Therefore, Butler et al. [67] used DEXA and a whole-room respiration chamber to determine the relationship among body composition, activity levels, and metabolic rates by measuring body composition, total energy expenditure (TEE), resting energy expenditure (REE), physical activity, and mechanical work (MW) during an 8-h monitoring period in non-GH-treated PWS ($N = 27$) and obese ($N = 24$) subjects greater than 10 years of age with an average

age of 23 years. The chamber consisted of a live-in whole-room indirect calorimeter equipped with a force platform floor to allow simultaneous measurement of energy expenditure, physical activity, and work efficiency during spontaneous activities and observed standardized exercise. PWS subjects had significantly decreased TEE by 20% and reduced LBM compared to obese subjects. Similarly, REE was significantly reduced by 16% in PWS individuals relative to the comparison obese subjects. Total MW performed during the 8-h monitoring period was significantly reduced by 35% in the PWS group. After adjusting for subject group differences, LBM, TEE, and REE were no longer significantly different between the two groups. The data indicated a significant reduction in energy expenditure in PWS individuals resulting from reduced activity and lower energy utilization due to reduced muscle mass.

6.9 *GNAS*, a Complex and Imprinted Locus

GNAS is an imprinted locus on chromosome 20q13.11 that produces multiple transcripts through the use of alternative promoters and alternative splicing, and if altered, leads to pathophysiology of several disorders through complex mechanisms and pathways. The most well-characterized transcript derived from *GNAS* is G protein subunit alpha (Gs-alpha) which encodes the stimulatory guanine nucleotide-binding protein (G protein). Gs-alpha is expressed biallelically in most tissues and plays essential roles in a multitude of physiologic processes, but expressed monoallelically from only the maternal *GNAS* allele in a small number of tissues including the gonads, pituitary and thyroid glands, and renal proximal tubules. Other transcripts produced by *GNAS* are expressed exclusively from either the paternal or the maternal *GNAS* allele [73, 74].

The *GNAS* locus is imprinted and encodes four main transcripts, Gs-alpha, *XLAS*, *NESP55*, and the A/B transcript, as well as an antisense *GNAS* transcript (*GNASAS*). The four main transcripts are produced through alternative promoters and splicing of four unique first exons of exons 2–13 of the gene. Gs-alpha is ubiquitously expressed. It encodes a protein that stimulates adenyl cyclase when activated by an agonist-occupied G protein-coupled receptor, thereby generating the second messenger cyclic AMP (cAMP). Many hormones, neurotransmitters, and autocrine/paracrine factors exert their actions through receptors coupled to Gs-alpha.

The *XLAS* transcript is a large variant of the Gs-alpha subunit and expressed exclusively from the paternal *GNAS* allele. This occurs primarily in neuroendocrine tissues and the nervous system. The XLAS and Gs-alpha proteins are identical over their C-terminal portions but have distinct N-termini.

The *NESP55* transcript is exclusively expressed from the maternal *GNAS* allele and encodes a chromogranin-like neuroendocrine secretory protein. It shares no amino acid sequence with Gs-alpha due to a stop codon in its unique first exon. The *A/B* transcript, which uses the alternative first exon *A/B* or exon 1A or 1-prime, and the antisense *GNAS* transcript consist of exons that do not overlap with any other *GNAS* exons and are noncoding transcripts ubiquitously expressed from the paternal *GNAS* allele. The promoters of the *XLAS*, *NESP55*, *A/B*, and antisense transcripts are located in the genome within differentially methylated regions (DMRs). When the promoter is unmethylated, expression of the transcripts occurs; however, the promoter for Gs-alpha lacks methylation and is biallelically expressed in most tissues [73].

Furthermore, genetic defects affecting even a single *GNAS* allele are associated with human disease [75]. Somatic mutations that constitutively activate Gs-alpha are found in various endocrine tumors, such as growth hormone-secreting adenomas, and somatic mutations are found in individuals with McCune–Albright syndrome. Heterozygous mutations within *GNAS* that impair either the activity or the expression of Gs-alpha are associated with pseudohypoparathyroidism (PHP), a disorder of target-organ resistance affecting predominantly, but not exclusively, the actions of parathyroid hormone (PTH). While imprinting of the *GNAS* locus is predicted to influence the molecular mechanisms of all these disorders, its role has been best documented in the development of PHP, which includes various different clinical types that are caused by related, but distinct, genetic defects and show parent-of-origin-specific inheritance.

6.10 Albright Hereditary Osteodystrophy (AHO), Pseudohypoparathyroidism (PHP), and Pseudopseudohypoparathyroidism (PPHP)

In 1942, Albright [76] first reported an osteodystrophy condition which was due to an end-organ resistance to the actions of parathyroid and other hormones. Two major variants are now recognized including PHP (PHP-Ia, PHP-Ib) and PHPP. Those with PHP-Ia have features of Albright hereditary osteodystrophy (AHO). They present with hypocalcemia and hyperphosphatemia despite elevated parathyroid hormone levels. Resistance to thyroid-stimulating hormone, gonadotropins, growth hormone-releasing hormone, and calcitonin can also occur in affected individuals. In contrast, individuals with PPHP have characteristic physical features of AHO, but do not show evidence of resistance to parathyroid or other hormones and with normal calcium levels. PHP-Ia and PPHP have been reported in the same families, but are dependent on the parent of origin. Both variants result from decreased activity of the Gs-alpha subunit and therefore decreased ability to couple membrane receptors to adenyl cyclase to stimulate cAMP formation [75].

PHP is divided into two subgroups, PHP-Ia and PHP-Ib, depending on the presence and absence of additional hormone resistance and the AHO phenotype. Those individuals with PHP-Ia and features of AHO are reported with mutations of the *GNAS* gene as well as cytogenetic deletions of chromosome 20q including *GNAS*. PHP-Ia with AHO is characterized by short stature (final adult height 54–60 in.), moderate obesity, mental deficiency (average IQ of 60), round face with a short nose and short neck, delayed dental eruption and enamel hypoplasia, short metacarpals and metatarsals (especially of fourth and fifth digits), short distal phalanx of the thumb, osteoporosis, areas of mineralization in subcutaneous tissues including the basal ganglia, variable hypocalcemia and/or hyperphosphatema, and seizures. Occasional findings include hypothyroidism, hypogonadism, lens opacity or cataracts, optic atrophy, ocular degeneration, and vertebral anomalies [77, 78]. Those patients with PHP who present with PTH resistance but lack other AHO features are defined as having the PHP-Ib subtype. Most PHP-Ib cases are sporadic, but have occurred in families with an autosomal dominant inheritance pattern with incomplete penetrance. Individuals with PHP-Ib typically lack *GNAS* gene mutations; however, studies show that the inheritance comes from a female exhibiting alteration in imprinting of the *GNAS* locus. Loss of methylation in controlling elements regulating the imprinting of the *GNAS* gene is the most consistent defect. However, one case of PHP-Ib was found with paternal disomy of chromosome 20 [74, 75].

Patients with PHPP also carry heterozygous inactivating *GNAS* mutations, but of paternal inheritance which yields AHO alone. These differences in the imprinted mode of inheritance for hormone resistance could be explained by the predominantly maternal expression of *GNAS* in certain tissues. Those with PHP-Ia lacking *GNAS* mutations, but displaying the gene disturbance, are due to an imprinting defect and loss of imprint at the exon A/B differentially methylated region of the gene. A unique 3-kb microdeletion has been reported that disrupts the neighboring *STX16* which is close to the differentially methylated domain and can cause PHP-I as well and loss of imprint [74].

In summary, the pattern of inheritance of the *GNAS* gene with multiple transcriptional units is located at chromosome 20q13.11. It stimulates adenyl cyclase activity and is responsible for both PHP-Ia and PPHP variants of the AHO syndrome. PHP-Ia and PPHP are caused by heterozygous inactivating mutations in exons of the *GNAS* gene encoding the alpha subunit of the stimulatory guanine nucleotide-binding protein (Gs-alpha), while the autosomal dominant form of PHP-Ib is caused by heterozygous mutations disrupting a long-range imprinting control element of *GNAS*. Both disorder variants are dependent on parent of origin, therefore due to imprinting, and reported in the same family. If the altered gene is inherited from the affected father with either PHP-Ia or PPHP, then PHPP occurs in the offspring. If the inheritance of the same *GNAS* mutation is present in the mother with either PHP-Ia or PHPP, then the child will present with PHP-Ia.

6.11 McCune–Albright Syndrome

McCune–Albright syndrome (MAS) is a unique condition reported in 1937 by McCune, Albright, and colleagues [79, 80]. It consists of polyostotic fibrous dysplasia, irregular skin pigmentation patterns, various endocrine tumors, and sexual precocity. More females than males (3:2) are diagnosed with this disorder. The main abnormalities in MAS include multiple areas of fibrous dysplasia leading to bone thickening which is usually unilateral. It most commonly involves the long bones and pelvis. However, other areas may include the cranium, facial bones (leading to facial asymmetry), ribs, and occasionally the spine. The involvement of the skull and facial bones can be extreme and may lead to deafness and blindness. The bone dysplasia may progress during childhood and result in fractures or deformities most commonly in the upper femur. Rarely, malignancy transformation occurs at these bone sites. Bone thickening in the calvarium can lead to cranial nerve compression, blindness, or deafness. Cutaneous abnormalities may be unilateral and generally include irregular brown pigmentation (café au lait spots) with most common areas including the sacrum, buttocks, and upper spine. The pigmentary changes are usually evident during infancy [78].

Endocrine system disturbances include sexual precocity (occurs in over one-half of affected females), hyperthyroidism (second most common form of endocrinopathy), hyperparathyroidism, and pituitary adenomas that secrete excessive growth hormone leading to acromegaly or gigantism. Cushing syndrome and hyperprolactinemia are occasionally seen, but concentrations of tropic hormones are generally normal or reduced. Sexual precocity in the female can be rapid and may induce menstruation before pubic hair development. This accelerated maturation may result in early epiphyseal fusion, with adult height being relatively short. When endocrine problems occur in infancy, it can be life-threatening [81].

The cause of MAS is due to postzygotic somatic activating gain-of-function mutations of the *GNAS* gene yielding a monoclonal population of mutated cells in various affected tissues, which encode the alpha subunit of G proteins involved in signal transduction pathways and affect the production of cAMP in affected tissues. An overactive cAMP pathway stimulates the growth and function of the gonads, adrenal cortex, specific pituitary cell populations, osteoblasts, and melanocytes. The nonmosaic state for activating mutations is presumably lethal in the developing embryo [82, 83]. Thus, variable clinical expression is determined by the relative number of mutant cells in a mosaic fashion as well as the tissues involved.

In a study by Lumbroso et al. [83], 43% of MAS subjects had a *GNAS* mutation involving the Arg201 amino acid position, with a preponderance of the R201H, and a minority of patients exhibiting, R201C. No difference in clinical findings or severity was noted between these mutations.

Somatic mutations of the *GNAS* gene have been reported in pituitary adenomas, including acromegaly and Cushing syndrome. In a series of 32 corticotroph adenomas of the pituitary, Williamson et al. [84] found two with somatic mutations in the *GNAS* gene at codon 227. Hayward et al. [85] noted that approximately 40% of growth hormone-secreting pituitary adenomas contain somatic mutations in the *GNAS* gene at Arg201 or Glu227 which activate the alpha subunit of *GNAS*. Although transcripts encoding Gs-alpha are biallelically derived in most human tissues, Hayward et al. [85] showed that the mutation had occurred on the maternal allele in 21 of 22 *GNAS*-positive somatotroph adenomas. They also showed that Gs-alpha is monoallelically expressed from the maternal allele in normal adult pituitary tissue, but this monoallelic expression of Gs-alpha was frequently relaxed in somatotroph tumors regardless of *GNAS* mutation status implicating a possible role for loss of Gs-alpha imprinting during pituitary somatotroph tumorigenesis.

6.12 Applications to Other Areas of Health and Disease Related to Epigenetics and Obesity

Basic research and the delineation of clinical findings in clinical epigenetic disorders with obesity as a major feature are important to understand health and disease. Obesity has reached epidemic levels and is a major public health problem in our industrialized society. There is a sense of urgency for better understanding of the causal relationships among genetic and environmental factors in the development of obesity. Research on obesity syndromes such as PWS should lead to a better understanding of this disorder as well as genetics of exogenous obesity. The complexity of the genetic mechanisms in PWS discovered during the past 20 years informs us about the influence of genes on growth and development in other genetic disorders as well as in the general population. In PWS, the experience with growth hormone therapy has implications for pharmacotherapy of other genetic disorders. Stefan and Nicholls [86] have proposed that a number of aspects of the genetics of PWS could provide insights into etiologic mechanisms in obesity. First, they point out that PWS likely involves multiple genes, with the primary etiologic genes being clustered in the genome. Epigenetics may also play a role in exogenous obesity and the effects of nutrition on genetics (nutrigenomics). Possibly other undiscovered clusters of obesity-causing genes that are related to nonsyndromic obesity in human populations may be identified or characterized. Second, investigation of the genetic pathways in PWS might also add to the number of candidate genes associated with obesity leading to treatment modalities. Finally, PWS is among several conditions in which imprinted genes are involved and many of the loci are associated with overgrowth or obesity in animals. Research on PWS during the past three decades has strongly suggested that genetic mechanisms identified in PWS and other rare obesity-related genetic syndromes will ultimately be counted among the multiple genes and pathways that contribute to nonsyndromic obesity.

The diagnosis of PWS used to be based primarily on clinical criteria, but completion of the Human Genome Project and other technical advances has changed the means of diagnosis for this condition. Current studies in genetics have revealed complexities that we could only imagine 30 years ago, such as imprinted genes that are now often associated with human diseases and known to contribute to cellular growth and development in PWS and a number of other genetic disorders. In PWS, abnormalities of this imprinting mechanism lead to the early failure-to-thrive phenotype observed in human infants and mouse models of PWS. An important gene in the 15q11–q13 region is the paternally expressed *SNURF–SNRPN* gene and other imprinted genes and transcripts including the snoRNAs (*SNORDs*). Paternally expressed genes in general influence growth and development. Mutations have been identified in the imprinting center and *SNORDs* alone contributing to PWS on the

PWS phenotype. There may be selection for imprinting genes in this region due to the postnatal growth advantage conferred by paternally derived genes. Other known clinical epigenetic disorders with obesity including those involving the complex *GNAS* imprinted locus follow similar patterns by disturbance of maternally or paternally expressed alleles. Similar mechanisms are being explored in other conditions involving failure-to-thrive and growth anomalies and/or obesity.

The introduction of growth hormone therapy during the 1980s has profoundly altered the phenotypic outcomes in PWS, especially the lean-to-fat body mass ratio and linear growth. Questions have been raised about its use involving dosage, timing, and monitoring for side effects and safety in individuals with PWS and other genetic disorders. However, the experience with growth hormone in PWS has generally been positive. It is clear that the experience with growth hormone therapy in PWS and other conditions will provide models for the evaluation of future therapeutic interventions.

The complexities of managing genetic disorders can never be underestimated, and PWS is no exception. The array of physical and behavioral problems encountered in individuals with PWS coupled with the introduction of growth hormone therapy and other medical and behavioral interventions has necessitated the development of multidisciplinary team management in clinical settings. Approaches like those being introduced for PWS, including natural history studies and genotype–phenotype correlations, may serve as guides for the management of other genetic disorders and the more common diseases as their genetic components are elucidated and appropriate interventions developed.

Acknowledgments I thank Carla Meister for expert preparation of the manuscript. Partial funding support was provided by the NIH rare disease grant (1U54HD061222) and a grant from Prader–Willi Syndrome Association (USA).

References

1. Butler MG. Prader-Willi syndrome: current understanding of cause and diagnosis. Am J Med Genet. 1990; 35(3):319–32.
2. Butler MG, Lee PDK, Whitman BY. Management of Prader-Willi syndrome. 3rd ed. In: Butler MG, Lee PDK, Whitman BY, editors. New York, NY: Springer; 2006. pp. 1–550.
3. Cassidy SB, Driscoll DJ. Prader-Willi syndrome. Eur J Hum Genet. 2009; 17(1):3–13.
4. Bittel DC, Butler MG. Prader-Willi syndrome: clinical genetics, cytogenetics and molecular biology. Expert Rev Mol Med. 2005; 7(14):1–20.
5. Cattanach BM, Beechey CV, Peters J. Interactions between imprinting effects: summary and review. Cytogenet Genome Res. 2006; 113(1–4):17–23.
6. Delaval K, Wagschal A, Feil R. Epigenetic deregulation of imprinting in congenital diseases of aberrant growth. Bioessays. 2006; 28(5):453–9.
7. Zakharova IS, Shevchenko AI, Zakian SM. Monoallelic gene expression in mammals. Chromosoma. 2009; 118(3):279–90.
8. Murphy SK, Jirtle RL. Imprinting evolution and the price of silence. Bioessays. 2003; 25(6):577–88.
9. Butler MG. Genomic imprinting disorders in humans: a mini-review. J Assist Reprod Genet. 2009; 26(9–10):477–86.

10. Prader A, Labhart A, Willi H. Ein syndrome von adipositas, kleinwuchs, kryptorchismus and oligophrenie nach myatonieartigem zustand im neugeborenenalter. Schweizerische Medzinische Wochenschrift. 1956; 86:1260–1.
11. Ledbetter DH, Riccardi VM, Airhart SD, Strobel RJ, Keenan BS, Crawford JD. Deletions of chromosome 15 as a cause of the Prader-Willi syndrome. N Engl J Med. 1981; 304(6): 325–29.
12. Butler MG, Palmer CG. Parental origin of chromosome 15 deletion in Prader-Willi syndrome. Lancet. 1983; 1(8336):1285–6.
13. Nicholls RD, Knoll JH, Butler MG, Karam S, Lalande M. Genetic imprinting suggested by maternal heterodisomy in nondeletion Prader-Willi syndrome. Nature. 1989; 342(6247): 281–5.
14. Cassidy SB, Lai LW, Erickson RP, et al. Trisomy 15 with loss of the paternal 15 as a cause of Prader-Willi syndrome due to maternal disomy. Am J Hum Genet. 1992; 51(4):701–8.
15. Christian SL, Smith AC, Macha M, et al. Prenatal diagnosis of uniparental disomy 15 following trisomy 15 mosaicism. Prenat Diagn. 1996; 16(4):323–32.
16. Butler MG, Sturich J, Myers SE, Gold JA, Kimonis V, Driscoll DJ. Is gestation in Prader-Willi syndrome affected by the genetic subtype? J Assist Reprod Genet. 2009; 26(8):461–6.
17. Viville S, Surani MA. Towards unravelling the Igf2/H19 imprinted domain. Bioessays. 1995; 17(10):835–8.
18. Eggermann T. Silver-Russell and Beckwith-Wiedemann syndromes: opposite (epi) mutations in 11p15 result in opposite clinical pictures. Horm Res. 2009; 71 Suppl 2 :30–5.
19. Lau AW, Brown CJ, Penaherrera M, Langlois S, Kalousek DK, Robinson WP. Skewed X-chromosome inactivation is common in fetuses or newborns associated with confined placental mosaicism. Am J Hum Genet. 1997; 61(6):1353–61.
20. Butler MG, Theodoro MF, Bittel DC, Kuipers PJ, Driscoll DJ, Talebizadeh Z. X-chromosome inactivation patterns in females with Prader-Willi syndrome. Am J Med Genet A. 2007; 143(5):469–75.
21. Krepischi AC, Kok F, Otto PG. X chromosome-inactivation patterns in patients with Rett syndrome. Hum Genet. 1998; 102(3):319–21.
22. Ledbetter DH, Zachary JM, Simpson JL, et al. Cytogenetic results from the U.S. Collaborative Study on CVS. Prenat Diagn. 1992; 12(5):317–45.
23. Verdine BN, Troseth GL, Hodapp RM, Dykens EM. Strategies and correlates of jigsaw puzzle and visuospatial performance by persons with Prader-Willi syndrome. Am J Ment Retard. 2008; 113(5):343–55.
24. Butler MG, Thompson T. Prader-Willi syndrome: clinical and genetics findings. Endocrinologist. 2000; 10:3S–16S.
25. Butler MG, Fischer W, Kibiryeva N, Bittel DC. Array comparative genomic hybridization (aCGH) analysis in Prader-Willi syndrome. Am J Med Genet A. 2008; 146(7):854–60.
26. Nicholls RD, Knepper JL. Genome organization, function, and imprinting in Prader-Willi and Angelman syndromes. Annu Rev Genomics Hum Genet. 2001; 2:153–75.
27. Miller NL, Wevrick R, Mellon PL. Necdin, a Prader-Willi syndrome candidate gene, regulates gonadotropin-releasing hormone neurons during development. Hum Mol Genet. 2009; 18(2):248–60.
28. Mercer RE, Wevrick R. Loss of magel2, a candidate gene for features of Prader-Willi syndrome, impairs reproductive function in mice. PLoS One. 2009; 4(1):e4291.
29. Kozlov SV, Bogenpohl JW, Howell MP, et al. The imprinted gene Magel2 regulates normal circadian output. Nat Genet. 2007; 39(10):1266–72.
30. Gray TA, Hernandez L, Carey AH, et al. The ancient source of a distinct gene family encoding proteins featuring RING and C(3)H zinc-finger motifs with abundant expression in developing brain and nervous system. Genomics. 2000; 66(1):76–86.
31. Buiting K, Nazlican H, Galetzka D, Wawrzik M, Gross S, Horsthemke B. C15orf2 and a novel noncoding transcript from the Prader-Willi/Angelman syndrome region show monoallelic expression in fetal brain. Genomics. 2007; 89(5):588–95.

32. Ding F, Li HH, Zhang S, et al. SnoRNA Snord116 (Pwcr1/MBII-85) deletion causes growth deficiency and hyperphagia in mice. PLoS One. 2008; 3(3):e1709.
33. Bittel DC, Kibiryeva N, Talebizadeh Z, Butler MG. Microarray analysis of gene/transcript expression in Prader-Willi syndrome: deletion versus UPD. J Med Genet. 2003; 40(8):568–74.
34. Bittel DC, Kibiryeva N, Talebizadeh Z, Driscoll DJ, Butler MG. Microarray analysis of gene/transcript expression in Angelman syndrome: deletion versus UPD. Genomics. 2005; 85(1):85–91.
35. Ebert MH, Schmidt DE, Thompson T, Butler MG. Elevated plasma gamma-aminobutyric acid (GABA) levels in individuals with either Prader-Willi syndrome or Angelman syndrome. J Neuropsychiatry Clin Neurosci. Winter 1997; 9(1):75–80.
36. Ji Y, Rebert NA, Joslin JM, Higgins MJ, Schultz RA, Nicholls RD. Structure of the highly conserved HERC2 gene and of multiple partially duplicated paralogs in human. Genome Res. March 2000; 10(3):319–29.
37. Chai JH, Locke DP, Greally JM, et al. Identification of four highly conserved genes between breakpoint hotspots BP1 and BP2 of the Prader-Willi/Angelman syndromes deletion region that have undergone evolutionary transposition mediated by flanking duplicons. Am J Hum Genet. 2003; 73(4):898–925.
38. Butler MG, Jenkins BB. Analysis of chromosome breakage in the Prader-Labhart-Willi syndrome. Am J Med Genet. 1989; 32(4):514–9.
39. Butler MG, Bittel DC, Kibiryeva N, Talebizadeh Z, Thompson T. Behavioral differences among subjects with Prader-Willi syndrome and type I or type II deletion and maternal disomy. Pediatrics. 2004; 113(3 Pt 1):565–73.
40. Bittel DC, Kibiryeva N, Butler MG. Expression of 4 genes between chromosome 15 breakpoints 1 and 2 and behavioral outcomes in Prader-Willi syndrome. Pediatrics. 2006; 118(4):e1276–e83.
41. Roof E, Stone W, MacLean W, Feurer ID, Thompson T, Butler MG. Intellectual characteristics of Prader-Willi syndrome: comparison of genetic subtypes. J Intellect Disabil Res. 2000; 44 (Pt 1):25–30.
42. Zarcone J, Napolitano D, Peterson C, et al. The relationship between compulsive behaviour and academic achievement across the three genetic subtypes of Prader-Willi syndrome. J Intellect Disabil Res. 2007; 51(Pt. 6):478–87.
43. Kanber D, Giltay J, Wieczorek D, et al. A paternal deletion of MKRN3, MAGEL2 and NDN does not result in Prader-Willi syndrome. Eur J Hum Genet. 2009; 17(5):582–90.
44. Sahoo T, del Gaudio D, German JR, et al. Prader-Willi phenotype caused by paternal deficiency for the HBII-85 C/D box small nucleolar RNA cluster. Nat Genet. 2008; 40(6):719–21.
45. Smith AJ, Purmann C, Walters RG, et al. A deletion of the HBII-85 class of small nucleolar RNAs (snoRNAs) is associated with hyperphagia, obesity and hypogonadism. Hum Mol Genet. 2009; 18(17):3257–65.
46. Kishore S, Stamm S. The snoRNA HBII-52 regulates alternative splicing of the serotonin receptor 2C. Science. 2006; 311(5758):230–2.
47. Bittel DC, Kibiryeva N, Sell SM, Strong TV, Butler MG. Whole genome microarray analysis of gene expression in Prader-Willi syndrome. Am J Med Genet A. 2007; 143(5):430–42.
48. Hall BD, Smith DW, Prader-Willi S. A resumé of 32 cases including an instance of affected first cousins, one of whom is of normal stature and intelligence. J Pediatr. 1972; 81(2):286–93.
49. Bray GA, Dahms WT, Swerdloff RS, Fiser RH, Atkinson RL, Carrel RE. The Prader-Willi syndrome: a study of 40 patients and a review of the literature. Medicine (Baltimore). 1983; 62(2):59–80.
50. Cassidy SB. Prader-Willi syndrome. Curr Probl Pediatr. 1984; 14(1):1–55.
51. Butler MG, Meaney FJ, Palmer CG. Clinical and cytogenetic survey of 39 individuals with Prader-Labhart-Willi syndrome. Am J Med Genet. 1986; 23(3):793–809.
52. Butler MG. Prader-Willi syndrome: an example of genomic imprinting. In: Butler MG, Meaney FJ editors. Genetics of developmental disabilities. 1st ed. Boca Raton, FL: Taylor & Francis; 2005. pp. 279–318.

53. Hirsch HJ, Eldar-Geva T, Benarroch F, Rubinstein O, Gross-Tsur V. Primary testicular dysfunction is a major contributor to abnormal pubertal development in males with Prader-Willi syndrome. J Clin Endocrinol Metab. July 2009; 94(7):2262–8.
54. Eldar-Geva T, Hirsch HJ, Rabinowitz R, Benarroch F, Rubinstein O, Gross-Tsur V. Primary ovarian dysfunction contributes to the hypogonadism in women with Prader-Willi syndrome. Horm Res. 2009; 72(3):153–9.
55. Stevenson DA, Heinemann J, Angulo M, et al. Gastric rupture and necrosis in Prader-Willi syndrome. J Pediatr Gastroenterol Nutr. 2007; 45(2):272–4.
56. Goldstone AP, Holland AJ, Hauffa BP, Hokken-Koelega AC, Tauber M. Recommendations for the diagnosis and management of Prader-Willi syndrome. J Clin Endocrinol Metab. Nov 2008; 93(11):4183–97.
57. Meaney FJ, Butler MG. The developing role of anthropologists in medical genetics: anthropometric assessment of the Prader-Labhart-Willi syndrome as an illustration. Med Anthropol. 1989; 10(4):247–53.
58. Meaney FJ, Butler MG. Characterization in obesity in the Prader-Labhart-Willi syndrome: fatness patterning. Med Anthropol Q. 1989; 3:294–305.
59. Talebizadeh Z, Butler MG. Insulin resistance and obesity-related factors in Prader-Willi syndrome: comparison with obese subjects. Clin Genet. 2005; 67(3):230–9.
60. Goldstone AP, Thomas EL, Brynes AE, et al. Visceral adipose tissue and metabolic complications of obesity are reduced in Prader-Willi syndrome female adults: evidence for novel influences on body fat distribution. J Clin Endocrinol Metab. 2001; 86(9):4330–8.
61. Theodoro MF, Talebizadeh Z, Butler MG. Body composition and fatness patterns in Prader-Willi syndrome: comparison with simple obesity. Obesity (Silver Spring). 2006; 14(10): 1685–90.
62. Cummings DE, Clement K, Purnell JQ, et al. Elevated plasma ghrelin levels in Prader Willi syndrome. Nat Med. 2002; 8(7):643–4.
63. Haqq AM, Stadler DD, Rosenfeld RG, et al. Circulating ghrelin levels are suppressed by meals and octreotide therapy in children with Prader-Willi syndrome. J Clin Endocrinol Metab. 2003; 88(8):3573–6.
64. Butler MG, Bittel DC, Talebizadeh Z. Plasma peptide YY and ghrelin levels in infants and children with Prader-Willi syndrome. J Pediatr Endocrinol Metab. 2004; 17(9): 1177–84.
65. Butler MG, Bittel DC. Plasma obestatin and ghrelin levels in subjects with Prader-Willi syndrome. Am J Med Genet A. 2007; 143(5):415–21.
66. Holsen LM, Zarcone JR, Brooks WM, et al. Neural mechanisms underlying hyperphagia in Prader-Willi syndrome. Obesity (Silver Spring). 2006; 14(6):1028–37.
67. Butler MG, Theodoro MF, Bittel DC, Donnelly JE. Energy expenditure and physical activity in Prader-Willi syndrome: comparison with obese subjects. Am J Med Genet A. 2007; 143(5):449–59.
68. Scheimann A, Butler MG, Stevenson D, Miller JL, Cuffari C, Klish WJ. Efficacy of laparoscopic sleeve gastrectomy as a stand-alone technique for children with morbid obesity and BioEnterics intragastric balloon for treatment of morbid obesity in Prader-Willi syndrome: specific risks and benefits. Obes Surg. 2009; 19(5):671–2.
69. Holm VA, Pipes PL. Food and children with Prader-Willi syndrome. Am J Dis Child. 1976; 130(10):1063–7.
70. Holm VA, Sulzbacher SJ, Pipes PL. Prader-Willi Syndrome. In: Holm VA, Sulzbacher SJ, Pipes PL, editors. Baltimore, MD: University Park Press; 1981. pp. 1–349.
71. Butler MG. Management of obesity in Prader-Willi syndrome. Nat Clin Pract Endocrinol Metab. 2006; 2(11):592–3.
72. Butler MG, Meaney FJ. Standards for selected anthropometric measurements in Prader-Willi syndrome. Pediatrics. 1991; 88(4):853–60.
73. Bastepe M, Juppner H. GNAS locus and pseudohypoparathyroidism. Horm Res. 2005; 63(2):65–74.

74. Bastepe M. The GNAS locus and pseudohypoparathyroidism. Adv Exp Med Biol. 2008; 626:27–40.
75. GNAS complex locus. www.ncbl/nlm.nih.gov/OMIM. Accessed 12 Mar 2010.
76. Albright F, Burnett CH, Smith PH, Parson W. Pseudo-hypoparathyroidism – an example of "Seabright-Bantam syndrome": report of three cases. Endocrinology. 1942; 30:922–32.
77. Levine MA. Clinical spectrum and pathogenesis of pseudohypoparathyroidism. Rev Endocr Metab Disord. 2000; 1(4):265–74.
78. Jones KL (editor.). Smith's recognizable patterns of human malformation. 5th ed. Philadelphia, PA: W.B. Saunders Company 2006.
79. McCune DJ, Bruch H. Progress in pediatrics: osteodystrophia fibrosa. Am J Dis Child. 1937; 54:806–48.
80. Albright F, Butler AM, Hampton AO, Smith P. Syndrome characterized by osteitis fibrosa disseminata, areas of pigmentation and endocrine dysfunction, with precocious puberty in females: report of five cases. New Eng J Med. 1937; 216:727–46.
81. McCune-Albright syndrome. www.ncbl/nlm.nih.gov/OMIM. Accessed 12 Mar 2010.
82. Aldred MA, Bagshaw RJ, Macdermot K, et al. Germline mosaicism for a GNAS1 mutation and Albright hereditary osteodystrophy. J Med Genet. 2000; 37(11):E35.
83. Lumbroso S, Paris F, Sultan C. Activating Gsalpha mutations: analysis of 113 patients with signs of McCune-Albright syndrome – a European Collaborative Study. J Clin Endocrinol Metab. 2004; 89(5):2107–13.
84. Williamson EA, Ince PG, Harrison D, Kendall-Taylor P, Harris PE. G-protein mutations in human pituitary adrenocorticotrophic hormone-secreting adenomas. Eur J Clin Invest. 1995; 25(2):128–31.
85. Hayward BE, Barlier A, Korbonits M, et al. Imprinting of the G(s)alpha gene GNAS1 in the pathogenesis of acromegaly. J Clin Invest. 2001; 107(6):R31–6.
86. Stefan M, Nicholls RD. What have rare genetic syndromes taught us about the pathophysiology of the common forms of obesity? Curr Diab Rep. 2004; 4(2):143–50.

Chapter 7
Evidence for Epigenetic Changes as a Cause of Clinical Obesity

Graham C. Burdge and Karen A. Lillycrop

7.1 Introduction

Obesity together with type 2 diabetes mellitus (T2DM), dyslipidemia, and hypertension is a major risk factor for cardiovascular disease, osteoarthritis, and certain forms of cancer including breast, colon, and prostate. The global prevalence of obesity has been predicted to increase to between 30 and 80% by 2030, with the greatest disease burden in developing counties such as India [1]. Obesity is routinely thought to be caused by lifestyle choices in which a poor quality yet high calorie diet and low levels of activity play major roles. In developing nations the increasing prevalence of obesity largely reflects migration from low-energy diets in rural communities to urban calorie-rich, westernized diets as nations move toward industrial and technology-driven economies rather than traditional agriculture. However, there is differential risk within populations of developing obesity and its associated conditions, which implies an underlying vulnerability in some individuals that limits their ability to maintain energy balance when presented with excessive calorie intake. The role of genetic variation in determining such differential susceptibility is unclear. As with other complex disease traits, while some candidate genes have been reported [2], the contribution of individual polymorphisms to pathogenesis may be small [3]. There is increasing evidence that the prenatal environment acts through developmental plasticity which involves induced changes in the epigenetic regulation of non-imprinted genes and underlies differential risk of obesity and associated conditions including cardiometabolic disease and some cancers. The role of altered epigenetic regulation of imprinted genes in obesity is described in detail in Chapter 6. This chapter will instead focus on the role of altered epigenetic processes in non-imprinted genes in humans and in animal models in determining differential susceptibility to obesity.

G.C. Burdge (✉)
Institute of Human Nutrition, University of Southampton School of Medicine, Southampton SO16 6YD, UK
e-mail: g.c.burdge@southampton.ac.uk

R.H. Lustig (ed.), *Obesity Before Birth*, Endocrine Updates 30,
DOI 10.1007/978-1-4419-7034-3_7, © Springer Science+Business Media, LLC 2011

7.2 Developmental Plasticity

Development represents a period of rapid change in the expression of the genome during which environmental cues may induce persistent changes in the phenotype of an organism. The developmental program tends to follow a path in which the characteristics of the wild type or typical phenotype are buffered against genetic and epigenetic change, termed canalization [4]. It has been known for almost 100 years that the environment in which an embryo and fetus develops can induce variations in the phenotype of the offspring without changing the genome. This is illustrated by experiments such as those described by Stockard, which show that modest, graded variations in the concentration of dissolved oxygen during specific periods in the development of trout embryo induced a range of changes in the phenotype of the offspring including conjoined fry [5]. Many organisms undergo adaptations during development in response to cues about the future environment, including nutrition and endocrine factors, which alter the developmental program in a manner which generates markedly different phenotypes from a single genotype. Crowding of typically nocturnal, solitary adult desert locusts (*Schistocerca gregaria*) induces in their offspring gregarious, diurnal, and migratory behavior [6]. The offspring of *Daphnia* are born with a defensive "helmet" structure if their mother has been exposed to chemicals produced by predators [7]. The duration of daylight to which meadow voles (*Microtus pennsylvanicus*) are exposed during pregnancy determines coat thickness in the offspring in anticipation of winter or spring temperatures [8]. Feeding Royal Jelly to larval honeybees (*Apis mellifera*) determines whether they will develop into fertile queens or infertile workers [9]. For some species, such rapid changes in phenotype may facilitate short-term survival, but may also be assimilated and so produce stable phenotypes on which natural selection may act [10]. Gluckman and Hanson have suggested that the phenotypic changes induced in mammals, including humans, by poor prenatal nutrition or maternal stress reflect an adaptive response to environmental cues acting through developmental plasticity which induce phenotypes that predict the future environment and thus may confer a Darwinian fitness advantage [11]. For example, poor nutrition of the pregnant mother may signal to the fetus that nutrients are scarce in the postnatal environment and so induces metabolic adaptations in the offspring which changes its homeostatic range and reduces energy demands (Fig. 7.1). However, prediction of a nutrient-poor environment and induction of a phenotype adaptive to conserve energy, but subsequent high calorie intake, would result in excessive storage of energy (Fig. 7.1). Such a mismatch has been suggested to underlie cardiometabolic disease in humans [11]. Inaccurate prediction of the future environment may arise if maternal nutrition is adequate but placental function is suboptimal, or if maternal nutrition is poor, but the offspring migrate to a region where food is abundant. One important feature of adaptive processes during development is that underlying changes in gene transcription are stabilized through the life course by epigenetic processes.

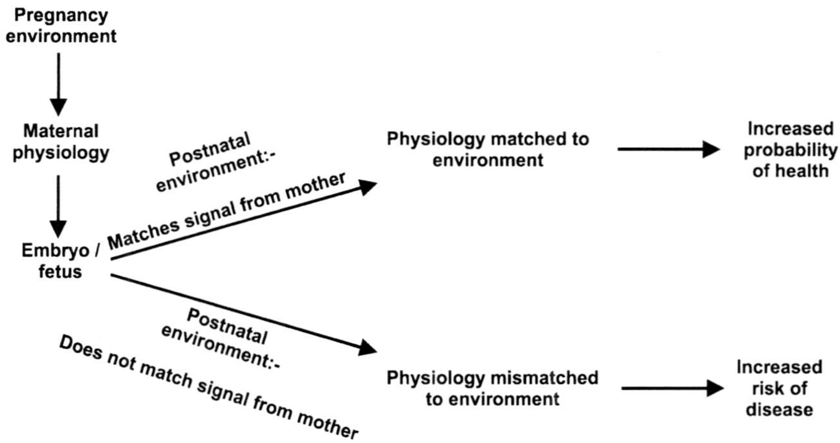

Fig. 7.1 Predictive adaptive response in mammals and future risk of disease [11]. In mammals, signals about the future environment, for example, nutrition, are transmitted to the offspring via the mother. Such environmental cues induce changes in the phenotype of the offspring which may be adaptive and, if correct, confer a fitness advantage. However, an incorrect signal from the mother may induce adaptations in the fetus which are mismatched to the future environment and which may be disadvantageous. Such mismatch has been implicated as a causal pathway toward increased risk of cardiometabolic disease in humans [11]

7.3 Developmental Plasticity and Human Metabolic Disease

It is perhaps not surprising that the quality of the environment to which human embryos are exposed induces lifelong variation in the phenotype of the offspring. Gross morphological variation in response to insults during the early life environment is relatively rare. Examples of such teratogenic effects include the dysmorphia and neurological impairment characteristic of fetal alcohol syndrome [12] and failure of limb growth in individuals exposed prenatally to thalidomide [13]. However, variation in the quality of intrauterine environment, for example, the availability of nutrients and oxygen and exposure of hormones, has been demonstrated repeatedly as a causal factor in differential risk of cardiometabolic disease including obesity as well as other chronic non-communicable diseases, including osteoporosis, some forms of cancer, and affective disorders [14, 15].

The first clear evidence of an association between the quality of the early life environment and subsequent risk of cardiometabolic disease was described in a series of epidemiological studies by David Barker and colleagues in the UK. They found a strong geographical relationship between infant mortality and risk of cardiovascular disease (CVD) 50–60 years later [16]. Subsequent retrospective studies in cohorts across the globe in developed and developing nations including the UK, North America, India, and the Far East have shown consistently that lower birthweight within the normal range for a particular population is associated with an increased risk in later life of CVD and the metabolic syndrome [14, 16, 17]. However, at the highest birthweights, which exceeded the normal range and may reflect macrosomia, the risk of cardiometabolic disease increased again, resulting in a U- or J-shaped relationship between birthweight and later disease risk [18, 19].

The timing of the nutritional constraint during pregnancy is important in determining the future risk of disease. Studies of individuals exposed in utero to the Dutch Famine, which occurred during the winter of 1944, showed that risk of obesity and its associated conditions was related to the timing of nutrient constraint. Individuals whose mothers were exposed to famine periconceptually and in the first trimester of pregnancy did not have reduced birthweights compared to unexposed individuals, but as adults exhibited increased risk of obesity and CVD. Individuals whose mothers were exposed in the later stages of gestation had reduced birthweights and showed an increased incidence of insulin resistance and hypertension [20]. This is in agreement with a study in sheep which showed that prenatal or postnatal undernutrition induces different changes in growth and vascular function [21]. One implication of the findings of these studies is that the activity of the mechanism which underlies the induction of an altered phenotype must vary as development proceeds and so producing periods of vulnerability to developing specific diseases in later life.

Overnutrition in early life also induces increased risk of future obesity which may account for the U-shaped or J-shaped relationships observed between birthweight and risk of obesity or insulin resistance in later life. Children born to mothers with gestational diabetes are frequently macrosomic, have increased gain in body mass by 4 years of age, and have increased risk of cardiometabolic disease [22, 23]. However, irrespective of gestational diabetes, children born to obese women are themselves more likely to become over weight and develop insulin resistance in later life [24]. Gestational weight gain irrespective of pre-pregnancy weight is positively associated with obesity at 3 years [25]. Moderate weight gain between successive pregnancies has been shown to result in a significant increase in large for gestational age births [26], although maternal weight loss as a result of bariatric surgery prevents or reduces risk of obesity in subsequent offspring [27].

In humans, weight gain up to 25-week gestation is due primarily to linear growth. Accumulation of body fat is initiated at about 25-week gestation [28]. Approximately 40% of the variation in birthweight reflects differences in the magnitude of fat deposition [29]. Thus infants born with a lower birthweight are likely to have a reduced fat mass. Small babies who undergo early catch-up growth that is characterized by a greater accumulation of fat mass relative to lean body mass have an increased risk of becoming obese in later life as compared to those born at higher birthweights [30–32]. Early catch-up growth in infants born preterm, who also have a reduced fat mass at birth, and who were fed formula milk also show increased risk of cardiometabolic disease including obesity in later life [33–35], although not all studies have found this association [36]. Fat mass is important for the onset of reproductive function, particularly in females [37]. In an evolutionary context, it seems logical that catch-up growth in children born with a lower birthweight is characterized by greater adiposity relative to lean body mass, possibly as a mechanism to reach puberty at a similar age to peers born at greater weights [37]. Although obesity is a risk factor for cardiometabolic disease, it has little negative effect in terms of potential reproductive success and so the trade-off associated with this strategy in terms of fitness is small.

7.4 Experimental Models

Animal models have been used extensively to investigate the mechanism by which the early life environment induces persistent alterations in metabolism and physiology of the offspring. These studies have generally been performed using sheep or rodents and have involved feeding either a low-protein diet, global dietary restriction, or even a high-fat or junk food diet through pregnancy and/or lactation. To varying extents, the offspring exhibit characteristics of humans with cardiometabolic disease, including obesity, insulin resistance, hypertension, and hyperlipidemia.

Perhaps the most studied animal model of nutritional induction of an altered metabolic phenotype is feeding rats a protein-restricted (PR) diet from conception throughout pregnancy. In some studies, this nutritional constraint continued during lactation. Offspring of PR dams show a number of features of human cardiometabolic disease, including graded hypertension dependent on dietary protein intake [38], increased fat deposition and altered feeding behavior [39–41], impaired glucose homeostasis and dyslipidemia [42], vascular dysfunction [39, 43], impaired immunity [44], and increased susceptibility to oxidative stress [45]. However, the offspring consistently have birthweights within the normal range which emphasizes the point that lower birthweight in humans marks risk of future non-communicable disease, but is not a major part of the causal process.

7.5 Nutrition in Early Life and Gene Transcription

There is substantial evidence that changes in activity of specific genes underlie induction of altered metabolism by variations in the early life environment. The range of genes which have been studied in detail is largely limited to those involved in metabolic processes associated with cardiometabolic disease (reviewed in [46]) although there are some recent reports of transcriptome-wide analysis (see below). In particular these include increased glucocorticoid receptor (GR) expression and 11β-hydroxysteroid dehydrogenase type 2 (11βHSD)-2, in liver, lung, kidney, and brain which suggests greater sensitivity in the offspring to corticosteroids [47]. In the liver, increased GR activity upregulates phosphoenolpyruvate carboxykinase (PEPCK) expression and activity which is consistent with gluconeogenesis [48] and which may contribute to the induction of insulin resistance in this model.

Restricting maternal protein intake during pregnancy and/or lactation in rats alters the expression of specific genes involved in lipid homeostasis. Expression of acetyl-CoA carboxylase and fatty acid synthase was increased in the liver of the offspring of rats fed a PR diet during pregnancy and lactation [49]. Peroxisomal proliferator-activated receptor (PPAR)-α expression was increased in the liver of the offspring of rats fed a PR diet during pregnancy and was accompanied by upregulation of its target genes acyl-CoA oxidase (AOX) and carnitine palmitoyltransferase-1 indicating greater capacity for fatty acid β-oxidation [50, 51] (Fig. 7.2). In contrast, in adipose tissue the expression of PPARγ_2 was reduced [50].

The nature of the induced changes in gene expression appears to be contingent on the nature of the nutritional constraint during pregnancy. In rats, global nutrient restriction to 30% of ad libitum throughout gestation is comparable to intrauterine growth retardation in humans and induces a more severe change in phenotype as compared to the maternal PR diet [52]. The offspring are significantly smaller at birth than controls and exhibit hypertension, hyperinsulinemia, hyperleptinemia,

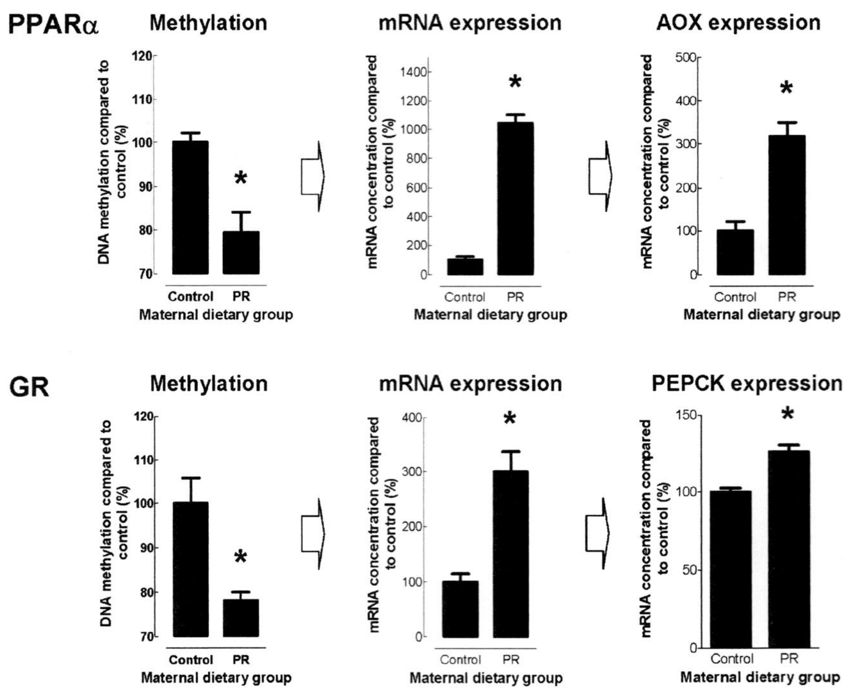

Fig. 7.2 Induction of altered methylation of the hepatic glucocorticoid receptor (GR) and PPARα promoters in the rat. Feeding a protein-restricted diet (PR) during pregnancy induced hypomethylation of the GR and PPARα promoters in 34-day-old offspring compared to controls. This was associated with reciprocal changes in the mRNA expression of these genes and of their targets acyl-CoA oxidase (AOX) and phosphoenolpyruvate carboxykinase (PEPCK) [51]

hyperphagia, reduced locomotion, and obesity. Although the nutritional constraint in this model is more severe than the PR diet, the overall reduction in energy intake is comparable to that to which pregnant women were exposed during the Dutch famine [53]. Gluckman et al. have showed that, in contrast to the PR model, PPARα and GR expression are downregulated in adult offspring born to dams fed a global nutrient-restricted diet of 30% of ad libitum during pregnancy (Fig. 7.3) [54].

Genome-wide analysis shows that approximately 1.3% of the liver transcriptome was altered in d84 rats whose dams were fed a PR diet during pregnancy and that this was reduced by 50% by supplementation of the PR diet with folic acid [55]. Others have shown a similar number of genes to be altered in the liver of rats exposed to global undernutrition in utero [56]. Seventy percent of the genes altered by the PR

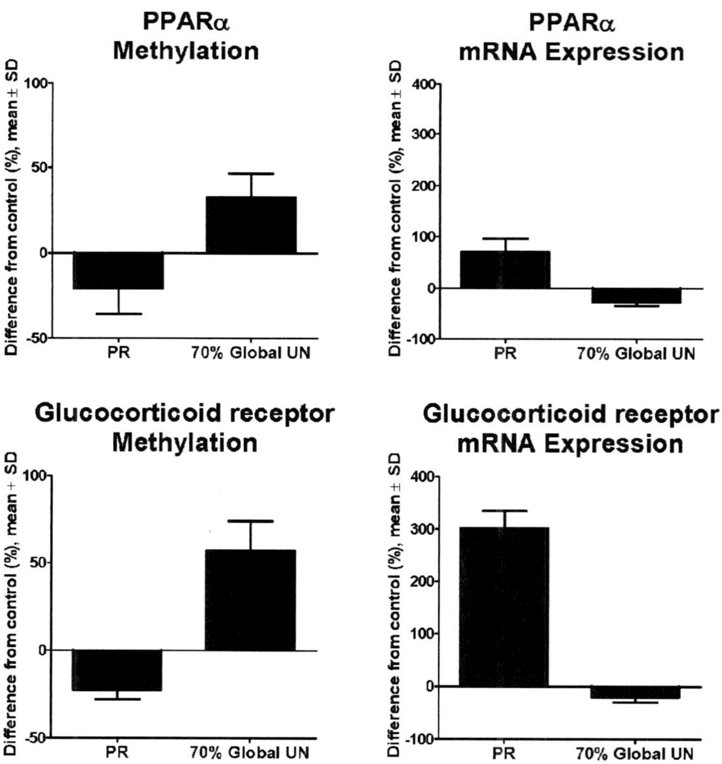

Fig. 7.3 The effect of different maternal diets during pregnancy on the methylation and mRNA expression of the hepatic glucocorticoid receptor (GR) and PPARα promoters. Dams were exposed during pregnancy to either a moderate reduction in dietary protein content (PR) or 70% total undernutrition. The GR and PPARα promoters were hypermethylated in the liver of adult offspring of dams exposed to 70% undernutrition, but were hypomethylated in offspring of dams fed the PR diet. This was accompanied by reciprocal changes in mRNA expression. These data suggest that maternal diet is an important determinant of the nature of induced epigenetic change [54, 84]

diet were increased, while of those which differed between offspring of dams fed the PR diet supplemented with folic acid 76% were downregulated. Only 16 genes were altered in both offspring of dams fed the PR diet and PR diet supplemented with folic acid (Fig. 7.4). These findings suggest that the altered hepatic phenotype induced by the PR diet involves persistent alteration of a discrete subset of genes and that the process is sensitive to the availability of specific nutrients in the mother's diet. The genes which showed the greatest difference between PR and control offspring covered a wide range of metabolic processes including protein glycosylation, G protein signaling, olfaction, ion transport, and cAMP signaling. The diversity of the pathways which are altered suggests that the PR diet induces a greater range of phenotypic effects than those studied as a model of human cardiometabolic disease and suggests further characterization of the induced phenotype is needed. These findings also suggest that induced changes in phenotype may reflect altered transcription of single genes leading to an overall shift in the activity of a metabolic pathway.

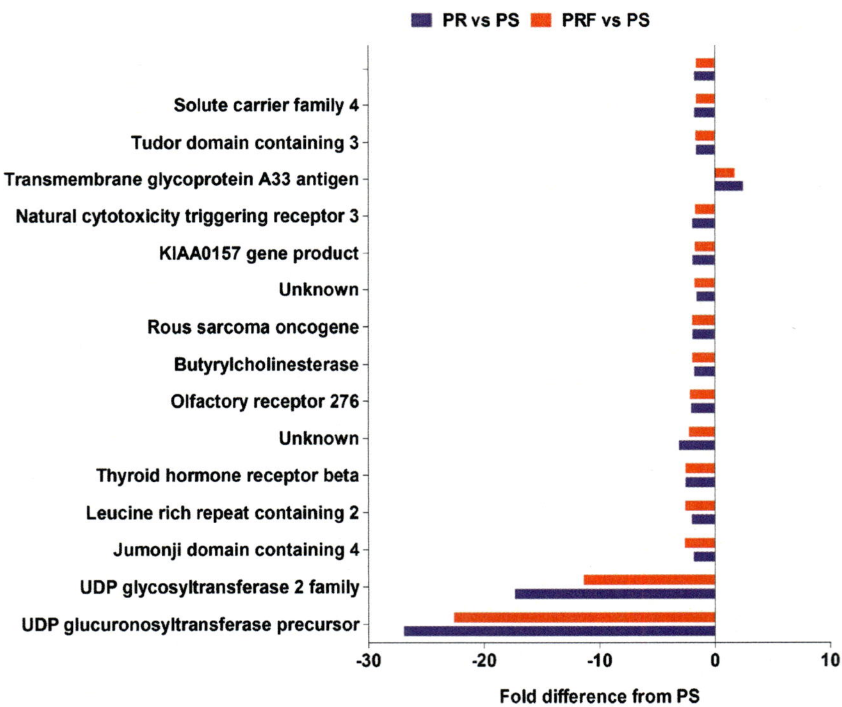

Fig. 7.4 Analysis of the effect of maternal nutrition on hepatic gene expression by microarray. Genes that differed between both adult offspring of dams fed a protein-restricted (PR) diet and those of dams fed the PR diet supplemented with folic acid (PRF) during pregnancy compared to offspring of dams fed a protein-sufficient (PS) diet

7.6 Epigenetic Mechanisms in Induced Risk of Obesity

There is increasing evidence that epigenetic processes are central to the mechanism by which the early nutritional environment can persistently alter the phenotype of the offspring. Epigenetic processes are integral to determining when and where specific genes are expressed [57]. The major epigenetic processes are DNA methylation, histone modification, and microRNAs. To date, most studies on the effect of early life nutrition on the epigenetic regulation of genes have focussed on DNA methylation.

7.6.1 Epigenetic Mechanisms and Gene Regulation

Methylation at the 5-position of cytosine within a CpG dinucleotide (the p denotes the intervening phosphate group) is a common modification in mammalian genomes and constitutes a stable epigenetic mark that is transmitted through DNA replication and cell division [58]. Methylation of CpG dinucleotides de novo is catalyzed by DNA methyltransferases (Dnmt) 3a and 3b and is maintained through mitosis by gene-specific methylation of hemimethylated DNA by Dnmt1 [59, 60]. CpG dinucleotides are not randomly distributed throughout the genome, but instead are clustered at the 5′-ends of genes/promoters in regions known as CpG islands. Hypermethylation of these CpG islands is associated with transcriptional repression, while hypomethylation of CpG islands is associated with transcriptional activation [61]. DNA methylation can induce transcriptional silencing by blocking the binding of transcription factors and/or through promoting the binding of the methyl CpG-binding protein (MeCP2) [62] which binds to methylated cytosines and, in turn, recruits histone-modifying complexes which include histone deacetylases (HDACs) and histone methyl transferases (HMTs) to the DNA [63–67], resulting in a closed chromatin structure and transcriptional silencing. Recent studies have shown that Dnmt1 is recruited by a number of histone-modifying enzymes such as HDAC1 and HDAC2 and the histone methyl transferases SUV39 and EZH2 [63, 68–70], suggesting that chromatin structure may also determine DNA methylation status and that there is a reciprocal relationship between these two processes.

DNA methylation is important for asymmetrical silencing of imprinted genes [71] (see Chapter 6). DNA methylation is also critical for cell differentiation by silencing the expression of specific genes during the development and differentiation of individual tissues [58]. Following fertilization, maternal and paternal genomes undergo extensive demethylation followed by global methylation de novo just prior to blastocyst implantation [72, 73]. Cell lineage-specific methylation occurs throughout during prenatal development and early postnatal life. For example, Oct-4 is permanently silenced by hypermethylation around E6.5 in the mouse [74], while HoxA5 and HoxB5 are not methylated and silenced until early postnatal life [75]. In contrast, PEPCK and δ-crystallin-2 are methylated in early embryos, but undergo progressive demethylation during development [76, 77]. The extent to which epigenetic marks are maintained throughout life is unclear. While the methylation status of genes associated with cell phenotype appears to be stable, the epigenetic regulation of other genes may be more plastic leading to specific periods of epigenetic instability during the life course. These include genome-wide hypomethylation or gene-specific hypermethylation associated with aging [78] which has been implicated in tumorigenesis [15]. However, environmental perturbations during periods when methylation patterns are induced may impair the program of gene silencing or activation with potential long-term adverse consequences. Furthermore, the temporal program of epigenetic changes during the life course suggests a mechanism for discrete periods of vulnerability when the epigenetic regulation of individual genes may be altered and thus for the induction of differential risk of specific diseases.

7.6.2 Evidence for the Involvement of Altered Epigenetic Regulation in Human Cardiometabolic Disease

Cell differentiation involves lineage-specific changes in the methylation of individual genes. This presents a challenge for identifying genes with altered epigenetic regulation in living humans because the limited range of tissues available for collection from a sufficient number subjects for robust statistical analysis, and hence the need to use proxy tissues. However, it is also possible that an altered epigenetic mark in a proxy tissue may be related to a disease process, and so may serve as a biomarker of disease risk, but is not part of the causal pathway. Thus the results of such studies should be interpreted with caution. Nevertheless, evidence is emerging that altered epigenetic regulation of specific genes is an important process for determining risk of cardiometabolic disease in humans. Heijmans et al. have reported hypomethylation of the imprinted insulin-like growth factor (IGF)-2 gene in genomic DNA isolated from whole blood from individuals who were exposed to the Dutch famine in utero as compared to unexposed same-sex siblings consistent [79]. The same group also found that IGF-2 was hypomethylated in individuals whose mothers were exposed periconceptually to famine while interleukin-10, leptin, ATP-binding cassette A1, guanine nucleotide-binding protein, and maternally expressed-3 were hypermethylated [80]. Unfortunately, whether the differences in promoter methylation were associated with altered levels of transcription was not investigated. Analysis of the epigenome and transcriptome of abdominal adipose tissue from adults undergoing caloric restriction showed that before starting the dietary intervention, the methylation status of 35 loci differed between individuals who were subsequently shown to be high or low responders in terms of weight loss [81]. These loci were associated with genes which were either known to be involved in weight loss or were imprinted. One implication of these findings is that capacity of individuals to successfully lose weight may be determined in part by epigenetic marks established earlier in life. After weight loss, three genes (PLCL4, phospholipase Cη-2; PRDM8, PR-domain-containing protein 8; unknown) were hypomethylated after the period of calorie restriction. While this suggests that at least for some genes DNA methylation is sensitive to calorie intake, the value of this finding in terms of future ability to lose or maintain weight is unclear.

Intrauterine growth retardation is associated with increased risk of T2DM and cardiovascular disease (seeChapter 8). A recent genome-wide discovery study using microarray followed by sequencing validation identified 56 differentially methylated loci including hepatocyte nuclear factor-4α (HNF4α) [82], which has been implicated in type 2 diabetes mellitus [83]. Although the study was limited by small number of samples in each group and lack of evidence that the methylation status altered the regulation of HNF4α, these findings at least demonstrate an association between phenotypic changes induced by an adverse intrauterine environment, altered epigenetic regulation, and future risk of cardiometabolic disease.

7.6.3 Epigenetic Regulation in Animal Models

Animal models are useful for identifying genes which are altered in tissues related to a disease process and for understanding mechanisms leading to altered epigenetic marks. Feeding a PR diet to pregnant rats induced hypomethylation of the GR and PPARα promoters in the livers of juvenile and adult offspring, which were associated with increased GR and PPARα mRNA expression, and an increased expression of their target genes PEPCK and AOX [51, 84] (Fig. 7.2). This was associated with histone modifications at the GR promoter which facilitate transcription, while those that suppress gene expression were reduced or unchanged [85]. Decreased methylation status of the liver PPARα promoter was due to hypomethylation of four specific CpG dinucleotides in juvenile offspring which persisted in adults [86] (Fig. 7.5). Of these four CpGs, two predicted the level of the mRNA transcript and were located proximal to putative transcription factor-binding sites. In addition, the angiotensin receptor 1b promoter is also hypomethylated in adrenal glands from PR offspring [87]. In contrast to the effect of the maternal PR diet, adult female offspring of dams which experienced 70% reduction in total nutrient intake during pregnancy showed hypermethylation and decreased expression of the hepatic GR and PPARα promoters [54] (Fig. 7.3). This suggests that the effects of maternal nutrition on the epigenome of the offspring depend upon the nature of the maternal nutrient challenge. This provides a mechanism by which changes in the epigenetic regulation of genes established during development determine the transcriptional response to specific stimuli, and thus the capacity of the tissue to respond to metabolic challenge.

Overnutrition can also alter epigenetic regulation. Plagemann et al. showed that neonatal over-feeding, produced by raising rat pups in small litters, induces hypermethylation of two CpG dinucleotides within the POMC promoter, which are essential for POMC induction by leptin and insulin [88]. Consequently POMC expression is not upregulated in these rats despite hyperinsulinemia and hyperleptinemia. Thus over-feeding during early postnatal life when the hypothalamic

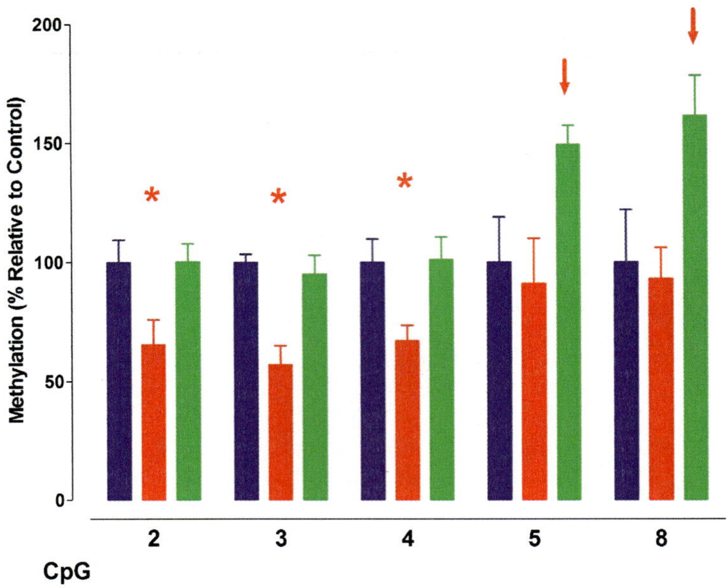

Fig. 7.5 Methylation of individual CpG dinucleotides in the hepatic PPARα promoter. The methylation of 16 CpGs was measured in a region 306 bp upstream of the PPARα transcription start site in rat liver. *Four CpGs (three shown) were hypomethylated in the liver of the offspring of dams fed a protein-restricted (PR) diet (*red bars*) during pregnancy compared to the offspring of protein-sufficient (*blue bars*) dams. Supplementation of the PR diet with folic acid (*green bars*) prevented hypomethylation of these four CpGs, but induced hypermethylation of two CpGs (*arrows*) [86]

circuitry is still developing can alter the methylation of genes critical for body weight regulation, resulting in altered programming of this regulatory system and an increased disposition toward obesity in later life.

Furthermore, feeding adult rats a high-fat cafeteria diet induced hypermethylation of a single CpG dinucleotide in the leptin promoter in retroperitoneal adipose tissue in male rats [89]. Although gene expression or leptin concentrations were not measured, this finding suggests that even in adult animals overnutrition may induce changes in the epigenetic regulation of genes involved in energy balance, which may contribute to development of an obesity phenotype.

7.6.4 Mechanisms for Induced Changes in the Epigenome

De novo methylation of CpG dinucleotides is catalyzed by DNA methyltransferases (Dnmt) 3a and 3b and is maintained through mitosis by gene-specific methylation of hemimethylated DNA by Dnmt1 [46]. A number of DNA demethylases have been proposed, including MBD2b [90], MBD4 [91], the DNA repair endonucleases XPG (Gadd45a) [92], and a G/T mismatch repair DNA glycosylase [93] although evidence that they fulfill this role is at present limited. However, there is clear evidence that demethylase activity exists including active demethylation of paternal genomic DNA in the newly fertilized zygote, the myogenin gene in differentiating myoblasts [94], IL2 upon T-cell activation [95], and IFNγ upon antigen exposure of memory CD8 T cells [96]. Syzf has proposed that the methylation status of CpG in post-mitotic cells may also represent an equilibrium state dependent upon the relative activities of Dnmt1 and demethylases, and that a shift in this equilibrium induced by an environmental signal may lead to either hyper- or hypomethylation of a gene [97, 98].

Feeding a PR diet to rats during pregnancy induced a reduction in Dnmt1 expression and in binding of Dnmt1 at the GR promoter in the liver of the offspring, while the expression of Dnmt3a, Dnmt3b, and MBD2 and the binding of Dnmt3a were unaltered [85]. This suggests that hypomethylation of the GR promoter in the liver of the offspring, and probably other genes including PPARα, is induced by the maternal diet as a result of reduced capacity to maintain patterns of cytosine methylation during mitosis. Although a reduction in Dnmt1 might be expected to result in global demethylation, loss of Dnmt1 has been shown to result in only a subset of genes being demethylated [99]. These data indicate that Dnmt1 is targeted to specific genes. There are now a number of reports which have shown that Dnmt1 interacts with a number of histone-modifying enzymes and is targeted to specific DNA sites [63, 68–70]. In human umbilical cord, variation in the level of Dnmt1 mRNA expression accounts for about 40% of the difference between individuals in methylation of the $GR1C_{\text{-total}}$ promoter [85]. Hyperglycemia and hyperinsulinemia have been reported to enhance homocysteine remethylation, leading to increased intracellular concentrations of *S*-adenosylmethionine and enhanced DNA methyltransferase activity [100] supporting findings from previous undernutrition studies that the methylation balance and regulation of DNA methyltransferases are sensitive to nutritional environmental cues.

7.6.5 Prevention and Reversal of an Altered Epigenotype and Phenotype

Despite the apparent stability of methylation marks, alterations in offspring DNA methylation induced by maternal diet can be prevented and even reversed by interventions in postnatal life. Supplementation of the maternal PR diet with folic acid prevents hypertension, vascular dysfunction, and dyslipidemia in the adult offspring [42]. Increasing the folic acid content of the PR diet also prevented the hypomethylation of the PPARα and GR promoters and restored levels of GR and PPAR expression to levels seen in control offspring. Folic acid supplementation of PR diet during pregnancy also upregulated Dnmt1 expression [51]. This suggests that impaired 1-carbon metabolism plays a central role in the induction of altered epigenetic regulation of GR and PPARα by the maternal PR diet. Detailed sequence analysis of the PPARα promoter showed that although increased maternal folic acid intake prevented hypomethylation of the majority of CpG dinucleotides induced by the PR diet alone, two CpGs were hypermethylated [86] (Fig. 7.4). Thus, increasing maternal folic acid intake does not simply prevent the effects of the PR diet, but may itself induce subtle changes in gene regulation. Supplementation of the maternal diet with methyl donors also prevented the transgenerational amplification of obesity observed in Agouti mice [101].

Folic acid supplementation during the juvenile–pubertal period altered both the phenotype and epigenotype induced by a maternal PR diet and induced a phenotype characterized by increased adiposity, hepatosteatosis, and dyslipidemia (Fig. 7.6) [102]. The altered phenotype was associated with increased methylation of the insulin receptor promoter in adipose tissue and of the PPARα promoter in liver, with reciprocal changes in the expression of these genes and of specific targets (Fig. 7.6). These findings suggest that the period between weaning and adulthood in rats represents a period of increased plasticity and that it may be possible to reverse the adverse effects of prenatal nutrition by nutritional interventions before adulthood. However, the design of any supplementation regimen for use in humans is far off and would need to consider carefully the timing and magnitude of the intervention.

In another paradigm, administration of leptin between postnatal days 3 and 13 to neonatal rats born to dams exposed to 70% global reduction in food intake during pregnancy normalized caloric intake on a high-fat diet, locomotor activity, body weight, fat mass and fasting plasma glucose, insulin and leptin concentrations in adult offspring in contrast to saline-treated offspring of undernourished dams [103].

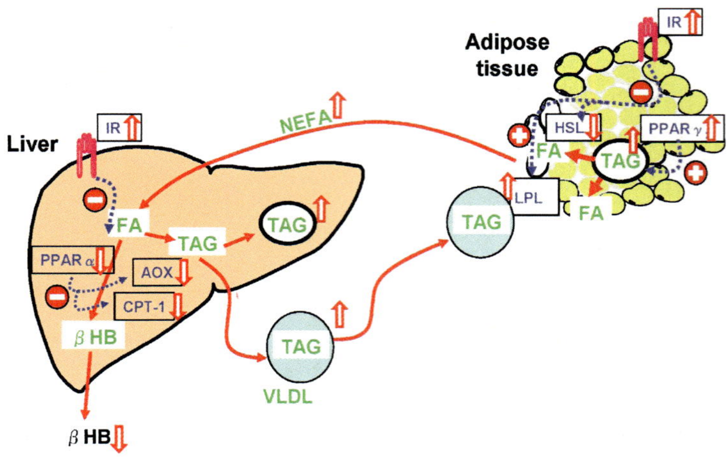

Fig. 7.6 Induction of altered regulation of liver metabolism in rats by supplementation with folic acid during their juvenile–pubertal period. Adult offspring fed a diet supplemented with folic acid showed increased weight gain, higher concentrations of non-esterified fatty acids (NEFA) and triacylglycerol (TAG) in plasma, and hepatosteatosis. This was accompanied by increased mRNA expression of the insulin receptor and lipoprotein lipase (LPL) in adipose tissue and liver, and PPARγ in adipose tissue, and decreased expression of hormone-sensitive lipase (HSL) in adipose tissue, and PPARα, acyl-CoA oxidase (AOX) and carnitine palmitoyltransferase (CPT)-1 in liver

Furthermore, leptin treatment normalized PPARα promoter methylation in adult female liver, but did not alter the methylation status of GR promoter [54].

In summary, dietary or hormonal interventions during specific postnatal periods appear to be able to alter the epigenotype and phenotype induced by prenatal nutrient constraint. However, substantial further work is needed to identify optimal periods for intervention, the precise nature of the intervention, and to prevent induction of harmful epigenetic and phenotypic changes.

7.7 Conclusions

There is substantial evidence in animal models that the early environment determines future disease risk and that induced changes in the epigenome are part of the causal process. However, research to apply the findings of animal studies to understand the role of epigenetics in human obesity and related co-morbidities is still in its early stages. Nevertheless, identification of periods of epigenetic plasticity after birth and demonstration that the epigenome can be manipulated by relatively simple interventions strongly support the feasibility of future therapeutic strategies to reverse the adverse effects of prenatal constraint on risk of disease throughout the life course.

References

1. Hossain P, Kawar B, El NM. Obesity and diabetes in the developing world–a growing challenge. N Engl J Med. 2007;356:213–5.
2. Andreasen CH, Andersen G. Gene-environment interactions and obesity–further aspects of genomewide association studies. Nutrition. 2009;25:998–1003.
3. Manolio TA. Cohort studies and the genetics of complex disease. Nat Genet. 2009;41:5–6.
4. Waddington CH. Canalization of development and the inheritance of acquired characters. Nature. 1942;150:563–5.
5. Stockard CR. Developmental rate and structural expression: an experimental study of twins, double monsters and single deformities, and the interaction among embryonic organs during their origin and development. Am J Anatomy. 1921;28:115–277.
6. Pener MP, Yerushalmi Y. The physiology of locust phase polymorphism: an update. J Insect Physiol. 1998;44:365–77.
7. Laforsch C, Tollrian R. Embryological aspects of inducible morphological defenses in Daphnia. J Morphol. 2004;262:701–7.
8. Lee TM, Zucker I. Vole Infant Development is influenced perinatally by maternal photoperiodic history. Am J Physiol. 1988;255:R831–8.
9. Kucharski R, Maleszka J, Foret S, Maleszka R. Nutritional control of reproductive status in honeybees via DNA methylation. Science. 2008;319:1827–30.
10. Waddington CH. Canalization of development and genetic assimilation of acquired characters. Nature. 1959;183:1654–5.
11. Gluckman PD, Hanson MA. Living with the past: evolution, development, and patterns of disease. Science. 2004;305:1733–6.
12. Jones KL, Smith DW. Recognition of the fetal alcohol syndrome in early infancy. Lancet. 1973;302:999–1001.
13. McBride WG. Thalidomide embryopathy. Teratology. 1977;16:79–82.

14. Gluckman PD, Hanson MA, Cooper C, Thornburg KL. Effect of in utero and early-life conditions on adult health and disease. N Engl J Med. 2008;359:61–73.
15. Burdge GC, Lillycrop KA, Jackson AA. Nutrition in early life, and risk of cancer and metabolic disease: alternative endings in an epigenetic tale? Br J Nutr. 2009;101:619–30.
16. Barker DJ, Osmond C. Infant mortality, childhood nutrition, and ischaemic heart disease in England and Wales. Lancet. 1986;1:1077–81.
17. Godfrey KM, Barker DJ. Fetal programming and adult health. Public Health Nutr. 2001;4:611–24.
18. Curhan GC, Chertow GM, Willett WC, et al. Birth weight and adult hypertension and obesity in women. Circulation. 1996;94:1310–5.
19. McCance DR, Pettitt DJ, Hanson RL, Jacobsson LT, Knowler WC, Bennett PH. Birth weight and non-insulin dependent diabetes: thrifty genotype, thrifty phenotype, or surviving small baby genotype? BMJ. 1994;308:942–5.
20. Painter RC, Roseboom TJ, Bleker OP. Prenatal exposure to the Dutch famine and disease in later life: an overview. Reprod Toxicol. 2005;20:345–52.
21. Cleal JK, Poore KR, Boullin JP, et al. Mismatched pre- and postnatal nutrition leads to cardiovascular dysfunction and altered renal function in adulthood. Proc Natl Acad Sci USA. 2007;104:9529–33.
22. Silverman BL, Rizzo TA, Cho NH, Metzger BE. Long-term effects of the intrauterine environment. The Northwestern University Diabetes in Pregnancy Center. Diabetes Care. 1998;21 Suppl 2:B142–9.
23. Boney CM, Verma A, Tucker R, Vohr BR. Metabolic syndrome in childhood: association with birth weight, maternal obesity, and gestational diabetes mellitus. Pediatrics. 2005;115:e290–6.
24. Dorner G, Plagemann A. Perinatal hyperinsulinism as possible predisposing factor for diabetes mellitus, obesity and enhanced cardiovascular risk in later life. Horm Metab Res. 1994;26:213–21.
25. Oken E, Taveras EM, Kleinman KP, Rich-Edwards JW, Gillman MW. Gestational weight gain and child adiposity at age 3 years. Am J Obstet Gynecol. 2007;196:322–8.
26. Villamor E, Cnattingius S. Interpregnancy weight change and risk of adverse pregnancy outcomes: a population-based study. Lancet. 2006;368:1164–70.
27. Kral JG, Biron S, Simard S, et al. Large maternal weight loss from obesity surgery prevents transmission of obesity to children who were followed for 2 to 18 years. Pediatrics. 2006;118:e1644–9.
28. Poissonnet CM, LaVelle M, Burdi AR. Growth and development of adipose tissue. J Pediatr. 1988;113:1–9.
29. Catalano PM, Kirwan JP. Maternal factors that determine neonatal size and body fat. Curr Diab Rep. 2001;1:71–7.
30. Rolland-Cachera MF, Deheeger M, Bellisle F, Sempe M, Guilloud-Bataille M, Patois E. Adiposity rebound in children: a simple indicator for predicting obesity. Am J Clin Nutr. 1984;39:129–35.
31. Ong KK, Ahmed ML, Emmett PM, Preece MA, Dunger DB. Association between postnatal catch-up growth and obesity in childhood: prospective cohort study. BMJ. 2000;320:967–71.
32. Ong KK. Size at birth, postnatal growth and risk of obesity. Horm Res. 2006;65 Suppl 3: 65–9.
33. Singhal A, Lucas A. Early origins of cardiovascular disease: is there a unifying hypothesis? Lancet. 2004;363:1642–5.
34. Singhal A. Early nutrition and long-term cardiovascular health. Nutr Rev. 2006;64: S44–9.
35. Harder T, Bergmann R, Kallischnigg G, Plagemann A. Duration of breastfeeding and risk of overweight: a meta-analysis. Am J Epidemiol. 2005;162:397–403.
36. Owen CG, Martin RM, Whincup PH, vey-Smith G, Gillman MW, Cook DG. The effect of breastfeeding on mean body mass index throughout life: a quantitative review of published and unpublished observational evidence. Am J Clin Nutr. 2005;82:1298–307.

37. Gluckman PD, Hanson MA. Changing times: the evolution of puberty. Mol Cell Endocrinol. 2006;254–255:26–31.
38. Langley SC, Jackson AA. Increased systolic blood pressure in adult rats induced by fetal exposure to maternal low protein diets. Clin Sci (Lond). 1994;86:217–22.
39. Lucas A, Baker BA, Desai M, Hales CN. Nutrition in pregnant or lactating rats programs lipid metabolism in the offspring. Br J Nutr. 1996;76:605–12.
40. Bellinger L, Lilley C, Langley-Evans SC. Prenatal exposure to a maternal low-protein diet programmes a preference for high-fat foods in the young adult rat. Br J Nutr. 2004;92: 513–20.
41. Bellinger L, Sculley DV, Langley-Evans SC. Exposure to undernutrition in fetal life determines fat distribution, locomotor activity and food intake in ageing rats. Int J Obes (Lond). 2006;30:729–38.
42. Burdge GC, Lillycrop KA, Jackson AA, Gluckman PD, Hanson MA. The nature of the growth pattern and of the metabolic response to fasting in the rat are dependent upon the dietary protein and folic acid intakes of their pregnant dams and post-weaning fat consumption. Br J Nutr. 2008;99:540–9.
43. Torrens C, Brawley L, Anthony FW, et al. Folate supplementation during pregnancy improves offspring cardiovascular dysfunction induced by protein restriction. Hypertension. 2006;47:982–7.
44. Calder PC, Yaqoob P. The level of protein and type of fat in the diet of pregnant rats both affect lymphocyte function in the offspring. Nutr Res. 2000;20:995–1005.
45. Langley-Evans SC, Sculley DV. Programming of hepatic antioxidant capacity and oxidative injury in the ageing rat. Mech Ageing Dev. 2005;126:804–12.
46. Burdge GC, Hanson MA, Slater-Jefferies JL, Lillycrop KA. Epigenetic regulation of transcription: a mechanism for inducing variations in phenotype (fetal programming) by differences in nutrition during early life? Br J Nutr. 2007;97:1036–46.
47. Bertram C, Trowern AR, Copin N, Jackson AA, Whorwood CB. The maternal diet during pregnancy programs altered expression of the glucocorticoid receptor and type 2 11beta-hydroxysteroid dehydrogenase: potential molecular mechanisms underlying the programming of hypertension in utero. Endocrinology. 2001;142:2841–53.
48. Burns SP, Desai M, Cohen RD, et al. Gluconeogenesis, glucose handling, and structural changes in livers of the adult offspring of rats partially deprived of protein during pregnancy and lactation. J Clin Invest. 1997;100:1768–74.
49. Maloney CA, Gosby AK, Phuyal JL, Denyer GS, Bryson JM, Caterson ID. Site-specific changes in the expression of fat-partitioning genes in weanling rats exposed to a low-protein diet in utero. Obes Res. 2003;11:461–8.
50. Burdge GC, Phillips ES, Dunn RL, Jackson AA, Lillycrop KA. Effect of reduced maternal protein consumption during pregnancy in the rat on plasma lipid concentrations and expression of peroxisomal proliferator–activated receptors in the liver and adipose tissue of the offspring. Nutr Res. 2004;24:639–46.
51. Lillycrop KA, Phillips ES, Jackson AA, Hanson MA, Burdge GC. Dietary protein restriction of pregnant rats induces and folic acid supplementation prevents epigenetic modification of hepatic gene expression in the offspring. J Nutr. 2005;135:1382–6.
52. Woodall SM, Johnston BM, Breier BH, Gluckman PD. Chronic maternal undernutrition in the rat leads to delayed postnatal growth and elevated blood pressure of offspring. Pediatr Res. 1996;40:438–43.
53. Roseboom T, de RS, Painter R. The Dutch famine and its long-term consequences for adult health. Early Hum Dev. 2006;82:485–91.
54. Gluckman PD, Lillycrop KA, Vickers MH, et al. Metabolic plasticity during mammalian development is directionally dependent on early nutritional status. Proc Natl Acad Sci USA. 2007;104:12796–800.
55. Lillycrop KA, Rodford J, Garratt ES, et al. Maternal diet during pregnancy induces specific changes in the hepatic transcriptome of the adult male offspring. Br J Nutr. 2010; doi:10.1017/S0007114509993795.

56. Morris TJ, Vickers M, Gluckman P, Gilmour S, Affara N. Transcriptional profiling of rats subjected to gestational undernourishment: implications for the developmental variations in metabolic traits. PLoS One. 2009;4:e7271.
57. Goldberg AD, Allis CD, Bernstein E. Epigenetics: a landscape takes shape. Cell. 2007;128:635–8.
58. Bird A. DNA methylation patterns and epigenetic memory. Genes Dev. 2002;16:6–21.
59. Razin A, Szyf M. DNA methylation patterns. Formation and function. Biochim Biophys Acta. 1984;782:331–42.
60. Bird AP. Functions for DNA methylation in vertebrates. Cold Spring Harb Symp Quant Biol. 1993;58:281–5.
61. Bird A, Macleod D. Reading the DNA methylation signal. Cold Spring Harb Symp Quant Biol. 2004;69:113–8.
62. Bird AP, Wolffe AP. Methylation-induced repression–belts, braces, and chromatin. Cell. 1999;99:451–4.
63. Fuks F, Hurd PJ, Wolf D, Nan X, Bird AP, Kouzarides T. The methyl-CpG-binding protein MeCP2 links DNA methylation to histone methylation. J Biol Chem. 2003;278: 4035–40.
64. Strahl BD, Ohba R, Cook RG, Allis CD. Methylation of histone H3 at lysine 4 is highly conserved and correlates with transcriptionally active nuclei in Tetrahymena. Proc Natl Acad Sci USA. 1999;96:14967–72.
65. Lachner M, O'Carroll D, Rea S, Mechtler K, Jenuwein T. Methylation of histone H3 lysine 9 creates a binding site for HP1 proteins. Nature. 2001;410:116–20.
66. Zegerman P, Canas B, Pappin D, Kouzarides T. Histone H3 lysine 4 methylation disrupts binding of nucleosome remodeling and deacetylase (NuRD) repressor complex. J Biol Chem. 2002;277:11621–4.
67. Nakayama J, Rice JC, Strahl BD, Allis CD, Grewal SI. Role of histone H3 lysine 9 methylation in epigenetic control of heterochromatin assembly. Science. 2001;292:110–3.
68. Fuks F, Burgers WA, Brehm A, Hughes-Davies L, Kouzarides T. DNA methyltransferase Dnmt1 associates with histone deacetylase activity. Nat Genet. 2000;24:88–91.
69. Rountree MR, Bachman KE, Baylin SB. DNMT1 binds HDAC2 and a new co-repressor, DMAP1, to form a complex at replication foci. Nat Genet. 2000;25:269–77.
70. Vire E, Brenner C, Deplus R, et al. The Polycomb group protein EZH2 directly controls DNA methylation. Nature. 2006;439:871–4.
71. Li E, Beard C, Jaenisch R. Role for DNA methylation in genomic imprinting. Nature. 1993;366:362–5.
72. Reik W, Dean W, Walter J. Epigenetic reprogramming in mammalian development. Science. 2001;293:1089–93.
73. Bird A. Molecular biology. Methylation talk between histones and DNA. Science. 2001;294:2113–5.
74. Gidekel S, Bergman Y. A unique developmental pattern of Oct-3/4 DNA methylation is controlled by a cis-demodification element. J Biol Chem. 2002;277:34521–30.
75. Hershko AY, Kafri T, Fainsod A, Razin A. Methylation of HoxA5 and HoxB5 and its relevance to expression during mouse development. Gene. 2003;302:65–72.
76. Benvenisty N, Szyf M, Mencher D, Razin A, Reshef L. Tissue-specific hypomethylation and expression of rat phosphoenolpyruvate carboxykinase gene induced by in vivo treatment of fetuses and neonates with 5-azacytidine. Biochemistry. 1985;24:5015–9.
77. Grainger RM, Hazard-Leonards RM, Samaha F, Hougan LM, Lesk MR, Thomsen GH. Is hypomethylation linked to activation of delta-crystallin genes during lens development? Nature. 1983;306:88–91.
78. Dolinoy DC, Das R, Weidman JR, Jirtle RL. Metastable epialleles, imprinting, and the fetal origins of adult diseases. Pediatr Res. 2007;61:30R–7R.
79. Heijmans BT, Tobi EW, Stein AD, et al. Persistent epigenetic differences associated with prenatal exposure to famine in humans. Proc Natl Acad Sci USA. 2008;105:17046–9.

80. Tobi EW, Lumey LH, Talens RP, et al. DNA Methylation differences after exposure to prenatal famine are common and timing- and sex-specific. Hum Mol Genet. 2009;18:4046–53.
81. Bouchard L, Rabasa-Lhoret R, Faraj M, et al. Differential epigenomic and transcriptomic responses in subcutaneous adipose tissue between low and high responders to caloric restriction. Am J Clin Nutr. 2009;91:309–20.
82. Einstein F, Thompson RF, Bhagat TD, et al. Cytosine methylation dysregulation in neonates following intrauterine growth restriction. PLoS One. 2010;5:e8887.
83. Yamagata K, Furuta H, Oda N, et al. Mutations in the hepatocyte nuclear factor-4alpha gene in maturity-onset diabetes of the young (MODY1. Nature. 1996;384:458–60.
84. Burdge GC, Slater-Jefferies J, Torrens C, Phillips ES, Hanson MA, Lillycrop KA. Dietary protein restriction of pregnant rats in the F0 generation induces altered methylation of hepatic gene promoters in the adult male offspring in the F1 and F2 generations. Br J Nutr. 2007;97:435–9.
85. Lillycrop KA, Slater-Jefferies JL, Hanson MA, Godfrey KM, Jackson AA, Burdge GC. Induction of altered epigenetic regulation of the hepatic glucocorticoid receptor in the offspring of rats fed a protein-restricted diet during pregnancy suggests that reduced DNA methyltransferase-1 expression is involved in impaired DNA methylation and changes in histone modifications. Br J Nutr. 2007;97:1064–73.
86. Lillycrop KA, Phillips ES, Torrens C, Hanson MA, Jackson AA, Burdge GC. Feeding pregnant rats a protein-restricted diet persistently alters the methylation of specific cytosines in the hepatic PPARalpha promoter of the offspring. Br J Nutr. 2008;100:278–82.
87. Bogdarina I, Welham S, King PJ, Burns SP, Clark AJ. Epigenetic modification of the renin-angiotensin system in the fetal programming of hypertension. Circ Res. 2007;100:520–6.
88. Plagemann A, Harder T, Brunn M, et al. Hypothalamic proopiomelanocortin promoter methylation becomes altered by early overfeeding: an epigenetic model of obesity and the metabolic syndrome. J Physiol. 2009;587:4963–76.
89. Milagro FI, Campion J, Garcia-Diaz DF, Goyenechea E, Paternain L, Martinez JA. High fat diet-induced obesity modifies the methylation pattern of leptin promoter in rats. J Physiol Biochem. 2009;65:1–9.
90. Bhattacharya SK, Ramchandani S, Cervoni N, Szyf M. A mammalian protein with specific demethylase activity for mCpG DNA. Nature. 1999;397:579–83.
91. Zhu B, Zheng Y, Angliker H, et al. 5-Methylcytosine DNA glycosylase activity is also present in the human MBD4 (G/T mismatch glycosylase) and in a related avian sequence. Nucleic Acids Res. 2000;28:4157–65.
92. Barreto G, Schafer A, Marhold J, et al. Gadd45a promotes epigenetic gene activation by repair-mediated DNA demethylation. Nature. 2007;445:671–5.
93. Jost JP. Nuclear extracts of chicken embryos promote an active demethylation of DNA by excision repair of 5-methyldeoxycytidine. Proc Natl Acad Sci USA. 1993;90:4684–8.
94. Lucarelli M, Fuso A, Strom R, Scarpa S. The dynamics of myogenin site-specific demethylation is strongly correlated with its expression and with muscle differentiation. J Biol Chem. 2001;276:7500–6.
95. Bruniquel D, Schwartz RH. Selective, stable demethylation of the interleukin-2 gene enhances transcription by an active process. Nat Immunol. 2003;4:235–40.
96. Kersh EN. Impaired memory CD8 T cell development in the absence of methyl-CpG-binding domain protein 2. J Immunol. 2006;177:3821–6.
97. Szyf M. The dynamic epigenome and its implications in toxicology. Toxicol Sci. 2007;100:7–23.
98. Szyf M. Epigenetics, DNA methylation, and chromatin modifying drugs. Annu Rev Pharmacol Toxicol. 2008;49:243–63.
99. Jackson-Grusby L, Beard C, Possemato R, et al. Loss of genomic methylation causes p53-dependent apoptosis and epigenetic deregulation. Nat Genet. 2001;27:31–9.
100. Chiang EP, Wang YC, Chen WW, Tang FY. Effects of insulin and glucose on cellular metabolic fluxes in homocysteine transsulfuration, remethylation, S-adenosylmethionine

synthesis, and global deoxyribonucleic acid methylation. J Clin Endocrinol Metab. 2009;94:1017–25.

101. Waterland RA, Travisano M, Tahiliani KG, Rached MT, Mirza S. Methyl donor supplementation prevents transgenerational amplification of obesity. Int J Obes (Lond). 2008;32:1373–9.

102. Burdge GC, Lillycrop KA, Phillips ES, Slater-Jefferies JL, Jackson AA, Hanson MA. Folic acid supplementation during the juvenile-pubertal period in rats modifies the phenotype and epigenotype induced by prenatal nutrition. J Nutr. 2009;139:1054–60.

103. Vickers MH, Gluckman PD, Coveny AH, et al. Neonatal leptin treatment reverses developmental programming. Endocrinology. 2005;146:4211–6.

Chapter 8
Epigenetic Changes Associated with Intrauterine Growth Retardation and Adipogenesis

Sara E. Pinney and Rebecca A. Simmons

8.1 Introduction

Obesity is a growing threat worldwide, and its prevalence has risen dramatically over the past decade. Several studies have shown that early life exposures are important in promoting adult obesity. There are a number of critical periods during childhood that appear to influence the later development of obesity, including early infancy, 5–7 years of age (the adiposity rebound period), and puberty [1]. It is becoming increasingly evident that the prenatal stage also represents a window of susceptibility to the influence of early life exposures (reviewed in [2, 3]). The period from conception to birth is a time of rapid growth, cellular replication and differentiation, and functional maturation of organ systems. These processes are very sensitive to alterations in the nutritional milieu and the metabolic milieu of the mother. For instance, obesity in pregnancy can have long-lasting effects on the development of obesity and diabetes in the offspring [4–9]. Environmental contributions to the development of childhood obesity may include a suboptimal in utero environment, diabetes and/or obesity in pregnancy, and pre- and postnatal exposure to environmental chemicals, also known as obesogens. Epigenetic modifications may be one mechanism by which exposure to an altered intrauterine milieu or metabolic perturbation may influence the phenotype of the organism much later in life. This chapter highlights our current knowledge of epigenetic gene regulation and the evidence that chromatin remodeling and histone modifications play key roles in adipogenesis and the development of obesity.

S.E. Pinney (✉)
Division of Endocrinology and Diabetes, Department of Pediatrics, The Children's Hospital of Philadelphia, University of Pennsylvania School of Medicine, Philadelphia, PA, USA
e-mail: pinneys@email.chop.edu

R.H. Lustig (ed.), *Obesity Before Birth*, Endocrine Updates 30,
DOI 10.1007/978-1-4419-7034-3_8,

8.2 Chromatin Structure, DNA Methylation, and Gene Expression

Epigenetic modifications of the genome provide a mechanism that allows the stable propagation of gene expression from one generation of cells to the next [10–13]. Epigenetic states can be modified by environmental factors, which may contribute to the development of abnormal phenotypes. There are at least three distinct categories through which epigenetic information can be inherited: histone modifications, DNA methylation, and noncoding RNAs.

8.2.1 Histone Modifications

In eukaryotes, the nucleosome is formed when DNA is wrapped around an octameric complex of two molecules of each of the four histones H2A, H2B, H3, and H4. The amino-termini of histones can be modified by acetylation, methylation, sumoylation, phosphorylation, glycosylation, and ADP ribosylation. The most common histone modifications involve acetylation and methylation of lysine residues in the amino-termini of H3 and H4. Increased acetylation induces transcription activation, whereas decreased acetylation usually induces transcription repression. Methylation of histones, on the other hand, is associated with both transcription activation and repression. Moreover, lysine residues can be mono-, di-, or trimethylated in vivo, providing an additional node of regulation [10].

8.2.2 DNA Methylation

The second class of epigenetic regulation is DNA methylation, in which a cytosine base is modified by a DNA methyltransferase at the C5 position of cytosine, a reaction that is carried out by various members of a single family of enzymes. Approximately 70% of CpG dinucleotides in human DNA are constitutively methylated, whereas most of the unmethylated CpGs are located in CpG islands. CpG islands are CG-rich sequences located near coding sequences and serve as promoters for their associated genes. Approximately half of mammalian genes have CpG islands. The methylation status of CpG islands within promoter sequences works as an essential regulatory element by modifying the binding affinity of transcription factors to DNA-binding sites. In normal cells, most CpG islands remain unmethylated; however, under circumstances such as cancer [14–17] or oxidative stress, they can become methylated de novo. This aberrant methylation is accompanied by local changes in histone modification and chromatin structure, such that the CpG island and its embedded promoter take on a repressed conformation that is incompatible with gene transcription. It is not known why particular CpG islands are susceptible to aberrant methylation.

There is a stepwise passive loss of DNA methylation in the embryonic nucleus that occurs as DNA replicates between two-cell and morula stages, with somatic cell levels of methylation being reestablished by, or after the blastocyst stage when differentiated lineages are formed [18, 19]. Differential DNA methylation is established through two opposing mechanisms: first, through the wave of de novo methylation at the time of blastocyst implantation and second, through a mechanism that protects CpG islands from DNA methylation. The specifics of these mechanisms have yet to be elucidated [20]. DNA methylation is commonly associated with gene silencing and contributes to X-chromosomal inactivation, genomic imprinting, as well as transcriptional regulation of tissue-specific genes during cellular differentiation (reviewed in [21, 22]).

Histone methylation can affect DNA methylation patterns and vice versa [20]. For example, methylation of lysine 9 on the histone H3 promotes DNA methylation, while CpG methylation stimulates lysine 9 methylation on H3 [21]. Recent evidence indicates that this dual relationship between histone methylation and DNA methylation might be accomplished by direct interactions between histone and DNA methyltransferases [20]. Thus, chromatin modifications induced by adverse stimuli are self-reinforcing and can propagate.

8.2.3 Noncoding RNAs

New evidence from a variety of model systems indicates that noncoding RNAs such as microRNAs, small RNAs, and long or large RNAs play a significant role in epigenetic gene regulation and chromosomal dynamics, including processes such as dosage compensation, imprinting, and gene silencing by RNA interference. Noncoding RNAs with different regulatory functions are a common feature of mammalian transcriptomes, especially after the discovery that most of the eukaryotic genomes are transcribed into RNAs that have no protein-coding potential (reviewed in [23]). Noncoding RNAs are able to direct the cytosine methylation and histone modifications that are related to regulation of gene expression in complex organisms, in addition to having several other unrelated functions [24]. Recent reports suggest that gene silencing, mediated through DNA methylation, can be induced by promoter-directed silencing RNAs (siRNAs) in mammalian cells (reviewed in [25, 26]). Kawasaki et al. found that siRNAs targeted to a promoter could induce H3K9 methylation in various mammalian cell lines [25]. It is becoming clear that these molecules are very important in various epigenetic mechanisms such as heterochromatin silencing, transposon activity and silencing, and X chromosome inactivation; however, much remains to be learned about their specific epigenetic roles.

8.3 Epigenetic Regulation of Gene Expression in Intrauterine Growth Retardation

A number of studies suggest that uteroplacental insufficiency, the most common cause of intrauterine growth retardation (IUGR) in the developed world, induces epigenetic modifications in the offspring [27–30]. IUGR can be induced by bilateral uterine artery ligation in the pregnant rat [31]. Following ligation, pups are born spontaneously and have decreased levels of glucose, insulin, IGF-1, and amino acids [31]. Their birthweights are decreased compared to controls, but they have increased fat mass by 2 weeks of age, and by 26 weeks of age the fat pad mass of the IUGR animals is 1.8 times greater than controls [31]. In this model, diabetes develops in animals at approximately 15–26 weeks of age, with underlying β-cell secretory defects and insulin resistance, the salient features of most forms of type 2 diabetes mellitus (T2DM) in humans [31, 32]. Epigenetic modifications affecting processes important to glucose regulation and insulin secretion have been described in the pancreatic β-cells and muscle of the IUGR offspring, characteristics essential to the pathophysiology of T2DM. Although no specific experiments have looked at the epigenetic control of gene expression in adipose tissue to date, the data presented here suggest that in the IUGR model, epigenetic regulation of gene expression plays an important role in the development of adult disease. The following sections describe specific epigenetic modifications induced in the IUGR model and their relationship to the development of T2DM.

8.3.1 Chromatin Remodeling in the β-Cell of IUGR Rats

Pdx-1 is a homeodomain-containing transcription factor that plays a critical role in the early development of both the endocrine and exocrine pancreas and in the later differentiation and function of the β-cell. As early as 24 h after the onset of growth retardation, *Pdx-1* mRNA levels are reduced by more than 50% in IUGR fetal rats. Suppression of *Pdx-1* expression persists after birth and progressively declines in the IUGR animal, implicating an epigenetic mechanism.

A change in histone acetylation is the first epigenetic modification found in β-cells of IUGR animals. Islets isolated from IUGR fetuses show a significant decrease in H3 and H4 acetylation at the proximal promoter of *Pdx-1* [29]. These changes in H3 and H4 acetylation are associated with a loss of binding of USF-1 to the proximal promoter of *Pdx-1* [29]. USF-1 is a critical activator of *Pdx-1* transcription and its decreased binding markedly decreases *Pdx-1* transcription [33, 34]. After birth, histone deacetylation progresses and is followed by a marked decrease in H3K4 trimethylation and a significant increase in dimethylation of H3K9 in IUGR islets [29]. H3K4 trimethylation is usually associated with active gene transcription while H3K9 dimethylation is usually a repressive chromatin mark. Progression of these histone modifications parallels the progressive decrease in *Pdx-1* expression that manifests as defective glucose homeostasis and increased oxidative stress in aging IUGR animals [29]. Nevertheless, at 2 weeks of age, the silencing histone modifications in the IUGR pup are responsible for suppression of *Pdx-1* expression, since there is no appreciable methylation of CpG islands in mice at this age [29]. Reversal of histone deacetylation in IUGR islets at 2 weeks of age is sufficient to nearly normalize *Pdx-1* mRNA levels permanently, perhaps due to active β-cell replication present in the neonatal rodent [29].

In the IUGR model, *Pdx-1* is first silenced due to recruitment of corepressors, including histone deacetylase-1 (HDAC1) and mSin3A [12]. These repressors catalyze histone deacetylation. Binding of these deacetylases facilitates loss of trimethylation of H3K4, further repressing *Pdx-1* expression [29]. We found that inhibition of HDAC activity by trichostatin A (TSA) treatment normalizes H3K4me3 levels at *Pdx-1* in IUGR islets [29]. These data suggest that the association of HDAC1 at *Pdx-1* in IUGR islets likely serves as a platform for the recruitment of a demethylase, which catalyzes demethylation of H3K4.

The molecular mechanism responsible for DNA methylation in IUGR islets is likely dependent on the methylation status of lysine 9 on H3 (H3K9). Previous studies have shown that changes in methylation of H3K9 precede changes in DNA methylation [35, 36]. It has also been suggested that DNA methyltransferases may act only on chromatin that is methylated at H3K9 [37]. Another class of enzymes, e.g., DNA methyltransferase 3A (DNMT3A) and DNA methyltransferase 3B (DNMT3B), binds to DNA methylases to initiate DNA methylation [27].

These results demonstrate that IUGR induces a self-propagating epigenetic cycle in which the mSin3A/HDAC complex is first recruited to the *Pdx-1* promoter, histone tails are subjected to deacetylation, and Pdx-1 transcription is repressed (Fig. 8.1). At the neonatal stage, this epigenetic process is reversible and may define an important developmental window for therapeutic approaches. However, as dimethylated H3K9 accumulates, DNMT3A is recruited to the promoter and initiates de novo DNA methylation, which locks in the silenced state in the IUGR adult pancreas resulting in diabetes.

How do these epigenetic events lead to diabetes? Targeted homozygous disruption of *Pdx-1* in mice results in pancreatic agenesis, and homozygous mutations yield a similar phenotype in humans [38]. Milder reductions in Pdx-1 protein levels, as occurs in the $Pdx^{+/-}$ mice, allow for the development of a normal β-cell mass [38], but result in the impairment of several events in glucose-stimulated insulin secretion [38]. These results indicate that Pdx-1 plays a critical role in the normal function of β-cells [38], in addition to its role in β-cell lineage development. This may be the reason that humans with heterozygous missense mutations in *Pdx-1* exhibit early- and late-onset forms of diabetes, known as Mature Onset of Diabetes in Youth-4 (MODY4) [38].

The discovery of a theoretical time period during which aberrant epigenetic modifications may be reversed represents a therapeutic window for the use of novel agents that could prevent common diseases with late-onset phenotypes 29]. T2DM and perhaps obesity are such diseases, whereby predisposed individuals could be treated with agents that normalize the epigenetic programming of key genes, thus providing protection against development of the adult disease phenotype.

8.3.2 Chromatin Remodeling in the Muscle of IUGR Rats

A reduction in glucose transport in muscle is a central mechanism for insulin resistance in the IUGR offspring [39, 40]. Glucose transport, a rate-limiting step in glucose utilization under normal physiological circumstances, occurs by facilitated diffusion [41]. This process is mediated by a family of structurally related membrane-spanning glycoproteins, termed the facilitative glucose transporters

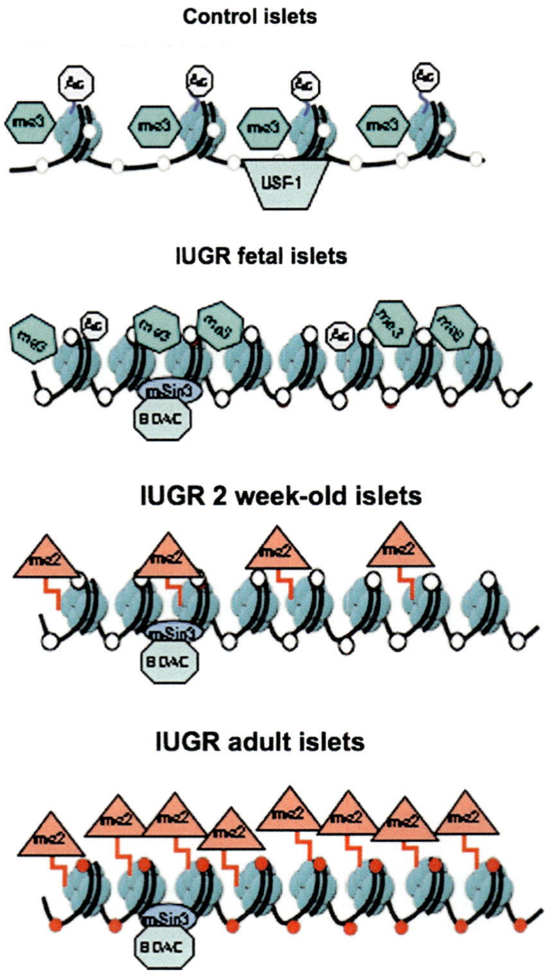

Fig. 8.1 Summary of epigenetic changes at *Pdx-1* in IUGR rats during the development of type 2 diabetes. In pancreatic β-cells (*top*), the *Pdx-1* proximal promoter is normally found in an unmethylated (*white circles*) open chromatin state allowing access to transcription factors such as USF-1 and associated with nucleosomes characterized by acetylated (Ac, *blue octagons*) histones H3 and H4 and with trimethylated H3K4 (Me, *green hexagons*). In IUGR fetal and 2-week islets (*middle*), histone acetylation is progressively lost through association with an mSin3A–HDAC1–DNMT1 repressor complex, with trimethylated H3K4 disappearing and dimethylated H3K9 (Me, *red hexagons*) appearing after birth. IUGR adult islets are characterized by inactive chromatin with dimethylated H3K9 and extensive DNA methylation (*red circles*) locking in the transcriptionally silent state of *Pdx-1*

(GLUT; Slc2 family of transport proteins) (reviewed in [42]). Of the isoforms cloned to date, GLUT4 is the major insulin-responsive isoform expressed in insulin-sensitive tissues such as skeletal muscle, adipose tissue, and cardiac muscle [42]. The promoter region of *glut4* has been well characterized, and disruption of the myocyte enhancer factor 2 (MEF2)-binding site ablates tissue-specific *glut4* expression in transgenic mice [42]. On the other hand, MyoD is responsible for *glut4* expression in vitro during differentiation of myoblasts to myocytes [42]. MyoD binding with that of MEF2 and TR 1 spans the 502–420-bp region of the *glut4* gene in skeletal muscle. These two proteins synergistically enhance skeletal muscle *glut4* gene expression and transcription [43].

It has recently been shown by Raychaudhuri et al. [30] that IUGR is associated with an increase in MEF2D (a form of MEF2 that acts as an inhibitor) and a decrease in both MEF2A (a form of MEF2 that acts as an activator) and MyoD (a coactivator) binding to the *glut4* promoter in skeletal muscle. Interestingly, differential methylation of these three CpG clusters in the *glut4* promoter was not observed. This study also found that various isoforms of DNA methyltransferase (DNMT) bind to the *glut4* gene at different ages: DNA methyltransferase 1 (DNMT1) binds postnatally, whereas DNMT3a and DNMT3b bind in adults. The increase in DNMT binding was associated with exposure to increased methyl CpG-binding protein 2 (MeCP2) concentrations. Covalent modifications of the histone code consisted of histone 3 lysine 14 (H3K14) deacetylation mediated by recruitment of HDAC-1 and enhanced association of histone deacetylase-4 (HDAC-4) enzymes. This set the stage for Suv39H1 methylase-mediated dimethylation of H3K9 and increased recruitment of heterochromatin protein-1, which partially inactivates postnatal and adult IUGR *glut4* gene transcription. These studies demonstrate that perinatal nutrient restriction resulting in IUGR leads to silencing histone modifications in skeletal muscle and decreased *glut4* gene expression, effectively creating a metabolic knockdown of this important regulator of peripheral glucose transport and insulin resistance and contributing to the adult T2DM phenotype [30]. Hence, these studies show that histone modifications can be stably inherited in a calorie-restricted model of IUGR, mimicking the Dutch Famine experience [10].

The cascade of epigenetic modifications at specific genes in the IUGR β-cell (e.g., *Pdx-1*) and muscle (e.g., *glut4*) and their relationship to changes in gene expression that ultimately lead to the adult diabetic phenotype are well studied and thoroughly described. In the case of IUGR-induced obesity, specific epigenetic mechanisms leading to changes in the expression of key genes relating to the development of obesity and adipogenesis have not yet been established. However, recent advances in the understanding of the adipocyte as an independent endocrine organ, and the process of adipogenesis itself, have led to research revealing the important roles of chromatin and chromatin remodeling proteins and histone modifications to the process of adipogenesis. The following sections will briefly review adipogenesis in general and what is currently known about the role that epigenetic modifications play in the regulation of gene expression in the developing adipocyte.

8.4 Epigenetics of the Adipocyte

For many years the adipose tissue was considered to be a depot of stored energy that was rather inert, mainly functioning as an insulating agent and providing mechanical support for various structures. The discovery of leptin in 1994 led to the knowledge that adipocytes play important roles in the regulation of whole-body energy homeostasis [44]. Adipocytes were found to secrete proteins known as adipokines that regulate diverse processes such as hemostasis, immune function, angiogenesis, and energy balance (reviewed in [45]). Adipocytes are unique in the amount of lipid they can store and release rapidly for use by other organs in response to metabolic cues. Adipocytes are found in various depots in the body including subcutaneous locations, visceral locations, and fat pads of extremities and the orbital socket. Adipocytes can also be found mixed within other cell types, especially in loose connective tissue.

The factors determining fat mass in adult humans are not completely understood, but increased lipid storage in already developed adipocytes is thought to be an important component in the development of obesity. Spalding et al. showed that adipocyte number is a major determinant for fat mass in adults, and that the number of fat cells stays constant in adulthood in lean and obese individuals, even after marked weight loss, indicating that the number of adipocytes is set during childhood and adolescence [46]. The authors measured adipocyte turnover using ^{14}C derived from nuclear bomb tests in genomic DNA to establish the dynamics within the stable population of adipocytes in adults. They determined that approximately 10% of adipocytes are renewed annually at all ages and levels of body mass index. Neither adipocyte death nor the rate of adipogenesis is altered in early-onset obesity, suggesting a tight regulation of fat cell number in the obese state [46]. If the number of adipocytes is set to a higher level in obese people before adulthood, this could be because (1) cell number expansion begins at an earlier age in obese individuals; (2) expansion proceeds at a faster pace in obese individuals; or (3) expansion ends at a later age in obese individuals. The authors used a birth and death model to determine that the age of onset of adipocyte number expansion is significantly low in obese individuals [46]. Perhaps the early onset of adipocyte number expansion is the window during which alterations in the epigenetic regulation of gene expression lead to the earlier onset of adipocyte expansion. Studies testing this hypothesis have not yet been performed.

Mammals have two types of adipocytes, termed brown and white adipocytes. Both brown and while adipose tissues are involved in energy balance, but they assume opposite functions. Brown adipose tissue is specialized in energy dissipation as heat during cold and diet-induced thermogenesis. White adipose tissue is mainly involved in energy storage and mobilization in the form of triacylglycerols (reviewed in [47]). Brown adipocytes store less lipid and have more mitochondria than white adipocytes. Brown adipocytes express almost all the genes and proteins that are expressed in white adipocytes, but they also express some distinct ones, including uncoupling protein-1 (UCP-1), which allows energy to be dissipated as heat without generating ATP (reviewed in [45]). Most brown adipose tissue in rodents is stored in the interscapular region. Humans have a large amount of brown adipose tissue as infants, but as adults only small amounts of brown adipose tissue remain and it is dispersed within the white adipose tissue depots (reviewed in [45]). Unlike white adipose tissue differentiation, which occurs in the postnatal period in rodents, brown adipose tissue differentiation occurs before birth. Lineage tracing studies show that UCP-1-expressing cells do not contribute to the pool of white adipocytes [48]. However, there is evidence that white adipose tissue can acquire some of the heat-dissipating qualities of brown adipose tissue when exposed to conditions of cold or catecholamine excess [49].

8.5 Stages of the Developing Adipocyte: Determination and Differentiation

Until recently, the developmental origin of fat tissues has received very little attention. Adipocytes, like muscle and bone cells, are generally described as arising from the mesoderm. However, precise lineage tracing studies to define the origin of mesenchymal stem cell (MSC) adipocytes have not been performed [47]. In a review of the developmental origin of adipocytes, Billion et al. note that in higher vertebrates the mesoderm is not the only germ-layer source of MSCs [47]. The authors point out that within the head, the facial bones, jaw, and associated connective tissues are derived from neural crest cells, a cell population that arises from neuroectoderm. In the head and neck, the neural crest cells yield mesenchymal precursors, which have been shown to differentiate into connective tissue cells, vascular smooth muscle cells, dermis, odontoblasts, cartilage, and bone. The authors propose that these cells, being of mesenchymal origin, could also differentiate into adipose tissue. Different depots of adipose tissue have different patterns of gene expression and varying molecular and physical properties, and one possible explanation for these variations is that they are ultimately derived from differently derived pools of MSCs. There have been attempts to more clearly define the intermediate steps between pluripotent stem cells and mature adipocytes, but one complication to these studies is that many of the experiments were performed under in vitro conditions. Billion et al. described various studies that attempted to pinpoint the origin of the various pools of MSCs, citing pools that may be derived from neural crest cells, hematopoietic pluripotent cells, and mesoderm [47].

Adipogenesis is generally described as a two-step process. The first step is called determination, the process by which pluripotent MSCs are committed to the adipocyte lineage. Determination results in the conversion of stem cells into preadipocytes, which cannot be distinguished morphologically from pluripotent MSCs, but they have lost the potential to differentiate into other cell types (reviewed in [45]). The second step is called terminal differentiation. Here, preadipocytes acquire the characteristics of mature adipocytes, obtaining the cellular machinery necessary for the functions of lipid synthesis and transport, insulin sensitivity, and the ability to secrete adipocyte-specific proteins or adipokines. The molecular processes necessary for terminal differentiation have been more extensively studied and described due to the availability of in vitro experimental systems of preadipocyte 3T3-L1 and 3T3-F442A cell lines, which are described extensively below.

8.6 Experimental Systems for Studying Adipogenesis

Much of our understanding of the complex network of transcription factor activation and cell signaling processes, as well the epigenetic regulation of adipogenesis, comes from the use of various experimental systems that were established for the study of the processes by which preadipocytes are differentiated into mature adipocytes. The in vitro experimental systems involve the use of various cocktails of hormones and other drugs to stimulate the preadipocyte into differentiation into adipocytes. However, the general applicability of these in vitro models to the in vivo situation has been questioned. More recently, several knockout mouse models have been developed to study transcription factor roles in adipocyte development, which will be described below. Given that many of the transcription factors are obligate for embryo survival, alternative strategies were developed to obtain knockout models, but with their own limitations. Regardless of these concerns, most of the research in the field of adipogenesis has been preformed with the experimental systems that are described below.

The preadipocyte cell lines, 3T3-L1 and 3T3-F422A, were originally established by Green et al. in 1975–1976 [50, 51]. Although these cell lines were already committed to the adipocyte lineage, they provide a basic model to study the processes involved in terminal differentiation of the adipocyte. Confluent 3T3-L1 cells differentiate upon exposure to a cocktail of adipogenic inducers including fetal bovine serum (FBS), dexamethasone, isobutylmethylxanthine (a cyclic AMP inducer), and insulin. This combination of hormonal inducers activates the adipogenic program, which occurs in two well-defined stages. The stimulated cells immediately reenter the cell cycle and progress through at least two cell cycle divisions, a phase referred to as clonal expansion. It is during this time that the cells express specific adipogenic transcription factors as well cell cycle regulators. Following the clonal expansion, the cells undergo terminal differentiation defined by the production of lipid droplets and the expression of multiple metabolic programs characteristic of mature fat cells [51]. Mouse (C3H10T1/2) and human preadipocyte cell lines do not undergo the clonal expansion step and are able to differentiate without post-confluence mitosis. C3H10T1/2 is an adipogenic cell line that was derived from murine bone marrow [45]. It is an appropriate cell line for use in studying adipose cell commitment because these cells can differentiate in vitro into adipocytes, chondrocytes, and myotubes after being treated with 5-azacytidine (a general inhibitor of mammalian methyltransferases) and then stimulated with the appropriate adipogenic, chondrogenic, or myogenic signals. Multipotent adipocyte precursors were isolated only recently in 2006 by Nakagami et al., and this area remains relatively unexplored ([52]; reviewed in [53]).

Embryonic stem (ES) cells can be differentiated directly into adipocytes using a combination of retinoic acid and proadipogenic hormones. Mouse embryonic fibroblasts (MEFs) can be isolated after disaggregation of embryos at embryonic day E12–14 and can be differentiated into adipocytes or can be immortalized by several methods including serial passaging, the introduction of SV40 large T antigen, or chemical treatment prior to differentiation. Primary MEFs differentiate with variable efficiency (usually 10–70%) whereas most immortalized MEF lines do not differentiate unless a proadipogenic transcription factor cocktail is introduced. Multipotent precursor cells isolated from several adult tissues including adipose tissue, skeletal muscle, and bone marrow provide another source of cells, which can be useful for mesenchymal-cell-fate studies.

8.7 Adipogenesis

Here we briefly review the hormonal and transcriptional regulation of adipocyte differentiation that will serve as a platform by which we can further describe the epigenetic regulation of adipogenesis. Our review will focus on the transcription factor cascade involving CAAT/enhancer-binding proteins (C/EBPs) and PPARγ, although additional transcription factors and signaling pathways involved in adipogenesis will be highlighted in Chapter 17. Limited research has been performed on the events directing the commitment of pluripotent cells to the adipose lineage. One recent discovery involving the process of differentiating pluripotent cells to adipocytes involves bone morphogenetic protein-4 (BMP-4) and its ability to induce white adipose tissue development in C3H10T1/2 cells (reviewed in [53–55]), while treatment with bone morphogenetic protein-7 (BMP-7) specifically triggers commitment into the brown adipose lineage (reviewed in [56, 57]). The role of the BMP factors in adipocyte development remains an active area of research.

8.7.1 CAAT/Enhancer-Binding Proteins (C/EBPs)

One of the first steps in terminal differentiation is the increased expression and protein accumulation of C/EBPs, specifically C/EBPβ and C/EBPδ, stimulated in vitro by isobutylmethylxanthine and dexamethasone, respectively [58]. The C/EBP family is a group of basic leucine zipper transcription factors that include six members (α, β, δ, γ, ε, and ξ), three of which play crucial roles in adipogenesis (α, β, and δ) (reviewed in [53]). Early induction of C/EBPβ and C/EBPδ leads to induction of C/EBPα. C/EBPβ and C/EBPδ begin to accumulate within 4 h of adipocyte induction but are initially inactive (reviewed in [53, 59]). C/EBPβ-deficient mice have reduced adiposity but this effect may be due to reduced lipogenesis and has not been shown to be due to reduced adipogenesis specifically. C/EBPβ and C/EBPδ function in part by inducing the transcription of C/EBPα and PPARγ. After induction of C/EBPβ and C/EBPδ, the cells reenter the cell cycle and undergo mitotic expansion, a step that requires C/EBPβ (reviewed in [53, 60]). C/EBPβ is hypophosphorylated and thus activated by MAPK and GSK3B, which then goes on to induce the transcription of C/EBPα and PPARγ. By day 2 of the differentiation process, C/EBPα protein begins to accumulate and is phosphorylated by the Cyclin D3–CDK2 complex. Phosphorylated C/EBPα exerts an inhibitory effect on the growth of the cells which can then exit the cell cycle and begin the process of terminal differentiation to adipocytes (reviewed in [53,61,62]).

C/EBPα induces many adipogenic genes directly. Analysis of *c/ebpα*$^{-/-}$ mice is complicated by perinatal hypoglycemia and requires restoration of hepatic *c/ebpα* levels by a liver-specific rescue. Once the hepatic *c/ebpα* levels are restored, the mice display normal liver function but have reduced amounts of white adipose tissue [63]. *C/ebpα*$^{-/-}$ mice are almost completely devoid of white adipose tissue except for the mammary gland [64]. In the *c/ebpα*$^{-/-}$ model, the development of brown adipose tissue is delayed but eventually results in relatively normal amounts or brown adipose tissue in the adult. Other isoforms of C/EBP, including C/EBPγ and CHOP, appear to suppress adipogenesis, perhaps through heterodimerization and inactivation of C/EBPβ.

8.7.2 PPARγ – A Master Regulator of Adipogenesis

PPARγ is a member of the nuclear receptor superfamily and is both necessary and sufficient for adipogenesis (reviewed in [45]). Forced expression of PPARγ is sufficient to induce adipocyte differentiation from fibroblasts; yet, no additional factors have been identified to promote adipogenesis in the absence of PPARγ (reviewed in [45, 51]). Most additional proadipogenic transcription factors have been found to function at least in part by activating *pparγ* gene expression or activity. Both C/EBPs and Kruppel-like factors (KLFs) have been shown to induce at least one of the two PPARγ promoters. Antiadipogenic GATA factors (GATA2 and GATA3) function in part by repressing PPARγ expression. There are two existing isoforms of PPARγ generated by alternative splicing and promoter usage, and both are induced during adipogenesis (reviewed in [45]). PPARγ1 is found in other cell types besides adipocytes, including colonic epithelium and macrophages. PPARγ2 has been shown to be more efficient than PPARγ1 in promoting adipogenesis, although two selective *pparγ2* knockout mouse models have displayed different results. One model shows impaired adipogenesis in the absence of PPARγ2, while the other showed normal adipose tissue mass in the absence of PPARγ2 (reviewed in [45]). Although it is clear that PPARγ is necessary for adipogenesis, it is not clear whether PPARγ2 is the dominant isoform needed (reviewed in [53]). PPARγ is not only required for adipogenesis, but necessary for maintenance of the differentiated state (reviewed in [45]). Adenoviral introduction of a dominant-negative PPARγ into mature 3T3-L1 adipocytes caused dedifferentiation with loss of lipid accumulation and decreased expression of adipocyte markers (reviewed in [45, 65]).

8.8 Epigenetic Regulation of Adipogenesis

PPARγ and C/EBP are transcription factors that play key roles in adipogenesis. Epigenetic events regulating these transcription factors have been described in the regulation of preadipocyte determination as well as in the later stages of adipocyte differentiation.

8.8.1 Epigenetic Regulation of Preadipocyte Determination

Differentiation of pluripotent cells requires selective silencing and activation of subsets of genes at appropriate time points, usually accomplished by the induction of expression of a number of transcription factors (Fig. 8.2). In addition, gene

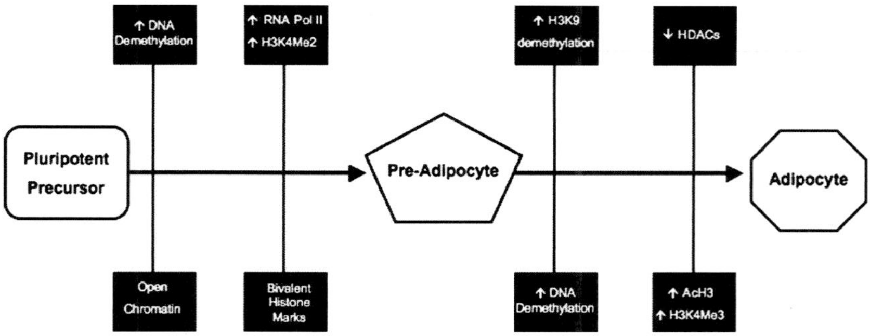

Fig. 8.2 Epigenetic modifications contributing to adipocyte development. Pluripotent adipocyte precursors have been shown to associate with loosely related chromatin proteins. During determination, DNA demethylation of key genes such as *BMP-4* takes place, directing cells toward adipogenesis [54]. RNAPol II and the active transcription mark H3K4me2 can be detected at the promoters of genes that are transcriptionally silent at this stage including *glut4* and *lep*. This signal is not found in pluripotent cells and is therefore a sign of cells committed to the adipocyte lineage [53]. During differentiation of the committed adipocyte precursors, further DNA demethylation takes place [71–73]. H3K9 is demethylated at the promoter of late adipogenic genes and H3 acetylation and H3K4 trimethylation increase [54, 89]. In addition, there is global decrease in histone deacetylase enzymes as this stage [89]

activity is determined by chromatin structure and the intervention of chromatin-binding proteins (Fig. 8.3). Studies on embryonic stem cells have shown that the binding of several architectural chromatin proteins to chromatin is not as tight as in more developed cells, leading to what has been described as "hyperdynamic chromatin" (reviewed in [53, 66]). Hyperdynamic chromatin has been found in the mesenchymal pluripotent cell line C3H10T1/2, which maintains the ability to give rise to chrondroblasts, myoblasts, and preadipocytes. However, hyperdynamic heterochromatin is not found in the undifferentiated but already committed C2C12 myoblast cell line (reviewed in [53]). This feature has not been studied to date in the 3T3-L1 preadipocyte cell line. Increased chromatin plasticity is a hallmark of pluripotent cells establishing that these cells maintain a large number of genes that, although currently are silenced, remain in the poised position and are available for transcription [53].

Another characteristic of pluripotent stem cells is the presence of a bivalent histone mark. Bivalent histone marks describe when both the activating mark of H3 and H4 acetylation and the repressing mark of H3K27 hypermethylation are present at the same time (reviewed in [53, 67]). These two bivalent histone marks are present both in mouse embryonic stem cells and in human embryonic fibroblasts. The negative mark of H3K27 hypermethylation is particularly enriched at the promoters of developmentally important genes such as the adipogenic genes adiponectin, leptin (*lep*), UCP1, and DLK1 (PREP1) (reviewed in [53, 68]), insuring that these genes are silenced in the pluripotent state, but poised for activation if the appropriate differentiation signals are eventually received.

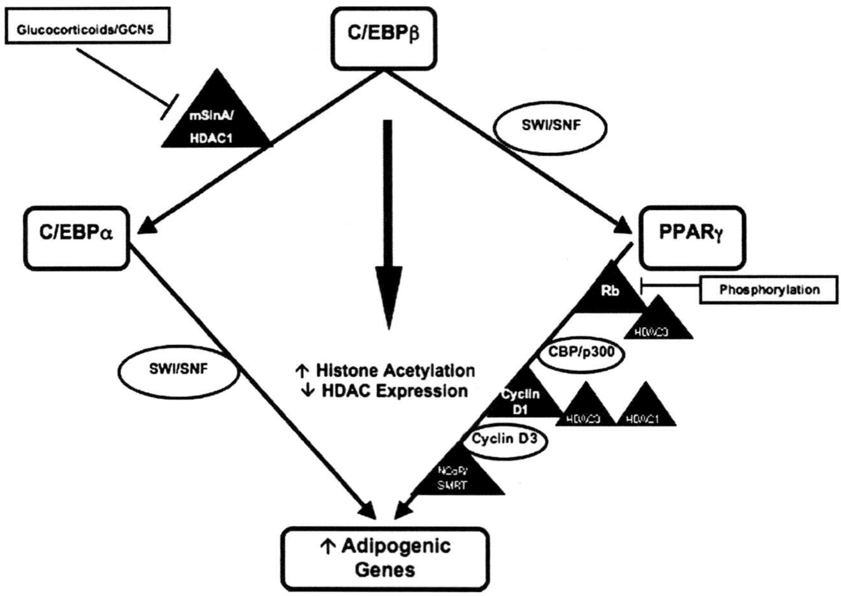

Fig. 8.3 Summary of the role of chromatin-modifying proteins in adipogenesis. Transcription factor C/EBPβ in bound to both *ppar*γ and the *cebp*α promoters in undifferentiated adipocytes 1–4 h after adipocyte induction but prior to initiation of transcription [75]. On day 2 of the differentiation process, the chromatin remodeling complex SWI/SNF is recruited to the *ppar*γ promoter allowing transcription to begin [76]. Glucocorticoids can displace the repressive mSin3a/HDAC1 complex from the *cebp*α promoter, thus permitting C/EBPβ to activate C/EBPα transcription [78]. C/EBPα interacts with an activating SWI/SNF complex and therefore goes on to further activate its adipogenic targets [53]. In undifferentiated cells, PPARγ binds to the promoters of its target genes but is also in association with repressor complexes including Rb and HDAC3. Phosphorylation of Rb breaks this specific complex and prevents its repressive activity [81]. PPARγ can also interact with corepressors NCoR/SMRT in undifferentiated adipocytes [84]. Cell cycle regulators have both positive and negative effects on adipocyte differentiation. Cyclin D1 is recruited to PPARγ target promoters and represses transcriptional activity by associating with HDAC3 and HDAC1 in the early stages of adipogenesis [87]. Cyclin D3, whose expression increases throughout adipogenesis, interacts with PPARγ acting as an activator and enhancing expression of PPARγ's target genes [86]. White ovals represent activating complexes and black triangles represent repressing complexes

As described earlier, C3H10T1/2 cells need to be treated with 5-azacytidine (a general DNA-demethylating agent) in order to differentiate into adipocytes, suggesting that DNA methylation may be involved in the process of preadipocyte determination [69]. Noer et al. performed a study in isolated adipose tissue stromal cells and described hypomethylation of several adipogenic promoters including *ppar*γ*2* and *lep* even though the promoters of several myogenic and endothelial genes were methylated (reviewed in [53, 70]). The results of this study may indicate that the stromal cells used were not pluripotent but were already committed to the adipocyte cell lineage. Several studies using 3T3-L1 cells have found that the promoters of late adipogenic genes such as leptin or the adipose and muscle-specific glucose transporter *glut4* are methylated in preadipocytes but become demethylated during the process of adipogenesis (reviewed in [53, 71–73]). Similarly, the *myod1* promoter has been shown to be methylated in C3H10T1/2 cells, but after 5-azacytidine treatment this promoter is demethylated and the cells are committed to the myogenic lineage. Another study found that the C3H109T1/2 clonal line spontaneously undergoes adipogenesis correlated with demethylation after treatment with 5-azacytidine and expression of the *bmp4* gene [74]. Although some results from 5-azacytidine treatment appear conflicting, it appears that demethylation plays an important role in the adipocyte determination process.

Musri et al. have studied the posttranslational modifications of histones taking place throughout adipogenesis at the promoters of several adipogenic genes such as *glut4*, *lep*, and adiponectin [53]. The promoters of these genes display significant levels of histone H3K4 dimethylation in undifferentiated 3T3-L1 fibroblasts prior to the induction of differentiation. In the predifferentiated 3T3-L1 cells, the H3K4 dimethylation mark was present in association with recruitment of RNA polymerase II (RNAPol II) to the promoters of *glut4*, *lep*, and adiponectin before expression of these genes was detected. In the pluripotent C3H10T1/2 fibroblasts, neither H3K4 dimethylation nor RNAPol II binding was detected at the promoters of the same genes, indicating that cells bearing the H3K4 dimethylation mark along with RNAPol II binding are poised to become adipocytes even at this early stage of development [53].

8.8.2 Chromatin Remodeling and C/EBP Transcription Factors

Although adipocyte-specific genes are not expressed prior to differentiation, gene expression is likely prevented in part by regulatory sequences controlling the expression of these genes by the incorporation of a repressive chromatin structure. Eukaryotic cells have evolved two classes of enzymes that can alter chromatin structure to control the accessibility to transcriptional machinery. These enzymes include (1) histone-modifying enzymes, which posttranslationally modify the N-terminal and C-terminal domains of the individual histone proteins that compromise the nucleosome and (2) ATP-dependent chromatin-remodeling enzymes, which alter structure by disrupting the histone:DNA contacts of the nucleosome, thereby altering the nucleosome.

In the first few hours after induction of the terminal differentiation process, C/EBPβ and C/EBPδ proteins bind the *cebpα* and *pparγ2* promoters (reviewed in [53, 75]). At the *pparγ2* promoter, C/EBPβ and RNAPol II are bound by day 1 of adipocyte differentiation, well in advance of the start of gene expression [76]. The mammalian SWI/SNF family of ATP-dependent chromatin remodeling enzymes includes members containing Brg1 and Brm ATPases. By day 2 of terminal differentiation, the SWI/SNF complex binds to the *pparγ2* promoter and results in chromatin remodeling at both the promoter and the transcription start site. Ini1 is common to all SWI/SNF complexes but Brg1 and Brm are the ATPase subunits of two different complexes, and thus the presence of both subunits indicates that more than one complex is bound. Experiments with cell lines expressing dominant-negative versions of Brg1 and Brm indicate that both complexes are necessary for *ppar*γ*2* activation [76]. The SWI/SNF complex is not stable and it dislodges from the *ppar*γ*2* promoter by day 4 of the differentiation process [76]. Coinciding with the detachment of the SWI/SNF complex, expression of PPARγ2 is decreased by day 4 of differentiation and was almost undetectable by day 5 and thereafter [76]. In these experiments it appears that the remodeling of the chromatin by the binding of the SWI/SNF complex allows for a chromatin structure that favors *ppar*γ*2* gene transcription during the adipocyte differentiation process.

As described earlier, C/EBPβ can bind to the *cebpα* promoter as early as 4 h after induction of the terminal differentiation of the adipocyte. However, its activation can be blocked by the presence of the repressive complex composed of histone deacetylases mSin3A and histone deacetylase-1 (HDAC1) (mSin3A/HDAC1). As the PPARγ protein begins to accumulate after induction, it is able to facilitate degradation of the HDAC1 protein, thus permitting C/EBPβ to bind to the *cebpα* promoter and activate gene expression (reviewed in [53, 77]). C/EBPβ is initially associated with HDAC1, preventing its ability to bind to the *cepbα* promoter. Treatment with glucocorticoids activates GCN5, a histone acetyltransferase, resulting in the dissociation of HDAC1 and C/EBPβ and the activation of the *cebpα* promoter by C/EBPβ (reviewed in [53, 78]).

In addition to regulating the expression of adipogenic genes, one of the main function of C/EBPα is to promote cells to exit the cell cycle, a crucial event for any model of differentiation (reviewed in [53, 79]). In order to accomplish this, C/EBPα depends on the Brm-containing SWI/SNF complex to promote growth arrest by suppressing E2F-dependent promoters (reviewed in [53, 62, 80]). Studies with mutated constructs of NIH-3T3 cells, a mouse embryonic fibroblast cell line, have shown that C/EBPα requires interaction with a functional and active SWI/SNF complex in order to exert its well-established effect arrest of cell proliferation (reviewed in [53, 80]).

8.8.3 Epigenetic Regulation of PPARγ: The Role of Histone Acetylation

The epigenetic regulation of PPARγ has been studied in detail and involves many coactivators and corepressors (Fig. 8.3). The protein Rb, known to exert a repressive effect on the initial phases of adipogenesis, has been found to be associated with histone deacetylase-3 (HDAC3) in 3T3-L1 fibroblasts (reviewed in [53, 81]). While Rb is active and dephosphorylated, the complex Rb–HDAC3 interacts with PPARγ, resulting in the recruitment of deacetylase activity to the target promoters of PPARγ and resulting in the repression of gene transcription. When Rb becomes phosphorylated, the Rb–PPARγ interaction is disrupted. PPARγ is then free to associate with histone acetyltransferases such as CREB-binding protein (CBP) and p300, which results in increased gene transcription. CBP and p300 establish an important interaction with PPARγ, and the downregulation of CBP and p300 results in decreased adipogenesis in 3T3-L1 cells [82, 83].

PPARγ may also recruit corepressors to the promoters of adipogenic genes, including NCoR and SMRT, which result in the downregulation of transcriptional activity and decreased expression of the target gene. In 3T3-L1 cells, the addition of pioglitazone (a PPARγ ligand) breaks the PPARγ–NCoR association and results in increased PPARγ transcriptional activity [84]. At the same time, when PPARγ binds to a ligand, this also increases the interaction of PPARγ with the histone acetyltransferases CBP and p300, which results in increased transcriptional activity [85].

PPARγ also interacts with Cyclin D3, which plays a role in regulating adipogenesis independent from its main role as a cell cycle regulator. Cyclin D3 along with its cyclin-dependent kinase, CDK6, binds to and phosphorylates PPARγ [86]. Cyclin D3, whose expression increases throughout adipogenesis, acts as a ligand-dependent PPARγ coactivator and plays an important stimulatory role in adipogenesis. Cyclin D1 has the opposite effect on regulating the transcriptional activating activity of PPARγ by enhancing the recruitment of HDAC1 and HDAC3 to the target promoters, as well as recruiting the histone methyltransferase SUV39H1. Cyclin D1's ultimate effect results in the decreased acetylation of the target promoters of PPARγ, including lipoprotein lipase, leading to decreased expression of adipose-specific target genes [87].

As seen from the examples described above, histone acetylation plays a central role in the regulation of adipogenesis and the activity of key adipogenic transcription factors. Most HDAC inhibitors cause cell cycle arrest and increase differentiation, and for this reason many histone deacetylases are being targeted as anticancer therapies [88]. Histone acetylation increases throughout the process of adipogenesis at the promoter regions of adipogenic genes, and decreased HDAC expression occurs during the terminal differentiation process [53, 89]. Inhibition of HDAC activity increases adipogenesis and the overexpression of HDAC1 blocks adipocyte development [78, 81, 89].

Histone acetylation also plays an important role in the function of mature adipocytes. Sirt1 is a NAD-dependent class III histone deacetylase that is activated by caloric restriction. Sirt1 promotes fat mobilization by docking with NCor-SMRT and repressing PPARγ [90]. Sirt1 expression increases throughout adipogenesis. SiRNA experiments depleting Sirt1 result in enhanced adipocyte formation, whereas overexpression of Sirt1 results in decreased adipogenesis [90].

8.8.4 Histone Methylation in Adipogenesis

Methylation of H3K4 is related to active gene transcription in a manner similar to histone acetylation. As mentioned earlier, the promoters of adipogenic genes have increased dimethyl H3K4 in the preadipocyte state, marking those genes that are poised for transcription, even though they are silent in preadipocytes [53]. Although increased dimethyl H3K4 is seen *only* at the promoters of the preadipogenic genes, during the differentiation phase H3K4 dimethylation is increased both at the promoters and at the coding regions of those genes, coinciding with the initiation of transcription [53]. Increased H3K4 trimethylation is seen at the promoters of *amp1*, *lep*, and *glut4* only after the start of transcription, whereas the increased H3K4 trimethyl mark is only seen in the coding region of these genes in fully differentiated adipocytes [53].

Musri et al. treated 3T3-L1 fibroblasts with a low dose of a methylthioadenosine (a methytransferase inhibitor) in order to erase histone methylation at gene promoters and noted decreased adipogenesis, thereby indicating that histone methylation is an important aspect regulating adipogenesis [53]. To date no transcription factor or other proteins have been identified as the agents responsible for initiating and/or maintaining appropriate levels of histone methylation at the promoters of adipogenic genes.

8.8.5 DNA Methylation and Gene Expression

Okada et al. sought to identify the role of chromatin and chromatin-modifying proteins in the regulation of gene expression related to adipocyte hypertrophy in the differentiated adipocyte [91]. The authors maintained C57BL/6 J mice on a high-fat diet for 16 weeks and found markedly increased gene expression of leptin (*lep*), mesoderm-specific transcript, also known as paternally expressed gene-1 (*Mest* or *Peg1*), and secreted frizzled-related protein 5 (*sFRP5*) in white adipose tissue. Treatment of 3T3-L1 adipocytes with 5-aza-2′-deoxycytidine increased the amount of Mest/Peg1 mRNA, but there was no increase in leptin or sFRP5 mRNA. Maintenance of mice on the high-fat diet for various times did not affect the level of DNA methylation at specific CpG sites within the promoters of *lep*, *Mest/Peg1*, and *sFRP5* in white adipose tissues as measured by matrix-assisted laser desorption ionization time-of-flight (MALDI-TOF) mass spectrometry [91]. These results indicate that diet-induced upregulation of gene expression of *lep*, *Mest/Peg1*, and *sFRP5* in white adipose tissue is not mediated directly by changes in DNA methylation, suggesting that there are additional factors involved in the upregulation of gene expression that must be identified and studied.

8.9 Conclusions

Epigenetic regulation has been clearly noted to play an important role in gene expression both in the β-cell and in the muscle of the IUGR animal model. In addition, epigenetics contributes to the regulation of both adipocyte determination and differentiation in in vitro models. The contributions of histone acetylation, histone methylation, and DNA methylation to the process of adipogenesis in vivo remain to be evaluated. In theory, the IUGR animal model could play a critical part in elucidating the epigenetic mechanisms crucial to appropriate gene regulation in the adipocyte and in determining specific epigenetic modifications that contribute to the phenotype of adiposity and obesity. Furthermore, pharmaceuticals are in development for treating and restoring aberrant epigenetic marks that contribute to disease. The role of histone acetyltransferases (HATs) in the pathology of cancer, asthma, and viral infections has been described. The potential for specific HAT inhibitors in disease treatment or prevention is an active area of pharmaceutical research, especially with the development of small-molecule inhibitors of HATs as potential drug therapies [92]. Once these agents have well-established, defined, and specific targets, they may also be useful for preventative treatment. These agents would be especially useful in conditions such as diabetes and obesity, where such drugs may be able to rectify an exposure to an abnormal intrauterine environment if they are administered within the appropriate developmental window.

References

1. Dietz WH. Overweight in childhood and adolescence. N Engl J Med. 2004;350:855–7.
2. Taylor PD, Poston L. Developmental programming of obesity in mammals. Exp Physiol. 2007;92:287–98.
3. Simmons R. Perinatal programming of obesity. Semin Perinatol. 2008;32:371–4.
4. Bayol SA, Bigboy SH, Stickland NC. A maternal cafeteria diet during gestation and lactation promotes adiposity and impairs skeletal muscle development and metabolism in rat offspring at weaning. J Physiol. 2005;567:951–61.
5. Catalano PM. Obesity and pregnancy – the propagation of a viscous cycle? J Clin Endocrinol Metab. 2003;88:3500–6.
6. Levin BE, Dunn-Meynell AA. Maternal obesity alters adiposity and monoamine function in genetically predisposed offspring. Am J Physiol Regul Integr Comp Physiol. 2002;283:R1087–R93.
7. Levin BE, Govek E. Gestational obesity accentuates obesity in obesity-prone progeny. Am J Physiol Regul Integr Comp Physiol. 1998;275:R1375–9.
8. Guo F, Jen K-L. High-fat feeding during pregnancy and lactation affects offspring metabolism in rats. Physiol Behav. 2005;57:681–6.
9. Reifsnyder PC, Churchill G, Leiter EH. Maternal environment and genotype interact to establish diabesity in mice. Genome Res. 2000;10:1568–78.
10. Bannister AJ, Kouzarides T. Reversing histone methylation. Nature. 2005;436:1103–6.
11. Bernstein E, Allis CD. RNA meets chromatin. Genes Dev. 2005;19:1635–55.
12. Mellor J. The dynamics of chromatin remodeling at promoters. Mol Cell. 2005;19:147–57.
13. Sproul D, Gilbert N, Bickmore WA. The role of chromatin structure in regulating the expression of clustered genes. Nat Rev Genet. 2005;6:775–81.
14. Yoshida H, Broaddus R, Cheng W, et al. Deregulation of the HOXA10 homeobox gene in endometrial carcinoma: role in epithelial-mesenchymal transition. Cancer Res. 2006;66: 889–97.
15. So K, Tamura G, Honda T, et al. Multiple tumor suppressor genes are increasingly methylated with age in non-neoplastic gastric epithelia. Cancer Sci. 2006;97:1155–8.
16. Takahashi T, Shigematsu H, Shivapukas N, et al. Aberrant promoter methylation of multiple genes during multistep pathogenesis of colorectal cancers. Int J Cancer. 2006;118:924–31.

17. Grady WM, Carethers JM. Genomic and epigenetic instability incolorectal cancer pathogenesis. Gastroenterology. 2008;135:1079–99.
18. Kafri T, Ariel M, Brandeis M, et al. Developmental pattern of gene-specific DNA methylation in the mouse embryo and germline. Genes Dev. 1992;6:705–14.
19. Monk M, Boubelik M, Lehnert S. Temporal and regional changes in DNA methylation in the embryonic, extra-embryonic and germ cell lineages during mouse embryo development. Development. 1987;99:371–82.
20. Cedar H, Bergman Y. Linking DNA methylations and histone modifications: patterns and paradigms. Nat Rev Genet. 2009;10:295–304.
21. Schubeler D, Lorincz MC, Cimbora DM, et al. Genomic targeting of methylated DNA: influence of methylation on transcription, replication, chromatin structure, and histone acetylation. Mol Cell Biol. 2000;20:9103–12.
22. Gopalakrishnan S, Van Emburgh BO, Robertson KD. DNA methylation in development and human disease. Mutat Res. 2008;647:30–83.
23. Costa FF. Non-coding RNAs, epigenetics and complexity. Gene. 2008;410:9–17.
24. Costa FF. Non-coding RNAs: new players in eukaryotic biology. Gene. 2005;2:83–94.
25. Kawasaki H, Taira K. Induction of DNA methylation and gene silencing by short interfacing RNAs in human cells. Nature. 2004;431:211–7.
26. Morris KV, Chan SW, Jacobsen SE, Looney DJ. Small interfering RNA-induced transcriptional gene silencing in human cells. Science. 2004;305:1289–92.
27. MacLennan NK, James SJ, Melnyk S, et al. Uteroplacental insufficiency alters DNA methylation, one-carbon metabolism, and histone acetylation in IUGR rats. Physiol Genomics. 2004;18:43–50.
28. Fu Q, McKnight RA, Yu X, et al. Uteroplacental insufficiency induces site-specific changes in histone H3 covalent modifications and affects DNA-histone H3 positioning in day 0 IUGR rat liver. Physiol Genomics. 2004;20:108–16.
29. Park JH, Stoffers DA, Nichols RD, et al. Development of type 2 diabetes following intrauterine growth retardation in rats is associated with progressive epigenetic silencing of Pdx-1. J Clin Invest. 2008;118:2316–24.
30. Raychaudhuri N, Raychaudhari S, Thamotharan M, et al. Histone code modifications repress glucose transporter 4 expression in the intrauterine growth-restricted offspring. J Biol Chem. 2008;283:13611–26.
31. Simmons RA, Templeton LJ, Gertz SJ. Intrauterine growth retardation leads to type II diabetes in adulthood in the rat. Diabetes. 2001;50:2279–86.
32. Stoffers DA, Desai BM, DeLeon DD, et al. Neonatal exendin-4 prevents the development of diabetes in the intrauterine growth retarded rat. Diabetes. 2003;52:734–40.
33. Qian J, Kaytor ED, Towle HC, et al. Upstream stimulatory factor regulates *Pdx*-1 gene expression in differentiated pancreatic β-cells. Biochem J. 1999;341:315–22.
34. Sharma S, Leonard J, Lee S, et al. Pancreatic islet expression of the homeobox factor STF-1 (*Pdx*-1) relies on an E-box motif that binds USF. J Biol Chem. 1996;271: 2294–9.
35. Li H, Rauch T, Chen ZX, et al. The histone methyltransferase SETDB1 and the DNA methyltransferase DNMT3A interact directly and localize to promoters silenced in cancer cells. J Biol Chem. 2006;281:19489–500.
36. Bachman KE, Park BH, Rhee I, et al. Histone modifications and silencing prior to DNA methylation of a tumor suppressor gene. Cancer Cell. 2003;3:89–95.
37. Kouzarides T. Histone methylation in transcriptional control. Curr Opin Genet Dev. 2002;12:198–209.
38. Bernardo AS, Hay CW, Docherty K. Pancreatic transcription factors and their role in the birth, life and survival of the pancreatic beta cell. Mol Cell Endocrinol. 2008;294:1–9.
39. Thamotharan M, Shin BC, Suddirikku DT, et al. GLUT4 expression and subcellular localization in the intrauterine growth-restricted adult rat female offspring. Am J Physiol Endocrinol Metab. 2004;288:E935–47.

40. Ozanne SE, Jensen CB, Storgaard H, et al. Low birthweight is associated with specific changes in muscle insulin-signalling protein expression. Diabetologia. 2005;48:547–52.
41. Fueger PT, Shearer J, Krueger TM, et al. Control of muscle glucose uptake: test of the rate-limiting step paradigm in conscious, unrestrained mice. J Physiol. 2005;562:925–35.
42. Karnieli E, Armoni M. Transcriptional regulation of the insulin-responsive glucose transporter GLUT4 gene: from physiology to pathology. Am J Physiol Endocrinol Metab. 2008;295: E38–45.
43. Moreno H, Serrano AL, Santaucia T, et al. Differential regulation of the muscle-specific GLUT4 enhancer in regenerating and adult skeletal muscle. J Biol Chem. 2003;278: 40557–64.
44. Zhang Y, Proenca R, Maffei M, et al. Positional Clonging of the mouse *obese* gene and its human homologue. Nature. 1994;372:425–31.
45. Rosen ED, MacDougald OA. Adipocyte differentiation from the inside out. Nat Rev Mol Cell Biol. 2006;7(12):886–96.
46. Spalding KL, Arner E, Westermark PO, et al. Dynamics of fat cell turnover in humans. Nature. 2008;453:783–7.
47. Billion N, Monteiro MC, Dani C. Developmental origin of adipocytes: new insights into a pending question. Biol Cell. 2008;100(10):563–75.
48. Moulin K, Truel N, Andre M, et al. Emergence during development of the white-adipose cell phenotype is independent of the brown-adipose cell phenotype. Biochem J. 2001;356: 659–64.
49. Himms-Hagen J, Melnyk A, Zingaretti MC, et al. Multilocular fat cells in WAT of CL-316243-treated rats derive directly from white adipocytes. Am J Physiol Cell Physiol. 2000;279: C670–81.
50. Green H, Kehinde O. Spontaneous heritable changes leading to increased adipose conversion in 3T3 cells. Cell. 1976;7:105–13.
51. Farmer SR. Transcriptional control of adipocyte formation. Cell Metab. 2006;4:263–73.
52. Nakagami H, Morishita R, Maeda K, et al. Adipose tissue-derived stromal cells as a novel option for regenerative cell therapy. J Atheroscler Thromb. 2006;13:77–81.
53. Musri MM, Gomis R, Parrozas M. Chromatin and chromatin-modifying proteins in adipogenesis. Biochem Cell Biol. 2007;85:397–410.
54. Bowers RR, Kim JW, Otto TC, Lane MD. Stable stem cell commitment to the adipocyte lineage by inhibition of DNA methylation: role of the BMP-4 gene. Proc Natl Acad Sci USA. 2006;103:13022–7.
55. Tang QQ, Otto TC, Lane MD. Commitment of Ch310T1/2 pluripotent stem cells to the adipocyte lineage. Proc Natl Acad Sci USA. 2004;101:9607–11.
56. Schulz TJ, Tseng YH. Emerging role of bone morphogenetic proteins in adipogenesis and energy metabolism. Cytokine Growth Factor Rev. 2009;20:523–31.
57. Tseng YH, Kokkotou E, Schulz TJ, et al. New role of bone morphogenetic protein 7 and energy expenditure. Nature. 2008;454(7207):1000–4.
58. Yeh WC, Cao Z, Classon M, Mc Knight SL. Cascade regulation of terminal adipocyte differentiation by three members of the C/EBP family of leucine zipper proteins. Genes Dev. 1995;9:168–81.
59. Tang QQ, Lane MD. Activation and centromeric localization of CCAAT/enhancer-binding proteins during the mitotic clonal expansion of adipocyte differentiation. Genes Dev. 1999;13:2231–41.
60. Tang QQ, Otto TC, Lane MD. Mitotic clonal expansion: a synchronous process required for adipogenesis. Proc Natl Acad Sci USA. 2003;100:44–9.
61. Reichard M, Eick D. Analysis of cell cycle arrest in adipocyte differentiation. Oncogene. 1999;18:459–66.
62. Wang GL, Shi X, Salisbury E, Sun Y, Albrecht JH, Smith RG, et al. Cyclin D3 maintains growth inhibitory activity of C/EBPα by stabilizing C/EBPα-cdk2 and C/EBPα-Brm complexes. Mol Cell Biol. 2006;26:2570–82.

63. Chen SS, Chen JF, Johnson PF, Muppala V, Lee YH. C/EBPβ when expressed from the C/EBPα gene locus can functionally replace C/EBPα in liver but not adipose tissue. Mol Cell Biol. 2000;20:7292–9.
64. Linhart HG, Ishimura-Oka K, DeMayo F, et al. C/EBPα is required for differentiation of white but not brown adipose tissue. Proc Natl Acad Sci USA. 2001;98:12532–7.
65. Tamoir Y, Masugi J, Nishine N, Kasuga M. Role of peroxisome proliferator-activated receptor γ in maintenance of the characteristics of mature 3T3-11 adipocytes. Diabetes. 2002;51: 2045–55.
66. Meshorer E, Yellajoshula D, George E, et al. Hyperdynamic plasticity of chromatin proteins in pluripotent embryonic stem cells. Dev Cell. 2006;10:105–16.
67. Bernstein BE, Mikkelson TS, Xie X, Kamal M, et al. A bivalent chromatin structure marks key developmental genes in embryonic stem cells. Cell. 2006;125:315–25.
68. Bracken AP, Dietrich N, Pasini D, Hansen KH, et al. Genome-wide mapping of Polycomb target genes unravels their roles in cell fate transitions. Genes Dev. 2006;20: 1123–36.
69. Taylor SM, Jones PA. Multiple new phenotypes induced in 10T1/2 and 3T3 cells treated with 5-azacytidine. Cell. 1979;17:771–9.
70. Noer A, Sorensen AL, Boquet AC, Collas P. Stable CpG hypomethylation of adipogenic promoters in freshly isolated, cultured and differentiated mesenchymal stem cells from adipose tissue. Mol Cell Biol. 2006;17:3543–56.
71. Melzner I, Scott V, Dorsch K, Fischer P, et al. Leptin gene expression in human preadipocytes is switched on by maturation-induced demethylation of distinct CpGs in its proximal promoter. J Biol Chem. 2002;277:45420–7.
72. Yokomori N, Tawata M, Onaya T. DNA demethylation during differentiation of the 3T3-L1 cells affects the expression of the mouse GLUT4 gene. Diabetes. 1999;48:685–90.
73. Yokomori N, Tawata M, Onaya T. DNA demethylation modulates mouse leptin promoter activity during differentiation of the 3T3-L1 cells. Diabetologia. 2002;45:140–8.
74. Bowers RR, Kim JW, Otto TC, Lane MD. Stable stem cell commiment to the adipocyte lineage by inhibition of DNA methylation: role of the BMP-4 gene. Proc Natl Acad Sci USA. 2006;103:13022–7.
75. Salma N, Xiao H, Imbalzano AN. Temporal recruitment of C/EBPs to early and late adipogenic promoters in vivo. J Mol Endocrinol. 2006;36:139–51.
76. Salma N, Xiao H, Mueler E, Imbalzano AN. Temporal recruitment of transcription factors and SWI/SNF chromatin-remodeling enzymes during adipogenic induction of the PPARγ nuclear hormone receptor. Mol Cell Biol. 2004;24:4651–63.
77. Zuo Y, Qiang L, Farmer SR. Activation of C/EBPα expression by C/EBPβ during adipogenesis requires a PPARγ-associated repression of HDAC1 at the C/EBPα gene promoter. J Biol Chem. 2006;281:7960–7.
78. Wiper-Bergeron N, Salem HA, Tomilson JJ, Wu D, Hache RJ. Glucocorticoid-stimulated preadipocyte differentiation is mediated through acetylation of C/EBPβ by GCN5. Proc Natl Acad Sci USA. 2007;104:2703–8.
79. Johnson PF. Molecular stop signs: regulation of cell-cycle arrest by C/EBP transcription factors. J Cell Sci. 2005;118:2545–55.
80. Mueller C, Calkhoven CF, Sha X, Leutz A. C/EBPα requires a SWI/SNF complex for proliferation arrest. J Biol Chem. 2004;279:7353–8.
81. Fajas L, Egler V, Reiter R, Hansen J, et al. The retinoblastoma-histone deacetylase 3 complex inhibits PPARγ and adipocyte differentiation. Dev. Cell. 2002;3:903–10.
82. Chen Z, Johnson BA, Li Y, Aster S, et al. Both co-activators of LxxLL motif-dependent and independent interactions are required for PPARγ function. J Biol Chem. 2000;275: 3733–6.
83. Takahashi N, Kawada T, Yamamoto T, et al. Overexpression and ribozyme-mediated targeting of transcriptional coactivators CBP and p300 revealed their indispensable roles in adipocyte differentiation through the regulation of PPARγ. J Biol Chem. 2002;277:16906–12.

84. Yu C, Markan K, Temple KA, et al. The nuclear receptor corepressors NCoR and SMRT decrease PPARγ transcriptional activity and repress 3T3-L1 adipogenesis. J Biol Chem. 2005;280:13600–5.
85. Gelman L, Zhou G, Fajas L, et al. p300 interacts with the N- and C-terminal part of PPARγ 2 in a ligand-independent and -dependent manner, respectively. J Biol Chem. 1999;274:7681–8.
86. Sarruf DA, Iankova I, Abella A, et al. Cyclin D3 promotes adipogenesis through activation of PPARγ. Mol Cell Biol. 2005;25:9985–95.
87. Fu M, Rao M, Bouras T, et al. Cyclin D1 inhibits PPARγ-mediated adipogenesis through histone deacetylase recruitment. Biol Chem. 2005;280:16934–41.
88. Huang L. Targeting histone deacetylases for treatment of cancer and inflammatory diseases. J Cell Physiol. 2006;209:611–6.
89. Yoo EJ, Chung JJ, Choe SS, et al. Down-regulation of histone deacetylases stimulates adipocyte differentiation. J Biol Chem. 2006;281:6608–15.
90. Picard F, Kurtev M, Chung N, et al. Sirt1 promotes fat mobilization in white adipocytes by repressing PPARγ. Nature. 2004;429:771–6.
91. Okada Y, Sakaue H, Nagare T, Kasuga M. Diet-induced up-regulation of gene expression in adipocytes without changes in DNA methylation. Kobe J Med Sci. 2008;54(5):E241–9.
92. Dekker FJ, Haisma HJ. Histone acetyl transferases as emerging drug targets. Drug Discov Today. 2009;14:942–8.

Part III
Developmental Programming and the Development of Obesity

Chapter 9
Exposure to Diabetes In Utero, Offspring Growth, and Risk for Obesity

Tessa Crume and Dana Dabelea

9.1 Introduction

The late Norbert Freinkel, in his 1980 Banting Lecture, introduced the concept of "fuel-mediated teratogenesis," which described a causal relationship between exposure to a metabolic insult during fetal life and immediate, but also long-term, postnatal consequences [1]. In the past three decades, evidence has accumulated from animal models, human clinical research, and epidemiological studies in support of this hypothesis. The possibility that intrauterine exposure to maternal diabetes could place the offspring at increased risk for obesity and related metabolic consequences later in life has generated considerable interest. Several mechanisms that are not mutually exclusive have been suggested to explain these associations, including shared genetic susceptibility, shared postnatal lifestyles, and specific intrauterine effects operating through fetal overnutrition. More research is necessary to determine the mechanisms through which exposure to overnutrition in the intrauterine period increases the risk of obesity and related metabolic conditions in childhood and adulthood. An improved understanding of the critical periods for development of obesity and its consequences may serve to focus preventive and therapeutic interventions that can be both cost-effective and maximize clinical utility.

This chapter reviews the evidence that exposure to maternal diabetes during gestation delivers a specific metabolic insult to the fetus at a critically important period of development, thus increasing offspring's risk for future obesity and T2DM.

9.2 Maternal Hyperglycemia and Fetal Growth

Gestational diabetes mellitus (GDM) occurs in 3–5% of pregnant women [2]. Recent studies have shown that GDM is increasing in the United States among

T. Crume (✉)
Department of Epidemiology, Colorado School of Public Health, University of Colorado, Denver, CO, USA
e-mail: tessa.crume@ucdenver.edu

R.H. Lustig (ed.), *Obesity Before Birth*, Endocrine Updates 30,
DOI 10.1007/978-1-4419-7034-3_9, © Springer Science+Business Media, LLC 2011

all racial/ethnic groups (1.9–3.4% among non-Hispanic whites, 2.8–5.1% among Hispanics, 2.5–5.1% among African-Americans, and 6.3–8.6% among Asians) [3, 4]. In addition, incident T2DM is increasing rapidly and among younger individuals, and as a result, more women are being diagnosed during their reproductive years [5, 6]. Risk factors for GDM include increasing maternal age, obesity, parity, previous delivery of a macrosomic infant, and family history of diabetes [2].

Development in a diabetic intrauterine environment results in excessive fetal growth. While maternal glucose freely crosses the placenta to the fetus, maternal insulin does not [1]. The developing fetal pancreas responds to the glucose load by producing additional insulin, which in turn, acts as a fetal growth hormone promoting growth and adiposity. Maternal hyperglycemia, extreme enough to be diagnosed as GDM, is a recognized risk factor for macrosomia. However, most macrosomic infants are not born to mothers with a diagnosis of GDM, but rather to mothers with obesity or with unrecognized glucose intolerance [7]. Health-care providers disagree about several aspects of GDM, including criteria for diagnosis, associated perinatal and maternal morbidity, and optimal therapeutic strategies [8–10]. The current screening approach in the United States, recommended by the American Diabetes Association [11] and the American College of Obstetricians and Gynecologists [12], starts with an initial 50 g oral glucose tolerance test (OGTT) in a non-fasting state, at 24–28 weeks gestation to determine plasma glucose levels at 1 h. For women with glucose levels $\geq$140 mg/dl, a second diagnostic 3-h 100 g glucose tolerance test is performed in a fasting state. GDM is diagnosed when two or more plasma glucose values meet or exceed the criteria for a positive test. The plasma glucose thresholds recommended by the National Diabetes Data Group (NDDG) for fasting 5.8 mmol/l (105 mg/dl), 1-h 10.5 mmol/l (190 mg/dl), 2-h 9.1 mmol/l (165 mg/dl), and 3-h 8.0 mmol/l (145 mg/dl) [13]. In 1982, Carpenter and Coustan [14] published a different set of diagnostic criteria to reflect a new enzymatic method for measuring plasma glucose levels, resulting in a lower diagnostic threshold that effectively subtracts 0.28 mmol/l (5 mg/dl) from the NDDG cutoff. Both criteria are used in the United States, though the prevalence of GDM has been estimated to be as much as 50% higher with the Carpenter and Coustan thresholds [15].

Women with lesser degrees of glucose intolerance, who exhibit one abnormal glucose screening test but do not meet diagnostic criteria for GDM, may also be at risk for delivering a macrosomic infant. Mello et al. [16] reported increased macrosomia among women with an abnormal screening result, but not meeting criteria for GDM diagnosis. A large retrospective analysis in Singapore found that women with impaired glucose tolerance, but not overt diabetes, during pregnancy had significantly higher risk of fetal macrosomia and obstetric complications than those with normal glucose tolerance [17].

Several recent studies suggest the relationship between glycemia during pregnancy and infant body size may be linear. In a study of 6,854 pregnant women screened for GDM, increased glucose concentration at screening was associated with higher prevalence of macrosomia [18]. In a large community-based study in Mysore, south India, maternal fasting glucose at 30 weeks of gestation was positively associated with infant birthweight (79 g increase per 1 mmol/l increase in glucose), ponderal index, and head circumference, even among mothers who did not fulfill the criteria for GDM diagnosis [19]. There were similar findings in a study of 917 non-diabetic women in Scotland, in which birthweight, length, head circumference, and skin folds were positively related to maternal fasting plasma glucose concentrations measured in the third trimester of pregnancy [20].

Since maternal fuel supply across a population is a continuum, the relationship between glycemia and offspring size at birth should be present across the entire distribution of maternal glucose concentrations. Recently, the Hyperglycemia and Adverse Pregnancy Outcomes [21] (HAPO) study, a major international effort including over 20,000 pregnant women, specifically tested and confirmed the hypothesis that maternal glucose levels during pregnancy showed a linear association with adverse pregnancy outcomes (including birthweight), thus indicating the need to reconsider current GDM diagnostic criteria [21]. In HAPO, an increase by 1 SD (30.9 mg/dl) of fasting glucose levels at 24–32 weeks of gestation was associated with 1.38-fold higher odds (95% CI=1.32–1.44) for neonatal macrosomia (birthweight above the 90th percentile) and 1.55-fold higher odds (95% CI= 1.47–1.64) for neonatal hyperinsulinemia (cord blood C-peptide above the 90th percentile).

There is also evidence that infants born to diabetic mothers have increased adiposity, regardless of their birthweight. Using total body electrical conductivity estimates of body composition, Catalano et al. [22] reported that infants of mothers whose pregnancies were complicated by diabetes had 20% higher body fat mass than infants of mothers with normal glucose tolerance during pregnancy. Controlling for birthweight did not attenuate the relationship. They also reported that fasting maternal glucose level was the strongest single predictor of neonatal adiposity. Hammami et al. [23] conducted dual-energy x-ray absorptiometry (DXA) on large and average for gestational age infants at 1.8 ± 1.0 days after birth to assess body composition. They reported that infants born large for gestational age had higher proportions of total body fat, but less lean body mass than infants born average size for gestational age ($p < 0.001$).

9.3 Early Life Growth Patterns and Risk for Obesity in Offspring of Diabetic Mothers

In 1953, White et al. [24] at the Joslin Clinic reported "superiority of growth in stature and weight" in the offspring of women with diabetes. Subsequently, reports from many parts of the world confirmed and documented excessive growth in the offspring of diabetic women after the first few years of life. In 1959, Hagbard et al. [25] reported the stature of 239 children with an average age of 5 years, who were born after the onset of their mothers' diabetes and 68 with an average age of 16 years, who were born before the onset of the diabetes. Those born after the mothers got diabetes were significantly shorter and heavier than expected for their age while those born before showed no deviation from normal. Vohr et al. [26] examined the 7-year-old offspring of diabetic and control women and found that the offspring of diabetic women were significantly more likely to have a weight for height index above 1.2. Gerlini et al. [27] looked at heights and weights of infants of diabetic mothers at birth, during the first year of life and annually up to 4 years. They found that by 4 years, the children of mothers with poor metabolic control during pregnancy were significantly heavier and had a significantly higher weight for height ratio than the offspring of women who had been well controlled. The difference was smallest at 6 months and increased progressively during the 4 years of observation.

Several studies have suggested that offspring of diabetic women often experience a period of "catchdown weight" between birth and 1–2 years of age. Stenhouse et al. [28] found a significant association between increasing maternal glucose levels at 26–28 weeks gestation, even within the normal range, and higher birthweight but a negative effect on child's growth trajectory in both weight and height by 96–120 weeks of age postnatal. More recently, Touger et al. [29] studied early childhood growth patterns among Pima Indians and reported that children exposed to diabetes in utero had higher birthweight (BWT) than those not exposed (BWT z-score =0.49 vs. –0.01, $p < 0.01$) and experienced "catch-down growth" between birth and 1.5 years (weight $\Delta_{0\text{–}1.5}$ z-score = –0.56 for exposed and 0.12 for non-exposed offspring, $p < 0.01$), yet still had a higher weight and relative weight at 7.7 years than the non-exposed children (weight z-score 0.89 vs. –0.07, $p < 0.01$; relative weight z-score 1.26 vs. 0.00, $p < 0.01$) [25]. Silverman et al. [30] also observed a period of catch-down growth among a multiethnic population of offspring of diabetic pregnancies compared to offspring of non-diabetic pregnancies in Chicago. This finding remained even after stratification by birthweight status (large vs. average weight for gestational age). Thus, the initial period of poor growth or catch down weight observed among offspring of diabetic mothers during the first year of life seems to be followed by a period of accelerated weight gain relative to non-exposed peers [30, 31].

The Diabetes in Pregnancy Center (DPC) at Northwestern University in Chicago followed a multiethnic population of offspring of diabetic pregnancies, including GDM and pre-existing diabetes requiring insulin treatment [30]. They examined children at birth, 6 months, and then annually up to 8 years of age and found that the children exposed to DM in utero were, on average, 30% heavier by age 8 than expected for their height. Unfortunately, they did not include an internal comparison group. A second analysis of this study was published in 1995, this time including an unexposed group, and found that the offspring of diabetic mothers at ages 10–16 had higher 2-h glucose levels (6.8 $\pm$ 1.4 vs. 5.7 $\pm$ 0.9 mmol/l, $p < 0.001$) and insulin levels (660$\pm$720 vs. 455 $\pm$ 285 pmol/l, $p < 0.03$), when compared to unexposed youth [31]. A third publication from the DPC reported that by age 17 years, the offspring of DM pregnancies had a mean body mass index (BMI) of 26.0 kg/m^2 compared with 20.9 kg/m^2 in control subjects [32].

The four-decade epidemiologic study of the Pima Indians of Arizona has provided some of the most dramatic evidence of fetal programming for future obesity. A series of articles by Pettitt et al. has demonstrated that the offspring of Pima Indian women with pre-existing T2DM or GDM were heavier at birth and at every age throughout childhood and adolescence than offspring of non-diabetic or prediabetic mothers [33–36]. Moreover, they found that even normal birthweight offspring exposed to maternal diabetes in utero were heavier throughout childhood than those not exposed, suggesting that the effect of exposure to diabetes in utero on childhood obesity risk is not confined to macrosomic infants [36]. Up to 20 years of age, offspring of diabetic mothers had a much higher prevalence of severe obesity than those of prediabetic and non-diabetic mothers. After age 20 years, the differences between the offspring of diabetic women and the other two groups are much less, reflecting the high rates of obesity that are present in this population regardless of the intrauterine environment [37]. However, at older ages, the obese offspring of the diabetic women were likely to have been obese much longer than the obese offspring of the non-diabetic and prediabetic women, further increasing the risk for diabetes in the offspring of diabetic women.

Recently, Hiller et al. [38] reported a dose–response relationship between maternal hyperglycemia in pregnancy and obesity in the offspring in a retrospective cohort study of 9,439 mother–child pairs enrolled in Kaiser Permanente Hawaii and Northwest. The authors reported the risk of childhood obesity by 5–7 years was nearly double in offspring of mothers with an elevated fasting glucose value of >5.3 mmol/l (95 mg/dl) on the OGTT compared with those whose mothers had a normal fasting glucose but other abnormal post-OGTT values ($p < 0.0001$).

9.4 Abnormal Glucose Tolerance and T2DM in Offspring of Diabetic Mothers

The Pima Indians of Arizona experience the highest prevalence and incidence of T2DM in the world. For more than 30 years, Pima Indian women have had routine OGTT's approximately every 2 years as well as during pregnancy [33]. Women who had diabetes before or during pregnancy were termed diabetic mothers; those who developed diabetes only after pregnancy were termed prediabetic mothers. Presence of T2DM in their offspring was compared according to maternal diabetes status during the index pregnancy. By age 5–9 and 10–14, T2DM was present almost exclusively among the offspring of diabetic women. In all age groups there was significantly more diabetes in the offspring of diabetic women than in those of prediabetic and non-diabetic women, and there were much smaller differences in diabetes prevalence between offspring of prediabetic and non-diabetic women [39]. Intrauterine exposure to maternal hyperglycemia was the strongest single risk factor for T2DM in Pima Indian youth (odds ratio 10.4, $p < 0.0001$) [40].

Recently, the SEARCH Case–Control Study (SEARCH CC) [41] provided novel evidence that intrauterine exposure to maternal diabetes and obesity are important determinants of T2DM in youth of other racial/ethnic groups (non-Hispanic white, Hispanic, and African-American) as well. In this study, youth with T2DM were significantly more likely to have been exposed to maternal diabetes in utero than were non-diabetic controls (OR=7.3, $p < 0.0001$).

9.5 The Role of Fetal Hyperinsulinemia

In the study conducted by the Diabetes in Pregnancy Center (DPC) at Northwestern University in Chicago, amniotic fluid insulin concentrations collected at 32–38 weeks of gestation were compared to a symmetry index of offspring obesity at 6 years of age [42]. They reported the amniotic fluid insulin concentrations in 6-year-old children who had a symmetry index of less than 1.0 (86.1 pmol/l) or between 1.0 and 1.2 (69.9 pmol/l) were only half that of the more obese children with a symmetry index greater than 1.2 (140.5 pmol/l, $p < 0.05$ for each) (Fig. 9.1). Amniotic fluid insulin is of fetal origin and is directly correlated with the amount of fetal insulin produced. Fetal insulin, in turn, is correlated with the amount of the circulating glucose, which is of maternal origin and is directly related to the mother's diabetes control. Thus, this study demonstrates a direct correlation between an objective measure of the diabetic intrauterine environment and the degree of obesity in children and adolescents.

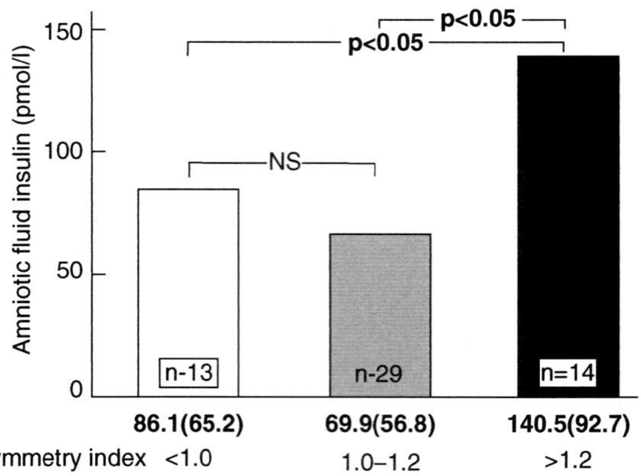

Fig. 9.1 Association between symmetry index at age 6 and amniotic fluid insulin concentration during late gestation. The bars denote the mean amniotic fluid insulin concentration for each group; the values under each bar are mean (SD). Significance of the differences between groups was determined by the Duncan method

9.6 Less Conclusive Findings

Other studies have addressed the issue of fetal programming of future obesity with less conclusive results. Gillman et al. [43] assessed the risk of adolescent obesity among 14,811 children aged 9–14 in the Growing up Today Study (465 of whom were exposed to GDM in utero) through a survey administered to parents to assess parental-reported BMI of offspring and self-reported GDM during pregnancy. The authors reported a crude OR of 1.4 (95% CI 1.1–2.0) for the association between adolescent overweight and in utero GDM exposure. The association, however, was attenuated by adjustment for birthweight (OR = 1.3, 95% CI 0.9–1.9) and additionally attenuated by adjustment for mother's current BMI (OR = 1.2, 95% CI 0.8–1.7). In another study, Boney et al. [44] examined a cohort of children born either appropriate for gestational age (AGA) or large for gestational age (LGA) who were either exposed or not exposed to maternal diabetes in utero, to determine if fetal exposure increased the risk of metabolic syndrome in adolescence. They found increased overweight (BMI >85th percentile) at age 11 years among the LGA-GDM offspring compared to the AGA controls (35% vs. 24%). They also found the presence of both LGA status and maternal GDM exposure was significantly associated with an increased risk of adolescent insulin resistance (OR = 4.3, 95% CI 1.4–11.9; and OR = 10.4, 95% CI 1.5–74.4, respectively); however, the associations were not independent of each other. The authors reported that the prevalence of more than two components of the metabolic syndrome was 50% for the LGA-GDM group compared to 29% for the LGA control group, and 21% for the AGA-GDM group compared to 18% for the AGA-non-GDM group.

9.7 An Independent Effect of Intrauterine Exposure: Beyond Genetics and Postnatal Environment

GDM is highly predictive of future diagnosis of T2DM, with as many 50% of women developing T2DM within 5 years of the index pregnancy [45]. T2DM has a strong genetic component, and because GDM is considered a strong risk factor for T2DM, a woman with either condition could transmit an increased risk of diabetes to their offspring in the form of greater genetic susceptibility. How much of the excess diabetes in the offspring of diabetic mothers that can be attributed to heredity and how much can be attributed to the environment are not clear, but there is strong evidence that the intrauterine environment plays an important role.

First, excessive growth in the offspring of diabetic mothers is not seen in the offspring of diabetic fathers [46]. Second, a comparison of two groups that would presumably inherit similar diabetes risk genes from their mothers (i.e., offspring of diabetic and offspring of prediabetic mothers) shows different levels of childhood obesity. Pettitt et al. [34] found that offspring of diabetic mothers were heavier than offspring of prediabetic mothers by 5–9 years and that the difference persisted through adolescence and teenage years. Interestingly, prevalence of obesity was similar among the offspring of prediabetic mothers and offspring of non-diabetic mothers. Third, within Pima Indian families with non-diabetic offspring, BMI was significantly higher (+2.6 kg/m^2) in the 62 siblings exposed to their mother T2DM during pregnancy (born after the mother was diagnosed with diabetes) than in the 121 unexposed siblings (born before the mother was diagnosed) [47]. In contrast, there was no significant difference between siblings born before or after their father was diagnosed with T2DM (mean BMI difference: 0.4 kg/m^2). These data support the hypothesis that exposure to diabetes in utero has effects on offspring body size that are in addition to genetic susceptibility to obesity. These results are powerful because they mitigate both shared genetic risk and postnatal environment, emphasizing the importance of the in utero environment.

9.8 The Long-Term Consequences Are Independent of Maternal Diabetes Type

Further evidence for an independent role of the intrauterine environment is the observation that the long-term consequences of exposure to diabetes in utero are not influenced by maternal diabetes type (pre-existing type 1, type 2, or GDM) [30, 33, 48]. In the cohort followed by Silverman et al. [49] at Northwestern University, there was an increased prevalence of impaired glucose tolerance among 10- to 16-year-old offspring who were exposed to diabetes in utero, compared with unexposed youth. And, in another study of this population, Silverman et al. [30] reported that impaired glucose tolerance among offspring of diabetic pregnancies was associated with maternal hyperglycemia, but not diabetes type (pre-existent type 1 diabetes and GDM). Weiss et al. [48] followed a cohort of offspring of women with type 1 diabetes during pregnancy and reported higher BMI, cholesterol, LDL, post-load glucose, insulin, and C-peptide levels by age 5–15 compared to offspring of non-diabetic women.

9.9 Public Health Consequences

The effects of maternal diabetes on the child appear to generate a "vicious cycle" [32]. Children whose mothers had diabetes during pregnancy are at increased risk of becoming obese. Many of these female offspring already have abnormal glucose tolerance or diabetes by the time they reach their childbearing years, thereby perpetuating the cycle. Among the Pima Indian children, the dramatic increases in the prevalence of diabetes (a twofold to threefold increase over the past three decades) were statistically accounted for by the increase in gestational diabetes and exposure to diabetes in utero [40], thus closing this postulated vicious cycle.

If exposure to diabetes in pregnancy is an important risk factor for future obesity, the recent findings of significant increases in GDM over the past decade among all racial/ethnic groups [3, 50] raise the issue of a potential worsening in the obesity epidemic yet to come. The cycle of diabetes during pregnancy fueling more diabetes and obesity in future generations, initially described in Pima Indians, is likely operating within other populations. For example, in the recent SEARCH Case–Control Study (SEARCH CC), intrauterine exposure to maternal diabetes and obesity contributed together to 47% of T2DM in the offspring of non-Hispanic white, Hispanic, and African-American origin [41]. This suggests that preventive efforts aiming at halting the obesity epidemic may need to target the increasing number of pregnancies complicated by obesity and diabetes.

9.10 Prevention and Risk Reduction Strategies

An important clinical goal is to maintain strict glycemic control during pregnancy in women with diabetes through a combination of pharmacologic treatment and diet. Intensive glucose control among GDM women resulted in lower pregnancy weight gain and lower incidence of macrosomia compared with routine clinical care [51]. Limiting excessive pregnancy weight gain among women with diabetes may also help attenuate the risk of fetal overgrowth. In 2009, the Institute of Medicine and National Research Council issued new guidelines for weight gain during pregnancy according to prepregnancy BMI category [52]. However, it is not known whether intensive glycemic control and limiting excessive weight gain during pregnancy would also result in mitigating the long-term metabolic disturbances in the offspring and reducing the increased risks of obesity and diabetes in the next generation.

Nutrition in the first postnatal weeks of life may also represent a powerful tool for attenuating the risk associated with fetal overnutrition. Enzi et al. [53] provided evidence that the excess obesity seen in the offspring of women with diabetes during the pregnancy may not be inevitable. They followed infants of diabetic mothers who received strict low-calorie diets since birth. The normal birthweight infants of mothers with DM during pregnancy who had received the controlled diets did not have increased fat mass by 1 year. They concluded that overnutrition in utero, such as it occurs with maternal diabetes, does not have long-lasting effects on adiposity if the birthweight is normal and infant overfeeding early in life is prevented.

The protective effect of breast-feeding on long-term obesity risk has been extensively studied and is now well supported as an important preventive strategy with considerable public health benefits. Gillman et al. [54] reported a protective, dose-dependent effect of breast-feeding on risk of overweight among adolescents in the Growing Up Today Study. Mayer-Davis et al. [55] also reported a lower prevalence of overweight among adolescent offspring of the Nurses' Health Study II, an effect that became more pronounced as the duration and exclusivity of breast-feeding increased. The findings were not altered by controlling for maternal overweight and diabetes during pregnancy, an important finding that further supports the recommendation by the American Academy of Pediatrics to encourage breast-feeding through the first year of life. It is possible that breast-feeding may offer an opportunity to break the cycle of overweight and diabetes that occurs among offspring of diabetic mothers.

References

1. Freinkel N. Of pregnancy and progeny (review). Banting lecture 1980. Diabetes. 1980;29:1023–36.
2. Ben-Haroush A, Yogev Y, Hod M. Epidemiology of gestational diabetes mellitus and its association with Type 2 diabetes. Diabet Med. 2003;21:103–13.
3. Dabelea D, Snell-Bergeon J, Hartsfield C, Bischoff K, Hamman R, McDuffie R. Increasing prevalence of gestational diabetes mellitus (GDM) over time and by birth cohort: Kaiser Permanente of Colorado GDM Screening Program. Diabetes Care. 2005;28:579–84.

4. Ferrara A, Kahn H, Quesenberry C, Riley C, Hedderson M. An increase in the incidence of gestational diabetes mellitus: Northern California, 1991–2000. Obstet Gynecol. 2004;103:526–33.
5. Hussain A, Claussen B, Ramachandran A, Williams R. Prevention of type 2 diabetes: A review. Diabetes Res Clin Pract. 2007;76:317–26.
6. Dabelea D, Pettitt D, Jones K, Arslanian S. Type 2 diabetes mellitus in minority children and adolescents. An emerging problem. Endocrinol Metab Clin North Am. 1999;28:709–29.
7. Langer O, Conway D. Level of glycemia and perinatal outcome in pregestational diabetes. J Matern Fetal Med. 2000;9(1):35–41.
8. Ratner R. Clinical review 47: gestational diabetes mellitus: after three international workshops do we know how to diagnose and manage it yet?. J Clin Endocrinol Metab. 1993;77(1):1–4.
9. Buchanan T, Kjos S. Gestational diabetes: risk or myth? J Clin Endocrinol Metab. 1999;84(6):1854–7.
10. Dornhorst A, Chan S. The elusive diagnosis of gestational diabetes. Diabet Med. 1998;15(1):7–10.
11. American Diabetes Association. Gestational diabetes mellitus. Diabetes Care. 2000;23 Suppl 1:S77–9.
12. ACOG Practice Bulletin. Clinical management guidelines for obstetrician-gynecologists. Obstet Gynecol. 2001;98(30):525–38.
13. National Diabetes Data Group. Classification and diagnosis of diabetes mellitus and other categories of glucose intolerance. Diabetes. 1979;28:1039–57.
14. Carpenter MW, Coustan DR. Criteria for screening tests for gestational diabetes. Am J Obstet Gynecol. 1982;144:768–73.
15. Ferrara A, Hedderson MM, Quesenberry CP, Selby JV. Prevalence of gestational diabetes mellitus detected by the national diabetes data group or the Carpenter and Coustan plasma glucose thresholds. Diabetes Care. 2002;25(9):1625–30.
16. Mello G, Parretti E, Mecacci F, Lucchetti R, Cianciulli D, Lagazio C. Anthropometric characteristics of full-term infants: effects of varying degrees of 'normal' glucose metabolism. J Perinat Med. 1997;25:197–204.
17. Tan Y, Yeo G. Impaired glucose tolerance in pregnancy–is it of consequence? Aust NZ J Obstet Gynaecol. 1996;36:248–55.
18. Yogev Y, Langer O, Xenakis E, Rosenn B. The association between glucose challenge test, obesity and pregnancy outcome in 6390 non-diabetic women. J Matern Fetal Neonatal Med. 2005;17:29–34.
19. Hill J, Krishnaveni G, Annamma I, Leary S, Fall C. Glucose tolerance in pregnancy in South India: relationships to neonatal anthropometry. Acta Obstet Gynecol Scand. 2005;84(2): 159–65.
20. Simmons D, Breier B. Adult obesity and growth in childhood. Fuel mediated teratogenesis driven by maternal obesity may be responsible for pandemic of obesity. BMJ. 2002;324(7338):674.
21. Group HSCR, Metzger B, Lowe L, Dyer A, Trimble E, Chaovarindr U, et al. Hyperglycemia and adverse pregnancy outcomes. N Engl J Med. 2008;358(19):1991–2002.
22. Catalano P, Thomas A, Huston-Presley L, Amini S. Increased fetal adiposity: a very sensitive marker of abnormal in utero development. AM J Obstet Gynecol. 2003;189:1698–704.
23. Hammami M, Walters J, Hockman E, Koo W. Disproportionate alterations in body composition of large for gestational age neonates. J Pediatr. 2001;138:817–21.
24. White P, Koshy P, Duckers J. Management of pregnancy complicating diabetes and of children of diabetic mothers. Med Clin North Am. 1953;1:1481–96.
25. Hagbard L, Olow I, Reinand T. A follow-up study of 514 children of diabetic mothers. Acta Paediatr. 1959;48(2):184–97.
26. Vohr B, Lipsitt L, Oh W. Somatic growth of children of diabetic mothers with reference to birth size. J Pediatr. 1980;97(2):196–9.

27. Gerlini G, Arachi S, Gori M, Gloria F, Bonci E, Pachi A, et al. Developmental aspects of the offspring of diabetic mothers. Acta Endocrinol. 1986;277 Suppl Copenh:150–5.
28. Stenhouse E, Wright D, Hattersley A, Millward B. Maternal glucose levels influence birth weight and 'catch-up' and 'catch-down' growth in a large contemporary cohort. Diabet Med. 2006;23:1207–12.
29. Touger L, Looker H, Krakoff J, Lindsay R, Cook V, Knowler W. Early growth in offspring of diabetic mothers. Diabetes Care. 2005;28(3):585–9.
30. Silverman B, Rizzo T, Green O, Cho N, Winter R, Ogata E, et al. Long-term prospective evaluation of offspring of diabetic mothers. Diabetes. 1991;40 Suppl 2:121–5.
31. Silverman B, Metzger B, Cho N, Loeb C. Impaired glucose tolerance in adolescent offspring of diabetic mothers. Diabetes Care. 1995;18(5):611–9.
32. Silverman B, Rizzo T, Cho N, Metzger B. Long-term effects of the intrauterine environment. The Northwestern University Diabetes in Pregnancy Center. Diabetes Care. 1998;21 Suppl 2:B142–9.
33. Pettitt D, Bennett P, Knowler W, Baird H, Aleck K. Gestational diabetes mellitus and impaired glucose tolerance during pregnancy: long-term effects on obesity and glucose tolerance in the offspring. Diabetes. 1985;34 Suppl 2:119–23.
34. Pettitt D, Nelson M, Saad R, Bennett P, Knowler W. Diabetes and obesity in the offspring of Pima Indian women with diabetes during pregnancy. Diabetes Care. 1993;16:310–5.
35. Pettitt D, Baird H, Aleck K, Bennett P, Knowler W. Excessive obesity in offspring of Pima Indian women with diabetes during pregnancy. N Engl J Med. 1983;308:242–6.
36. Pettitt D, Aleck K, Baird H, Carraher M, Bennett P, Knowler W. Congenital susceptibility to NIDDM: role of intrauterine environment. Diabetes. 1988;37(5):622–8.
37. Dabelea D, Knowler W, Pettitt D. Effect of diabetes in pregnancy on offspring: follow-up research in the Pima Indians. J Matern Fetal Med. 2000;9:83–9.
38. Hiller T, Pedula K, Schmidt M, Mullen J, Charles M, Pettitt D. Childhood obesity and metabolic imprinting: the ongoing effects of maternal hyperglycemia. Diabetes Care. 2007;30:2287–97.
39. Dabelea D, Pettitt D. Intrauterine diabetic environment confers risks for type 2 diabetes mellitus and obesity in the offspring, in addition to genetic susceptibility. J Pediatr Endocrinol Metab. 2001;14:1085–91.
40. Dabelea D, Hanson R, Bennett P, Roumain J, Knowler W, Pettitt D. Increasing prevalence of type II diabetes in American Indian children. Diabetologia. 1988;41:904–10.
41. Dabelea D, Mayer-Davis E, Lamichhane A, D'Agostino RJ, Liese A, Vehik K, et al. Association of intrauterine exposure to maternal diabetes and obesity with type 2 diabetes in youth: the SEARCH Case-Control Study. Diabetes Care. 2008;31(7):1422–7.
42. Metzger B, Silverman B, Freinkel N, Dooley S, Ogata E, Green O. Amniotic fluid insulin concentration as a predictor of obesity. Arch Dis Child. 1990;65:1050–3.
43. Gillman M, Rifas-Shiman S, Berkey C, Field A, Colditz G. Maternal gestational diabetes, birth weight, and adolescent obesity. Pediatrics. 2003;111(3):e221–7.
44. Boney CM, et al. Metabolic syndrome in childhood: association with birth weight, maternal obesity, and gestational diabetes mellitus. Pediatrics. 2005;115(3):e290–5.
45. Kim C, Newton K, Knopp R. Gestational diabetes and the incidence of type 2 diabetes: a systematic review. Diabetes Care. 2002;25:1862–8.
46. Pettitt D, Knowler W. Long-term effects of the intrauterine environment, birth weight, and breast-feeding in Pima Indians. Diabetes Care. 1988;21 Suppl 2:B138–41.
47. Dabelea D, Hanson R, Lindsay R, Pettitt D, Imperatore G, Gabir M, et al. Intrauterine exposure to diabetes conveys risks for type 2 diabetes and obesity: a study of discordant siblings. Diabetes. 2000;49:2208–11.
48. Weiss P, Scholz H, Haas J, Tamussino K, Seissler J, Borkenstein M. Long-term follow-up of infants of mothers with type 1 diabetes: evidence for hereditary and nonhereditary transmission of diabetes and precursors. Diabetes Care. 2000;23:905–11.

49. Silverman B, Metzger B, Cho N, Loeb C. Impaired glucose tolerance in adolescent offspring of diabetic mothers: relationship to fetal hyperinsulinism. Diabetes Care. 1995;18(5):611–7.
50. Lawrence JM, Contreras R, Chen W, Sacks DA. Trends in the prevalence of preexisting diabetes and gestational diabetes mellitus among a racially/ethnically diverse population of pregnant women, 1999–2005. Diabetes Care. 2008;31:899–904.
51. Crowther C, Hiller J, Moss J, McPhee A, Jeffries W, Robinson J. Effect of treatment of gestational diabetes mellitus on pregnancy outcomes. N Engl J Med. 2005;352:2477–86.
52. Institute of Medicine (U.S.). Subcommittee on nutritional status and weight gain during pregnancy. Weight gain during pregnancy: reexamining the guidelines. Washington, DC: National Academy Press; 2009.
53. Enzi G, Inelmen E, Rubaltelli F, Zanardo V, Favaretto L. Postnatal development of adipose tissue in normal children on strictly controlled calorie intake. Metabolism. 1982;31(10):1029–34.
54. Gillman M, Rifas-Shiman S, Camargo C, Berkey C, Frazier A, Rockett H, et al. Risk of overweight among adolescents who were breastfed as infants. JAMA. 2001;285(19):2461–9.
55. Mayer-Davis E, Rifas-Shiman S, Zhou L, Hu F, Colditz G, Gillman M. Breastfeeding and risk for childhood obesity: does maternal diabetes status matter? Diabetes Care. 2006;29(10):2231–8.

Chapter 10
Maternal Weight Gain During Pregnancy and Obesity in the Offspring

Naomi E. Stotland and Janet C. King

10.1 Introduction

A woman's pre-pregnancy weight and adiposity, and weight gain during pregnancy are related to the weight of the offspring through multiple mechanisms. Most simply, the weight of the fetus will be measured as part of a woman's overall pregnancy weight gain, which will explain some of the observed association between higher gestational weight gain and obesity in the child. However, a growing literature supports an association between mother's pre-pregnancy obesity, excessive gestational weight gain, and higher childhood weight and risk of obesity in later life. While it would be optimal to have every woman achieve her ideal body weight and metabolic status prior to conception, healthful and sustained weight loss is extremely difficult to achieve. In addition, pre-conception weight loss interventions are challenging to implement in part because approximately half of all pregnancies in the United States are unplanned. Unlike pre-pregnancy obesity, gestational weight gain may be modifiable, and the frequency of prenatal visits presents an opportunity to support women in making healthful lifestyle changes. Such efforts may help prevent obesity in the next generation, as well as reduce the risk of further long-term weight gain in the mother. This chapter will discuss the topic of weight gain during human pregnancy and how it relates to obesity in the offspring.

10.2 The Physiology of Weight Gain During Pregnancy Among Obese and Non-obese Women

The amount of weight a woman gains during pregnancy varies considerably, depending on the woman's body mass index (BMI), age, ethnicity, and whether it is a singleton or multiple pregnancy. The "normal" gestational weight gain of normal weight adult women delivering full-term, singleton infants in the USA ranges from

N.E. Stotland (✉)
Department of Obstetrics and Gynecology, University of California, San Francisco, CA, USA
e-mail: stotlandn@obgyn.ucsf.edu

R.H. Lustig (ed.), *Obesity Before Birth*, Endocrine Updates 30,

DOI 10.1007/978-1-4419-7034-3_10,

10 to 16.7 kg [1]. Adolescents tend to gain more weight than do adult women. Data from US studies report mean gains for adolescents ranging from 14.6 to 18.0 kg. All studies consistently report that women with higher BMIs tend to gain less weight, but the amount of weight gained by obese women still varies widely.

Typically, women gain less weight in the first trimester of pregnancy than in the second or third trimesters. In a large cohort of women from the University of California, San Francisco [2, 3], the rate of weight gain averaged 0.169 kg/week in the first, 0.563 kg/week in the second, and 0.518 kg/week in the third trimester among normal and underweight women. Birthweight was correlated most strongly with weight gain in the second trimester. Obese women gained 0.41 kg/week in the second and 0.45 kg/week in the third trimesters. It is interesting to note that obese women had larger babies on average despite having lower rates of second trimester weight gain, compared to normal-weight women.

Components of total gestational weight gain can be divided into the baby, the products of conception (placenta, fetus, amniotic fluid), and maternal tissue (blood, uterus, mammary gland, and extracellular, extravascular fluid). At term, the products of conception comprise about one-third of the total gain [4]. In addition to these tissues, most women gain some adipose tissue stores during gestation. Fat gain occurs primarily in the first half of pregnancy. As fetal growth reaches a peak in the last 10 weeks of gestation, maternal fat storage slows down. Fat is preferentially deposited over the abdomen, the back and the upper thighs. The gain seems to be greatest over the abdomen [4]. In general, the amount of fat gained during pregnancy is influenced by maternal BMI. In a study of 200 healthy women, a careful measurement of body fat gain between 14 and 37 weeks of gestation showed that obese women gained significantly less fat than underweight or normal weight women (8.7 versus 12.6 and 12.2 kg, respectively) [5]. Since the rate of fat gain tends to be highest during the second trimester, the lower fat gains of obese women may explain why they tend to gain less weight in the second trimester than do normal weight women.

Total body water gain during pregnancy is highly variable and is positively correlated with birthweight [1]. On average, healthy women gain about 7–8l of water [4]. This may increase to about 12l of water in women with generalized edema. Expansion of maternal blood volume accounts for about 15% of the total fluid gain in pregnancy. Since plasma volume expansion improves the nutrient transfer to placenta and fetus, it is not surprising that maternal plasma volume expansion correlates positively with birthweight [6].

It is predicted that protein gain during pregnancy averages about 925 g or only about 7% of the total gain [4]. However, actual estimates of protein retention from measurements of total body potassium and assuming a potassium/nitrogen ratio of 2.15 mEq potassium/g nitrogen predicts that the actual protein gain is about 690 g or 25% less than that predicted by Hytten and Chamberlain [1]. These studies confirm that pregnant women do not store protein for lactational needs, as was thought to be the case about 60 years ago [7]. About half of the protein gained is deposited in the fetus; the remainder primarily represents proteins accumulated in the placenta, uterine muscle, and maternal blood.

10.3 The Institute of Medicine (IOM) Weight Gain Guidelines

In 1990, the IOM released a report that included BMI-specific weight gain guidelines for pregnant women [8]. These recommendations were based on a review of epidemiologic studies associating maternal pregnancy weight gain with birth outcomes and data that showed interactions between maternal pre-pregnancy BMI, weight gain, and outcomes. At that time, the main focus of the IOM was the prevention of low birthweight (LBW), and it was especially noted that lower pregnancy weight gain was associated with an increased risk of preterm birth and small for gestational age (SGA) infants. Despite wide dissemination and acceptance of the 1990 IOM guidelines, data generated over the subsequent 20 years showed that a large percentage of women were gaining above the IOM guidelines [9]. Additionally, the percent of women entering pregnancy already overweight or obese increased during this time period. The 1990 IOM weight gain guidelines did not give an upper limit of gain for obese women (BMI≥30) as there were not adequate data to establish the optimal range. Since 1990 there have been many more cohort and population-based studies examining optimal weight gain and including larger percentages of obese women. The IOM decided to re-visit the issue of maternal weight gain during pregnancy and in 2009 issued a new report which included new weight gain guidelines for obese women (Table 10.1) [9].

Table 10.1 2009 Institute of medicine guidelines for weight gain during pregnancy [9]

	Total weight gain		Rates of weight gain[a] second and third trimester	
Pre-pregnancy BMI	Range (kg)	Range (lbs)	Mean (range) (kg/week)	Mean (range) (lbs/week)
Underweight (<18.5 kg/m^2)	12.5–18	28–40	0.51 (0.44–0.58)	1 (1–1.3)
Normal weight (18.5–24.9 kg/m^2)	11.5–16	25–35	0.42 (0.35–0.50)	1 (0.8–1)
Overweight (25.0–29.9 kg/m^2)	7–11.5	15–25	0.28 (0.23–0.33)	0.6 (0.5–0.7)
Obese (≥30.0 kg/m^2)	5–9	11–20	0.22 (0.17–0.27)	0.5 (0.4–0.6)

[a]Calculations assume a 0.5–2 kg (1.1–4.4 lbs) weight gain in the first trimester (based on Siega-Riz et al., 1994; Abrams et al., 1995; Carmichael et al., 1997)
Source: Reprinted with permission, National Academies Press

10.4 Epidemiology and Trends of Pregnancy Weight Gain

Average pregnancy weight gain varies by pre-pregnancy weight, with obese women gaining less weight than normal and underweight women [9]. Mean weight gains by pre-pregnancy BMI are seen in Fig. 10.1. However, the trends are different when weight gain is categorized by the IOM guidelines, with overweight women having the highest rates of gain above the guidelines (Fig. 10.2). Data from the

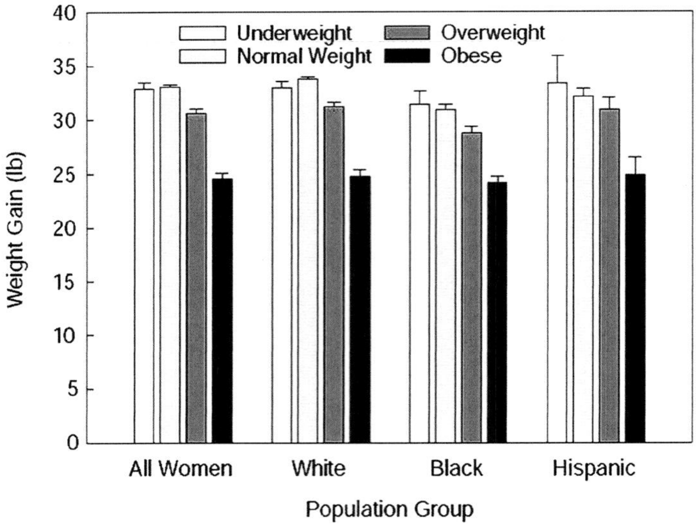

Fig. 10.1 Mean gestational weight gain by BMI category and race/ethnicity, PRAMS 2002–2003 [9]. The WHO BMI categories were used (underweight, <18.5 kg/m^2; normal, 18.5–24.9 kg/m^2; overweight, 25.0–29.9 kg/m^2; obese, $\geq$30 kg/m^2). Reprinted with permission, National Academies Press

CDC PRAMS (Pregnancy Risk Assessment Monitoring System) cohort, representing nine US states, show that many women are gaining above the IOM guidelines and that overweight women are the most likely to gain above these guidelines [9].

10.5 Association Between Gestational Weight Gain (GWG) and Childhood Obesity

In the preponderance of epidemiologic studies, higher GWG is associated with a higher risk of childhood obesity. Two US studies examined the relationship between GWG and child weight at age 3. Oken et al. studied 1,044 mother–child pairs in a prospective cohort study. Higher GWG was associated with a higher offspring BMI *z*-score (0.13 units per 5 kg of weight gain, 95% CI, 0.08, 0.19). Women with adequate or excessive weight gain in pregnancy (according to the 1990 IOM guidelines) had an approximately 4-fold elevated odds of a child with a BMI $\geq$95th percentile compared to women gaining below the IOM guidelines. Olson et al. examined 208 mother–child pairs in rural upstate New York and found a significant interaction between maternal pre-pregnancy BMI, GWG, and child weight at age 3 years. While they did not find an independent effect of GWG on child weight in the overall multivariate model, they attributed this to their small sample size. The authors modeled the risk of child obesity based on maternal weight gain and pre-pregnancy BMI.

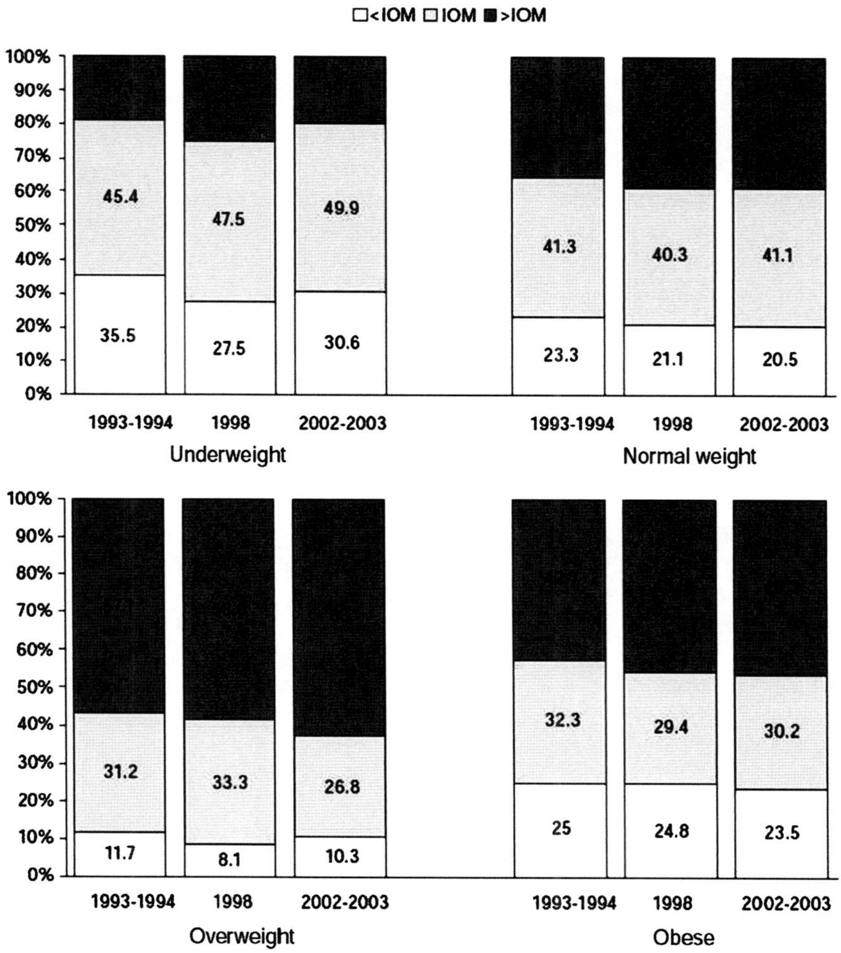

Fig. 10.2 Distribution of gestational weight gain by pre-pregnancy BMI category and 1990 IOM weight gain guidelines [9]. Reprinted with permission, National Academies Press

A normal weight woman gaining above IOM guidelines had a 4-fold increased odds of having an obese child, compared to a normal weight woman gaining within the guidelines. Among overweight women, gaining above IOM guidelines increased the odds of child obesity 2.5-fold. For obese women, excessive GWG increased the odds of child obesity 6-fold.

Three studies have examined GWG and obesity in older children/adolescents. Oken et al. examined approximately 12,000 children aged 9–14 years and found that each 5-lb increment in GWG was associated with an odds ratio of 1.09 (95% CI 1.06–1.13) for obesity. Compared to GWG within the 1990 IOM guidelines, gain above the guidelines was associated with an adjusted odds ratio of 1.42 (95% CI 1.19–1.70) for obesity. Maternal pre-pregnancy BMI did not modify the association between GWG and child obesity, in contrast to the Olson study. Wrotniak et al. studied 10,000 7-year olds from a cohort born in the 1950s and 1960s, when mean maternal BMI, GWG, and birthweight were lower than in the current era. Excessive GWG was associated with an adjusted odds ratio of 1.48 (95% CI 1.06–2.06) for child obesity. Among a cohort of Portugese children aged 6–12, GWG $\geq$16 kg versus <9 kg was associated with an adjusted odds ratio of 1.27 (95% CI 1.01–1.61) for child obesity.

However, not all studies demonstrate such an independent relationship between GWG and child obesity. In a cohort of 1,103 male Swedish army conscripts, maternal pre-pregnancy BMI but not GWG was predictive of obesity in a multivariate analysis [10]. Likewise, among 8,494 low-income US children born between 1994 and 2001, GWG had a U-shaped association with child weight at age 2 and 3 years, but was no longer a statistically significant predictor in a multivariate analysis. However, maternal pre-pregnancy obesity had an adjusted odds ratio of 4.31 (95% CI 3.17–5.87) for child obesity in this cohort [11].

While these studies attempt to control for confounding variables such as infant feeding practices, lifestyle and behavioral factors are difficult to measure and thus may still play some role in the observed association. Findings from animal studies, where the diet and physical activity can be controlled, show that overnutrition during pregnancy and early postnatal life has long-term effects on the weight and metabolism of the offspring. Overall, the preponderance of data suggests that gestational weight gain exerts an independent effect on child obesity.

10.6 Optimal Weight Gain for Obese Women – an Ongoing Controversy

Nearly 30% of reproductive age women are obese, according to data from NHANES 2003–2004, and 8% had a BMI > 40 (class 3 obesity) [12]. Since children of obese women are more likely to be obese themselves, modifying weight gain in this group may be an important target of childhood obesity prevention efforts. As noted above, the 1990 IOM guidelines for pregnancy weight gain did not provide much guidance for obese women, recommending a gain of "at least 15 lbs." The 2009 guidelines recommend a total GWG of 11–20 lbs for women of BMI $\geq$30 [9]. Immediately after publication, a firestorm ensued in the literature about the appropriateness of this weight gain range [13]. The controversy centers on the balancing of risks between restricted weight gain, which is associated with preterm birth and low LBW, and excessive weight gain, which is associated with several morbidities in obese women including GDM, preeclampsia, cesarean birth, macrosomia, and long-term weight retention. Artal et al. argued that "poor gestational weight gain is unlikely to affect birthweights in overweight and obese women." [13] There is conflicting evidence about the risk of low GWG among obese women, and several studies support an increased risk of SGA as well as preterm birth among obese women who gain below IOM guidelines [9]. Of course, since these data are all observational, the relationship between GWG and LBW may not be causal; or it may be that some underlying condition (independent of nutrition and possibly epigenetic) is causing both the SGA and the low weight gain. Additionally, there are little data that separate risk by obesity class and it is likely that the optimal weight gain will be lower for class 2 and 3 obesity as compared to class 1. At the time of this writing, there are at least two large ongoing clinical trials of weight gain restriction among obese pregnant women, and the data from such trials will shed light on both the safety and efficacy of such interventions.

10.7 Interventions to Prevent Excessive Pregnancy Weight Gain

Several studies have tested interventions implemented during prenatal care to reduce excessive GWG among diverse populations of women. Polley et al. tested a behavioral intervention during pregnancy to decrease the percentage of women gaining above the IOM recommendations [14]. The intervention decreased the percentage of normal weight women who exceeded the IOM recommendations relative to controls; no effect was found in overweight but a trend in the opposite direction was observed. Gray-Donald et al. examined the effects of periodic dietary counseling on weight gain in a non-randomized study of the Cree population [15]. The intervention was found to have only a minor impact; the authors noted that cultural factors likely limited the intervention's efficacy in this population [16]. Olson et al. [17] conducted a study evaluating the effects of periodic weight monitoring, graphing, and education to prevent excessive weight gain during pregnancy in a sample of women from upstate New York. This intervention, although small and non-randomized, appeared effective in both overweight and normal weight low-income women; 32% exceeded weight gain recommendations in the intervention groups as compared with 59% in the historical control group. Asbee et al. randomized 100 pregnant women to either intensive dietary and lifestyle counseling or no intervention and found a decreased mean weight gain in the intervention group, although there was no difference in the percentage gaining above the IOM guidelines [18]. Two studies showed that intensive behavioral counseling could improve diet and exercise behaviors and reduce GWG specifically among obese pregnant women. Wolff et al. randomized 50 obese women to 10 h of dietary counseling versus usual care [19]. Women in the intervention group reduced their caloric intake and exhibited a mean GWG of 6.6 kg versus 13.3 kg in the usual care group. Claesson et al. conducted a prospective case–control intervention study of 348 obese pregnant women [20]. The intervention group had weekly motivational talks and attended water aerobics classes. The intervention group gained a mean of 8.7 kg during pregnancy versus 11.3 kg in the control group ($p < 0.001$).

While the effects of these interventions have been modest, the overall body of literature demonstrates that diet and physical activity interventions do have an impact on GWG. However, research shows that prenatal care providers often fail to counsel women adequately about weight gain, diet, and exercise during pregnancy. Cogswell surveyed 2,237 predominantly white, middle-class pregnant women, and 27% reported receiving no advice about weight gain. Of those receiving advice, 22% were told to gain more than the guidelines recommend [21]. Similarly, in a multicenter study in the San Francisco Bay Area, a third of pregnant women surveyed reported receiving no advice about how much weight they should gain during pregnancy and overweight women who received weight gain information were often advised to gain more than the IOM guidelines [22]. A national survey of US obstetrician–gynecologists revealed that only 36% of respondents modified their GWG counseling based on the patient's BMI at least "most of the time" [23]. A qualitative focus group study of prenatal care providers revealed several barriers to effective counseling on diet, exercise, and weight gain [24]. Many obstetricians felt they had inadequate training in nutrition and weight management to effectively counsel women. Clinicians were often fearful of causing anxiety or embarrassment in patients by raising the issue of weight during pregnancy and so many avoided the topic. This resulted in many patients not receiving a baseline assessment or goal-setting with regard to weight gain early in pregnancy. Public health efforts should encourage and support efforts of prenatal care providers and primary care clinicians to discuss the risks of excessive weight gain, both prior to conception and early in pregnancy.

10.8 Special Diets for Obese Women During Pregnancy

Currently, special diets are not prescribed for obese pregnant women. Maternal obesity increases the risk of metabolic complications during pregnancy and increases the risk for later obesity in the child. Maternal diet could contribute to the risk, but may also assist in the prevention of these problems. A diet composed primarily of low glycemic load carbohydrates may reduce the risk of impaired glucose tolerance and fetal overgrowth in obese women. Several small studies of low glycemic load diets fed to normal weight women showed that those diets reduced the glycemic response to meals, improved insulin sensitivity in mid and late pregnancy, and reduced birthweights and neonatal fat mass [25–28]. It has also been shown that a low glycemic load breakfast was effective in reducing the insulin and glucose response in obese as well as normal weight women, suggesting that obese pregnant women may benefit from a low glycemic diets as do normal weight women [29]. The efficacy of low glycemic load diets for reducing pregnancy complications and fetal overgrowth in obese women is currently being tested.

Whenever dietary carbohydrate is lowered, dietary fat increases. Studies in experimental animals show that high-fat diets increase the risk of obesity in the offspring [30, 31] (see Chapter 12). The type of dietary fat consumed also appears to influence pregnancy outcomes. A diet high in saturated fat from whole fat dairy products, meats, and butters appears to increase insulin resistance and the risk for GDM

[32], whereas high intakes of polyunsaturated oils appear to be protective against impaired glucose tolerance [33]. An evaluation of the benefits of a diet high in polyunsaturated fatty acids has not been performed in obese pregnant women. Data are insufficient at the present time to define the optimal diet for obese pregnant women. However, preliminary data suggest that they may benefit from limiting refined, high glycemic load carbohydrates and saturated fats, and increasing their intake of low glycemic load carbohydrates and polyunsaturated fatty acids.

References

1. Rasmussen K, Yaktine A. Weight gain during pregnancy: reexamining the guidelines. Washington, DC: The National Academies Press; 2009.
2. Abrams B, Selvin S. Maternal weight gain pattern and birth weight. Obstet Gynecol. 1995;86(2):163–9.
3. Carmichael S, Abrams B, Selvin S. The pattern of maternal weight gain in women with good pregnancy outcomes. Am J Public Health. 1997;87:1984–8.
4. Hytten F, Chamberlain G. Clinical physiology in obstetrics. Oxford: Blackwell Scientific Publications; 1980.
5. Lederman SA, Paxton A, Heymsfield SB, Wang J, Thornton J, Pierson RN. Body fat and water changes during pregnancy in women with different body weight and weight gain. Obstet Gynecol. 1997;90:483–8.
6. Rosso P. Nutrition and metabolism in pregnancy. Mother and fetus. New York, NY: Oxford University Press; 1990.
7. Naismith DJ. Adaptations in the metabolism of protein during pregnancy and their nutritional implications. Nutr Rept Int. 1973;7:383–399.
8. Institute of Medicine (U.S.). Subcommittee on nutritional status and weight gain during pregnancy, Institute of Medicine (U.S.). Subcommittee on dietary intake and nutrient supplements during pregnancy. Nutrition during pregnancy: part I, weight gain: part II, nutrient supplements. Washington, DC: National Academy Press; 1990.
9. Institute of Medicine (U.S.). Subcommittee on nutritional status and weight gain during pregnancy, Weight gain during pregnancy: reexamining the guidelines. Washington, DC: National Academy Press; 2009.
10. Koupil I, Toivanen P. Social and early-life determinants of overweight and obesity in 18-year-old Swedish men. Int J Obes (Lond). Jan 2008;32(1):73–81.
11. Whitaker RC. Predicting preschooler obesity at birth: the role of maternal obesity in early pregnancy. Pediatrics. Jul 2004;114(1):e29–36.
12. Kim SY, Dietz PM, England L, Morrow B, Callaghan WM. Trends in pre-pregnancy obesity in nine states, 1993–2003. Obesity (Silver Spring). Apr 2007;15(4):986–93.
13. Artal R, Lockwood CJ, Brown HL. Weight gain recommendations in pregnancy and the obesity epidemic. Obstet Gynecol. Jan 2010;115(1):152–5.
14. Polley BA, Wing RR, Sims CJ. Randomized controlled trial to prevent excessive weight gain in pregnant women. Int J Obes Relat Metab Disord. Nov 14 2002;26(11):1494–502.
15. Gray-Donald K, Robinson E, Collier A, David K, Renaud L, Rodrigues S. Intervening to reduce weight gain in pregnancy and gestational diabetes mellitus in Cree communities: an evaluation. CMAJ. Nov 2000;163(10):1247–51.
16. Gray-Donald K, Robinson E, Collier A, David K, Renaud L, Rodrigues S. Intervening to reduce weight gain in pregnancy and gestational diabetes mellitus in Cree communities: an evaluation. Can Med Assoc J. 2000;163(10):1247–51.
17. Olson CM, Strawderman MS, Reed RG. Efficacy of an intervention to prevent excessive gestational weight gain. Am J Obstet Gynecol. 2004;191(2):530–6.

18. Asbee SM, Jenkins TR, Butler JR, White J, Elliot M, Rutledge A. Preventing excessive weight gain during pregnancy through dietary and lifestyle counseling: a randomized controlled trial. Obstet Gynecol. Feb 2009;113(2 Pt 1):305–12.
19. Wolff S, Legarth J, Vangsgaard K, Toubro S, Astrup A. A randomized trial of the effects of dietary counseling on gestational weight gain and glucose metabolism in obese pregnant women. Int J Obes (Lond). Mar 2008;32(3):495–501.
20. Claesson IM, Sydsjo G, Brynhildsen J, Cedergren M, Jeppsson A, Nystrom F, et al. Weight gain restriction for obese pregnant women: a case-control intervention study. BJOG. Jan 2008;115(1):44–50.
21. Cogswell ME, Scanlon KS, Fein SB, Schieve LA. Medically advised, mother's personal target, and actual weight gain during pregnancy. Obstet Gynecol. Oct 1999;94(4):616–22.
22. Stotland NE, Haas JS, Brawarsky P, Jackson RA, Fuentes-Afflick E, Escobar GJ. Body mass index, provider advice, and target gestational weight gain. Obstet Gynecol. Mar 2005;105(3):633–8.
23. Power ML, Cogswell ME, Schulkin J. Obesity prevention and treatment practices of U.S. obstetrician-gynecologists. Obstet Gynecol. Oct 2006;108(4):961–8.
24. Stotland NE, Gilbert P, Bogetz A, Harper CC, Abrams B, Gerbert B. Preventing excessive weight gain in pregnancy: how do prenatal care providers approach counseling? J Women's Health (Larchmt). Apr 2010;19(4):807–14.
25. Clapp JF, 3rd. Effect of dietary carbohydrate on the glucose and insulin response to mixed caloric intake and exercise in both nonpregnant and pregnant women. Diabetes Care. 1998;21:B107–12.
26. Clapp JF, 3rd. Maternal carbohydrate intake and pregnancy outcome. Proc Nutr Soc. 2002;61:45–50.
27. Moses RG, Barker M, Winter M, Petocz P, Brand-Miller JC. Can a low-glycemic index diet reduce the need for insulin in gestational diabetes mellitus? A randomized trial. Diabetes Care. Jun 2009;32(6):996–1000.
28. Moses RG, Luebcke M, Davis WS, Coleman KJ, Tapsell LC, Petocz P, et al. Effect of a low-glycemic-index diet during pregnancy on obstetric outcomes. Am J Clin Nutr. Oct 2006;84(4):807–12.
29. Bronstein MN, Mak RP, King JC. The thermic effect of food in normal weight and overweight pregnant women. Br J Nutr. 1995;75(1):261–75.
30. McCurdy CE, Bishop JM, Williams SM, Grayson BE, Smith MS, Friedman JE, et al. Maternal high-fat diet triggers lipotoxicity in the fetal livers of nonhuman primates. J Clin Invest. Feb 2009;119(2):323–35.
31. Metges CC. Early nutrition and later obesity: animal models provide insights into mechanisms. Adv Exp Med Biol. 2009;646:105–12.
32. Bo S, Menato G, Lezo A, Signorile A, Bardelli C, De Michieli F, et al. Dietary fat and gestational hyperglycaemia. Diabetologia. 2001;44:972–8.
33. Wang Y, Storlien LH, Jenkins AB, Tapsell LC, Jin Y, Pan JF, et al. Dietary variables and glucose tolerance in pregnancy. Diabetes Care. 2000;23(4):460–4.

Chapter 11
Intrauterine Growth Restriction, Small for Gestational Age, and Experimental Obesity

Michael G. Ross, Ivan Huber, and Mina Desai

11.1 Introduction

As summarized in Chapter 8, epidemiologic studies demonstrate a paradoxical effect of low birth weight (LBW) on the expression of offspring obesity, coronary heart disease, type 2 diabetes, and metabolic syndrome [1–5]. LBW infants commonly exhibit intrauterine growth restriction (IUGR) and are small for gestational age (SGA), though preterm LBW infants are also at risk for developmental programming of adult metabolic syndrome. Evidence indicates that that a striking 25–63% of adult diabetes, hypertension and coronary heart disease can be attributed to the effects of LBW with accelerated newborn-to-adolescent weight gain [6].

IUGR has contributed in important ways to the population shift toward obesity. Briefly (Fig. 11.1), in past generations, normal weight mothers most commonly gave birth to normal weight infants, which predominantly developed into normal weight adults. The current increased incidence of prematurity and IUGR has resulted in an increase in LBW offspring. When combined with markedly improved neonatal survival and exposure to Western diets, these offspring are frequently programmed to develop adult obesity. This process has accounted to a significant degree for the continuing population shift toward an obese phenotype, with these obese mothers in turn ultimately giving birth to macrosomic newborns.

In order to understand the origins of these problems, animal models have been used to explore mechanisms as well as the impact of varying types and timing of prenatal insults. Our focus in this chapter will be on the developmental processes (programming) beginning in embryonic and fetal life and beyond, which result in obesity in adulthood. In humans, programmed obesity also includes the "thin-fat" phenotype, representing those who are neither overweight nor obese in their body mass index but rather demonstrate an increased percent body fat and reduced percent lean mass [7]. Unfortunately, few animal models exist for the specific study of

M.G. Ross (✉)
Department of Obstetrics and Gynecology, Harbor-UCLA Medical Center, Torrance, CA, USA
e-mail: mikeross@ucla.edu

R.H. Lustig (ed.), *Obesity Before Birth*, Endocrine Updates 30,
DOI 10.1007/978-1-4419-7034-3_11, © Springer Science+Business Media, LLC 2011

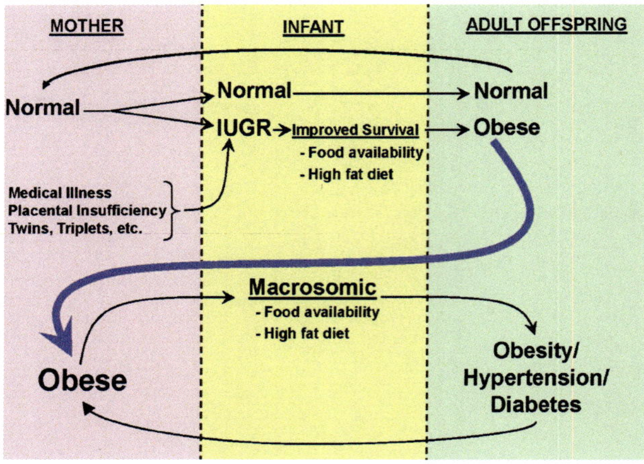

Fig. 11.1 Obesity population shift due to programming

"thin-fat" offspring. Nevertheless, both animal and human studies of developmental programming can assess both body mass and body composition sequelae.

11.2 Programming of Obesity

Evidence is rapidly accumulating for a major role of epigenetic environmental factors in the early onset of body weight dysregulation [8–10]. Aside from genotype, fetal and neonatal nutrition may play key roles in the development of obesity, type 2 diabetes mellitus (T2DM), abnormal lipid and carbohydrate metabolism, cardiovascular disease, and hypertension, termed "metabolic syndrome" [11–13]. Paradoxically, both maternal caloric deprivation [14–17] and maternal obesity [18] produce obese offspring. One of the first clinical documentations was among men born during the Dutch Famine of 1944–1945. Those exposed to famine during the first half of gestation had a markedly increased risk of developing obesity in adulthood [16]. During the neonatal/postnatal periods, excess intake [19] of infant formula feeding is associated with increased obesity [20], likely a result of the contribution of rapid catch-up growth to programming mechanisms. There is increasing evidence that the in utero environment programs fetal development and alters a diversity of adult regulatory mechanisms [21–24] (see [25] for a review). Mothers with gestational diabetes [26] tend to have macrosomic babies, which become obese progeny. Conversely, LBW babies are at increased risk of developing obesity, especially when they exhibit catch-up growth in the first few years of life [27, 28]. Several studies have addressed the association of small size at birth with measures of later central adiposity [29–31], insulin resistance [32, 33], and metabolic syndrome [34, 35]. Thus, we note an apparent paradox of increased adiposity at both ends of the birth weight spectrum (i.e., higher BMI following high birth weight and increased central adiposity following LBW). It may be that similar underlying mechanism(s) predispose both LBW/high birth weight newborns to adult obesity. These may include lasting changes in proportions of fat and lean body mass, central nervous system appetite control, adiposity structure and function, adipokine secretion and regulation, and vascular responsiveness. Thus, elucidating the relationship between early life experiences and later body proportions is critical in preventing obesity, particularly because it can have a lifelong and perhaps multigenerational impact.

11.3 Effects of the In Utero Environment on Fetal Development

Since the pioneering work of McCance and Widdowson and Winick and Nobel [36–39] studies relating developmental physiology to nutrition have repeatedly demonstrated that minor alterations to the diets of pregnant animals can produce lasting changes in physiology and metabolism of the offspring. This phenomenon of "developmental plasticity" enables one genotype to give rise to a range of different physiological or morphological states in response to different environmental conditions during development [10, 40, 41]. Such gene–environment interactions are ubiquitous in the development of all living things. The benefit of developmental plasticity is the production of phenotypes that are better matched to a changing environment than would be possible by the production of the same phenotype in all environments.

Another milestone in these earlier studies was the delineation of "critical periods" which demonstrated that the cellular effects of undernutrition were dependent upon the phase of growth of the animal at the time of onset of the undernutrition. Very early in life, undernutrition may irreversibly impede cell division, organ growth, and differentiation [42, 43]. Later in life, undernutrition may alter cell composition and cell size [43, 44]. Conversely, overfeeding rats (raising animals in litters of 3–4 vs. 8–10) during the proliferative phase of growth causes acceleration of the rate of cell division and produces higher DNA content per organ [45, 46]. These studies indicate that a reduced supply of nutrients during prenatal and postnatal life interferes with the rate of cell multiplication in various organs, and the effect is proportionally more deleterious in tissues with a faster rate of cell multiplication [47, 48]. Furthermore, the earlier the undernutrition, the less likely will be the recovery after the insult is discontinued.

"Developmental programming" refers to an unfavorable prenatal environment believed to trigger adaptations that improve fetal survival or prepare the fetus in expectation of a particular range of postnatal environments [49]. These "predictive adaptive responses" [50] may, however, later prove to be disadvantageous when the pre- and postnatal environments are widely discrepant or mismatched. IUGR/SGA infants "perceive" undernutrition in utero, a result of either uteroplacental insufficiency (developed countries) or maternal undernutrition (developing countries). When exposed to a surfeit of food postnatally, development of obesity is likely.

11.4 Animal Models

Animal models have provided opportunities to examine mechanisms of developmental programming and explore possible preventive/therapeutic strategies. Obviously, there are experiments that would be impossible or unethical with humans. Second, a much greater degree of control is possible with animal models as to both genetics and environment, as the heterogeneity of human populations and environments makes unraveling the causes of complex syndromes daunting. Finally, animal models allow us to test preventative and other strategies.

We will emphasize our laboratory rat studies and refer to other studies and other animal models for contrast or concordance. In our model of SGA offspring, maternal rats are fed a 50% food-restricted (FR) diet from day E10 to term, determined by quantification of normal intake in ad libitum (AdLib) fed rats. At postnatal day P1, litter size is culled to 4 males and 4 females per litter. All maternal diets are maintained during lactation (i.e., all dams are designated AdLib/AdLib or FR/FR, reflecting both pregnancy and lactation periods). We have studied three offspring groups: FR/AdLib, FR/FR (offspring do not develop obesity), and AdLib/AdLib, reflecting the maternal diet during the pregnancy/lactation periods. Offspring from FR dams which are intended for FR/AdLib are cross-fostered to rat dams fed AdLib during pregnancy, in order to eliminate the effect of pregnancy FR on lactation [51]. FR/FR and AdLib/AdLib offspring have also been cross-fostered to control study design. Table 11.1 shows the design of a typical experiment [27].

Table 11.1 Conditions of prenatal programming. All pups were cross-fostered. All dams are FR or AdLib. Offspring diet postweaning was lab chow

Pregnancy	Lactation	Offspring Group	Name
FR	FR	FR/FR	Delayed catch-up growth
FR	AdLib	FR/AdLib	Immediate catch-up growth
AdLib	FR	AdLib/FR	Lactation control
AdLib	AdLib	AdLib/AdLib	Control

We have demonstrated that 50% food restriction during the rat pregnancy (E10–E21) results in IUGR newborns with reduced plasma insulin, glucose and triglyceride levels [27, 48, 52]. When nursed by AdLib fed control dams, IUGR pups exhibit hyperphagia with rapid catch-up growth at 3 weeks, though with normal percent body fat, in presence of hypoinsulinemia, hyperglycemia, and hypotriglyceridemia. Offspring continue accelerated growth, resulting in increased weight and percent body fat with development of adult hyperinsulinemia, hyperglycemia, and hypertriglyceridemia.

Several methods have been used to produce IUGR in animal models, including maternal food restriction described above [49, 53], maternal low protein [47, 54], calorie restriction [17, 55, 56], and iron restriction [57, 58]. Other approaches include hormonal insults, such as glucocorticoids (GCs) [59, 60], and surgical interventions, including uterine artery ligation [61, 62], meso-ovarian vessel cautery [63], placental embolization [64, 65], and carunculectomy [66].

11.5 Animal Species

A diversity of animal species have been utilized for studies of SGA and fetal programming [49]. Ovine models have been useful for analyzing placental/fetal interactions because of their larger size, their primarily singleton pregnancies, similar organogenesis to humans [67], and the applications to animal husbandry. Catheters can be inserted in both fetal and maternal compartments [68] for blood collection during fetal life. A variant model in the sheep is that of adolescent maternal overfeeding [64, 69], which has its equivalent in adolescent girls in which increased maternal weight gain decreases placental growth, resulting in IUGR [70, 71].

Among the rodents, the rat and mouse are the most popular models. The rodent model offers the advantage of large litter sizes which can be culled to a uniform offspring number to examine the effect of lactation. Large litter sizes also make possible an array of newborn and adult studies, and an examination of gender-specific effects. Rats and mice are also well characterized in terms of their biochemistry, physiology, brain function, and neuronal pathways, and many inbred strains are available. Rats have been extensively used to study the effect of catch-up growth in the newborn period which produces obesity and metabolic syndrome [27]. An important domain in which mice currently surpass rats is the development of genetic knockouts [72] as well as “humanized” mice in which human genes have been inserted.

Using mice, Coe et al. [73] developed a “crowded uterine horn” model to diminish fetal growth and produce IUGR offspring. Briefly, hemi-ovariectomized females were allowed to mate. The remaining ovary compensates with an increase in ovulation resulting in a crowded uterine horn, in which some fetuses are SGA. As this model avoids limiting maternal food intake, the offspring are the product of reduced placental blood flow, akin to uteroplacental insufficiency.

Pigs are perhaps more similar to humans than any other mammals, with the exception of apes [74]. A recent incomplete list of species comparisons (in nutrition and physiology) considers the following points of dissimilarity between pigs and humans [75]. Adipose tissue is the principal site of fatty acid synthesis in pigs (and ruminants), whereas adipose and liver are both important sites in rats. In humans, a great deal of lipogenesis takes place in the liver. Pigs and rats use both D-tryptophan and L-tryptophan, while mice and humans use the L-form primarily. The study of large animal models should lead to increased collaboration between biomedical and animal husbandry researchers [76, 77].

Notably, intensive development of pig farming has produced highly inbred lines of pigs characterized by extremely fast growth and reduced fat content. Some of the genetic diseases in these lines are similar to those seen in human obesity

[78]. Exogenous doses of porcine recombinant leptin shift energy away from lipid increase toward lean meat. This opens up the possibility of pharmacologically transforming metabolism to decrease adipose tissue growth. It will be important to identify the pig genes that channel metabolism to store excess energy in adipose tissue. Techniques to accomplish these aims include identifying quantitative trait loci, gene transcript profiling, and genetic polymorphisms of obesity-related genes in the porcine genome that might be useful targets in the study of human obesity. Among porcine models of obesity and the metabolic syndrome [79], the Ossabaw feral pig is a particularly compelling model animal. This pig has undergone selection for cyclical feast/famine over the 500 years that it has existed in isolation on an island off the coast of Georgia, USA [80]. Female Ossabaws fed a high cholesterol diet, develop at least five of the six criteria of the metabolic syndrome, including primary insulin resistance and coronary artery disease; symptoms which have been difficult to produce in other pig models.

A study of maternal FR in fetal baboons showed global methylation effects on a variety of organs at different gestational ages [81]. These are potential epigenetic mechanisms in which maternal FR exerts long-term programming alterations on fetal organs.

11.6 Programming Mechanisms and Results: Appetite and Adipogenesis

Our discussion focuses on the role of programmed appetite and adipogenesis as the primary contributors to programmed obesity. Orexigenic function and regulation develop in utero in the early newborn period. Programming of appetite/satiety mechanisms in response to an altered fetal/newborn environment thus may influence infant, childhood, and ultimately adult appetite "setpoints." Humans have well-developed orexigenic mechanisms, such that hunger and appetite are evoked (in response to nutrient restriction, hypoglycemia, etc.), initially with an unconscious drive, and subsequently with increasing symptoms and conscious behavior changes. Conversely, satiety pathways are markedly less functional, contributing to the difficulty of self-motivated dietary weight loss. As demonstrated by our studies and others, gestational programming may further reduce the efficacy of these satiety mechanisms, and perhaps enhance orexigenic drive resulting in an appetite–satiety imbalance and hyperphagia-induced obesity.

In addition to obesity, IUGR also leads to changes in other fetal and adult organ systems. For example, changes in renal and blood vessel development and decreased beta-cell function contribute to metabolic syndrome in adults. Depending on the origin of the IUGR, the effects of fetal programming may differ [82]. There is an increased risk of dementia, including Alzheimer's, in individuals with midlife obesity [71]. One potential link between obesity and Alzheimer's is altered insulin-like growth factor-1 (IGF-1) levels in both IUGR offspring and Alzheimer's patients. The authors postulate epigenetic changes are responsible for altered levels of gene expression. See also Chapter 8 for a discussion of epigenetics associated with IUGR and experimental obesity.

11.7 Appetite Physiology

Feeding is controlled by an interaction of diverse peripheral and central, endocrine and neuronal signals which influence short- and long-term orexigenic and anorexigenic responses (for review see [83]). The hypothalamus is a critical appetite regulatory center, primarily controlled by a circuit of hypothalamic nuclei which receive input from central and peripheral sources including ghrelin from the brain and stomach, leptin from adipocytes [84], stomach epithelia, placenta, and glands [85–88], and insulin from the pancreas. Together, these inputs provide neural and hormonal signals to adjust orexigenic drive to energy needs.

Within the hypothalamus, the arcuate (ARC) and the paraventricular (PVN) nuclei are key targets of appetite regulatory factors, processing orexigenic and anorexigenic signals. The ARC contains at least two distinct populations of neurons with opposing actions on food intake. The medial ARC orexigenic neurons contain neuropeptide Y (NPY) and agouti-related protein (AgRP) whereas lateral ARC anorexigenic neurons contain melanocortin (MC) products pro-opiomelanocortin (POMC) and cocaine- and amphetamine-regulated transcript (CART). ARC neurons highly express leptin receptors. Leptin increases POMC and decreases NPY and AgRP mRNA levels. ARC NPY/AgRP and POMC neurons project to the PVN [89–101], serving as an integrating center of appetite neural pathways. ARC neurons integrate a diverse variety of peripheral and central signals to modulate energy status. While most studies have examined mRNA expression of hypothalamic neuropeptides in the regulation of appetite, anatomical and functional intercell communication is increasingly recognized as critical. Release of downstream neurotransmitters is dependent in part, upon neuronal electrical activity, which itself is regulated by neuropeptide-mediated inhibitory and excitatory inputs.

The obese gene (*ob*) codes for leptin while the *db* gene codes for its receptor. Congenital leptin deficiency alters the innervation of the ARC, potentiating appetite and reducing satiety, as *ob/ob* mice demonstrate altered neuronal inputs at orexigenic and anorexigenic neurons: Increased inhibitory postsynaptic currents (IPSC) at POMC neurons and excitatory postsynaptic currents (EPSC) at NPY neurons [102] suppress anorexigenic responses and augment orexigenic function. These changes in tone are accompanied by corresponding changes in the number of excitatory and inhibitory synapses. Neuronal excitability of NPY/AgRP neurons is increased in these offspring [103] further potentiating appetite responses. These studies indicate that neuropeptides can modulate appetite/satiety both by direct receptor activation as well as by changing synapse number and electrical activity of cells. In our rat model of programmed obesity, we postulate that FR/AdLib offspring have reduced satiety responses that are secondary to programmed ARC neuronal intrinsic properties, as well reduced sensitivity and responses to anorexigenic neuropeptides.

11.8 Development of Appetite and Satiety Mechanisms

11.8.1 Role of Leptin

11.8.1.1 Animal Leptin Physiology

Although fetal growth is influenced by maternal nutritional, genetic and uteroplacental factors, orexigenic functions must develop in utero in precocial species, to prepare for newborn life. Both NPY and leptin are expressed during fetal development. Rats demonstrate a well-described leptin surge at P10–12 which correlates with the development of axonal projections from the ARC to PVN [104]. In mice, the development of these feeding circuits has been traced using DiI axonal labeling [105]. The development of axonal projections from ARC to PVN did not reach the target until P8–10 with maturity by P12. This process is dependent, in part, on leptin trophic effects during this critical period. A postnatal leptin surge is evidenced by a continual increase in plasma leptin from P12 to P20 with a decline on P21 [106]. Thus, appetitive modulation of ingestive behavior becomes functional during the rat suckling period, with maturation just prior to weaning [107]. In contrast, neonatal overnutrition inhibits ARC leptin responsiveness, likely due to local leptin resistance [108].

Normal development of orexigenic pathways results in an enhanced orexigenic vs anorexigenic function during early newborn life. In the newborn rat, NPY mRNA is observed in the ARC [109]. As early as P2, newborn rats are responsive to central NPY, with increasing weight gain [110]. Although peripheral or central administration of leptin induces satiation in adults, leptin does not appear to alter appetite in the fetus or newborn. In near term pig and rat fetuses, leptin receptors are weakly expressed in the hypothalamus compared with the adult, and leptin receptor expression remains at a low level during the suckling period [111, 112]. In rat pups from P5 to P10, chronic leptin administration downregulates leptin receptor and NPY mRNA, but does *not* alter food intake [113]. Although mouse leptin levels increase 5- to 10-fold during the second postnatal week, food intake during this period does not respond to treatment with exogenous leptin [114]. Thus central leptin "signaling responses" are developed in utero, though leptin does not regulate food intake during early development. Alternatively, central administration of leptin inhibits the fetal hypothalamus–pituitary–adrenal (HPA) axis during late gestation [115, 116], suggesting an interaction of fetal weight/body fat with the timing of parturition. In the newborn, the enhanced orexigenic vs. anorexigenic function likely serves to promote rapid newborn weight gain.

Animal studies demonstrate that maternal malnutrition may lead to offspring obesity [17, 117]. Similarly, both infant over- and underfeeding may result in adult obesity. Overfeeding in neonatal animals (i.e., diet-induced obesity) causes an increased early weight gain and fat deposition, followed by hyperphagia, obesity, hyperleptinemia, hyperinsulinemia, and insulin resistance [118–121]. Electrophysiological studies showed a reduced leptin inhibitory effect on appetite stimulatory neurons (assumed to be NPY) of the ARC in these offspring [108, 122–124]. Neurons in the ventromedial (VM) hypothalamic nucleus also have altered responses to NPY in the young adult after postnatal overfeeding [120–122, 125, 126]. That maternal FR induces offspring obesity in association with an increased appetite is well documented [15, 17, 117, 127].

Biochemical data support the concept of programming of orexigenic pathways. In IUGR fetuses, placental leptin mRNA and protein and cord blood leptin levels are decreased [128, 129] and preterm or LBW human, rat, or calf newborns have reduced plasma leptin levels [130–132]. At 2 months, leptin mRNA in subcutaneous fat is negatively correlated with birth weight [133]. As adults, leptin and insulin levels are related to birth weight, independent of adult obesity [128]. Among animal studies, sheep FR results in near term fetuses with increased hypothalamic NPY mRNA levels [134]. Similarly, in rats, maternal protein restriction significantly increased NPY levels in the PVN and lateral hypothalamic nuclei of the offspring [135].

As noted above, leptin signaling is active at the level of the ARC during the early postnatal period, though anorexigenic responses are not evoked. Leptin promotes the development of ARC neuronal projections, consistent with a role in brain development. ARC projections in mice are formed primarily during the second week of postnatal life [136] (developmentally similar to the human third trimester of pregnancy). In leptin-deficient, obese mice, these projection pathways regulating appetite are permanently disrupted, demonstrating axonal densities one-third to one-fourth that of controls [137]. Both anorexigenic and orexigenic pathways are disrupted, suggesting a greater reduction in the former as compared to the latter, potentiating increased food intake and obesity. Mice lacking leptin signaling also show additional brain abnormalities and reduced brain weight, as well as altered expression of neuronal and glial proteins [138]. Our studies indicate that maternal FR, associated with reduced plasma leptin in the offspring, upregulates newborn hypothalamic leptin receptors [27, 139].

As with other developmental factors, leptin acts primarily during a restricted, crucial postnatal period. In the rodent, this developmental window coincides with the natural surge in leptin, though intrauterine undernutrition in mice results in a premature neonatal leptin surge [140]. Treatment of adult *ob/ob* mice with leptin does not restore ARC projections to the PVN, but daily injections of leptin in *ob/ob* newborn mice from P4–12 rescues innervation of the PVN by ARC axons [137]. Leptin replacement beyond this critical window corrects changes in synaptic density and postsynaptic currents, but does not alter the neural pathways. Recent evidence indicates that leptin supplementation from P3–13 to offspring of rat dams who were 70% malnourished throughout gestation prevents obesity from developing in response to a high fat diet [141]. Despite the prevention of an obese phenotype with newborn leptin supplementation, it is unknown whether cellular signaling processes are normalized. Furthermore, the absence of physical obesity does *not* assure a normal body composition (e.g., percent body fat, plasma lipids), as demonstrated in our studies [27, 52, 142].

11.8.1.2 Human Leptin Physiology

In humans, leptin is measurable in fetal plasma as early as 126 days [143, 144]. In utero leptin levels are linked to fetal adiposity, as evidenced by the positive correlation between newborn serum leptin concentrations and birthweight [144]. Serum leptin in preterm newborns is lower than in term newborn infants [145], consistent with reduced preterm body fat. In infants, plasma leptin levels decrease with fasting and increase with feeding [146]. In contrast to the rodent, there is no evidence of a postnatal leptin surge in human infants [147]. The quality of nutrition in the neonatal period also impacts on leptin expression and function in later life, as infants born preterm and fed enriched formula had higher plasma leptin levels at P13–16 than controls fed standard formula [148].

11.8.1.3 Research on Neural Stem Cell Cultures (NSC)

The growth of fetal NSC provides an insight into development of hypothalamic appetite pathways. Because LBW offspring have reduced cord blood leptin and insulin levels, we hypothesized that reduced neurotrophic stimulation may alter the development of these pathways. Hypothalami from E20 control rat embryos were cultured in complete medium (CM) containing growth factors and heparin. On day 8–9 of culture, NSC were seeded in CM or differentiating medium (DM) for baseline studies. For neurotrophic proliferation studies, NSC cultured in CM were treated with leptin or insulin. For differentiation responses, NSC cultured in DM were treated as above. Signaling pathways were examined by measure of select molecules (e.g., Notch 1 and pSTAT3) and NSC responses in the presence of selective pathway antagonists. Our conclusion was that both hormones have strong effects on NSC proliferation, enhancing with selective effects on NSC differentiation, neuronal or glial cells, respectively. These results suggest a critical role of neural trophic factors in utero, and that excess or deficiency of these hormones associated with IUGR may permanently alter neural pathway development and behavior. Our recent studies have confirmed that NSC derived from 1-day-old offspring from maternally undernourished dams have a markedly reduced growth and differentiation potential [149].

11.8.2 Role of Adipose Tissue

Adipogenesis occurs primarily during the prenatal and postnatal periods, though some adipogenesis continues throughout adulthood [150]. The chronology of white adipose tissue appearance, however, is strictly dependent on the species as well as the adipose depot [151, 152]. In most species, adipose tissue formation begins before birth, as assessed by morphological studies performed on human [153], pig, mouse, and rat embryos [154]. In rats, growth of adipose tissue occurs in well-defined stages. From birth to 4 weeks, adipose tissue growth is hyperplastic. Overfeeding a rat during this period can lead to permanent increases in body weight and fat cell number [155]. From 4 to 14 weeks both adipocyte hypertrophy and hyperplasia occur. Following 14 weeks, adipose tissue growth occurs predominantly by hypertrophy. In humans and sheep [156–158], preadipocytes begin to differentiate into adipose tissue during late embryonic development, with a majority of the differentiation occurring shortly after birth [159]. This enables the newborn to cope more efficiently with intervals between nutrient intakes [160]. Rat and mouse preadipocytes do not begin conversion into adipose tissue until after birth [159]. Adipose tissue expansion takes place rapidly after birth as a result of hyperplasia as well as hypertrophy. This hypertrophic growth occurs primarily by lipid accumulation within the adipocyte. In humans, during the first year of extrauterine life, most adipose tissue growth occurs by hypertrophic growth rather than by hyperplastic growth, but after 2 years there is little additional increase in adipocyte volume in the non-obese child [161]. In obese children, there is continual enlargement of adipocytes without hyperplasia during the same period [162]. These data support the concept that during critical periods of adipose tissue growth, it is possible to program adipocyte development [163, 164].

11.9 Programming of Adiposity

Studies in our laboratory have demonstrated that in addition to an imbalance of appetite/satiety, programmed obesity results from enhanced adipogenesis and lipogenesis. Adipogenesis involves both cellular hypertrophy of adipocytes (increase in cell size) and hyperplasia (increase in cell number) and occurs predominantly in prenatal and postnatal periods [153, 165]. Nuclear hormone receptors regulate adipogenesis. In particular, the adipogenic transcription factor peroxisome proliferator-activated receptor gamma-2 (PPARγ_2) plays a pivotal role in adipogenesis [166, 167]. PPAR transactivation is induced by ligand-dependent and independent mechanisms. Ligand binding of fatty acids, arachidonic acid metabolites, and synthetic drugs used to treat metabolic disorders (e.g., thiazolidinediones) leads to the dissociation of corepressors and the recruitment of coactivators (Fig. 11.2).

11.9.1 Enhanced Adipogenesis and Lipogenesis

At 1 day of age, IUGR male offspring exhibit an upregulated adipogenic signaling cascade, including increased expression of PPARγ [168]. Furthermore, factors influencing adipocyte lipid storage and release indicate propensity to retain fat in IUGR adipocytes. These changes occur prior to development of obesity and suggest a programmed pathway of increased adipocyte differentiation and lipogenesis which likely promotes the development of obesity and metabolic abnormalities in IUGR offspring.

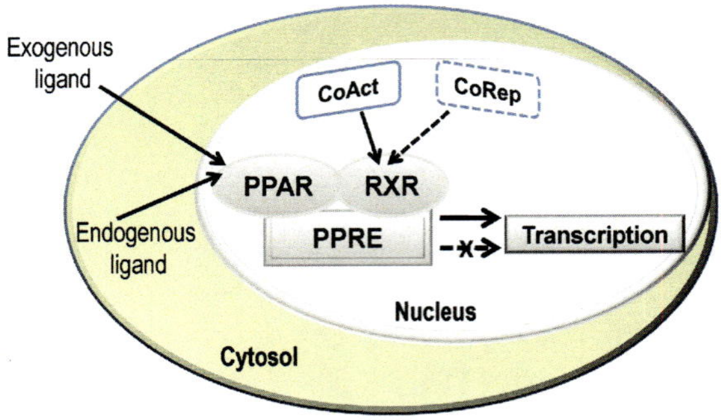

Fig. 11.2 Gene transcription mechanisms of PPAR. In the unliganded state, PPAR interacts with anti-repressor complex; the deacetylated state activity of corepressor, CoRep, inhibits gene transcription. Upon binding of exogenous (drugs) or endogenous (fatty acids) ligands, PPAR heterodimerizes with RXR and recruits the coactivator, CoAct, containing histone acetylase activity and facilitates transcription of genes

We have investigated the putative mechanism for the paradoxically increased PPARγ_2 activity and determined the adipose tissue (retroperitoneal) protein expression of stress–response and chromatin-silencing factor 1 (SIRT1), nuclear receptor corepressor (NCoR), and silencing mediator for retinoid and thyroid hormone receptor (SMRT) in IUGR and control males at P1 and at 9 months of age. At P1, IUGR newborns showed significantly increased protein expression of SIRT1 and SMRT, consistent with their growth-restricted status. In contrast, the expression of NCoR was significantly reduced in IUGR newborns. At 9 months, IUGR adults had decreased expression of SIRT1 and SMRT, consistent with their obese status. Notably, NCoR levels were unchanged in IUGR as compared to control adults. This suggests that dysregulation of NCoR at an early age in IUGR newborns may impact PPARγ_2 modulation and hence its activity [169].

We also investigated the adipose tissue (retroperitoneal) protein expression of PPARγ *coactivators*, SRC1 and transcriptional intermediary factor 2 (TIF2) in IUGR, and control male offspring at P1 and 9 months. TIF2 is associated with adipocyte differentiation and fat storage by potentiating PPARγ activity whereas steroid receptor coactivator 1 (SRC1) mediates fat storage principally in brown adipose tissue [170]. At P1, IUGR newborns had increased protein expression of SRC1 though the expression of TIF2 was comparable to controls. Conversely, IUGR adults at 9 months showed increased expression of both SRC1 and TIF2. This suggests that in IUGR offspring, upregulation of particularly TIF2 enhances activation of PPARγ, leading to increased lipid accumulation and programmed obesity [169].

Human sirtuin (SIRT1), expressed in white adipose tissue, is a factor that modulates endocrine signaling and regulates a number of transcription factors. It is an NAD(+)-dependent histone deacetylase [171] which is upregulated in adipose tissue during fasting, suggesting that SIRT1 may regulate fat storage in adipocytes. Importantly, SIRT1 binds to and represses PPARγ activity by docking PPARγ the

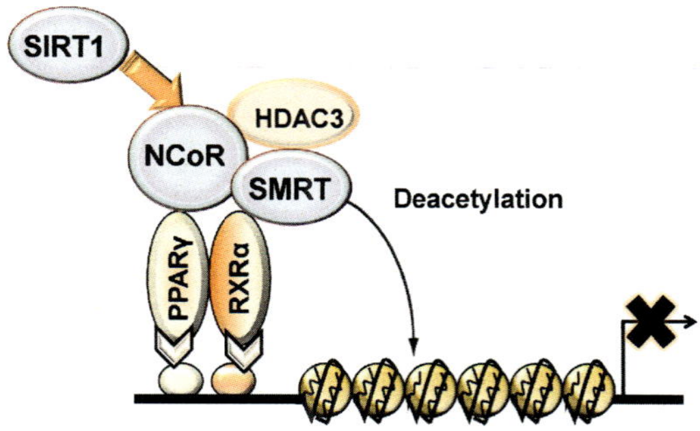

Fig. 11.3 SIRT1 Regulation of PPARγ. Chromatin-silencing factor SIRT1 responds to nutrient signal and recruits corepressors, NCoR and SMRT, and suppresses PPARγ via HDAC3

corepressors NCoR and SMRT. The complex SIRT1/PPARγ/NCoR is recruited to specific DNA sequences (PPRE) in the promoter region of PPARγ target genes and inhibits their transcription (Fig. 11.3). In particular, SIRT1-mediated repression of PPARγ_2 transactivation inhibits lipid accumulation in adipocytes and causes increased mobilization of fat depots for release into the circulation [172, 173].

In addition to adipogenesis, PPARγ modulates lipid homeostasis [174–176] through its role in adipocyte differentiation and lipid storage in adipose tissue. PPARγ activates lipogenic transcription factor (SREBP1) that [177] leads to induction of extracellular lipolytic enzyme (lipoprotein lipase) [178, 179] and lipogenic enzyme (fatty acid synthase). These promote fatty acid delivery to adipocytes and increased synthesis, respectively, leading to lipid accumulation within the adipocyte [180, 181].

11.9.1.1 Research in Primary Adipocyte Cultures

Although IUGR newborns exhibit acute upregulation of the adipogenesis signaling cascade prior to the development of obesity, we sought to determine whether this increased adipogenic potential was an intrinsic cellular response and thus maintained in adipose cell culture. IUGR had significantly increased mRNA and protein expression of PPARγ as compared to control adipocytes. Thus, an IUGR primary adipocyte cell culture exhibits basal phenotypic expression characteristic of programmed upregulation of adipogenic transcription factors which may promote adipose cell proliferation [182]. In response to the PPARγ antagonist Bisphenol A diglycidyl ether (BADGE), PPARγ expression was expectedly downregulated. Furthermore, the IUGR adipocytes showed a similar response to BADGE, as did the control adipocytes. The normal suppressive response to the inhibitor suggests that IUGR adipocytes may respond to pharmacologic approaches to prevent obesity during this period [182].

11.10 Programmed Obesity: Putative Causative Mechanisms

The underlying mechanisms responsible for perinatally acquired "malprogramming" still remain unclear. Studies indicate that endocrine regulatory systems may be programmable. It is well known that hormones regulate the fundamental processes of hemostasis and when present in nonphysiological concentrations during critical ontogenetic periods, can have adverse effects [183, 184]. For example, the effects on the offspring of maternal malnutrition could be related to disturbances in maternal and/or fetal GC status [185–187]. On the other hand, a deficiency in placental 11β-hydroxysteroid dehydrogenase-2 (11βHSD2), which converts active glucocorticoid to inactive 11-keto products (e.g., cortisol to cortisone; see Chapter 14) [188, 189], has been reported in babies with low birthweight [190]. Thus, low placental 11βHSD2 activity and consequent exposure of fetuses to high levels of GC of maternal origin could lead to disturbances in intrauterine development. Similarly, fetal and neonatal hyperinsulinism is a pathognomic feature in the offspring of diabetic mothers. Notably, several rat models, including ours, have shown that nutritional permutations during the perinatal period, resulting in adult obesity, also result in elevated fasting plasma leptin and insulin levels in the offspring [10, 27, 191]. Alternatively, abnormalities of adipocytes may affect later obesity, either through upregulation of cell proliferation and/or through differentiation, leading to abnormal adipocyte cell metabolism and regulation [192, 193]. Adipose tissue has evolved to efficiently store energy for times of caloric restriction. The large caloric excess common in many Western diets negated the need for this thrifty function, leaving adipose tissue ill equipped to handle this increased load. As an active participant in whole body-energy homeostasis, adipose tissue can negatively influence other systems when overloaded. Although adipocytes are capable of increasing in size, the cellular homeostasis and the secretory profile of larger adipocytes becomes altered and increasingly dysregulated compared with adipocytes of smaller size [194–197].

11.11 Therapies and Applications

The mechanism by which newborn leptin supplementation may prevent obesity remains controversial for several reasons. In contrast to the study above [141], leptin supplementation to pups from P1–10 programs adult hyperleptinemia and leptin resistance, increased food intake, and excess body weight [51, 198]. Furthermore, our studies have demonstrated that FR during *both* pregnancy and lactation, which results in further newborn growth restriction and continued plasma hypoleptinemia, prevented offspring hyperphagia and obesity [27]. *Thus, neonatal leptin excess may actually induce obesity while fetal/newborn leptin deficiency may prevent obesity.* These conflicting findings make it essential to understand the cellular mechanism(s) of leptin-mediated anorexigenic pathway development, rather than simply examining offspring phenotype.

A recent review [199] of leptin suggests that leptin in milk may be beneficial in developmental programming and that it should be considered as an additive to improve infant formula. However, Melnik [200] suggests that formula protein consumption induces postprandial hyperinsulinemia and permanently increases IGF-1 serum levels. In particular, milk intake by the mother may affect fetal programming leading to childhood and adult diseases. Though his policy is not endorsed, he recommends that obstetricians advise pregnant patients not to consume milk during pregnancy [200].

Like humans, rats are altricial and their period of lactation has been correlated with the third trimester in human pregnancy. Perhaps then, nutritional intervention in this trimester may be important as a corrective measure [27]. Recent work suggests that, at least in the rat, developmental metabolic programming is potentially reversible by an intervention late in the phase of developmental plasticity. Circulating leptin levels vary dramatically during intrauterine and early postnatal life, with a 5- to 10-fold increase in leptin occurring between P4–10 in female mice – the leptin surge [105]. Leptin treatment administered to neonatal female rats following maternal undernutrition prevented the development of the programmed phenotype in adulthood. The complete normalization of the "programmed" phenotype by neonatal leptin treatment implies that leptin can reverse the prenatal adaptations resulting from relative fetal undernutrition.

Nonetheless, the rodent data highlight the importance of this critical leptin window in reprogramming the postnatal phenotype. These results demonstrate that manipulation of postnatal diet can limit adverse outcomes of developmental programming, with programmed hyperleptinemia prevented by a postnatal diet enriched with omega-3 fatty acids. This raises the possibility that dietary supplementation with omega-3 fatty acids may provide a viable therapeutic option for preventing or reducing adverse programming outcomes in humans [201].

Interestingly, ghrelin receptor antagonists may improve glucose tolerance in rats without inducing weight gain by increasing insulin secretion. Antagonism of ghrelin function to treat diabetes may be applicable to treat IUGR postnatally. This review [202] concentrates on recent findings on ghrelin and its derivatives in metabolic disorders with emphasis on human studies.

11.12 Conclusions

A recent review [203] suggests that the twin challenges of studying and combating the obesity epidemic are ideally suited to the relatively new interdisciplinary field of complexity science. The obesity epidemic is an example of a complex adaptive system. Such a system is composed of multiple heterogeneous elements interacting in subtle and/or nonlinear ways, which can strongly influence the behavior of the entire system. This perspective has proven heuristic in systems ranging from political and economic to social and biological. When such systems are studied by complexity science, they often yield insights about their functioning, as well as suggesting strategies for intervention. As combating obesity will clearly require cross-disciplinary approaches, modeling with testable assumptions can advance our understanding of the system. When combined with empirical study, modeling can be a powerful tool as new hypotheses are generated in an iterative fashion. While these approaches have been successful in fields such as engineering and ecology, to date they have been minimally applied in the public health arena.

References

1. Barker DJ, Bagby SP, Hanson MA. Mechanisms of disease: in utero programming in the pathogenesis of hypertension. Nat Clin Pract Nephrol. 2006;2(12):700–7.
2. Barker DJ. Fetal programming of coronary heart disease. Trends Endocrinol Metab. 2002;13(9):364–8.
3. Godfrey KM, Barker DJ. Fetal programming and adult health. Public Health Nutr. 2001;4(2B):611–24.
4. Nilsson PM, Ostergren PO, Nyberg P, Soderstrom M, Allebeck P. Low birth weight is associated with elevated systolic blood pressure in adolescence: a prospective study of a birth cohort of 149378 Swedish boys. J Hypertens. 1997;15(12 Pt 2):1627–31.
5. Ozanne SE, Hales CN. Early programming of glucose-insulin metabolism. Trends Endocrinol Metab. 2002;13(9):368–73.
6. Barker DJ, Eriksson JG, Forsen T, Osmond C. Fetal origins of adult disease: strength of effects and biological basis. Int J Epidemiol. 2002;31(6):1235–9.
7. Yajnik CS. Early life origins of insulin resistance and type 2 diabetes in India and other Asian countries. J Nutr. 2004;134(1):205–10.
8. Desai M, Hales CN. Role of fetal and infant growth in programming metabolism in later life. Biol Rev Camb Philos Soc. 1997;72(2):329–48.
9. Hales CN, Barker DJ. The thrifty phenotype hypothesis. Br Med Bull. 2001;60:5–20.
10. Ross MG, Desai M. Gestational programming: population survival effects of drought and famine during pregnancy. Am J Physiol Regul Integr Comp Physiol. 2005;288(1):R25–R33.
11. Barker DJ. Intrauterine programming of adult disease. Mol Med Today. 1995;1(9):418–23.
12. Desai M, Crowther NJ, Ozanne SE, Lucas A, Hales CN. Adult glucose and lipid metabolism may be programmed during fetal life. Biochem Soc Trans. 1995;23(2):331–5.
13. Lucas A, Baker BA, Desai M, Hales CN. Nutrition in pregnant or lactating rats programs lipid metabolism in the offspring. Br J Nutr. 1996;76(4):605–12.
14. Barker M, Robinson S, Osmond C, Barker DJ. Birth weight and body fat distribution in adolescent girls. Arch Dis Child. 1997;77(5):381–3.
15. Jones AP, Simson EL, Friedman MI. Gestational undernutrition and the development of obesity in rats. J Nutr. 1984;114(8):1484–92.
16. Ravelli GP, Stein ZA, Susser MW. Obesity in young men after famine exposure in utero and early infancy. N Engl J Med. 1976;295(7):349–53.
17. Vickers MH, Breier BH, Cutfield WS, Hofman PL, Gluckman PD. Fetal origins of hyperphagia, obesity, and hypertension and postnatal amplification by hypercaloric nutrition. Am J Physiol Endocrinol Metab. 2000;279(1):E83–7.
18. Levin BE, Govek E. Gestational obesity accentuates obesity in obesity-prone progeny. Am J Physiol. 1998;275(4 Pt 2):R1374–9.
19. Faust IM, Johnson PR, Hirsch J. Long-term effects of early nutritional experience on the development of obesity in the rat. J Nutr. 1980;110(10):2027–34.
20. Gillman MW, Rifas-Shiman SL, Camargo CA Jr., Berkey CS, Frazier AL, Rockett HR, et al. Risk of overweight among adolescents who were breastfed as infants. JAMA. 2001;285(19):2461–7.
21. Barker DJ. In utero programming of chronic disease. Clin Sci (Lond). 1998;95(2):115–28.

22. Barker DJ. Intrauterine programming of adult disease. Mol Med Today. 1995;1(9):418–23.
23. Phillips DI, Barker DJ, Osmond C. Infant feeding, fetal growth and adult thyroid function. Acta Endocrinol (Copenh). 1993;129(2):134–8.
24. Dodic M, May CN, Wintour EM, Coghlan JP. An early prenatal exposure to excess glucocorticoid leads to hypertensive offspring in sheep. Clin Sci (Lond). 1998;94(2):149–55.
25. McMillen IC, Robinson JS. Developmental origins of the metabolic syndrome: prediction, plasticity, and programming. Physiol Rev. 2005;85(2):571–633.
26. Perseghin G, Ghosh S, Gerow K, Shulman GI. Metabolic defects in lean nondiabetic offspring of NIDDM parents: a cross-sectional study. Diabetes. 1997;46(6):1001–9.
27. Desai M, Gayle D, Babu J, Ross MG. Programmed obesity in intrauterine growth-restricted newborns: modulation by newborn nutrition. Am J Physiol Regul Integr Comp Physiol. 2005;288(1):R91–6.
28. Remacle C, Bieswal F, Reusens B. Programming of obesity and cardiovascular disease. Int J Obes Relat Metab Disord. 2004;28 Suppl 3:S46–S53.
29. Andrew R, Phillips DI, Walker BR. Obesity and gender influence cortisol secretion and metabolism in man. J Clin Endocrinol Metab. 1998;83(5):1806–9.
30. Ong KK, Ahmed ML, Emmett PM, Preece MA, Dunger DB. Association between postnatal catch-up growth and obesity in childhood: prospective cohort study. BMJ. 2000;320(7240):967–71.
31. Rogers I. The influence of birthweight and intrauterine environment on adiposity and fat distribution in later life. Int J Obes Relat Metab Disord. 2003;27(7):755–77.
32. Yajnik C. Interactions of perturbations in intrauterine growth and growth during childhood on the risk of adult-onset disease. Proc Nutr Soc. 2000;59(2):257–65.
33. Stocker CJ, Arch JR, Cawthorne MA. Fetal origins of insulin resistance and obesity. Proc Nutr Soc. 2005;64(2):143–51.
34. Jaquet D, Deghmoun S, Chevenne D, Collin D, Czernichow P, Levy-Marchal C. Dynamic change in adiposity from fetal to postnatal life is involved in the metabolic syndrome associated with reduced fetal growth. Diabetologia. 2005;48(5):849–55.
35. Vanhala M. Childhood weight and metabolic syndrome in adults. Ann Med. 1999;31(4):236–9.
36. Widdowson EM, McCance RA. A review: new thoughts on growth. Pediatr Res. 1975;9(3):154–6.
37. McCance RA, Widdowson EM. The effect of undernutrition upon the composition of the body and its tissues. Acta Med Scand. 1953;146(1):45–6.
38. Widdowson EM, McCance RA. The effect of finite periods of undernutrition at different ages on the composition and subsequent development of the rat. Proc R Soc Lond B Biol Sci. 1963;158:329–42.
39. Widdowson EM, McCance RA. Some effects of accelerating growth. I. General somatic development. Proc R Soc Lond B Biol Sci. 1960;152:188–206.
40. Gluckman PD, Cutfield W, Hofman P, Hanson MA. The fetal, neonatal, and infant environments-the long-term consequences for disease risk. Early Hum Dev. 2005;81(1): 51–9.
41. Horton TH. Fetal origins of developmental plasticity: animal models of induced life history variation. Am J Hum Biol. 2005;17(1):34–43.
42. Winick M. Cellular growth in intrauterine malnutrition. Pediatr Clin North Am. 1970;17(1):69–78.
43. Winick M, Rosso P, Brasel JA. Malnutrition and cellular growth in the brain: existence of critical periods. In: lipids, malnutrition and the developing brain. Ciba Found Symp. 1971;199–212.
44. Winick M, Noble A. Cellular response in rats during malnutrition at various ages. J Nutr. 1966;89(3):300–6.
45. Winick M, Noble A. Cellular response with increased feeding in neonatal rats. J Nutr. 1967;91(2):179–82.

46. Winick M, Noble A. Quantitative changes in DNA, RNA, and protein during prenatal and postnatal growth in the rat. Dev Biol. 1965;12(3):451–66.
47. Desai M, Crowther NJ, Lucas A, Hales CN. Organ-selective growth in the offspring of protein-restricted mothers. Br J Nutr. 1996;76(4):591–603.
48. Desai M, Gayle D, Babu J, Ross MG. Permanent reduction in heart and kidney organ growth in offspring of undernourished rat dams. Am J Obstet Gynecol. 2005;193 3 Suppl:1224–32.
49. Vuguin PM. Animal models for small for gestational age and fetal programming of adult disease. Horm Res. 2007;68(3):113–23.
50. Gluckman PD, Hanson MA, Spencer HG. Predictive adaptive responses and human evolution. Trends Ecol Evol. 2005;20(10):527–33.
51. Toste FP, de Moura EG, Lisboa PC, Fagundes AT, de OE, Passos MC. Neonatal leptin treatment programmes leptin hypothalamic resistance and intermediary metabolic parameters in adult rats. Br J Nutr. 2006;95(4):830–7.
52. Desai M, Gayle D, Babu J, Ross MG. The timing of nutrient restriction during rat pregnancy/lactation alters metabolic syndrome phenotype. Am J Obstet Gynecol. 2007;196(6):555–7.
53. Ozanne SE. Metabolic programming in animals. Br Med Bull. 2001;60:143–52.
54. Ozanne SE, Hales CN. The long-term consequences of intra-uterine protein malnutrition for glucose metabolism. Proc Nutr Soc. 1999;58(3):615–9.
55. Swenne I, Crace CJ, Milner RD. Persistent impairment of insulin secretory response to glucose in adult rats after limited period of protein-calorie malnutrition early in life. Diabetes. 1987;36(4):454–8.
56. Woodall SM, Johnston BM, Breier BH, Gluckman PD. Chronic maternal undernutrition in the rat leads to delayed postnatal growth and elevated blood pressure of offspring. Pediatr Res. 1996;40(3):438–43.
57. Shepard TH, Mackler B, Finch CA. Reproductive studies in the iron-deficient rat. Teratology. 1980;22(3):329–34.
58. Felt BT, Lozoff B. Brain iron and behavior of rats are not normalized by treatment of iron deficiency anemia during early development. J Nutr. 1996;126(3):693–701.
59. Reinisch JM, Simon NG, Karow WG, Gandelman R. Prenatal exposure to prednisone in humans and animals retards intrauterine growth. Science. 1978;202(4366):436–8.
60. Seckl. JR. Glucocorticoids, 11b-hydroxysteroid [beta] dehydrogenase and fetal programming. In: O'Brien PMS, Wheeler T, Barker DJP, editors. Fetal programming. Influences on development and disease in later life. London: Royal College of Obstetricians and Gynaecologists; 1999. pp. 430–9.
61. Wigglesworth JS. Fetal growth retardation. Animal model: uterine vessel ligation in the pregnant rat. Am J Pathol. 1974;77(2):347–50.
62. Simmons RA, Templeton LJ, Gertz SJ. Intrauterine growth retardation leads to the development of type 2 diabetes in the rat. Diabetes. 2001;50(10):2279–86.
63. Camprubi M, Ortega A, Balaguer A, Iglesias I, Girabent M, Callejo J, et al. Cauterization of meso-ovarian vessels, a new model of intrauterine growth restriction in rats. Placenta. 2009;30(9):761–6.
64. Morrison JL. Sheep models of intrauterine growth restriction: fetal adaptations and consequences. Clin Exp Pharmacol Physiol. 2008;35(7):730–43.
65. Anthony RV, Scheaffer AN, Wright CD, Regnault TR. Ruminant models of prenatal growth restriction. Reprod Suppl. 2003;61:183–94.
66. Luque A, Carpizo DR, Iruela-Arispe ML. ADAMTS1/METH1 inhibits endothelial cell proliferation by direct binding and sequestration of VEGF165. J Biol Chem. 2003;278(26):23656–65.
67. Wallace JM, Regnault TR, Limesand SW, Hay WW Jr., Anthony RV. Investigating the causes of low birth weight in contrasting ovine paradigms. J Physiol. 2005;565(Pt 1):19–26.
68. Barry JS, Anthony RV. The pregnant sheep as a model for human pregnancy. Theriogenology. 2008;69(1):55–67.

69. Wallace JM, Aitken RP, Milne JS, Hay WW Jr. Nutritionally mediated placental growth restriction in the growing adolescent: consequences for the fetus. Biol Reprod. 2004;71(4):1055–62.
70. Nielsen JN, O'Brien KO, Witter FR, Chang SC, Mancini J, Nathanson MS, et al. High gestational weight gain does not improve birth weight in a cohort of African American adolescents. Am J Clin Nutr. 2006;84(1):183–9.
71. Ross MG, Desai M, Khorram O, McKnight RA, Lane RH, Torday J. Gestational programming of offspring obesity: a potential contributor to Alzheimer's disease. Curr Alzheimer Res. 2007;4(2):213–7.
72. Crossey PA, Pillai CC, Miell JP. Altered placental development and intrauterine growth restriction in IGF binding protein-1 transgenic mice. J Clin Invest. 2002;110(3):411–8.
73. Coe BL, Kirkpatrick JR, Taylor JA, vom Saal FS. A new 'crowded uterine horn' mouse model for examining the relationship between foetal growth and adult obesity. Basic Clin Pharmacol Toxicol. 2008;102(2):162–7.
74. Tumbleson M. Swine in biomedical research. New York, NY: Plenum Press; 1986.
75. Baker DH. Animal models in nutrition research. J Nutr. 2008;138(2):391–6.
76. Stahl CH, Lei X, Larson B. Introduction to the symposium: appropriate animal models for nutritional research in health and disease. J Nutr. 2008;138(2):389–390.
77. Ireland JJ, Roberts RM, Palmer GH, Bauman DE, Bazer FW. A commentary on domestic animals as dual-purpose models that benefit agricultural and biomedical research. J Anim Sci. 2008;86(10):2797–805.
78. Brambilla G, Cantafora A. Metabolic and cardiovascular disorders in highly inbred lines for intensive pig farming: how animal welfare evaluation could improve the basic knowledge of human obesity. Ann Ist Super Sanita. 2004;40(2):241–4.
79. Spurlock ME, Gabler NK. The development of porcine models of obesity and the metabolic syndrome. J Nutr. 2008;138(2):397–402.
80. Brisbin IL Jr., Mayer JJ. Problem pigs in a poke: a good pool of data. Science. 2001;294(5545):1280–1.
81. Unterberger A, Szyf M, Nathanielsz PW, Cox LA. Organ and gestational age effects of maternal nutrient restriction on global methylation in fetal baboons. J Med Primatol. 2009;38(4):219–27.
82. Ross MG, Beall MH. Adult sequelae of intrauterine growth restriction. Semin Perinatol. 2008;32(3):213–8.
83. Arora S, Anubhuti. Role of neuropeptides in appetite regulation and obesity – a review. Neuropeptides. 2006;40:375–401.
84. Zhang Y, Proenca R, Maffei M, Barone M, Leopold L, Friedman JM. Positional cloning of the mouse obese gene and its human homologue. Nature. 1994;372(6505):425–32.
85. Oliver P, Pico C, De Matteis R, Cinti S, Palou A. Perinatal expression of leptin in rat stomach. Dev Dyn. 2002;223(1):148–54.
86. Cinti S, Matteis RD, Pico C, Ceresi E, Obrador A, Maffeis C, et al. Secretory granules of endocrine and chief cells of human stomach mucosa contain leptin. Int J Obes Relat Metab Disord. 2000;24(6):789–93.
87. Hoggard N, Hunter L, Duncan JS, Williams LM, Trayhurn P, Mercer JG. Leptin and leptin receptor mRNA and protein expression in the murine fetus and placenta. Proc Natl Acad Sci USA. 1997;94(20):11073–8.
88. Masuzaki H, Ogawa Y, Sagawa N, Hosoda K, Matsumoto T, Mise H, et al. Nonadipose tissue production of leptin: leptin as a novel placenta-derived hormone in humans. Nat Med. 1997;3(9):1029–33.
89. Pich EM, Messori B, Zoli M, Ferraguti F, Marrama P, Biagini G, et al. Feeding and drinking responses to neuropeptide Y injections in the paraventricular hypothalamic nucleus of aged rats. Brain Res. 1992;575(2):265–71.
90. Morley JE, Levine AS, Gosnell BA, Kneip J, Grace M. Effect of neuropeptide Y on ingestive behaviors in the rat. Am J Physiol. 1987;252(3 Pt 2):R599–R609.

91. Stanley BG, Leibowitz SF. Neuropeptide Y injected in the paraventricular hypothalamus: a powerful stimulant of feeding behavior. Proc Natl Acad Sci USA. 1985;82(11):3940–3.
92. Stanley BG, Chin AS, Leibowitz SF. Feeding and drinking elicited by central injection of neuropeptide Y: evidence for a hypothalamic site(s) of action. Brain Res Bull. 1985;14(6):521–4.
93. Stanley BG, Leibowitz SF, Neuropeptide Y. stimulation of feeding and drinking by injection into the paraventricular nucleus. Life Sci. 1984;35(26):2635–42.
94. Yokosuka M, Kalra PS, Kalra SP. Inhibition of neuropeptide Y (NPY)-induced feeding and c-Fos response in magnocellular paraventricular nucleus by a NPY receptor antagonist: a site of NPY action. Endocrinology. 1999;140(10):4494–500.
95. Vinuela MC, Larsen PJ. Identification of NPY-induced c-Fos expression in hypothalamic neurones projecting to the dorsal vagal complex and the lower thoracic spinal cord. J Comp Neurol. 2001;438(3):286–99.
96. Yokosuka M, Dube MG, Kalra PS, Kalra SP. The mPVN mediates blockade of NPY-induced feeding by a Y5 receptor antagonist: a c-FOS analysis. Peptides. 2001;22(3):507–14.
97. Niimi M, Sato M, Taminato T. Neuropeptide Y in central control of feeding and interactions with orexin and leptin. Endocrine. 2001;14(2):269–73.
98. Yokosuka M, Xu B, Pu S, Kalra PS, Kalra SP. Neural substrates for leptin and neuropeptide Y (NPY) interaction: hypothalamic sites associated with inhibition of NPY-induced food intake. Physiol Behav. 1998;64(3):331–8.
99. Xu B, Li BH, Rowland NE, Kalra SP. Neuropeptide Y injection into the fourth cerebroventricle stimulates c-Fos expression in the paraventricular nucleus and other nuclei in the forebrain: effect of food consumption. Brain Res. 1995;698(1–2):227–31.
100. Lambert PD, Phillips PJ, Wilding JP, Bloom SR, Herbert J. c-fos expression in the paraventricular nucleus of the hypothalamus following intracerebroventricular infusions of neuropeptide Y. Brain Res. 1995;670(1):59–65.
101. Li BH, Xu B, Rowland NE, Kalra SP. c-fos expression in the rat brain following central administration of neuropeptide Y and effects of food consumption. Brain Res. 1994;665(2):277–84.
102. Pinto S, Roseberry AG, Liu H, Diano S, Shanabrough M, Cai X, et al. Rapid rewiring of arcuate nucleus feeding circuits by leptin. Science. 2004;304(5667):110–5.
103. Takahashi KA, Cone RD. Fasting induces a large, leptin-dependent increase in the intrinsic action potential frequency of orexigenic arcuate nucleus neuropeptide Y/Agouti-related protein neurons. Endocrinology. 2005;146(3):1043–7.
104. Ahima RS, Prabakaran D, Flier JS. Postnatal leptin surge and regulation of circadian rhythm of leptin by feeding. Implications for energy homeostasis and neuroendocrine function. J Clin Invest. 1998;101(5):1020–7.
105. Bouret SG, Simerly RB. Developmental programming of hypothalamic feeding circuits. Clin Genet. 2006;70(4):295–301.
106. Herrera E, Lasuncion MA, Huerta L, Martin-Hidalgo A. Plasma leptin levels in rat mother and offspring during pregnancy and lactation. Biol Neonate. 2000;78(4):315–20.
107. Wirth JB, Epstein AN. Ontogeny of thirst in the infant rat. Am J Physiol. 1976;230(1):188–98.
108. Davidowa H, Plagemann A. Decreased inhibition by leptin of hypothalamic arcuate neurons in neonatally overfed young rats. Neuroreport. 2000;11(12):2795–8.
109. Singer LK, Kuper J, Brogan RS, Smith MS, Grove KL. Novel expression of hypothalamic neuropeptide Y during postnatal development in the rat. Neuroreport. 2000;11(5):1075–80.
110. Varma A, He J, Weissfeld L, Devaskar SU. Postnatal intracerebroventricular exposure to neuropeptide Y causes weight loss in female adult rats. Am J Physiol Regul Integr Comp Physiol. 2003;284(6):R1560–6.
111. Lin J, Richard BC, Kraeling RR, Rampacek GB. Developmental changes in the long form leptin receptor and related neuropeptide gene expression in the pig brain. Biol Reprod. 2001;64(6):1614–8.

112. Matsuda J, Yokota I, Tsuruo Y, Murakami T, Ishimura K, Shima K, et al. Development changes in long-form leptin receptor expression and localization in rat brain. Endocrinology. 1999;140(11):5233–8.
113. Proulx K, Richard D, Walker CD. Leptin regulates appetite-related neuropeptides in the hypothalamus of developing rats without affecting food intake. Endocrinology. 2002;143(12):4683–92.
114. Mistry AM, Swick A, Romsos DR. Leptin alters metabolic rates before acquisition of its anorectic effect in developing neonatal mice. Am J Physiol. 1999;277(3 Pt 2):R742–7.
115. Howe DC, Gertler A, Challis JR. The late gestation increase in circulating ACTH and cortisol in the fetal sheep is suppressed by intracerebroventricular infusion of recombinant ovine leptin. J Endocrinol. 2002;174(2):259–66.
116. Yuen BS, McMillen IC, Symonds ME, Owens PC. Abundance of leptin mRNA in fetal adipose tissue is related to fetal body weight. J Endocrinol. 1999;163(3):R11–4.
117. Anguita RM, Sigulem DM, Sawaya AL. Intrauterine food restriction is associated with obesity in young rats. J Nutr. 1993;123(8):1421–8.
118. Plagemann A, Heidrich I, Gotz F, Rohde W, Dorner G. Obesity and enhanced diabetes and cardiovascular risk in adult rats due to early postnatal overfeeding. Exp Clin Endocrinol. 1992;99(3):154–8.
119. Plagemann A, Harder T, Rake A, Voits M, Fink H, Rohde W, et al. Perinatal elevation of hypothalamic insulin, acquired malformation of hypothalamic galaninergic neurons, and syndrome x-like alterations in adulthood of neonatally overfed rats. Brain Res. 1999;836 (1–2):146–55.
120. Plagemann A, Harder T, Rake A, Waas T, Melchior K, Ziska T, et al. Observations on the orexigenic hypothalamic neuropeptide Y-system in neonatally overfed weanling rats. J Neuroendocrinol. 1999;11(7):541–6.
121. Heidel E, Plagemann A, Davidowa H. Increased response to NPY of hypothalamic VMN neurons in postnatally overfed juvenile rats. Neuroreport. 1999;10(9):1827–31.
122. Davidowa H, Li Y, Plagemann A. Altered neuronal responses to feeding-relevant peptides as sign of developmental plasticity in the hypothalamic regulatory system of body weight. Zh Vyssh Nerv Deiat Im I P Pavlova. 2003;53(5):663–70.
123. Davidowa H, Plagemann A. Different responses of ventromedial hypothalamic neurons to leptin in normal and early postnatally overfed rats. Neurosci Lett. 2000;293(1):21–4.
124. Schmidt I, Schoelch C, Ziska T, Schneider D, Simon E, Plagemann A. Interaction of genetic and environmental programming of the leptin system and of obesity disposition. Physiol Genomics. 2000;3(2):113–20.
125. Davidowa H, Li Y, Plagemann A. Altered responses to orexigenic (AGRP, MCH) and anorexigenic (alpha-MSH, CART) neuropeptides of paraventricular hypothalamic neurons in early postnatally overfed rats. Eur J Neurosci. 2003;18(3):613–21.
126. Davidowa H, Li Y, Plagemann A. Differential response to NPY of PVH and dopamine-responsive VMH neurons in overweight rats. Neuroreport. 2002;13(12):1523–7.
127. Jones AP, Friedman MI. Obesity and adipocyte abnormalities in offspring of rats undernourished during pregnancy. Science. 1982;215(4539):1518–9.
128. Geary M, Pringle PJ, Persaud M, Wilshin J, Hindmarsh PC, Rodeck CH, et al. Leptin concentrations in maternal serum and cord blood: relationship to maternal anthropometry and fetal growth. Br J Obstet Gynaecol. 1999;106(10):1054–60.
129. Hoggard N, Haggarty P, Thomas L, Lea RG. Leptin expression in placental and fetal tissues: does leptin have a functional role? Biochem Soc Trans. 2001;29(Pt 2):57–63.
130. Blum JW, Zbinden Y, Hammon HM, Chilliard Y. Plasma leptin status in young calves: effects of pre-term birth, age, glucocorticoid status, suckling, and feeding with an automatic feeder or by bucket. Domest Anim Endocrinol. 2005;28(2):119–33.
131. Kotani Y, Yokota I, Kitamura S, Matsuda J, Naito E, Kuroda Y. Plasma adiponectin levels in newborns are higher than those in adults and positively correlated with birth weight. Clin Endocrinol (Oxf). 2004;61(4):418–23.

132. McMillen IC, Muhlhausler BS, Duffield JA, Yuen BS. Prenatal programming of postnatal obesity: fetal nutrition and the regulation of leptin synthesis and secretion before birth. Proc Nutr Soc. 2004;63(3):405–12.
133. Eckert JE, Gatford KL, Luxford BG, Campbell RG, Owens PC. Leptin expression in offspring is programmed by nutrition in pregnancy. J Endocrinol. 2000;165(3):R1–6.
134. Warnes KE, Morris MJ, Symonds ME, Phillips ID, Clarke IJ, Owens JA, et al. Effects of increasing gestation, cortisol and maternal undernutrition on hypothalamic neuropeptide Y expression in the sheep fetus. J Neuroendocrinol. 1998;10(1):51–7.
135. Plagemann A, Waas T, Harder T, Rittel F, Ziska T, Rohde W. Hypothalamic neuropeptide Y levels in weaning offspring of low-protein malnourished mother rats. Neuropeptides. 2000;34(1):1–6.
136. Bouret SG, Draper SJ, Simerly RB. Formation of projection pathways from the arcuate nucleus of the hypothalamus to hypothalamic regions implicated in the neural control of feeding behavior in mice. J Neurosci. 2004;24(11):2797–805.
137. Bouret SG, Draper SJ, Simerly RB. Trophic action of leptin on hypothalamic neurons that regulate feeding. Science. 2004;304(5667):108–10.
138. Bouret SG, Simerly RB. Minireview: Leptin and development of hypothalamic feeding circuits. Endocrinology. 2004;145(6):2621–6.
139. Desai M, Gayle D, Han G, Ross MG. Programmed hyperphagia due to reduced anorexigenic mechanisms in intrauterine growth-restricted offspring. Reprod Sci. 2007;14(4):329–37.
140. Yura S, Itoh H, Sagawa N, Yamamoto H, Masuzaki H, Nakao K, et al. Role of premature leptin surge in obesity resulting from intrauterine undernutrition. Cell Metab. 2005;1(6):371–8.
141. Vickers MH, Gluckman PD, Coveny AH, Hofman PL, Cutfield WS, Gertler A, et al. Neonatal leptin treatment reverses developmental programming. Endocrinology. 2005;146(10):4211–6.
142. Desai M, Babu J, Ross MG. Programmed metabolic syndrome: prenatal undernutrition and postweaning overnutrition. Am J Physiol Regul Integr Comp Physiol. 2007;293(6):R2306–14.
143. Cetin I, Morpurgo PS, Radaelli T, Taricco E, Cortelazzi D, Bellotti M, et al. Fetal plasma leptin concentrations: relationship with different intrauterine growth patterns from 19 weeks to term. Pediatr Res. 2000;48(5):646–51.
144. Jaquet D, Leger J, Levy-Marchal C, Oury JF, Czernichow P. Ontogeny of leptin in human fetuses and newborns: effect of intrauterine growth retardation on serum leptin concentrations. J Clin Endocrinol Metab. 1998;83(4):1243–6.
145. Matsuda J, Yokota I, Iida M, Murakami T, Yamada M, Saijo T, et al. Dynamic changes in serum leptin concentrations during the fetal and neonatal periods. Pediatr Res. 1999;45(1):71–5.
146. Cinaz P, Sen E, Bideci A, Ezgu FS, Atalay Y, Koca E. Plasma leptin levels of large for gestational age and small for gestational age infants. Acta Paediatr. 1999;88(7):753–6.
147. Akcurin S, Velipasaoglu S, Akcurin G, Guntekin M. Leptin profile in neonatal gonadotropin surge and relationship between leptin and body mass index in early infancy. J Pediatr Endocrinol Metab. 2005;18(2):189–95.
148. Singhal A, Farooqi IS, O'Rahilly S, Cole TJ, Fewtrell M, Lucas A. Early nutrition and leptin concentrations in later life. Am J Clin Nutr. 2002;75(6):993–9.
149. Desai M, Li T, Ross MG. Developmental programming of dysfunctional hypothalamic neuralo stem cells in leptin deficient, low birth weight newborns. J DOHaD. 2009;1 Suppl 1:S77.
150. Wabitsch M. The acquisition of obesity: insights from cellular and genetic research. Proc Nutr Soc. 2000;59(2):325–30.
151. Slavin BG. Fine structural studies on white adipocyte differentiation. Anat Rec. 1979;195(1):63–72.

152. Gregoire FM, Smas CM, Sul HS. Understanding adipocyte differentiation. Physiol Rev. 1998;78(3):783–809.
153. Hausman DB, DiGirolamo M, Bartness TJ, Hausman GJ, Martin RJ. The biology of white adipocyte proliferation. Obes Rev. 2001;2(4):239–54.
154. Poissonnet CM, Burdi AR, Bookstein FL. Growth and development of human adipose tissue during early gestation. Early Hum Dev. 1983;8(1):1–11.
155. Sypniewska G, Bjorntorp P. Increased DNA synthesis in adipocytes and capillary endothelium in rat adipose tissue during overfeeding. Eur J Clin Invest. 1987;17(3):202–7.
156. Adams M, Montague CT, Prins JB, Holder JC, Smith SA, Sanders L, et al. Activators of peroxisome proliferator-activated receptor gamma have depot-specific effects on human preadipocyte differentiation. J Clin Invest. 1997;100(12):3149–53.
157. Gnanalingham MG, Mostyn A, Symonds ME, Stephenson T. Ontogeny and nutritional programming of adiposity in sheep: potential role of glucocorticoid action and uncoupling protein-2. Am J Physiol Regul Integr Comp Physiol. 2005;289:R1407–15.
158. Symonds ME, Mostyn A, Pearce S, Budge H, Stephenson T. Endocrine and nutritional regulation of fetal adipose tissue development. J Endocrinol. 2003;179(3):293–9.
159. Ailhaud G, Grimaldi P, Negrel R. Cellular and molecular aspects of adipose tissue development. Annu Rev Nutr. 1992;12:207–33.
160. MacDougald OA, Lane MD. Transcriptional regulation of gene expression during adipocyte differentiation. Annu Rev Biochem. 1995;64:345–73.
161. Johnson F. Sex differences in fat patterning in children and youth. In: Bouchard C, Johnson F, editors. Fat distribution during growth and later health outcomes. New York, NY: Liss; 1988. pp. 85–102.
162. Knittle JL, Timmers K, Ginsberg-Fellner F, Brown RE, Katz DP. The growth of adipose tissue in children and adolescents. Cross-sectional and longitudinal studies of adipose cell number and size. J Clin Invest. 1979;63(2):239–46.
163. Gaben-Cogneville AM, Swierczewski E. Studies on cell proliferation in inguinal adipose tissue during early development in the rat. Lipids. 1979;14(7):669–75.
164. Kirtland J, Harris PM. Changes in adipose tissue of the rat due early undernutrition followed by rehabilitation. 3. Changes in cell replication studied with tritiated thymidine. Br J Nutr. 1980;43(1):33–43.
165. Rosen ED, Spiegelman BM. Molecular regulation of adipogenesis. Annu Rev Cell Dev Biol. 2000;16:145–71.
166. Rosen ED, Spiegelman BM. PPARgamma: a nuclear regulator of metabolism, differentiation, and cell growth. J Biol Chem. 2001;276(41):37731–4.
167. Morrison RF, Farmer SR. Insights into the transcriptional control of adipocyte differentiation. J Cell Biochem. 1999; Suppl 32–33:75:59–67.
168. Desai M, Guang H, Ferelli M, Kallichanda N, Lane RH. Programmed upregulation of adipogenic transcription factors in intrauterine growth-restricted offspring. Reprod Sci. 2008;15(8):785–96.
169. Desai M, Lane RH, Han G, Ross MG. Failure to suppress adipogenic transcription factor (PPAR) activity leads to programmed obesity in IUGR offspring. Reprod Sci. 2008;15 Suppl:76A.
170. Powell E, Kuhn P, Xu W. Nuclear receptor cofactors in PPARgamma-mediated adipogenesis and adipocyte energy metabolism. PPAR Res. 2006;2007:53843.
171. Yang T, Fu M, Pestell R, Sauve AA. SIRT1 and endocrine signaling. Trends Endocrinol Metab. 2006;17(5):186–91.
172. Picard F, Kurtev M, Chung N, Topark-Ngarm A, Senawong T, hado De OR, et al. Sirt1 promotes fat mobilization in white adipocytes by repressing PPAR-gamma. Nature. 2004;429(6993):771–6.
173. Kloting N, Bluher M. Extended longevity and insulin signaling in adipose tissue. Exp Gerontol. 2005;40(11):878–83.

174. Walczak R, Tontonoz P. PPARadigms and PPARadoxes: expanding roles for PPARgamma in the control of lipid metabolism. J Lipid Res. 2002;43(2):177–86.
175. Bocher V, Pineda-Torra I, Fruchart JC, Staels B. PPARs: transcription factors controlling lipid and lipoprotein metabolism. Ann N Y Acad Sci. 2002;967:7–18.
176. Schoonjans K, Staels B, Auwerx J. The peroxisome proliferator activated receptors (PPARS) and their effects on lipid metabolism and adipocyte differentiation. Biochim Biophys Acta. 1996;1302(2):93–109.
177. Kim JB, Spiegelman BM. ADD1/SREBP1 promotes adipocyte differentiation and gene expression linked to fatty acid metabolism. Genes Dev. 1996;10(9):1096–107.
178. Ailhaud G, Amri EZ, Grimaldi PA. Fatty acids and adipose cell differentiation. Prostaglandins Leukot Essent Fatty Acids. 1995;52(2–3):113–5.
179. Schoonjans K, Peinado-Onsurbe J, Lefebvre AM, Heyman RA, Briggs M, Deeb S, et al. PPARalpha and PPARgamma activators direct a distinct tissue-specific transcriptional response via a PPRE in the lipoprotein lipase gene. EMBO J. 1996;15(19):5336–48.
180. Kim JB, Sarraf P, Wright M, Yao KM, Mueller E, Solanes G, et al. Nutritional and insulin regulation of fatty acid synthetase and leptin gene expression through ADD1/SREBP1. J Clin Invest. 1998;101(1):1–9.
181. Boizard M, Le LX, Lemarchand P, Foufelle F, Ferre P, Dugail I. Obesity-related overexpression of fatty-acid synthase gene in adipose tissue involves sterol regulatory element-binding protein transcription factors. J Biol Chem. 1998;273(44):29164–71.
182. Desai M, Lane RH, Han G, Ross MG. Response of IUGR primary cell culture adipocytes to PPARg activator-ligand and repressor-ligand mechanisms of programmed obesity. Reprod Sci. 2008;15 Suppl:194A.
183. Fowden AL, Giussani DA, Forhead AJ. Endocrine and metabolic programming during intrauterine development. Early Hum Dev. 2005;81(9):723–34.
184. Phillips DI. Fetal programming of the neuroendocrine response to stress: links between low birth weight and the metabolic syndrome. Endocr Res. 2004;30(4):819–26.
185. Lesage J, Blondeau B, Grino M, Breant B, Dupouy JP. Maternal undernutrition during late gestation induces fetal overexposure to glucocorticoids and intrauterine growth retardation, and disturbs the hypothalamo-pituitary adrenal axis in the newborn rat. Endocrinology. 2001;142(5):1692–702.
186. Benediktsson R, Lindsay RS, Noble J, Seckl JR, Edwards CR. Glucocorticoid exposure in utero: new model for adult hypertension. Lancet. 1993;341(8841):339–41.
187. O'Regan D, Kenyon CJ, Seckl JR, Holmes MC. Glucocorticoid exposure in late gestation in the rat permanently programs gender-specific differences in adult cardiovascular and metabolic physiology. Am J Physiol Endocrinol Metab. 2004;287(5):E863–E70.
188. Murphy BE, Clark SJ, Donald IR, Pinsky M, Vedady D. Conversion of maternal cortisol to cortisone during placental transfer to the human fetus. Am J Obstet Gynecol. 1974;118(4):538–41.
189. Brown RW, Chapman KE, Kotelevtsev Y, Yau JL, Lindsay RS, Brett L, et al. Cloning and production of antisera to human placental 11 beta-hydroxysteroid dehydrogenase type 2. Biochem J. 1996;313(Pt 3):1007–17.
190. Stewart PM, Rogerson FM, Mason JI. Type 2 11 beta-hydroxysteroid dehydrogenase messenger ribonucleic acid and activity in human placenta and fetal membranes: its relationship to birth weight and putative role in fetal adrenal steroidogenesis. J Clin Endocrinol Metab. 1995;80(3):885–90.
191. Symonds ME, Budge H, Stephenson T, Gardner DS. Leptin, fetal nutrition, and long-term outcomes for adult hypertension. Endothelium. 2005;12(1–2):73–9.
192. Rajala MW, Scherer PE. Minireview: The adipocyte – at the crossroads of energy homeostasis, inflammation, and atherosclerosis. Endocrinology. 2003;144(9):3765–73.
193. Shepherd PR, Crowther NJ, Desai M, Hales CN, Ozanne SE. Altered adipocyte properties in the offspring of protein malnourished rats. Br J Nutr. 1997;78(1):121–9.

194. Kubota N, Terauchi Y, Miki H, Tamemoto H, Yamauchi T, Komeda K, et al. PPAR gamma mediates high-fat diet-induced adipocyte hypertrophy and insulin resistance. Mol Cell. 1999;4(4):597–609.
195. Bluher M, Michael MD, Peroni OD, Ueki K, Carter N, Kahn BB, et al. Adipose tissue selective insulin receptor knockout protects against obesity and obesity-related glucose intolerance. Dev Cell. 2002;3(1):25–38.
196. Hara K, Kubota N, Tobe K, Terauchi Y, Miki H, Komeda K, et al. The role of PPARgamma as a thrifty gene both in mice and humans. Br J Nutr. 2000;84 Suppl 2:S235–9.
197. Kadowaki T, Hara K, Kubota N, Tobe K, Terauchi Y, Yamauchi T, et al. The role of PPARgamma in high-fat diet-induced obesity and insulin resistance. J Diabetes Complications. 2002;16(1):41–5.
198. Passos MC, Vicente LL, Lisboa PC, de Moura EG. Absence of anorectic effect to acute peripheral leptin treatment in adult rats whose mothers were malnourished during lactation. Horm Metab Res. 2004;36(9):625–9.
199. Djiane J, Attig L. Role of leptin during perinatal metabolic programming and obesity. J Physiol Pharmacol. 2008;59 Suppl 1:55–63.
200. Melnik BC. Milk–the promoter of chronic Western diseases. Med Hypotheses. 2009;72(6):631–9.
201. Vickers MH. Developmental programming and adult obesity: the role of leptin. Curr Opin Endocrinol Diabetes Obes. 2007;14(1):17–22.
202. Ukkola O. Ghrelin and metabolic disorders. Curr Protein Pept Sci. 2009;10(1):2–7.
203. Hammond RA. Complex systems modeling for obesity research. Prev Chronic Dis. 2009;6(3):A97.

Chapter 12
Experimental Models of Maternal Obesity and High-Fat Diet During Pregnancy and Programmed Obesity in the Offspring

Larissa Jane Prior, Geoffrey Albert Head, and James Andrew Armitage

12.1 Introduction

In the past 30–40 years, the prevalence of obesity has increased worldwide. So great is the anticipated burden of obesity and obesity-related disease, the World Health Organization predicts that obesity-related disease will exceed that of malnutrition and infection in the 21st century [1]. Globally, a 50% increase in obesity was reported in the incidence of obesity from 1995 to 2000 and current estimates from the International Obesity Task Force suggest that over 300 million adults are obese and a further 1 billion are overweight [2]. The marked rise in the prevalence of obesity in recent decades is explained by behavioral and environmental changes that have resulted from an increased availability of highly processed, high-fat, and energy-dense food and decreased physical activity through technological advances.

There is also emerging evidence that the environment encountered during fetal and neonatal life can alter fetal and neonatal developmental processes, rendering individuals more susceptible to adult disease. Evidence for the fetal or developmental programming of adulthood disease originated from epidemiological studies that related patterns of infant mortality and socioeconomic pressure with subsequent adult disease. One of the first studies to causally link poverty and infant mortality rates to subsequent disease examined the relationship between socioeconomic class at birth across a range of Norwegian counties in the early 20th century and arteriosclerotic heart disease 40–69 years later [3]. In 1986, a landmark study by Barker and Osmond found that the geographical distribution of infant mortality between 1921–1925 in England and Wales was closely related to mortality rates from stroke and cardiovascular disease in 1968–1978. Further studies supported the hypothesis that poor nutrition and living conditions encountered in early life were important determinants of stroke and ischemic heart disease [4] and glucose intolerance [5, 6]. Other epidemiological studies conducted worldwide have

J.A. Armitage (✉)
Department of Anatomy and Developmental Biology, School of Biomedical Sciences, Monash University, VIC, 3800, Australia
e-mail: james.armitage@monash.edu

R.H. Lustig (ed.), *Obesity Before Birth*, Endocrine Updates 30,
DOI 10.1007/978-1-4419-7034-3_12, © Springer Science+Business Media, LLC 2011

found associations between early growth patterns and an increased risk for developing hypertension, impaired glucose tolerance, type 2 diabetes, insulin resistance, obesity, and metabolic syndrome in adult life [7–10]. Although maternal dietary restriction in pregnancy can program offspring obesity and metabolic dysfunction, in many societies, maternal obesity and overnutrition are more prevalent today.

The rising prevalence of obesity, particularly among women of reproductive ages, is presenting a formidable challenge to health care. Within a decade, there has been a twofold rise in the number of pregnant women identified as obese at the time of registering for primary care within the UK, an increase from 9.4% obese women in 1990 to 18.9% in 2002/2004 [11]. Similar estimates are observed in the USA, where 18–35% of pregnant women are considered clinically obese [12], and in Australia, where 20% of pregnant women are overweight and 12% obese [13]. Overweight and obese pregnant women have a greater risk of obstetric complications compared to normal body weight mothers, including hypertensive disorders, gestational diabetes, thromboembolic events, and cesarean section [12–16].

Maternal obesity not only has direct implications for the health of a pregnancy but also impacts on the weight of the child in infancy and beyond, as heavier mothers tend to have heavier babies who subsequently become heavier as adults [17]. Several studies report a J-shaped or U-shaped relationship with birthweight and adult BMI, with highest prevalence of obesity in later life being associated with the lowest and highest birthweights [17–20]. The rate of large for gestational age (LGA) neonates that are 4,500 g or heavier (macrosomia) is higher among morbidly obese women than among normal weight women [16, 21, 22], and the finding of a Swedish birthweight cohort suggests that the 23% increase in macrosomia in the years 1991–2002 could be attributed mainly to increases in maternal weight (and a cessation in maternal smoking) [23].

12.2 Animal Models to Study the Role of Maternal Diet in Pregnancy on Offspring Health and Disease

Despite the evidence from long-term retrospective epidemiological studies supporting the developmental origins of health and disease hypothesis, such studies are limited in their ability to provide insight into the mechanisms that underlie the phenomenon, and not amenable to invasive sampling. Hence, animal models of developmental programming have been utilized to understand the mechanistic and molecular bases that link early nutrition and growth to risk for adult disease [7, 8].

Experimental models utilizing the rat, mouse, rabbit, guinea pig, pig, and sheep have many advantages, including a short life span, and genetic and environmental influences that can be carefully controlled [8]. These models also have inherent limitations; however it is the ability to tightly control environmental and genetic variables that makes contribution of animal studies to the developmental programming of adulthood disease invaluable. In fact, early studies, conducted in *Wistar* rats demonstrated that maternal dietary protein restriction in pregnancy was directly associated with programming of offspring hypertension; recapitulating the findings from human studies that implicated maternal nutrition in a controlled genetic and dietary environment [24]. Moreover, initial studies in rats proved useful in defining the so-called programming vectors [25], those factors that may cross from the maternal to fetal compartments and initiate changes in fetal development that lead to the eventual programmed phenotype.

The epidemiological data offer evidence that babies born of low (<5 lb) and very high (>10 lb) birthweight are at similar risk (odds ratios of 1.39 and 1.6, respectively, vs. the reference 8 lb population) for developing hypertension [19] in later life and a similar pattern is seen for diabetes risk [26]. Although animal models of maternal dietary insufficiency provided pivotal evidence that maternal dietary manipulation could induce programmed changes in offspring, the growing obesity epidemic in the Western world required the development of models in which to study the effects of maternal obesity, high-fat intake, and hypercaloric intake during pregnancy upon health and well-being of the offspring.

12.3 Animal Models of Maternal Obesity, Hypercaloric Diet, and High-Fat Feeding

In recent years, a number of studies have examined the effects of maternal hypercaloric diets, maternal obesity, or high-fat feeding in pregnancy and the programming consequences for offspring of such pregnancies.

Offspring of rat and mouse models of maternal high-fat feeding, maternal obesity, or maternal consumption of a highly palatable diet are characterized by a phenotype that includes increased adiposity [27–29], hyperleptinemia [27, 29], leptin resistance [30], hypertension [27, 29, 30], tachycardia [27, 30], vascular endothelial dysfunction [27, 31, 32], hyperglycemia [28, 29, 33], insulin resistance [28, 33], hepatic lipid accumulation [28, 34], non-alcoholic fatty pancreas [35], pancreatic islet cell exhaustion [36], and altered renal biochemical activity [30, 31, 37]. Appetite circuits in the hypothalamus are altered in offspring of high-fat fed or obese rodents, providing the neurobiological impetus for the development of obesity and related disease in later life [38].

Rodent models have the advantage of short life span, stable genetics, and can be studied in large numbers; however, lipid metabolism and handling in rats and mice differ from that in humans significantly. In addition, rodents, being altricial species are born with fused eyelids, an immature brain, peripheral nervous system and renal system, and significant maturation occurs in the early postnatal period. Moreover, rodents have multiparous pregnancies giving birth to 5–15 pups. Humans, on the other hand, are a precocial species born with open eyes, more mature peripheral nervous and renal systems, and usually have singleton or twin pregnancies.

Guinea pigs are a precocial species, and although multiparous, tend to have three to four pups per litter. Moreover gestation is relatively short (~70 days). Notwithstanding these apparent advantages, studies describing developmental programming in guinea pigs are few (compared with other rodent species) and we are not aware of studies of the programming effects of maternal obesity or overnutrition in this species. Newborn offspring of high-fat-fed guinea pigs demonstrate elevations in cell membrane phospholipids and plasma triglycerides that are commensurate with the level of maternal supplementation [39], but it is not clear whether such developmental changes are permanent; as animals remained on their mother's diet throughout life and therefore it is not possible to differentiate between programmed and current dietary factors.

Ovine models have been extensively used to understand the role of maternal obesity and overfeeding and are the subject of two excellent reviews [7, 40]. Gestation is moderately long (~147 days). Pregnancies are usually singleton or twin, although triplet pregnancies do also occur. The advantage of ovine models is the size and robustness of the fetal lamb which gives researchers the opportunity to chronically instrument to measure hemodynamics or take multiple blood samples in utero and then to follow animals into adulthood. Furthermore, sheep are a precocial species like humans and are born with relatively mature organ systems. Maternal obesity is produced by provision of increased ration volume or caloric load [41]. Thirty-day-old offspring of overnourished sheep fed a 40% increase in metabolizable energy from standard rations show increased adiposity, plasma glucose concentrations, and altered expression of hypothalamic appetite modulatory peptides [41]. Fetal offspring of ewes fed a 50% increase in metabolizable energy for 60 days prior to mating and during pregnancy demonstrate elevated inflammatory cytokine expression in placenta [42] and reduced insulin signaling [43] and insulin resistance [44] in skeletal muscle at fetal day 75. To date, there is a lack of data in ovine models describing the effect of maternal obesity on adult offspring with regard to obesity, hypertension, and insulin resistance. To the authors' knowledge there are no reports of programming in sheep following provision of a high-fat diet to ewes during pregnancy, although one study found a positive association between omega-3 fatty acid supplementation and length of gestation [45].

Non-human primates are likely the best approximation of an animal model to study the mechanistic processes that underlie human programming. Despite the cost, longer life span, gestational duration, and a host of other technical issues, a range of studies show that maternal fat intake in pregnancy can program offspring obesity, appetite [46], inflammation [46] in Macaque monkeys, which are accompanied by changes in metabolic profiles [47] and epigenetic marks [47]. Interestingly these animals appear to show altered behavior which is accompanied by dysregulation of serotonergic signaling [48].

12.4 What Is the Stimulus to Developmental Programming Following Maternal Obesity, Hypercaloric Diet, or High-Fat Feeding?

Despite the fact that many studies of maternal fat feeding report hypertension, obesity, or metabolic disturbances in the offspring, the resultant phenotype varies depending on the composition of the experimental diet and the duration of diet exposure. Indeed, this variability in offspring phenotype raises an important question: is maternal obesity or aspects of fat consumption the most important stimulus for programming of metabolic disease in the offspring? Although the programming vectors – molecules or factors that can cross from the maternal compartment to initiate offspring programming – have been discussed in several reviews [7–9, 49], one of the key unanswered issues is whether maternal obesity, maternal hypercaloric diet or maternal fat intake represent the same risk to developmental programming in offspring.

12.4.1 Elucidating the Programming Effects of Maternal Obesity and Fat Feeding

A wide range of animal studies supports the hypothesis that maternal hypercaloric feeding, high-fat feeding, and/or obesity are associated with developmental programming of an obesity-related hypertension phenotype [8, 9]. There is, however, no consensus as to whether these stimuli exert similar effects on the fetus. This is not an esoteric question. For example, are the offspring of lean pregnant women consuming a fat-rich diet at risk of developing obesity-related hypertension and can obese women decrease the likelihood of programmed obesity in their offspring by consuming a more balanced, moderate calorie diet during pregnancy?

Rodents are useful for these studies as they possess a relatively robust energy homeostatic system. Studies report that rats fed a high-fat diet for several weeks prior to mating and during pregnancy actually reduce food intake such that the overall caloric intake of high-fat fed animals is often the same or only slightly higher than that observed in controls [27, 50]. One study reports lower caloric intake in the high-fat fed dams [28]. The mothers consuming high-fat diets generally demonstrate subtle increases in body weight and plasma metabolic profiles [51]; however, this is not a universal finding. Nonetheless, the offspring of these dams were heavier or demonstrated elevated visceral fat deposits, suggesting that the maternal high-fat diet was the programming stimulus or vector. Offspring of mice fed a highly palatable diet in pregnancy (containing 16% fat and 33% sugar) also develop obesity and hypertension. These pregnant dams develop a phenotype consistent with gestational diabetes and obesity [29, 30]. It is possible that the high sucrose content produces a highly palatable diet that circumvents the hypophagia and calorie-matching observed in simple high-fat feeding. This combination of maternal obesity and high-fat intake in mice [29, 30] appears to produce a striking phenotype, suggesting that the coexistence of a high-fat diet and maternal obesity may exert independent or at least additive programming stimuli on offspring development and disease susceptibility.

The availability of simple sugars, sucrose, glucose, fructose, in the maternal diet is of interest with regard to the programming of obesity and metabolic disease in the offspring. The typical Western diet is high in processed carbohydrates and simple sugars and many experimental diets are high in sucrose and fat and are energy dense.

As such, most animal models of maternal obesity utilize a high-fat high-calorie, high-simple sugar diet but it is not well appreciated which component of the diet may be deleterious to offspring health. Although maternal hyperinsulinemia, hyperleptinemia, and hyperglycemia are often seen in obesity insulin and leptin do not readily cross the placental barrier. It is hypothesized that fetal hyperglycemia and subsequent hyperinsulinemia may stimulate increased fetal growth and alter fetal insulin signaling [52]. Indeed many experimental models of gestational diabetes involve the use of a high-sugar diet to the mother in order to produce fetal hyperglycemia. A small number of studies directly assess the role of maternal sucrose intake in pregnancy with offspring obesity-related disease. Maternal sucrose-rich diets (63% sucrose) promote hypertriglyceridemia in the mother [53] and fetus [54] and this may have an impact on the later cardiovascular health of offspring. Rats fed a 70% sucrose diet for 1 week prior to pregnancy and mice fed a 68.5% sucrose diet during pregnancy give birth to larger pups with elevated plasma glucose and triglycerides than those fed a 68.5% starch diet [55]. Moreover, pups cross-fostered to sucrose-fed dams also developed obesity and dyslipidemia [55]. Certainly, the weaning period is important in rodent life – particularly as many systems mature in the first weeks after births. Pre-weaning rats are able to discriminate between uniquely flavored solutions containing sucrose or saccharin and are conditioned to prefer, in later life, those flavors that were associated with sucrose intake rather than saccharin [56]. Mice fed a high-sucrose diet in the post-weaning period are more motivated to undertake tasks to receive a sugar-rich diet in later life and develop obesity [57]. Maternal fructose intake has differing effects than that of maternal sucrose intake. An early study by Jen et al. showed that offspring of rats fed a 50% fructose diet gave birth to offspring with elevated glucose concentration compared with controls and 50% sucrose-fed rats [58]. Notwithstanding this, a better understanding of the effects of high-sugar diets is warranted.

12.4.2 Programming Effects of Maternal Diets Differing in Types of Fatty Acids

The source of fat in the maternal diet is also an important factor in determining offspring phenotype. Most studies of maternal fat feeding employ diets that are rich in animal fats [8, 9]; however, mounting evidence suggests that fatty acid imbalance may be more important than the quantity of fat intake per se.

Essential omega-3 polyunsaturated fatty acid deprivation in the first 9 weeks of life results in permanent programming of greater blood pressure in 33-week-old *Sprague Dawley* rats, even if dietary omega-3 fatty acids are provided in adult life until brain omega-3 fatty acid levels appeared to be restored [59]. Moreover, consumption of omega-3 fatty acids in early life (to 9 weeks of age) protects against increased blood pressure induced by adult omega-3 fatty acid deprivation in 33-week-old Sprague Dawley rats [59]. Sixteen-week-old Sprague Dawley rats subjected to omega-3 fatty acid deprivation in pregnancy and suckling showed increased appetite and elevated appetite signaling [60]. This programming of hypertension occurred in the absence of maternal obesity, suggesting that even a moderate imbalance of essential fatty acids during gestation can result in offspring disease [61].

In addition to the programming effects of maternal fatty acid deprivation, programming by saturated fatty acids is seen in studies of Cpb-WU rats fed diets containing 18% soy oil (rich in omega-3 and omega-6 polyunsaturated fatty acids), coconut oil (rich in saturated fatty acids), or fish oil (rich in long-chain omega-3 polyunsaturated fatty acids) for 2 weeks prior to mating, during pregnancy, and during suckling. Twelve-week-old offspring of fish oil fed rats showed reduced body weight compared with the other groups, but the offspring of saturated fat-fed dams showed glucose intolerance and a reduction in pancreatic islet cell density [62]. Cardiovascular and renal function can also be programmed by exposure to saturated fatty acids in early life. Six-month-old offspring of Sprague Dawley rats fed a 20% lard diet in pregnancy and during suckling show greater body weight, low renin hypertension, aortic dysfunction, and a reduction in renal Na^+, K^+ ATPase activity compared with offspring of controls [31]; whereas 6-month-old offspring of Sprague Dawley rats fed a 20% omega-3 fatty acid diet showed normal Na^+, K^+ ATPase activity and body weight. These data further support the hypothesis that saturated fatty acid intake contributes to programming of obesity and hypertension in the offspring [37] in rat models.

Thus it appears that maternal diets high in saturated fatty acids or low in essential polyunsaturated fatty acids program offspring phenotypes consistent with a progression to disease. Perhaps maternal intake of diets that contain a high ratio of omega-3:6 polyunsaturated fatty acids are less of a risk to offspring health. Notwithstanding this fact, humans that consume high-fat diets are likely to be overweight or obese due to the fact that fat-rich diets are, by their very nature, energy dense. Thus it would be of interest to understand the programming effects of maternal obesity independent of fat intake and vice versa.

12.4.3 The Relative Importance of Maternal Obesity vs. Maternal Fat Intake in Pregnancy

A recent report in a unique non-human primate model (Macaque monkeys) indicates that maternal fat intake can act as a programming vector independently of obesity [63]. Monkeys fed a high-fat diet (15% vs. 5.5% control) for 2–4 years segregate into two groups: those that become obese and those that are resistant to the high-fat diet. Nonetheless, when these females become pregnant, significant elevation in liver triglyceride content (indicative of impending fatty liver disease) is manifest in fetuses of both obese and diet-resistant animals, suggesting that maternal obesity is not requisite for programming of offspring disease [63]. Further characterization of such a model would be of great interest and clinical relevance. Resistance to diet-induced obesity has been well described in Sprague Dawley rats [64] and offspring of fat-fed obese and obesity-resistant dams both demonstrate alterations in hypothalamic appetite pathways, suggesting that a lean maternal phenotype does not preclude offspring programming, provided a high-fat maternal diet [65].

Nonetheless, it appears that dietary modification in obese rats can minimize the programmed phenotype observed in the offspring. Zambrano et al. demonstrated that maternal obesity in Wistar rats (induced by 69 days of dietary lard supplementation that ceased before pregnancy) still programmed obesity, increased adipocyte size, and insulin resistance in the offspring relative to controls, but with an improved phenotype compared with offspring of rats that persisted with the high-fat diet during pregnancy and suckling [66].

Conversely, White et al. showed that maternal obesity is itself an important programming stimulus. Long Evans rats were fed an ad libitum diet of 30% fat, an ad libitum control diet of 5% fat, or the 30% fat diet but pair-fed to receive the same caloric load as the ad libitum control group (thus isocaloric but high fat) [67]. Offspring of the ad libitum high-fat group exhibited greater adiposity and insulin resistance than did offspring of control-fed rats, or rats fed the isocaloric high-fat diet. The authors suggested that maternal weight gain was more important than was fat intake. Interestingly, although offspring of isocaloric fat-fed rats had similar insulin sensitivity to controls, they still demonstrated greater fat mass compared with controls [67], indicating that fat intake can program adipocyte size independent of maternal adiposity. Fetal size is affected both by pre-pregnancy maternal obesity and by hypercaloric diet, but in differing patterns. Akyol et al. fed Wistar rats chow or a cafeteria diet for 8 weeks to induce obesity, and then, prior to mating, half of the group was crossed to examine the effects of obesity prior to pregnancy and an obesogenic diet during pregnancy [68]. Interestingly, fetal weight was reduced in offspring of pre-gravid obese rats irrespective of diet in pregnancy. Fetal:placental ratios were also reduced in pre-gravid obese rats irrespective of diet in pregnancy, but increased in offspring of rats fed the obesogenic diet in pregnancy alone [68]. The data from sheep studies (where offspring demonstrate programmed obesity and altered glucose homeostasis) clearly support the hypothesis that maternal obesity or hypercaloric feeding are sufficient stimuli for programming; however, these studies do not differentiate between the two stimuli [41–44].

Combined, these experimental strategies of cessation of fat feeding in obese rats and the exploitation of models of resistance to obesogenic diets have led to the hypothesis that consumption of a high-fat diet in pregnancy, even by lean individuals, may be deleterious to offspring health. In this light, a more thorough investigation of fatty acid transport across the placenta in models of maternal fat feeding is warranted.

12.4.4 *The Effect of Maternal Hypercholesterolemia in Developmental Programming*

Further evidence that fat intake (especially from animal sources) can program adult dysfunction independent of obesity can be found in studies of maternal hypercholesterolemia, which may manifest in either obesity or with consumption of a high-fat diet, but can be induced experimentally by maternal cholesterol supplementation. Data from the FELIC study indicated that normocholesterolemic children who died of trauma, cancer, or cerebral aneurysm exhibited an accelerated progression of aortic fatty streak cross-sectional area if they were born to mothers who were hypercholesterolemic during pregnancy as compared to normocholesterolemic mothers. Maternal weight was not reported; however, maternal diabetes and hypertension did not explain this acceleration in fatty streak development [69]. The authors conducted a follow-up study in New Zealand White rabbits fed a hypercholesterolemic or normal cholesterol diet for 2 weeks prior to mating, throughout gestation, and 2 weeks postpartum. Offspring were fed a control diet from weaning until 1 year of age. Maternal body weights and weight gain during pregnancy and offspring weights were invariant. However, 1-year-old offspring of hypercholesterolemic dams demonstrated greater area of aortic fatty streaks as compared with controls [70]. This same group also examined the effect of maternal hypercholesterolemia in LDL receptor knockout mice and showed a similar phenotype as did the human and rabbit studies [71]. Maternal obesity was not manifest in any of these studies, indicating that hypercholesterolemia can program dyslipidemia independently in the offspring.

12.5 The Postnatal Period Is Important and Implicates a Role for Altered Appetite Circuitry in the Development of Programmed Obesity

In altricial species such as rats and mice, postnatal nutrition is particularly important as significant maturation of most organs occurs rapidly in the early postnatal period [72, 73]. One classical model used to investigate the effects of early postnatal nutrition is the neonatal manipulation of litter size in rodents. This model was first described by McCance who demonstrated that altering litter sizes changes the milk intake of pups and results in an altered growth trajectory into adulthood [74]. Overfeeding during the suckling period of rodents, by reducing the litter sizes to 3–4 pups, has been shown to program dyslipidemia, hyperinsulinemia, hyperleptinemia, increased body weight, and adipose tissue mass [75–79]. Epigenetic changes appear to underlie this phenotype, with up-regulation of appetite stimulatory pathways and down-regulation of appetite inhibitory pathways in the hypothalamus of Wistar rat offspring that were raised in small litters and subject to neonatal overfeeding [80]. In contrast, increasing the number of pups per mother to 18–20 leads to lower growth trajectory and fat mass compared with those raised in a normal litter of 10–12 pups [75, 81].

Gestational diabetes mellitus (often seen with maternal obesity) is also associated with offspring macrosomia and an accelerated postnatal growth trajectory. There has been extensive study of the role of maternal hyperinsulinemia and hyperglycemia and readers are directed to studies by Plagemann and colleagues [82–84] (also see Chapter 9).

Whether the stimulus is the transfer of maternal lipids, hormones (such as leptin, ghrelin, insulin) or alteration in the availability of nutrition, converging lines of evidence point to early postnatal maturation of appetite circuitry in the hypothalamus as a key determinant of later obesity and/or cardiometabolic disease.

12.6 Development of the Appetite Regulatory System

Animal models have been critical in understanding the pathways and systems that regulate appetite and energy expenditure. Although the characterization of such pathways is well established in the adult (see Fig. 12.1), less is known about the

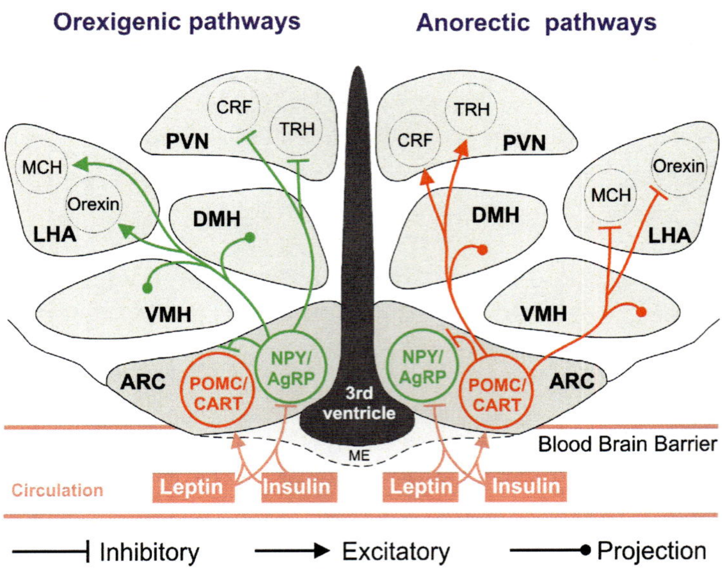

Fig. 12.1 Schematic of the hypothalamus illustrating neural pathways that stimulate appetite and reduce energy expenditure (orexigenic pathways, *green*) or that suppress appetite and increase energy expenditure (anorectic pathways, *red*). Signals from the circulation including leptin, insulin, and ghrelin access the brain in areas such as the median eminence (ME) that lacks a blood–brain barrier. Hormones such as leptin and insulin stimulate neurons co-expressing pro-opiomelanocortin (POMC)/cocaine and amphetamine transcript (CART) (colored *red*) and inhibit neurons co-expressing neuropeptide Y (NPY)/agouti-related transcript (AgRP) (colored *green*) within the arcuate nucleus (ARC). These neurons are proposed to relay these signals to the paraventricular nucleus (PVN), lateral hypothalamic area (LHA), ventromedial hypothalamus (VMH), and dorsomedial hypothalamus (DMH). Neurons in the PVN contain the anorexigenic neuropeptides corticotrophin releasing factor (CRF) and thyroid-releasing hormone (TRH), while neurons in the LHA contain the orexigenic neuropeptides melanin-concentrating hormone (MCH) as well as the orexin peptides. These areas project to higher cortical areas to modulate behavior such as hunger, satiety, and food seeking and hindbrain centers to increase sympathetic outflow to skeletal muscle, brown adipose tissue, and the kidney

development and maturation of these hypothalamic circuits. It has been suggested that an alteration in the environment during a "critical period" of maturation and growth may alter the normal development of the neuronal pathways regulating appetite and energy balance. In order to place this evidence in context, a short discussion of this energy-balance circuitry follows.

The hypothalamus was identified 70 years ago as a major brain region controlling energy homeostasis [85]. Lesion studies led to the proposal of a "dual center" model for regulation of appetite [86]. The ventromedial hypothalamus (VMH; consisting of the ventromedial (VMN) and arcuate (ARC) nuclei), paraventricular nucleus (PVN), and dorsomedial hypothalamus (DMH) were thought to be "satiety centers" as lesions in these areas induced hyperphagia and obesity in rats [85, 87]. Conversely, the lateral hypothalamic area (LHA) was thought to be a "hunger center," as lesions in this area promoted anorexia and starvation [88]. It is now known that these areas harbor leptin-responsive orexigenic and anorexigenic neurons (Fig. 12.1).

The pathways controlling appetite are discussed in significant detail in Chapter 3. In simple terms the ARC is ideally situated to respond to circulating hormones due to the absence of a blood–brain barrier in the median eminence [89]. Two separate populations of neurons mediate the appetite regulatory role of the ARC. One population of neurons are orexigenic and co-express neuropeptide Y (NPY) and agouti-related peptide (AgRP) [90, 91], while an adjacent population of neurons are anorectic and co-express pro-opiomelanocortin (POMC) and cocaine and amphetamine-related transcript (CART) [92, 93]. These two groups of first-order neurons are the primary targets for many peripheral metabolic feedback signals and play an important role in transforming hormonal signals to a neuronal signal. This neuronal signal is then transmitted to hypothalamic second-order neurons located in the VMH, LHA, DMH, and PVN [93].

In the rodent, NPY/AgRP neuronal projections within the ARC are low at birth and are formed primarily during the first and second week of life, innervating the PVN, DMH. and LHA at different time points [72, 94, 95]. Moreover, these projections are not mature until the third week of life, when pups begin to leave the microenvironment of the nest and search for solid food [96]. This indicates that the postnatal period in the rodent may be a particularly important period of development where appetite circuits may be susceptible to environmental and nutritional stimuli. Wistar rats suckled in small litters ($n = 3$ as compared with normal $n = 8$) demonstrate decreased electrophysiological responses to centrally applied NPY and MHC in adulthood [97]. Such small litter-raised rats demonstrate hypermethylation of the POMC promoter, consistent with a reduction in satiety signaling [80]. In contrast, development of NPY projections in ARC of non-humans primate is nearly complete at birth, forming predominantly during the third trimester [98]. This development is similar in the human fetus, where NPY neurons have been observed to first appear in the ARC in the late second trimester, with a progressive increase in NPY neurons during the third trimester [99]. Accordingly, fetal (third trimester) offspring of high-fat fed mothers demonstrate a reduction in POMC expression and elevated AgRP expression in the hypothalamus as compared with controls, indicating an elevation in appetite signaling pathways prior to birth [46]. Hence the "critical" period for hypothalamic circuits involved in appetite and energy balance in the human vs. rodent is likely to occur at different periods of gestation or lactation. Abnormalities in the formation of appetite circuits may underlie risk for obesity and diabetes in adulthood [73].

Recently leptin has been recognized as a trophic factor in the neural circuitry of energy homeostasis [73, 96, 100]. Development of ARC projections correlate with the postnatal leptin surge (1–2 weeks) in the rodent [101, 102]. Administration of leptin during this period is ineffective at reducing body weight, milk intake, or metabolic rate in C57BL/6 J mice [103]. This was originally interpreted as an indication that the neonatal brain is relatively insensitive to leptin as a mechanism to enhance survival by promoting feeding [103]. However, an alternate hypothesis is that this leptin surge functions as a developmental signal important for the growth of many hypothalamic circuits involved in appetite, energy expenditure, and the sympathetic nervous system (SNS) [104, 105]. Indeed, offspring of C57BL/6 mice fed an obesogenic diet for 6 weeks prior to mating and during pregnancy and suckling exhibit an exaggerated and prolonged leptin surge between postnatal days 6 and 18 [38]. In adulthood, these offspring demonstrate selective leptin resistance and alterations in hypothalamic AgRP expression [38]. Several lines of evidence support the hypothesis that leptin is a trophic factor for CNS development. For example, brain development is abnormal in leptin-deficient obese (*ob/ob*) and leptin receptor diabetic (*db/db*) mice [104, 105]. These *ob/ob* mice have profound disruptions in the development of the ARC projections to other downstream nuclei including the PVN. Interestingly this disruption can be normalized following leptin treatment during the first 2 weeks after birth, but not later in life [96]. This postnatal leptin treatment in *ob/ob* mice influences appetite in the long term, as feeding is reduced in leptin-treated *ob/ob* mice as compared to untreated *ob/ob* for weeks after leptin discontinuation [96]. Furthermore, leptin has been shown to directly promote the outgrowth of neurites from isolated ARC ex vivo cultures of 6-day-old mice [96], and exogenous leptin treatment during the postnatal period in Sprague Dawley rats has been shown to cause abnormal expression of NPY, AgRP, and POMC in the ARC [106]. Hence, an alteration in the timing or amplitude of the leptin surge during development as a consequence of exposure to overnutrition could alter the growth of hypothalamic circuits and lead to permanent changes to appetite and energy expenditure.

12.7 Programming of SNS Activity, Obesity, and Hypertension

Key to the neurobiological basis of obesity-related hypertension is the dual role of several hypothalamic nuclei that modulate energy homeostasis. Although there are complex behavioral inputs to energy homeostasis other inputs, such as non-exercise-associated thermogenesis (fidgeting) and sympathetically controlled thermogenesis, are also vital determinants [107]. Obesity is associated with increased blood pressure within the metabolic syndrome. Early hypotheses suggested that weight gain occurred due to low SNS activity [108]; however, direct SNS recording and noradrenaline spillover from sympathetic nerves indicate elevated sympathetic outflow to kidneys and skeletal muscle vasculature in obese humans, while SNS tone to the heart is reduced [109]. This disparity in SNS activity to different peripheral beds may explain why energy homeostasis and hemodynamics become deranged in obesity. In mouse models, SNS-mediated thermogenesis in brown adipose tissue has been found to be elevated in obesity [110, 111]. Landsberg hypothesized [112] that SNS activation occurs in obesity to facilitate energy wastage by thermogenesis in order to reduce body weight. The adverse consequence of chronic stimulation of the SNS is hypertension. The neurobiological basis of appetite control and elevated SNS activity most likely lies in the hypothalamic nuclei that control food intake, blood pressure, and renal sympathetic drive [113, 114] as well as their response to appetite controlling peptides leptin [113] and ghrelin [115].

Our studies [116] offer evidence that relatively short-term high-fat feeding can result in obesity-related hypertension and increased plasma noradrenaline concentrations. The mechanism underlying the hypertension may be increased adipose tissue release of leptin, which drives augmented renal sympathetic tone. Moreover, neural activity in the hypothalamus appears abnormal in high-fat fed rabbits, as evidenced by reduced *c-fos* immunoreactivity following leptin injection, but animals demonstrated enhanced sensitivity to the autonomic and cardiovascular actions of centrally administered leptin and selective leptin resistance. This apparently counterintuitive finding most likely occurs because of an imbalance of excitatory inputs (measured by *c-fos* immunohistochemistry) and inhibitory inputs which were not assessed. Nonetheless, even though the neurobiology of selective leptin resistance is yet to be fully elucidated, the hypothalamus appears central to the generation of obesity-related hypertension. Combined, these data suggest that relatively short-term high-fat feeding may result in obesity-related hypertension due to altered SNS activity [117]. Peripheral sympathetic nerves release NPY in response to stress; particularly chronic stress [118] which may manifest as increased basal SNS activity. NPY may contribute to increased adiposity because it causes proliferation of pre-adipocytes [119]. NPY may also act on the peripheral vasculature promoting atherosclerosis [120]. Igosheva et al. demonstrated increased NPY-mediated peripheral vasoconstriction in offspring of stress-affected rats [121], which is consistent with a role for both the SNS and the NPY. We and others hypothesize that maternal obesity or high-fat diet in pregnancy may disrupt hypothalamic/hindbrain pathways to induce increased SNS activity. There are, however, scarce data to support this hypothesis. Recently Samuelsson et al. showed that offspring of C57BL/6 mice fed an obesogenic diet in pregnancy and suckling have elevated renal noradrenaline content, consistent with increased renal SNS activity [30]. There is a clear need for further studies that examine the link maternal obesity and/or high-fat feeding with offspring obesity-related hypertension and SNS activity, as the relationship and underlying mechanisms remain largely undefined.

12.8 Perspectives

The worldwide epidemic of obesity and related cardiometabolic disease may, in some part, be determined by exposure to an early-life environment that is consistent with maternal obesity or a maternal high-fat diet in pregnancy or lactation. Although not all studies are supportive (particularly those in sheep), it appears likely that the consumption of a high-fat diet may be more deleterious to the offspring's health than maternal obesity per se. Moreover, diets that are high in saturated fat or cholesterol appear to carry the greatest likelihood of inducing programmed obesity and cardio metabolic disease. This has clear relevance to public health messages to women who are planning pregnancy. Although pre-existing obesity is one factor to be considered, a diet low in saturated fat may prove to be important in reducing the burden of programmed obesity for the next generation.

Although the validity of animal models for the study of mechanisms underlying developmental programming in humans is often questioned, nonetheless the data from rodent and non-human primate models are in remarkable concordance. A number of studies suggest that exposure to a high-fat diet during maturation of hypothalamic appetite circuits can result in a shifting in the balance of appetite stimulatory and inhibitory pathways to promote hyperphagia. The cellular mechanisms underlying this phenomenon are gradually being elucidated. Moreover, the complex relationship between obesity and hypertension suggests a dual role of hypothalamic nuclei in initiating feeding and sympathetic outflow. This promising avenue of research may prove pivotal in determining strategies to manage obesity-related hypertension and cardiovascular disease.

References

1. World Health Organisation. Obesity: preventing and managing the global epidemic. Report of a WHO consultation. World Health Organ Tech Rep Ser. 2000;894:i–xii, 1–253.
2. Pitkin RM, Institute of Medicine. Nutritional status and weight gain. In: editors. Subcommittee on nutritional status and weight gain during pregnancy, food and nutrition board. Nutrition during pregnancy. Washington, DC: National Academy Press, 1990. p. 27. International Obesity Task Force, 1990.
3. Forsdahl A. Are poor living conditions in childhood and adolescence an important risk factor for arteriosclerotic heart disease? Br J Prev Soc Med. 1977;31:91–5.
4. Barker DJ, Osmond C. Infant mortality, childhood nutrition, and ischaemic heart disease in England and Wales. Lancet. 1986;1:1077–81.
5. Hales C, Barker D, Clark P, et al. Fetal and infant growth and impaired glucose tolerance at age 64. BMJ. 1991;303:1019–22.
6. Barker DJ, Hales CN, Fall CH, et al. Type 2 (non-insulin-dependent) diabetes mellitus, hypertension and hyperlipidaemia (syndrome X): relation to reduced fetal growth. Diabetologia. 1993;36:62–7.
7. McMillen IC, Robinson JS. Developmental origins of the metabolic syndrome: prediction, plasticity, and programming. Physiol Rev. 2005;85:571–633.
8. Armitage JA, Khan IY, Taylor PD, et al. Developmental programming of the metabolic syndrome by maternal nutritional imbalance: how strong is the evidence from experimental models in mammals? J Physiol. 2004;561:355–77.

9. Armitage JA, Taylor PD, Poston L. Experimental models of developmental programming: consequences of exposure to an energy rich diet during development. J Physiol. 2005;565: 3–8.
10. Wells JC. Historical cohort studies and the early origins of disease hypothesis: making sense of the evidence. Proc Nutr Soc. 2009;68:179–88.
11. Kanagalingam MG, Forouhi NG, Greer IA, et al. Changes in booking body mass index over a decade: retrospective analysis from a Glasgow Maternity Hospital. BJOG. 2005;112: 1431–3.
12. Galtier-Dereure F, Boegner C, Bringer J. Obesity and pregnancy: complications and cost. Am J Clin Nutr. 2000;71:1242S–8S.
13. Callaway LK, Prins JB, Chang AM, et al. The prevalence and impact of overweight and obesity in an Australian obstetric population. Med J Aust. 2006;184:56–9.
14. Armitage JA, Poston L, Taylor PD. Developmental origins of obesity and the metabolic syndrome: the role of maternal obesity. Front Horm Res. 2008;36:73–84.
15. Ostlund I, Haglund B, Hanson U. Gestational diabetes and preeclampsia. Eur J Obstet Gynecol Reprod Biol. 2004;113:12–6.
16. Kumari AS. Pregnancy outcome in women with morbid obesity. Int J Gynaecol Obstet. 2001;73:101–7.
17. Parsons TJ, Power C, Manor O. Fetal and early life growth and body mass index from birth to early adulthood in 1958 British cohort: longitudinal study. BMJ. 2001;323:1331–5.
18. Seidman DS, Laor A, Gale R, et al. A longitudinal study of birth weight and being overweight in late adolescence. Am J Dis Child. 1991;145:782–5.
19. Curhan GC, Chertow GM, Willett WC, et al. Birth weight and adult hypertension and obesity in women. Circulation. 1996;94:1310–5.
20. Curhan GC, Willett WC, Rimm EB, et al. Birth weight and adult hypertension, diabetes mellitus, and obesity in US men. Circulation. 1996;94:3246–50.
21. Edwards LE, Hellerstedt WL, Alton IR, et al. Pregnancy complications and birth outcomes in obese and normal-weight women: effects of gestational weight change. Obstet Gynecol. 1996;87:389–94.
22. Perlow JH, Morgan MA, Montgomery D, et al. Perinatal outcome in pregnancy complicated by massive obesity. Am J Obstet Gynecol. 1992;167:958–62.
23. Surkan PJ, Hsieh CC, Johansson AL, et al. Reasons for increasing trends in large for gestational age births. Obstet Gynecol. 2004;104:720–6.
24. Langley SC, Jackson AA. Increased systolic blood pressure in adult rats induced by fetal exposure to maternal low protein diets. Clin Sci. 1994;86:217–22.
25. Taylor PD, Poston L. Developmental programming of obesity in mammals. Exp Physiol. 2007;92:287–98.
26. Catalano PM, Kirwan JP, Haugel-de Mouzon S, et al. Gestational diabetes and insulin resistance: role in short- and long-term implications for mother and fetus. J Nutr. 2003;133:1674S–83S.
27. Khan IY, Taylor PD, Dekou V, et al. Gender-linked hypertension in offspring of lard-fed pregnant rats. Hypertension. 2003;41:168–75.
28. Guo F, Jen KL. High-fat feeding during pregnancy and lactation affects offspring metabolism in rats. Physiol Behav. 1995;57:681–6.
29. Samuelsson AM, Matthews PA, Argenton M, et al. Diet-induced obesity in female mice leads to offspring hyperphagia, adiposity, hypertension, and insulin resistance: a novel murine model of developmental programming. Hypertension. 2008;51:383–92.
30. Samuelsson AM, Morris A, Igosheva N, et al. Evidence for sympathetic origins of hypertension in juvenile offspring of obese rats. Hypertension. 2010;55:76–82.
31. Armitage JA, Lakasing L, Taylor PD, et al. Developmental programming of aortic and renal structure in offspring of rats fed fat-rich diets in pregnancy. J Physiol. 2005;565:171–84.
32. Taylor PD, Khan IY, Hanson MA, et al. Impaired EDHF-mediated vasodilatation in adult offspring of rats exposed to a fat-rich diet in pregnancy. J Physiol. 2004;558:943–51.

33. Taylor PD, McConnell J, Khan IY, et al. Impaired glucose homeostasis and mitochondrial abnormalities in offspring of rats fed a fat-rich diet in pregnancy. Am J Physiol Regul Integr Comp Physiol. 2005;288:R134–9.
34. Bayol SA, Simbi BH, Fowkes RC, et al. A maternal "junk food" diet in pregnancy and lactation promotes nonalcoholic fatty liver disease in rat offspring. Endocrinology. 2010;151:1451–61.
35. Oben JA, Patel T, Mouralidarane A, et al. Maternal obesity programmes offspring development of non-alcoholic fatty pancreas disease. Biochem Biophys Res Commun. 2010;394:24–8.
36. Taylor PD, Persaud SJ, Jones PM, et al. Reduced insulin secretory capacity in the hypertensive adult offspring of rats exposed to a high fat diet in pregnancy. J Soc Gynecol Invest. 2004;11:305A.
37. Armitage JA, Gupta S, Wood C, et al. Maternal dietary supplementation with saturated, but not monounsaturated or polyunsaturated fatty acids, leads to tissue-specific inhibition of offspring Na^+, K^+-ATPase. J Physiol. 2008;586:5013–22.
38. Kirk SL, Samuelsson AM, Argenton M, et al. Maternal obesity induced by diet in rats permanently influences central processes regulating food intake in offspring. PLoS One. 2009;4:e5870.
39. Pavey DE, Widdowson EM, Robinson MP. Body lipids of guinea pigs exposed to different dietary fats from mid-gestation to 3 months of age. II. The fatty acid composition of the lipids of liver, plasma, adipose tissue, muscle and red cell membranes at birth. Nutr Metab. 1976;20:351–63.
40. McMillen IC, Rattanatray L, Duffield JA, et al. The early origins of later obesity: pathways and mechanisms. Adv Exp Med Biol. 2009;646:71–81.
41. Muhlhausler BS, Duffield JA, McMillen IC. Increased maternal nutrition increases leptin expression in perirenal and subcutaneous adipose tissue in the postnatal lamb. Endocrinology. 2007;148:6157–63.
42. Zhu MJ, Du M, Nathanielsz PW, et al. Maternal obesity up-regulates inflammatory signaling pathways and enhances cytokine expression in the mid-gestation sheep placenta. Placenta. 2010 vol. 31(5):387–91.
43. Zhu MJ, Han B, Tong J, et al. AMP-activated protein kinase signalling pathways are down regulated and skeletal muscle development impaired in fetuses of obese, over-nourished sheep. J Physiol. 2008;586:2651–64.
44. Yan X, Zhu MJ, Xu W, et al. Up-regulation of Toll-like receptor 4/nuclear factor-kappaB signaling is associated with enhanced adipogenesis and insulin resistance in fetal skeletal muscle of obese sheep at late gestation. Endocrinology. 2010;151:380–7.
45. Capper JL, Wilkinson RG, Mackenzie AM, et al. Polyunsaturated fatty acid supplementation during pregnancy alters neonatal behavior in sheep. J Nutr. 2006;136:397–403.
46. Grayson BE, Levasseur PR, Williams SM, et al. Changes in melanocortin expression and inflammatory pathways in fetal offspring of nonhuman primates fed a high-fat diet. Endocrinology. 2010;151:1622–32.
47. Aagaard-Tillery KM, Grove K, Bishop J, et al. Developmental origins of disease and determinants of chromatin structure: maternal diet modifies the primate fetal epigenome. J Mol Endocrinol. 2008;41:91–102.
48. Sullivan EL, Grayson B, Takahashi D, et al. Chronic consumption of a high-fat diet during pregnancy causes perturbations in the serotonergic system and increased anxiety-like behavior in nonhuman primate offspring. J Neurosci. 2010;30:3826–30.
49. McMillen IC, Adam CL, Muhlhausler BS. Early origins of obesity: programming the appetite regulatory system. J Physiol. 2005;565:9–17.
50. Khan IY, Dekou V, Douglas G, et al. A high-fat diet during rat pregnancy or suckling induces cardiovascular dysfunction in adult offspring. Am J Physiol Regul Integr Comp Physiol. 2005;288:R127–R33.
51. Taylor PD, Khan IY, Lakasing L, et al. Uterine artery function in pregnant rats fed a diet supplemented with animal lard. Exp Physiol. 2003;88:389–98.

52. Pederson J. The pregnant diabetic and her newborn. 2nd ed. Baltimore, MD: Williams and Wilkins; 1977.
53. Munilla MA, Herrera E. Maternal hypertriglyceridemia during late pregnancy does not affect the increase in circulating triglycerides caused by the long-term consumption of a sucrose-rich diet by rats. J Nutr. 2000;130:2883–8.
54. Soria A, Chicco A, Mocchiutti N, et al. A sucrose-rich diet affects triglyceride metabolism differently in pregnant and nonpregnant rats and has negative effects on fetal growth. J Nutr. 1996;126:2481–6.
55. Ghusain-Choueiri AA, Rath EA. Effect of carbohydrate source on lipid metabolism in lactating mice and on pup development. Br J Nutr. 1995;74:821–31.
56. Myers KP, Ferris J, Sclafani A. Flavor preferences conditioned by postingestive effects of nutrients in preweanling rats. Physiol Behav. 2005;84:407–19.
57. Frazier CR, Mason P, Zhuang X, et al. Sucrose exposure in early life alters adult motivation and weight gain. PLoS One. 2008;3:e3221.
58. Jen KL, Rochon C, Zhong SB, et al. Fructose and sucrose feeding during pregnancy and lactation in rats changes maternal and pup fuel metabolism. J Nutr. 1991;121:1999–2005.
59. Weisinger HS, Armitage JA, Sinclair AJ, et al. Perinatal omega-3 fatty acid deficiency affects blood pressure later in life. Nat Med. 2001;7:258–9.
60. Mathai ML, Soueid M, Chen N, et al. Does perinatal omega-3 polyunsaturated fatty acid deficiency increase appetite signaling? Obes Res. 2004;12:1886–94.
61. Armitage JA, Pearce AD, Sinclair AJ, et al. Increased blood pressure later in life may be associated with perinatal n-3 fatty acid deficiency. Lipids. 2003;38:459–64.
62. Siemelink M, Verhoef A, Dormans JA, et al. Dietary fatty acid composition during pregnancy and lactation in the rat programs growth and glucose metabolism in the offspring. Diabetologia. 2002;45:1397–403.
63. McCurdy CE, Bishop JM, Williams SM, et al. Maternal high-fat diet triggers lipotoxicity in the fetal livers of nonhuman primates. J Clin Invest. 2009;119:323–35.
64. Levin BE, Dunn-Meynell AA, Balkan B, et al. Selective breeding for diet-induced obesity and resistance in Sprague-Dawley rats. Am J Physiol. 1997;273:R725–R30.
65. Levin BE, Dunn-Meynell AA. Maternal obesity alters adiposity and monoamine function in genetically predisposed offspring. Am J Physiol Regul Integr Comp Physiol. 2002;283:R1087–R93.
66. Zambrano E, Martinez-Samayoa PM, Rodriguez-Gonzalez GL, et al. Dietary intervention prior to pregnancy reverses metabolic programming in male offspring of obese rats. J Physiol. 2010 vol. 588(Pt 10):1791–9.
67. White CL, Purpera MN, Morrison CD. Maternal obesity is necessary for programming effect of high-fat diet on offspring. Am J Physiol Regul Integr Comp Physiol. 2009;296: R1464–R72.
68. Akyol A, Langley-Evans SC, McMullen S. Obesity induced by cafeteria feeding and pregnancy outcome in the rat. Br J Nutr. 2009;102:1601–10.
69. Napoli C, Glass CK, Witztum JL, et al. Influence of maternal hypercholesterolaemia during pregnancy on progression of early atherosclerotic lesions in childhood: fate of early lesions in children (FELIC) study. Lancet. 1999;354:1234–41.
70. Napoli C, Witztum JL, Calara F, et al. Maternal hypercholesterolemia enhances atherogenesis in normocholesterolemic rabbits, which is inhibited by antioxidant or lipid-lowering intervention during pregnancy: an experimental model of atherogenic mechanisms in human fetuses. Circ Res. 2000;87:946–52.
71. Napoli C, de Nigris F, Welch JS, et al. Maternal hypercholesterolemia during pregnancy promotes early atherogenesis in LDL receptor-deficient mice and alters aortic gene expression determined by microarray. Circulation. 2002;105:1360–7.
72. Grove KL, Allen S, Grayson BE, et al. Postnatal development of the hypothalamic neuropeptide Y system. Neuroscience. 2003;116:393–406.
73. Grove KL, Grayson BE, Glavas MM, et al. Development of metabolic systems. Physiol Behav. 2005;86:646–60.

74. McCance RA. Food, growth, and time. Lancet. 1962;2:621–6.
75. Bassett DR, Craig BW. Influence of early nutrition on growth and adipose tissue characteristics in male and female rats. J Appl Physiol. 1988;64:1249–56.
76. Faust IM, Johnson PR, Hirsch J. Long-term effects of early nutritional experience on the development of obesity in the rat. J Nutr. 1980;110:2027–34.
77. Plagemann A, Harder T, Rake A, et al. Perinatal elevation of hypothalamic insulin, acquired malformation of hypothalamic galaninergic neurons, and syndrome x-like alterations in adulthood of neonatally overfed rats. Brain Res. 1999;836:146–55.
78. Schmidt I, Fritz A, Scholch C, et al. The effect of leptin treatment on the development of obesity in overfed suckling Wistar rats. Int J Obes Relat Metab Disord. 2001;25:1168–74.
79. Velkoska E, Cole TJ, Dean RG, et al. Early undernutrition leads to long-lasting reductions in body weight and adiposity whereas increased intake increases cardiac fibrosis in male rats. J Nutr. 2008;138:1622–7.
80. Plagemann A, Harder T, Brunn M, et al. Hypothalamic proopiomelanocortin promoter methylation becomes altered by early overfeeding: an epigenetic model of obesity and the metabolic syndrome. J Physiol. 2009;587:4963–76.
81. Aubert R, Suquet J-P, Lemonnier D. Long-term morphological and metabolic effects of early under- and over-nutrition in mice. J Nutr. 1980;110:649–61.
82. Plagemann A, Harder T, Dudenhausen JW. The diabetic pregnancy, macrosomia, and perinatal nutritional programming. Nestle Nutr Workshop Ser Pediatr Program. 2008;61:91–102.
83. Plagemann A. Perinatal nutrition and hormone-dependent programming of food intake. Horm Res. 2006;65 Suppl 3:83–9.
84. Plagemann A. Perinatal programming and functional teratogenesis: impact on body weight regulation and obesity. Physiol Behav. 2005;86:661–8.
85. Hetherington AW, Ranson SW. Hypothalamic lesions and adiposity in the rat. Anat Rec. 1940;78:149–72.
86. Stellar E. The physiology of motivation. Psychol Rev. 1954;61:5–22.
87. Brobeck J, Tepperman J, Long C. Experimental hypothalamic hyperphagia in the albino rat. Yale J Biol Med. 1943;15:831–53.
88. Anand BK, Brobeck JR. Localization of a "feeding center" in the hypothalamus of the rat. Proc Soc Exp Biol Med. 1951;77:323–4.
89. Peruzzo B, Pastor FE, Blazquez JL, et al. A second look at the barriers of the medial basal hypothalamus. Exp Brain Res. 2000;132:10–26.
90. Hahn TM, Breininger JF, Baskin DG, et al. Coexpression of Agrp and NPY in fasting-activated hypothalamic neurons. Nat Neurosci. 1998;1:271–2.
91. Broberger C, Johansen J, Johansson C, et al. The neuropeptide Y/agouti gene-related protein (AGRP) brain circuitry in normal, anorectic, and monosodium glutamate-treated mice. Proc Natl Acad Sci USA. 1998;95:15043–8.
92. Elias CF, Lee C, Kelly J, et al. Leptin activates hypothalamic CART neurons projecting to the spinal cord. Neuron. 1998;21:1375–85.
93. Schwartz MW, Woods SC, Porte D, et al. Central nervous system control of food intake. Nature. 2000;404:661–71.
94. Bouret SG, Draper SJ, Simerly RB. Formation of projection pathways from the arcuate nucleus of the hypothalamus to hypothalamic regions implicated in the neural control of feeding behavior in mice. J Neurosci. 2004;24:2797–805.
95. Nilsson I, Johansen JE, Schalling M, et al. Maturation of the hypothalamic arcuate agouti-related protein system during postnatal development in the mouse. Brain Res Dev Brain Res. 2005;155:147–54.
96. Bouret SG, Draper SJ, Simerly RB. Trophic action of leptin on hypothalamic neurons that regulate feeding. Science. 2004;304:108–10.
97. Davidowa H, Li Y, Plagemann A. Altered responses to orexigenic (AGRP, MCH) and anorexigenic (alpha-MSH, CART) neuropeptides of paraventricular hypothalamic neurons in early postnatally overfed rats. Eur J Neurosci. 2003;18:613–21.

98. Grayson BE, Allen SE, Billes SK, et al. Prenatal development of hypothalamic neuropeptide systems in the nonhuman primate. Neuroscience. 2006;143:975–86.
99. Koutcherov Y, Mai JK, Paxinos G. Hypothalamus of the human fetus. J Chem Neuroanat. 2003;26:253–70.
100. Louis GW, Myers MG Jr. The role of leptin in the regulation of neuroendocrine function and CNS development. Rev Endocr Metab Disord. 2007;8:85–94.
101. Ahima RS, Prabakaran D, Flier JS. Postnatal leptin surge and regulation of circadian rhythm of leptin by feeding. Implications for energy homeostasis and neuroendocrine function. J Clin Invest. 1998;101:1020–7.
102. Devaskar SU, Ollesch C, Rajakumar RA, et al. Developmental changes in ob gene expression and circulating leptin peptide concentrations. Biochem Biophys Res Commun. 1997;238:44–7.
103. Mistry AM, Swick A, Romsos DR. Leptin alters metabolic rates before acquisition of its anorectic effect in developing neonatal mice. Am J Physiol. 1999;277:R742–7.
104. Ahima RS, Bjorbaek C, Osei S, et al. Regulation of neuronal and glial proteins by leptin: implications for brain development. Endocrinology. 1999;140:2755–62.
105. Steppan CM, Swick AG. A role for leptin in brain development. Biochem Biophys Res Commun. 1999;256:600–2.
106. Proulx K, Richard D, Walker CD. Leptin regulates appetite-related neuropeptides in the hypothalamus of developing rats without affecting food intake. Endocrinology. 2002;143:4683–92.
107. Levine JA. Non-exercise activity thermogenesis. Proc Nutr Soc. 2003;62:667–79.
108. Bray GA. Obesity, a disorder of nutrient partitioning: the MONA LISA hypothesis. J Nutr. 1991;121:1146–62.
109. Esler M, Straznicky N, Eikelis N, et al. Mechanisms of sympathetic activation in obesity-related hypertension. Hypertension. 2006;48:787–96.
110. Sell H, Deshaies Y, Richard D. The brown adipocyte: update on its metabolic role. Int J Biochem Cell Biol. 2004;36:2098–104.
111. Bachman ES, Dhillon H, Zhang CY, et al. betaAR signaling required for diet-induced thermogenesis and obesity resistance. Science. 2002;297:843–5.
112. Young JB, Landsberg L. Suppression of sympathetic nervous system during fasting. Science. 1977;196:1473–5.
113. Elmquist JK, Flier JS. Neuroscience. The fat-brain axis enters a new dimension. Science. 2004;304:63–4.
114. Elmquist JK. Hypothalamic pathways underlying the endocrine, autonomic, and behavioral effects of leptin. Int J Obes Relat Metab Disord. 2001;25 Suppl 5:S78–S82.
115. Abizaid A, Horvath TL. Brain circuits regulating energy homeostasis. Regul Pept. 2008;149:3–10.
116. Prior LJ, Eikelis N, Armitage JA, et al. Exposure to a high-fat diet alters leptin sensitivity and elevates renal sympathetic nerve activity and arterial pressure in rabbits. Hypertension. 2010;55:862–8.
117. Prior LJ, Head GA, Morris MJ, et al. Maternal obesity in rabbits elevates offspring blood pressure and evokes selective leptin resistance in offspring. Hypertension. 2009;53:1117.
118. Zukowska-Grojec Z. Neuropeptide Y. A novel sympathetic stress hormone and more. Ann N Y Acad Sci. 1995;771:219–33.
119. Kuo LE, Kitlinska JB, Tilan JU, et al. Neuropeptide Y acts directly in the periphery on fat tissue and mediates stress-induced obesity and metabolic syndrome. Nat Med. 2007;13:803–11.
120. Zukowska Z. Atherosclerosis and angiogenesis: what do nerves have to do with it? Pharmacol Rep. 2005;57 Suppl:229–34.
121. Igosheva N, Taylor PD, Poston L, et al. Prenatal stress in the rat results in increased blood pressure responsiveness to stress and enhanced arterial reactivity to neuropeptide Y in adulthood. J Physiol. 2007;582:665–74.

Chapter 13
High-Carbohydrate Intake Only During the Suckling Period Results in Adult-Onset Obesity in Mother as well as Offspring

Mulchand S. Patel and Malathi Srinivasan

13.1 Introduction

The enormous increase in the worldwide incidence of obesity over the past several decades, particularly in Westernized societies, is not only a major health concern due to its association with several co-morbidities (such as type 2 diabetes (T2DM), cardiovascular disease, hypertension) but is also an economic burden because of the associated spiraling health-care costs. It is becoming increasingly clear that there are no easy solutions for already obese/overweight individuals. This recognition indicates a deficit in our understanding of the mechanisms which initiate and sustain these metabolic disorders.

Except for some rare types of genetic defects [1], increased intake of calorie-dense foods and sedentary lifestyles are traditionally viewed as important contributors to the etiology of the obesity epidemic. But the enormity and global nature of the obesity epidemic implies a role for other factors that contribute to this problem. That early life events can have long-term effects for the development of metabolic disorders in later life was recognized as early as in the 1930s [2], and further expanded by the studies of Dorner et al. [3]. The epidemiological studies by Barker and coworkers [4] led to the recognition of the role of the nutritional environment during early periods of life in predisposing an individual to later development of adult-onset metabolic disorders.

During early periods in life, development of the organism is plastic and vulnerable to environmental challenges in part because target tissues are in a high proliferating and differentiating phase. One such challenge is an altered nutritional environment experienced during gestation and/or lactation. Metabolic programming is the phenomenon by which a stress or stimulus experienced by an organism in utero or during the suckling period results in compensatory responses, which include among others (a) an altered development of a somatic structure; (b) resetting of

M.S. Patel (✉)
Department of Biochemistry, School of Medicine and Biomedical Sciences, University at Buffalo, State University of New York, Buffalo, NY, USA
e-mail: mspatel@buffalo.edu

R.H. Lustig (ed.), *Obesity Before Birth*, Endocrine Updates 30,
DOI 10.1007/978-1-4419-7034-3_13,

a physiologic system; and/or (c) imbalances in normal homeostatic mechanisms [5]. Such adaptations occur due to the overlap of the critical window of development of target organs with the duration of the stimulus or insult. These early responses enable the organism to survive under altered nutritional conditions, but in the long run such responses prove deleterious to the organism due to their impact on whole-body metabolic processes.

13.2 Metabolic Programming of the Fetus for Adult-Onset Disease

Barker's retrospective analysis of epidemiological data resulted in the hypothesis of "fetal origins of adult disease" [6]. These studies indicated an association between malnutrition during pregnancy and increased risk of cardiovascular disease, stroke, hypertension, and diabetes in the adult life of the offspring [7, 8]. Subsequently, several other cohort studies from different parts of the world corroborated Barker's hypothesis. An extension of the concept of "metabolic programming" is the "thrifty phenotype hypothesis" which postulates that undernutrition during pregnancy causes an altered physiologic and metabolic phenotype in the fetus to support its survival under sparse nutritional conditions [9]. Such programming is detrimental if the postweaning nutritional environment is one of plenty resulting in catch-up growth with eventual development of obesity [9]. The "developmental origins of health and disease (DOHaD)" hypothesis encompasses both metabolic programming and the thrifty phenotype hypotheses and is increasingly used to refer to the association between early life nutritional status and the development of adult-onset disease [10].

Animal models have been developed to mimic malnutrition in human pregnancy. The most extensively investigated model is the low-protein rodent model, in which dams are fed a low protein (8% protein) diet during both gestation and lactation to induce growth restriction in the offspring, resulting in small-sized pups that become progressively glucose intolerant, and develop diabetes by 17 months of age [11]. Functional alterations in pancreatic islets, liver, muscle, adipose tissue, and the hypothalamus are observed in the adult offspring of the low-protein diet-fed dams [11–13]. Similarly, restriction of total caloric intake during gestation and lactation results in retardation of fetal development, but with glucose intolerance in adulthood [14]. Gestational diabetes mellitus has been shown to have a detrimental effect on the offspring both clinically and experimentally [15, 16]. Clinical studies have shown that increased maternal body mass index prior to pregnancy and during pregnancy also result in the development of obesity in adulthood of their offspring [17] (see Chapter 10). Studies in animal models have shown that obesity during pregnancy induced by consumption of a high-fat (HF) diet in the immediate prepregnancy period and during pregnancy resulted in the development of obesity and related disorders in the offspring [18–20]. The reader is referred to Chapters 9, 10, 11, and 12 of this volume and to other reviews for detailed information on the topics discussed above [21–25].

13.3 Altered Dietary Experience in the Immediate Postnatal Period (Suckling Period)

The cellular development of several organs and many physiological and metabolic processes are not complete at birth. Maturation of these processes continues in the immediate period following birth (suckling period). For example, it has been reported that the maturation of rat pancreatic islets is complete only after the third postnatal week [26]. Neuronal development and the maturation of axonal connections between neurons in the rat hypothalamus continue in the immediate postnatal period [27]. Hence, it can be hypothesized that an insult or stimulus experienced in the immediate postnatal period can serve as an independent cue for metabolic programming effects, as observed by others during gestation.

In mammals, maternal breastfeeding is the natural source of nutrition for the newborn infant. Deviations from breastfeeding can be considered an altered nutritional experience for the newborn infant. The American Pediatric Society recommends infant breastfeeding for at least 6 months. Breastfeeding confers immunologic, developmental, and psychological benefits to the newborn [28, 29]. Further, it has been demonstrated that breastfeeding protects against the onset of obesity, diabetes, cardiovascular diseases, and the metabolic syndrome in later life [30, 31]. This protective effect is correlated with the duration of breastfeeding [32].

In animal models, McCance demonstrated that alterations in total caloric intake in the suckling period by reducing rat litter size resulted in permanent changes in the growth trajectory of these pups in the postweaning period [33]. Furthermore, Plagemann et al. using the small litter model (reducing litter size to three pups per dam) have shown that overnutrition in the immediate postnatal period also resulted in metabolic programming effects. During the suckling period, these pups were overweight, hyperinsulinemic, and hyperleptinemic; and in adulthood these rats were obese and demonstrated significant alterations in hypothalamic energy circuitry regulation [34–36]. The development of hyperphagia, increased body weight, and associated metabolic diseases in adulthood of pups born to normal dams but nursed by diabetic dams during the suckling period is further proof for the hypothesis that the animals in the immediate postnatal period are vulnerable to nutritional insult [37].

13.4 The High-Carbohydrate (HC) Rat Model

Although the effects of an altered early nutritional experience on the development of metabolic diseases in adulthood are well documented, a majority of these studies focused on the role of either undernutrition (total or specific nutrient) or overnutrition. Furthermore, aside the small litter model, investigation of the consequences of altered nutritional environments during early periods of life has been limited to pregnancy. There are limited studies on programming effects due to macronutrient redistribution (switch in the major source of calories) without changes in total caloric intake.

The HC rat model developed in our lab differs from other animal models in two aspects. First, the dietary modification is imposed only during the suckling period, and it is in the form of an alteration in the quality of nutrition without changes in quantity. Given the observation that decreases or increases in total caloric availability during early periods of life (fetal and immediate postnatal) results in adult-onset metabolic disorders, we asked the question whether an increase in carbohydrate-derived calories without altering total caloric intake would induce metabolic programming effects in suckling rats. In the HC rat model, rat milk (high in fat-derived calories) is replaced by a high-carbohydrate milk formula. The HC dietary intervention is imposed during the suckling period only (postnatal days 4–24). From the time of weaning, the newborn pups reared on the HC milk formula are given standard rodent chow ad libitum. The HC dietary intervention during suckling results in a phenotype of chronic hyperinsulinemia and adult-onset obesity in both male and female HC rats (F0 generation) [38–40]. Another important observation on this model was that female rat pups reared on the HC milk formula in their infancy (F0) spontaneously transmitted their phenotype (chronic hyperinsulinemia and adult-onset obesity) to their male and female offspring (HC offspring; F1 generation), thereby establishing a generational effect [41]. The generational effect observed in the HC rat model indicates the persistence of the effects of increased carbohydrate intake during the suckling period, not only in the adulthood of the same generation (F0) but also on the next generation (F1).

In order to demonstrate that our artificial rearing protocol per se does not induce the phenotype of chronic hyperinsulinemia and adult-onset obesity, newborn rat pups were reared away from their natural dams on a high-fat formula, whose macronutrient composition of which was similar to that of rat milk, and weaned on to a standard rodent chow on postnatal day 24. The rats reared on an HF milk formula were normoinsulinemic and did not develop adult-onset obesity, indicating that the development of the HC phenotype was a response to the HC milk formula imposed during the suckling period [42].

Unlike the low-protein diet rat model or the high-fat diet rat model, wherein the dietary intervention is imposed during pregnancy or just prior to and during pregnancy and/or lactation, the HC female rats do not undergo any dietary modification during these periods. The HC female rat (F0) is weaned onto a standard rodent chow and consumes this diet for life. Therefore, the altered intrauterine environment of the obese HC female rat (F0) that is responsible for the transmission of the HC phenotype to its offspring (F1) is not due to any dietary effect but is a consequence of the HC dietary intervention experienced in its immediate postnatal life. The offspring (F1) of HC female rats do not undergo any dietary manipulation at any time in their lives, but still develop adult-onset obesity on standard rodent chow.

In the following sections the HC rat model will be discussed. First, the immediate effects of the HC dietary modification will be briefly described to underscore the mechanisms that subsequently lead to the development of an adverse intrauterine environment in the HC female rat (F0). The long-term consequences of the HC milk formula observed in HC female rats in the prepregnancy and pregnancy periods as well as the effects of the obese/hyperinsulinemic HC maternal environment on the offspring (F1) at various stages of development such as term fetus, suckling rats, and postweaning period will then be reviewed. Lastly, the beneficial effects of dietary restriction imposed on HC female rats (F0) will also be discussed.

13.5 Effects of the HC Milk Formula Observed in Rat Pups (F0) During the Period of the Dietary Modification

Four-day-old rat pups were artificially reared on a high-carbohydrate (HC) milk formula by a non-surgically inserted intragastric cannula. The macronutrient calorie composition of the HC milk formula was 56% carbohydrate, 20% fat, and 24% protein, as compared to 8% carbohydrate, 68% fat, and 24% protein in rat milk. The immediate response observed in newborn rat pups (F0) given the HC milk formula was a steep increase in plasma insulin levels within 24 h [43]. On postnatal day 12, the plasma insulin level in HC rats was about sixfold higher compared to the level in age-matched control rats [mother-fed (MF)]. Several adaptive changes were observed in the islets of HC rats (F0) to support the hyperinsulinemia observed in these rats [38–40]. Some of these adaptations include higher number of small-sized islets with increased insulin content and molecular responses such as an increase in preproinsulin mRNA levels and insulin biosynthesis. On the biochemical front, HC islets demonstrated a marked leftward shift in their response to a glucose stimulus. Further, in vivo and in vitro studies indicated that the autonomic regulation of insulin secretion was dysregulated in HC rats (F0) with an increase in parasympathetic input and decrease in sympathetic input, driving insulin secretion [38–40].

During the period of the HC dietary modification, the body weight gain of HC rats (F0) was similar to that of age-matched MF rats. However, the plasma level of leptin was significantly reduced on postnatal day 12 [44]. Alterations in the hypothalamic melanocortin system, which contributes to appetite control, were observed in 12-day-old HC rats. Levels of mRNA for orexigenic neuropeptides such as neuropeptide Y, agouti-related polypeptide, and galanin were significantly increased, while the mRNA levels of anorexigenic neuropeptides such as pro-opiomelanocortin, corticotrophin releasing hormone, and cocaine–amphetamine-regulated transcript were markedly decreased in the hypothalamus of 12-day-old HC rats [44]. These observations indicate that the HC dietary modification resulted in metabolic programming for future hyperphagia. In this context, it is interesting to note that abnormal levels of leptin and insulin in the early periods of life have been reported to contribute to the malprogramming of the melanocortin appetite regulatory system [45, 46].

13.6 Long-Term Effects of the HC Dietary Modification Observed in Adulthood

After the withdrawal of the HC milk formula on postnatal day 24, the HC rats (F0) were weaned onto a standard rodent chow ad libitum. Hyperinsulinemia persisted into the postweaning period, accompanied by hyperphagia and increased body weight gains for HC rats (F0) compared to age-matched MF rats [38–40].

The mechanisms that supported the hypersecretory capacity of islets in 12-day-old HC rats persisted into adulthood (postnatal day 100), including alterations in the autonomic nervous system regulation of insulin secretion [38–40]. Further, hypothalamic mRNA levels of orexigenic neuropeptides were increased and mRNA levels of anorexigenic neuropeptides were decreased [44]. These observations suggest that the immediate responses to the HC milk formula as observed in 12-day-old rats become permanent despite the absence of the nutritional stimulus from the time of weaning and become the basis for the development of obesity in later life of these rats (F0).

13.7 The Transgenerational Effect of HC Dietary Modification

A notable observation from our studies on the HC rat model is the spontaneous transfer of the HC maternal phenotype to the offspring [41]. HC offspring (F1) were never subjected to any dietary modification in their postnatal life, which suggests that fetal development in the HC intrauterine environment programmed these offspring for adult-onset obesity and chronic hyperinsulinemia.

13.8 The HC Female Rat (F0) in the Prepregnancy Period

From the time of weaning, HC female rats demonstrated hyperphagia. There was a progressive increase in food intake ranging from 6% (postnatal week 5) to 18% (postnatal week 11) by HC female rats as compared to age-matched MF female rats [47]. There was a significant increase in body weight gain of HC female rats (F0) from postnatal day 40 onward, with a 10% increase being observed on postnatal day 90 [47]. Plasma insulin and leptin levels were markedly higher in the HC female rat starting at postnatal day 40 [47]. For example, on postnatal day 80, plasma insulin levels showed an increase of 60% and plasma leptin levels were increased by 1.8-fold in HC female rats (F0) compared to MF controls [47].

13.9 The HC Pregnant Rat (F0 Generation)

It is important to underscore that the HC female rat (F0) does not undergo any dietary modification during pregnancy. The development of an adverse pregnancy environment in the HC female rat is a direct effect of the HC dietary modification it experienced in its immediate postnatal life some months earlier.

Several differences were observed in the metabolic characteristics of the intrauterine environment between HC (F0) and age-matched control MF female rats

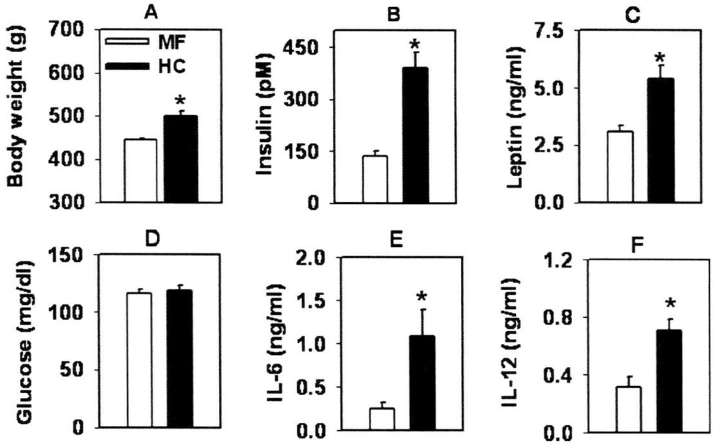

Fig. 13.1 Metabolic characteristics of the HC (F0) and age-matched MF control female rats on gestational day 21. Body weight (**a**), plasma insulin levels (**b**), plasma leptin levels (**c**), plasma glucose levels (**d**), plasma interleukin-6 levels (**e**), and plasma interleukin-12 levels (**f**). Results are means ± SEM ($n = 6$). *$p < 0.05$ (from [47])

(Fig. 13.1a–f) [47]. The total body weight gain during pregnancy was markedly higher in HC female rats. The major portion of body weight gain occurred in the third week of pregnancy in HC pregnant rat. Body weight of HC female rats (F0) on gestational day 21 was markedly higher than that of age-matched control MF rats (Fig. 13.1a). The HC pregnant rat also consumed significantly more food compared to the pregnant control rat. Plasma levels of both insulin and leptin showed significant increases during gestation in HC female rats compared to age-matched control female rat. On gestation days 7 and 14 a 40% increase in plasma insulin levels was observed in HC female rats and on gestation day 21, plasma insulin levels were approximately twofold higher in these rats (Fig. 13.1b). Plasma leptin levels were 98, 121, and 75% higher in HC pregnant rats at the end of the first, second, and third (Fig. 13.1c) weeks of pregnancy. These observations indicate that altered hormonal profiles characterize the HC pregnancy [47].

Plasma glucose levels (random) were not significantly different between HC (F0) and control female rats on gestation day 21 (Fig. 13.1d). However, plasma triglyceride levels were markedly increased while the levels of free fatty acids were decreased in the HC female rat on gestation day 21 [48].

Plasma levels of markers for inflammation and oxidative stress were significantly higher in HC female rats (F0) on gestational day 21 [47], including interleukin-6 (Fig. 13.1e), interleukin-12 (Fig. 13.1f), macrophage migration inhibitory factor-α, monocyte chemoattractant protein-1, and vascular endothelial growth factor. Also, an increase of approximately twofold was observed for the peroxidation products of linoleic acid, indicating the presence of oxidative stress in the pregnant HC rat [47].

13.10 The HC Fetus (F1 Generation)

Our initial investigation showed that the HC maternal phenotype of hyperinsulinemia and obesity were evident in the offspring (F1) in adulthood [41]. The question then arose if the expression of the maternal phenotype in adulthood of HC offspring rats (F1) was due to fetal development in the adverse intrauterine environment of the HC (F0) pregnant rat. Investigation of this question showed that there were no changes in either litter size or body weight in HC term fetuses. Further, there were no marked differences in the plasma levels of glucose (Fig. 13.2a), free fatty acids, and triglycerides in term HC fetuses (F1) compared to term control MF fetuses [48]. However, a marked increase in plasma insulin (82%; Fig. 13.2b) and leptin levels (150%; Fig. 13.2c) was observed in term HC fetuses suggesting endocrine abnormalities [47]. Interestingly, mechanisms that supported hypersecretory capacity of islets in HC rats (F0) were evident in HC term fetuses (F1). As observed in HC (F0) rats, pancreatic insulin content and mRNA levels of preproinsulin and pancreatic duodenal box transcription factor-1 (*Pdx-1*) were significantly higher in HC term fetuses (F1) [48]. Although it has been shown that fetal islets do not respond robustly to glucose, HC fetal islets secreted significantly more insulin in response to basal and high glucose, as well as in response to leucine and arginine, as compared to control MF term fetal islets, suggesting fetal programming of HC islets to hypersecrete insulin (Fig. 13.2d) [48].

During the period of fetal development, fetuses derive their nutrition from the maternal circulation. The regulation of food intake is not under the control of

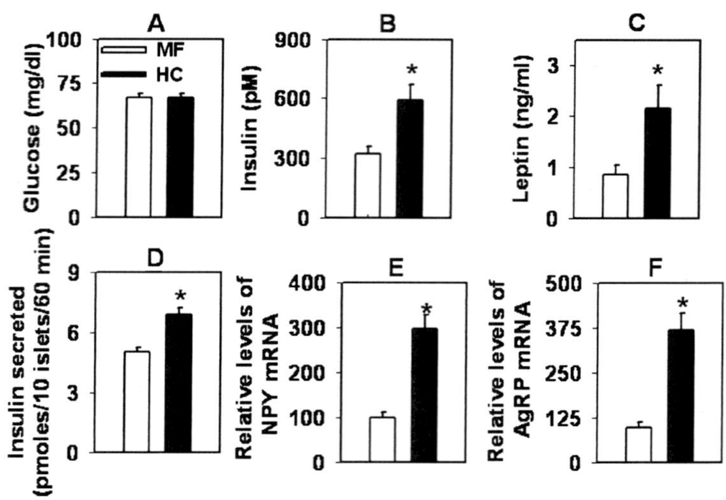

Fig. 13.2 Metabolic characteristics of the HC (F1) and age-matched MF control term fetuses. Plasma glucose levels (**a**), plasma insulin levels (**b**), plasma leptin levels (**c**), insulin secretion by fetal islets (**d**), neuropeptide mRNA levels in fetal brain (**e**), and agouti-related protein mRNA levels in fetal brain (**f**). Results are means ± SEM ($n = 6$). $^*p < 0.05$ (from [47, 48])

hypothalamic energy circuitry during this period. Interestingly, we observed that the mRNA levels of neuropeptide Y and agouti-related polypeptide were significantly higher in HC term fetal (F1) hypothalami (Fig. 13.2e and f) [47]. Although the effects of the increase in orexigenic signaling are not evident in HC (F1) rats until the postweaning period, the disposition for hyperphagia and increased body weight gain appear to have been already programmed during the fetal period. These observations on HC fetal islets and hypothalamus clearly demonstrate that fetal programming occurs in this rat model due to the intrauterine environment in the HC female rat (F0).

13.11 The HC Offspring (F1) in the Postnatal Period

During the suckling period there were no differences in the plasma insulin levels of HC offspring (F1) and age-matched control MF rats [49]. This was supported by a similar insulin secretory response to sub-basal, basal, and high glucose by HC offspring and age-matched control islets on postnatal days 12, 20, and 24 [49]. Preproinsulin and *Pdx-1* mRNA levels were also similar in 12-day-old HC offspring (F1) and control MF rats. The hypersecretory capacity of HC offspring (F1) islets (already evident in HC fetuses) was probably suppressed in the suckling period due to the high fat content of rat milk.

HC offspring rats (F1) were weaned onto a standard rodent chow on postnatal day 24. Thereafter plasma insulin levels were significantly higher in HC offspring rats (F1) (Fig. 13.3). A hypersecretory response to sub-basal, basal, and high glucose by islets isolated from 28-day-old HC offspring rats was observed [49]. mRNA levels of preproinsulin and *Pdx-1* were markedly higher in islets from HC rats (F1) compared to their expression in islets from age-matched control rats [49]. Further, the HC offspring (F1) demonstrated increased body weight gain in the postweaning

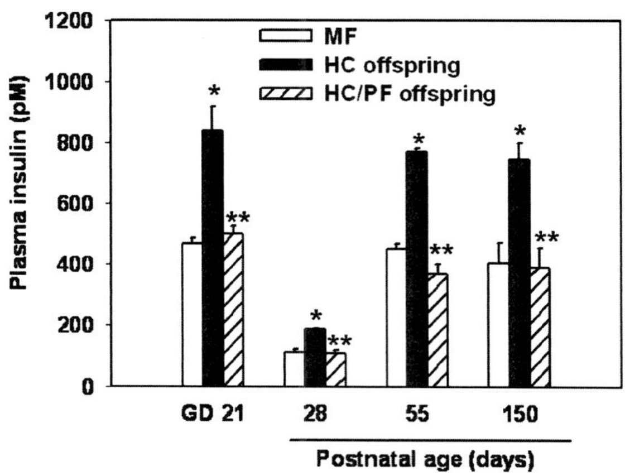

Fig. 13.3 Plasma insulin levels in HC (F1), age-matched MF control, and HC/pair-fed (F1) rats on fetal day 21 and postnatal days 28, 55, and 150. Results are means ± SEM ($n = 6$). $^*p < 0.05$. *HC versus MF and **HC/PF versus HC (from [48])

period and were obese by postnatal day 100. Obesity in adult HC offspring (F1) was associated with significant increase in the weight of the different adipose depots and in hypertrophy of the adipocytes [41]. The activities of lipogenic enzymes in both liver and epididymal adipose tissue were markedly higher in adult HC offspring (F1) as compared to control MF rats [41]. Development of insulin resistance in adult HC offspring rats was indicated by the marked decrease in glycogen content in both liver and skeletal muscle accompanied by a significant decrease in the activity of glycogen synthase [50].

These characteristics of the HC offspring (F1) are similar to those observed in the HC rat and indicate that the HC (F0) maternal intrauterine environment programs its offspring for expression of this metabolic phenotype. The contribution of the maternal pregnancy condition in the HC rat model to the observed transgenerational effect is underscored by the results obtained from the reciprocal embryo transfer experiment. Four-day-old control (normal) embryos developing in the HC uterus (F0) demonstrated marked increases in body weight in adulthood (Fig. 13.4) [47]. On the other hand, 4-day-old HC embryos (F1) developing in the control (normal) uterus did not develop adult-onset obesity (Fig. 13.4).

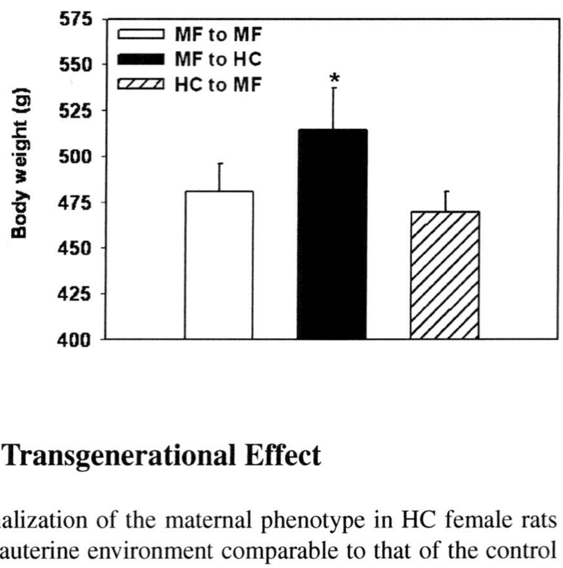

Fig. 13.4 The effect of transfer of 4-day-old embryos into the reciprocal maternal uterus on body weights of male progeny (F1) on postnatal day 80. Results are means ± SEM ($n = 6$). *$p < 0.05$ (from [47])

13.12 Reversal of the Transgenerational Effect

We hypothesized that normalization of the maternal phenotype in HC female rats (F0) would result in an intrauterine environment comparable to that of the control MF female rats and reverse the spontaneous transfer of the HC phenotype to its offspring (F1). For this purpose, HC female rats (F0) were pair fed (HC/PF) from the time of weaning to the quantity of food consumed by age-matched control MF rats. HC female rats (F0) fed ad libitum consume approximately 10–15% more chow than age-matched control rats. Therefore, the pair-feeding regimen was only a mild food restriction imposed on the HC/PF female rat (F0).

Pair feeding of HC female rats (F0) markedly improved the maternal phenotype in pregnant HC/PF rats [48]. On gestational day 21, pair feeding resulted in a significant reduction in body weight and plasma insulin levels in HC/PF rats (F0) compared to the HC female rat (F0) and were normalized to the body weight and plasma insulin levels in age-matched control MF female rats. The normalization of the intrauterine environment in the HC/PF female rat had important implications on the HC fetal (F1) development. Plasma insulin levels were significantly reduced in the HC/PF term fetus (F1) (Fig. 13.3; hatched bars). Insulin secretion by fetal islets isolated from HC/PF term fetuses (F1) in response to basal and high glucose, as well as to leucine and arginine, was similar to insulin secretion by control MF term fetal islets, and significantly reduced compared to HC term fetal (F1) islets. Fetal development in the normalized HC/PF (F0) intrauterine environment resulted in positive effects (normal development) for the HC/PF offspring (F1) in the postweaning period, indicating permanency of the effects. HC/PF rats (F1) had markedly reduced plasma insulin levels not only on fetal day 21 but also on postnatal days 28, 55, and 150 (Fig. 13.3; hatched bars) [48]. Furthermore, the body weight gains of HC/PF rats (F1) in the postweaning period were normalized to that of age-matched control MF rats and were significantly less as compared to age-matched HC rats(F1) [48].

13.13 Maternal Obesity due to High-Fat Diet Consumption and Programming Effects on the Offspring

Several reports have demonstrated that a high-fat diet-induced obesity in the mother results in an abnormal intrauterine environment for fetal development and promotes several adverse consequences for the offspring [51–53]. In these studies the duration of high-fat diet feeding and the percentage and nature of the fat in the diet were variable. Further, the programming effects were demonstrated in a majority of the studies only in the adult progeny. Nevertheless, these reports did underscore the observation that maternal obesity induced by consumption of an HF resulted in several metabolic and physiologic disturbances in the offspring. More recently, it has been demonstrated that programming effects are initiated in the fetal period [54, 55].

In addition to our investigations on the obese HC female rat, and as an alternate approach for the development of an obese pregnancy, we also investigated the long-term consequences of a high-fat diet (HF; 59.5% of total calories from fat) consumption in female rats from the time of weaning (postnatal day 24) for both the mother and her offspring. The HF-fed female rat was distinctly heavier in the prepregnancy and pregnancy periods, as well as hyperinsulinemic as compared to age-matched control rats [56]. Further, on gestational day 21 the HF-fed female rat was hyperglycemic and had an aberrant lipid profile. Term fetuses of the high-fat diet-fed mother were also hyperinsulinemic and their islets expressed a hypersecretory capacity to various secretogogues [56]. Further, alterations in the mRNA levels of neuropeptides and leptin and insulin signaling were observed in the hypothalami of HC term fetuses of HF-fed female rats [57]. In adulthood, the HF offspring rats were obese with perturbations in glucose and lipid metabolism [56]. The HF rat model developed in our lab demonstrated that consumption of a high-fat diet over a prolonged duration resulted in fetal programming for adult-onset disorders.

13.14 Mechanisms Supporting the Phenomenon of Metabolic Programming

The precise mechanisms that support the persistence of immediate effects in response to a nutritional insult or stimulus in the fetal or suckling periods are not well understood. An abnormal hormonal environment has been implicated in the altered development of regulatory mechanisms. Insulin and leptin have been suggested to function as teratogens during early developmental periods, unlike their functions in adulthood; hence, increases or decreases in the levels of these hormones could result in metabolic programming effects that persist in later life [45, 58, 59]. For example, leptin has been implicated in the development of the hypothalamus [46]. In the HC rat model, increased levels of insulin and leptin observed in both the mother and the term fetuses could be responsible for programming of the offspring for expression of the maternal obese phenotype in adulthood.

Except in the small proportion of the population who express inherited diseases, DNA mutations rarely determine phenotypes. Instead genes provide the background upon which a biological system develops based on its interactions with the environment it encounters during early periods in life. It is now being increasingly recognized that epigenetic processes contribute to the developmental origins of adult-onset diseases (see Chapters 6, 7, and 8), for instance, DNA methylation, acetylation, and phosphorylation, and changes in histone structure are central to cellular differentiation and developmental plasticity [60]. Heritable epigenetic modifications of genes associated with metabolism and endocrine function in response to the nutritional state of the mother have been observed in the offspring of a primate model [61]. Epigenetic silencing of *Pdx1* has been implicated in the development of diabetes in intrauterine growth retarded (IUGR) rats [62]. Histone code modifications have been reported to contribute to the programming of the repression of skeletal muscle *Glut4* transcription in rats that were growth retarded during fetal development [63]. Kuzawa and Sweet [64] recently reviewed evidence for developmental and epigenetic pathways that connect adult-onset cardiovascular diseases with the environment during early developmental periods and have evaluated their possible role in health disparities based on race in the USA.

13.15 Conclusions

Based on observations from epidemiological studies, several approaches have been employed in animal models to demonstrate that both quality and quantity of nutrition during early periods of development are critical components (via the process

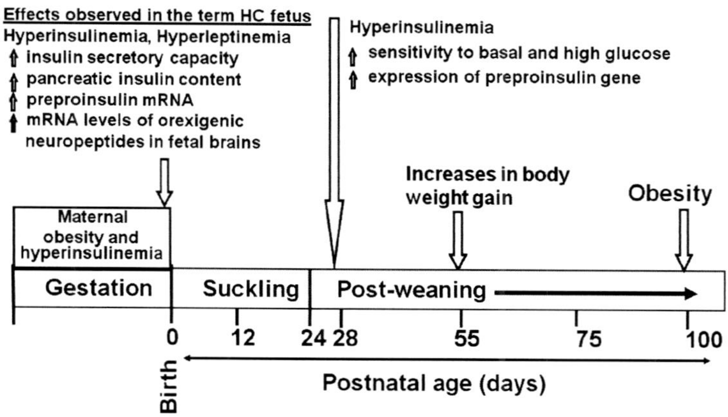

Fig. 13.5 Summary of the effects on the HC offspring (F1) due to fetal development in the adverse intrauterine environment of the HC female (F0) rat. HC mothers are obese and have an abnormal hormonal pattern during gestation. Fetal development in the HC intrauterine environment induces metabolic programming effects which are evident in term fetuses. These effects persist in the postweaning period resulting in adult-onset obesity and chronic hyperinsulinemia in the HC offspring (F1)

of metabolic programming) of the mechanisms which impact on the well-being of the adult offspring. The HC rat model is one such animal model, which particularly emphasizes the long-term effects of high carbohydrate consumption only in the immediate postnatal life for at least two generations of rats. Not only do the newborn rats consuming the HC milk formula become obese in adulthood, but the offspring of these obese HC mothers also acquire the maternal traits as summarized in Fig. 13.5. The presence of obesity in the pregnant HC rat is not the result of any maternal dietary manipulation, such as HF consumption, in the postweaning period (either prior to and/or during gestation), but rather is an effect of hyperphagia (dysregulation of the hypothalamic energy circuitry) induced in the newborn rats in response to the HC milk formula. Figure 13.5 shows that fetal development in the obese/hyperinsulinemic/hyperleptinemic HC mother (F0) (programming effects of the HC dietary modification in its suckling period) resulted in several adaptations in pancreatic islets and the hypothalamus of HC term fetuses (F1). It is further observed that despite weaning onto a standard rodent chow, hyperinsulinemia and increased body weight gains were evident in the HC offspring (F1) in the postweaning period. The transgenerational effect observed in the HC rat (F1) is a direct effect of the pregnancy environment (obesity and abnormal hormonal profile) encountered in the HC female rat (F0).

Although the increase in the prevalence of obese/overweight adults in the USA appears to be leveling off, a large fraction still belongs in this category. For the period 2007–2008, it has been reported that 60% of the women in the age group of 20–39 years (the childbearing years) are overweight/obese and 34% of the women in this age group are obese [65]. Similarly, it is estimated that more than one out of five pregnant women are obese in England [66]. Obesity during pregnancy increases morbidity and mortality for both the mother and the offspring [17]. In addition, maternal obesity results in higher birth weight for the offspring, which is associated with an increased risk for development of obesity and metabolic syndrome in later life, thereby perpetuating the cycle of obesity and its adverse consequences [67]. Further, gestational diabetes (see Chapter 9) has been reported to cause offspring obesity, possibly due to the altered intrauterine environment [68, 69]. More recently, it has been shown that both maternal overweight in the prepregnancy period and increased gestational weight gain by itself (see Chapter 10) result in increased risk of weight gain in children aged 2–14 years as well as in early adulthood [70].

Compared to the developmental origins of health and disease (DOHaD) hypothesis connection for the offspring of undernourished mothers, the establishment of the possible connection of maternal–fetal obesity is in its nascent period. In Western societies and in other parts of the developing world adapting the Western lifestyle, complications due to overnutrition during pregnancy are posing an equal if not a greater threat than a malnourished pregnancy. There is a sense of urgency for initiation of investigations not only on the etiology of obesity epidemic, but also on the mechanisms underlying the generational effect observed in overweight/obese pregnancies. The need for regulation of body weight gain in the prepregnancy and pregnancy periods is highlighted by our observations on the transgenerational effect in the HC rat model. Further, our findings also indicate the beneficial outcome for the progeny by maternal weight reduction by food restriction during the prepregnancy and pregnancy periods.

Extrapolating to humans, it is possible that early introduction of carbohydrate-rich supplementary foods to newborns could function as a cue for programming for hyperphagia and could provide a route to an obese intrauterine environment in females. Therefore, in addition to emphasis on the consequences of consumption of energy-dense foods, focus should also be directed on the quality of nutrition during the suckling period as an intervention strategy to curb the rise in the incidence of obesity and associated complications. The HC rat model developed in our lab simultaneously permits investigation of the role of nutritional environment in the immediate postnatal life on the development of obesity in adulthood and the contribution of an obese pregnancy to the spontaneous transfer of the maternal phenotype to the offspring.

Acknowledgments The work summarized in this review on the HC rat model was supported by National Institute of Diabetes and Digestive and Kidney Diseases Grants DK-51601 and DK-61518 awarded to MSP. We thank Dr. Gail Willsky (Department of Biochemistry, University at Buffalo) for critical reading of the manuscript.

References

1. Hirschhorn JN. Genomewide association studies–illuminating biologic pathways. N Engl J Med. 2009;360(17):1699–701.
2. Kermack W, McKendrick A, McKinely P. Death rates in Great Britain and Sweden: some general regularities and their significance. Lancet. 1934;223:698–703.

3. Dorner G, Plagemann A, Ruckert J, et al. Teratogenetic maternofoetal transmission and prevention of diabetes susceptibility. Exp Clin Endocrinol. 1988;91(3):247–58.
4. Barker DJ, Osmond C. Infant mortality, childhood nutrition, and ischaemic heart disease in England and Wales. Lancet. 1986;1(8489):1077–81.
5. Lucas A. Programming by early nutrition in man. Ciba Found Symp. 1991;156 (38–50):Discussion 50–35.
6. Barker DJ. In utero programming of chronic disease. Clin Sci (Lond). 1998;95(2):115–28.
7. Barker DJ. Fetal nutrition and cardiovascular disease in later life. Br Med Bull. 1997;53(1):96–108.
8. Barker DJ, Osmond C, Forsen TJ, et al. Trajectories of growth among children who have coronary events as adults. N Engl J Med. 2005;353(17):1802–9.
9. Hales CN, Barker DJ. The thrifty phenotype hypothesis. Br Med Bull. 2001;60:5–20.
10. Godfrey K. The developmental origins hypothesis: epidemiology. In: Gluckman PD, Hanson MA, editors. Developmental origins of health and disease. Cambridge, MA: Cambridge University Press; 2006. pp. 6–32.
11. Ozanne SE, Hales CN. The long-term consequences of intra-uterine protein malnutrition for glucose metabolism. Proc Nutr Soc. 1999;58(3):615–9.
12. Dahri S, Snoeck A, Reusens-Billen B, et al. Islet function in offspring of mothers on low-protein diet during gestation. Diabetes. 1991;40 Suppl 2:115–20.
13. Plagemann A, Harder T, Rake A, et al. Hypothalamic nuclei are malformed in weanling offspring of low protein malnourished rat dams. J Nutr. 2000;130(10):2582–9.
14. Garofano A, Czernichow P, Breant B. Beta-cell mass and proliferation following late fetal and early postnatal malnutrition in the rat. Diabetologia. 1998;41(9):1114–20.
15. Aerts L, Van Assche FA. Intra-uterine transmission of disease. Placenta. 2003;24(10):905–11.
16. Aerts L, Van Assche FA. Animal evidence for the transgenerational development of diabetes mellitus. Int J Biochem Cell Biol. 2006;38(5–6):894–903.
17. Nohr EA, Timpson NJ, Andersen CS, et al. Severe obesity in young women and reproductive health: the Danish National Birth Cohort. PLoS One. 2009;4(12):e8444. doi:10.1371/journal.pone.0008444.
18. Kahn BB, Flier JS. Obesity and insulin resistance. J Clin Invest. 2000;106(4):473–81.
19. Khan IY, Dekou V, Douglas G, et al. A high-fat diet during rat pregnancy or suckling induces cardiovascular dysfunction in adult offspring. Am J Physiol Regul Integr Comp Physiol. 2005;288(1):R127–R33.
20. Levin BE, Dunn-Meynell AA. Reduced central leptin sensitivity in rats with diet-induced obesity. Am J Physiol Regul Integr Comp Physiol. 2002;283(4):R941–8.
21. Fernandez-Twinn DS, Ozanne SE. Mechanisms by which poor early growth programs type-2 diabetes, obesity and the metabolic syndrome. Physiol Behav. 2006;88(3):234–43.
22. Guilloteau P, Zabielski R, Hammon HM, Metges CC. Adverse effects of nutritional programming during prenatal and early postnatal life, some aspects of regulation and potential prevention and treatments. J Physiol Pharmacol. 2009;60 Suppl 3:17–35.
23. Levin BE. Metabolic imprinting: critical impact of the perinatal environment on the regulation of energy homeostasis. Philos Trans R Soc Lond. 2006;361(1471):1107–21.
24. Petry CJ, Ozanne SE, Hales CN. Programming of intermediary metabolism. Mol Cell Endocrinol. 2001;185(1–2):81–91.
25. Umberto S, Barker D. Offspring of diabetic pregnancy: long-term consequences. Semin Fetal Neonatal Med. 2009;14:119–24.
26. Kaung HL. Growth dynamics of pancreatic islet cell populations during fetal and neonatal development of the rat. Dev Dyn. 1994;200(2):163–75.
27. Grove KL, Allen S, Grayson BE, Smith MS. Postnatal development of the hypothalamic neuropeptide Y system. Neuroscience. 2003;116(2):393–406.
28. Haisma H, Coward WA, Albernaz E, et al. Breast milk and energy intake in exclusively, predominantly, and partially breast-fed infants. Eur J Clin Nutr. 2003;57(12):1633–42.
29. Mortensen EL, Michaelsen KF, Sanders SA, Reinisch JM. The association between duration of breastfeeding and adult intelligence. JAMA. 2002;287(18):2365–71.

30. Baker JL, Michaelsen KF, Rasmussen KM, Sorensen TI. Maternal prepregnant body mass index, duration of breastfeeding, and timing of complementary food introduction are associated with infant weight gain. Am J Clin Nutr. 2004;80(6):1579–88.
31. Owen CG, Martin RM, Whincup PH, et al. The effect of breastfeeding on mean body mass index throughout life: a quantitative review of published and unpublished observational evidence. Am J Clin Nutr. 2005;82(6):1298–307.
32. Owen CG, Martin RM, Whincup PH, et al. Effect of infant feeding on the risk of obesity across the life course: a quantitative review of published evidence. Pediatrics. 2005;115(5):1367–77.
33. McCance RA. Food, growth, and time. Lancet. 1962;2:671–6.
34. Davidowa H, Li Y, Plagemann A. The main effect of cocaine- and amphetamine-regulated transcript (CART) peptide on hypothalamic neuronal activity depends on the nutritional state of rats. Neuroendocrinol Lett. 2005;26(1):29–34.
35. Davidowa H, Plagemann A. Hypothalamic neurons of postnatally overfed, overweight rats respond differentially to corticotropin-releasing hormones. Neurosci Lett. 2004;371(1):64–8.
36. Plagemann A. Perinatal programming and functional teratogenesis: impact on body weight regulation and obesity. Physiol Behav. 2005;86(5):661–8.
37. Fahrenkrog S, Harder T, Stolaczyk E, et al. Cross-fostering to diabetic rat dams affects early development of mediobasal hypothalamic nuclei regulating food intake, body weight, and metabolism. J Nutr. 2004;134(3):648–54.
38. Patel MS, Srinivasan M. Metabolic programming as a consequence of the nutritional environment during fetal and the immediate postnatal periods. In: Hay WW, Thureen, PJ, editors. Neonatal nutrition and metabolism. Cambridge, MA: Cambridge University Press; 2006. pp. 76–90.
39. Patel MS, Srinivasan M, Laychock SG. Metabolic programming: role of nutrition in the immediate postnatal life. J Inherit Metab Dis. 2009;32(2):218–28.
40. Srinivasan M, Patel MS. Metabolic programming in the immediate postnatal period. Trends Endocrinol Metab. 2008;19(4):146–52.
41. Vadlamudi S, Kalhan SC, Patel MS. Persistence of metabolic consequences in the progeny of rats fed a HC formula in their early postnatal life. Am J Physiol. 1995;269(4 Pt 1):E731–8.
42. Hiremagalur BK, Vadlamudi S, Johanning GL, Patel MS. Long-term effects of feeding high carbohydrate diet in pre-weaning period by gastrostomy: a new rat model for obesity. Int J Obes Relat Metab Disord. 1993;17(9):495–502.
43. Haney PM, Estrin CR, Caliendo A, Patel MS. Precocious induction of hepatic glucokinase and malic enzyme in artificially reared rat pups fed a high-carbohydrate diet. Arch Biochem Biophys. 1986;244(2):787–94.
44. Srinivasan M, Mitrani P, Sadhanandan G, et al. A high-carbohydrate diet in the immediate postnatal life of rats induces adaptations predisposing to adult-onset obesity. J Endocrinol. 2008;197(3):565–74.
45. Plagemann A, Harder T, Rake A, et al. Perinatal elevation of hypothalamic insulin, acquired malformation of hypothalamic galaninergic neurons, and syndrome x-like alterations in adulthood of neonatally overfed rats. Brain Res. 1999;836(1–2):146–55.
46. Bouret SG, Simerly RB. Developmental programming of hypothalamic feeding circuits. Clin Gen. 2006;70(4):295–301.
47. Srinivasan M, Dodds C, Ghanim H, et al. Maternal obesity and fetal programming: effects of a high-carbohydrate nutritional modification in the immediate postnatal life of female rats. Am J Physiol Endocrinol Metab. 2008;295(4):E895–E903.
48. Srinivasan M, Aalinkeel R, Song F, et al. Maternal hyperinsulinemia predisposes rat fetuses for hyperinsulinemia, and adult-onset obesity and maternal mild food restriction reverses this phenotype. Am J Physiol Endocrinol Metab. 2006;290(1):E129–E34.
49. Srinivasan M, Aalinkeel R, Song F, Patel MS. Programming of islet functions in the progeny of hyperinsulinemic/obese rats. Diabetes. 2003;52(4):984–90.
50. Srinivasan M, Vadlamudi S, Patel MS. Glycogen synthase regulation in hyperinsulinemic/obese progeny of rats fed a high carbohydrate formula in their infancy. Int J Obes Relat Metab Disord. 1996;20(11):981–9.

51. Cerf ME, Williams K, Nkomo XI, et al. Islet cell response in the neonatal rat after exposure to a high-fat diet during pregnancy. Am J Physiol Regul Integr Comp Physiol. 2005;288(5):R1122–8.
52. Levin BE, Govek E. Gestational obesity accentuates obesity in obesity-prone progeny. Am J Physiol. 1998;275(4 Pt 2):R1374–9.
53. Woods SC, Seeley RJ, Rushing PA, et al. A controlled high-fat diet induces an obese syndrome in rats. J Nutr. 2003;133(4):1081–7.
54. Chang GQ, Gaysinskaya V, Karatayev O, Leibowitz SF. Maternal high-fat diet and fetal programming: increased proliferation of hypothalamic peptide-producing neurons that increase risk for overeating and obesity. J Neurosci. 2008;28(46):12107–19.
55. Grayson BE, Levasseur PR, Williams SM, et al. Changes in melanocortin expression and inflammatory pathways in fetal offspring of nonhuman primates fed a high-fat diet. Endocrinology 2010;151:1622–32.
56. Srinivasan M, Katewa SD, Palaniyappan A, et al. Maternal high-fat diet consumption results in fetal malprogramming predisposing to the onset of metabolic syndrome-like phenotype in adulthood. Am J Physiol Endocrinol Metab. 2006;291(4):E792–9.
57. Gupta A, Srinivasan M, Thamadilok S, Patel MS. Hypothalamic alterations in fetuses of high fat diet-fed obese female rats. J Endocrinol. 2009;200(3):293–300.
58. Bouret SG, Simerly RB. Development of leptin-sensitive circuits. J Neuroendocrinol. 2007;19(8):575–82.
59. Plagemann A, Heidrich I, Rohde W, Gotz F, Dorner G. Hyperinsulinism during differentiation of the hypothalamus is a diabetogenic and obesity risk factor in rats. Neuroendocrinol Lett. 1992;5:373–8.
60. Reik W. Stability and flexibility of epigenetic gene regulation in mammalian development. Nature. 2007;447(7143):425–32.
61. Aagaard-Tillery KM, Grove K, Bishop J, et al. Developmental origins of disease and determinants of chromatin structure: maternal diet modifies the primate fetal epigenome. J Mol Endocrinol. 2008;41(2):91–102.
62. Park JH, Stoffers DA, Nicholls RD, Simmons RA. Development of type 2 diabetes following intrauterine growth retardation in rats is associated with progressive epigenetic silencing of Pdx1. J Clin Invest. 2008;118(6):2316–24.
63. Raychaudhuri N, Raychaudhuri S, Thamotharan M, Devaskar SU. Histone code modifications repress glucose transporter 4 expression in the intrauterine growth-restricted offspring. J Biol Chem. 2008;283(20):13611–26.
64. Kuzawa CW, Sweet E. Epigenetics and the embodiment of race: developmental origins of US racial disparities in cardiovascular health. Am J Hum Biol. 2009;21(1):2–15.
65. Flegal KM, Carroll MD, Ogden CL, Curtin LR. Prevalence and trends in obesity among US adults, 1999–2008. JAMA. 2010;303(3):235–41.
66. Heslehurst N, Rankin J, Wilkinson JR, Summerbell CD. A nationally representative study of maternal obesity in England, UK: trends in incidence and demographic inequalities in 619,323 births, 1989–2007. Int J Obes (Lond). 2010;34(3):420–8.
67. Gillman MW, Barker D, Bier D, et al. Meeting report on the 3rd international congress on developmental origins of health and disease (DOHaD). Pediatr Res. 2007;61(5 Pt 1):625–9.
68. Lawlor DA, Smith GD, O'Callaghan M, et al. Epidemiologic evidence for the fetal overnutrition hypothesis: findings from the mater-university study of pregnancy and its outcomes. Am J Epidemiol. 2007;165(4):418–24.
69. Dabelea D, Hanson RL, Lindsay RS, et al. Intrauterine exposure to diabetes conveys risks for type 2 diabetes and obesity: a study of discordant sibships. Diabetes. 2000;49(12):2208–11.
70. Schack-Nielsen L, Michaelsen KF, Gamborg M, et al. Gestational weight gain in relation to offspring body mass index and obesity from infancy through adulthood. Int J Obes (Lond). 2010:34(1):67–74.

Chapter 14
Prenatal Stress, Glucocorticoids, and the Metabolic Syndrome

Amanda J. Drake and Jonathan R. Seckl

14.1 Early Life Programming

There is now a well-established link between low birth weight and other early life anthropometric parameters, suggestive of exposure to an adverse intrauterine environment and a markedly elevated risk of subsequent hypertension, insulin resistance, type 2 diabetes, and hyperlipidemia, a cluster of cardiovascular risk factors that are termed the metabolic syndrome [1–5]. This relationship is largely independent of classical adult lifestyle risk factors, such as smoking, adult weight, social class, and excess alcohol intake [4, 6], and holds for the full range of birth weights, including those within the normal range rather than severely undersized, multiple, or premature babies [6, 7]. To explain this association between perinatal environmental events, altered fetal/postnatal growth, and development and later pathophysiology, the concept of developmental programming has been advanced [3, 8, 9]. Programming proposes that a stimulus or insult acting during critical developmental periods can permanently alter tissue structure and function, producing effects which persist throughout life. Different cells and tissues are sensitive at different developmental stages, so the effects of an environmental challenge will have distinct effects depending on its timing. Studies in inbred rodent models support the concept that early life environmental manipulations are associated with later physiology and disease risk and imply causation via non-genetic processes [10, 11]. Two major hypotheses have been proposed to explain this relationship: fetal malnutrition [6, 12] and overexposure of the fetus to glucocorticoids, for example, as a consequence of maternal stress [8]. Here we will focus on the role of glucocorticoids in programming of metabolic disease.

A.J. Drake (✉)
Centre for Cardiovascular Science, The Queen's Medical Research Institute, University of Edinburgh, Edinburgh, UK
e-mail: mandy.drake@ed.ac.uk

R.H. Lustig (ed.), *Obesity Before Birth*, Endocrine Updates 30,
DOI 10.1007/978-1-4419-7034-3_14,

14.2 The Role of Glucocorticoids

The programming effects of steroid hormones were initially best characterised for androgens. Neonatal exposure to androgens permanently programs the expression of hepatic steroid metabolising enzymes and the development of sexually dimorphic structures in the anterior hypothalamus, leading to lifelong changes in sexual behaviour [13, 14], irrespective of subsequent hormonal manipulation or the genetic sex of the animal. More recently, the programming effects of glucocorticoids have been extensively investigated. Secretion of glucocorticoids from the adrenal cortex is controlled by the hypothalamic–pituitary–adrenal (HPA) axis in a classical endocrine negative-feedback loop. Glucocorticoids exert their effects by binding intracellular glucocorticoid receptors (GR), members of the nuclear hormone superfamily of ligand-activated transcription factors. Additionally, in some tissues, glucocorticoids bind with high affinity to mineralocorticoid receptors (MR). GR and MR are activated upon ligand binding and the receptor–ligand complex translocates to the nucleus, binding to glucocorticoid response elements in the promoter region of target genes to influence gene transcription [15]. In addition, recent evidence suggests that rapid, non-genomic effects of these steroids may be mediated via cell membrane receptors [16] that appear to derive from the same genes as the nuclear receptors, since their genetic deletion abrogates "membrane" effects [17]. GR is found in the cells of virtually all vertebrate tissues. In adult mammals glucocorticoids regulate a variety of important cardiovascular, metabolic, immunologic, and other homeostatic functions. Excessive glucocorticoid levels, resulting either from exogenous administration or from endogenous overproduction (e.g. in Cushing's syndrome), have effects on many systems including well-characterised diabetogenic and hypertensive effects [18].

14.3 Glucocorticoids and Fetal Development

The GR is expressed in most fetal tissues from early embryonal stages [19, 20], whereas expression of the MR has a more limited tissue distribution in development and is only present at later gestational stages [21], at least in rodents. Additionally, GR is expressed in the placenta [22] where it mediates metabolic, anti-inflammatory, and parturitional effects. In the early human embryo, expression of GR mRNA has been identified in the metanephros, gut, muscle, spinal cord and dorsal root ganglia, periderm, sex chords of the testis, and adrenal by 8–10 weeks [23, 24] and in the human lung by 12 weeks of gestation. Thus, systems mediating glucocorticoid actions exist from early developmental stages, with complex cell-specific patterns of expression and presumable sensitivity to the widely accessible steroid ligands [20].

Many of the significant maturational changes in organ systems such as the lungs, heart, liver, gut, and kidneys [25–27] are glucocorticoid dependent and can be induced prematurely by exogenous glucocorticoid administration [28, 29], underpinning their widespread therapeutic use in threatened preterm labour, as a method to accelerate lung maturation [30]. Glucocorticoid treatment during pregnancy reduces birth weight in animals and in humans [31–36]. Furthermore, cortisol levels are increased in human fetuses with intrauterine growth retardation or in pregnancies complicated by pre-eclampsia, which may indicate a role for endogenous cortisol in fetal growth retardation [37, 38]. However, there may be significant differences between the effects of fetal exposure to endogenous glucocorticoids and those of synthetic glucocorticoids. For example, while endogenous glucocorticoids can bind both GR and MR, and the effects in tissues such as brain may be mediated by both of these receptors, synthetic glucocorticoids typically used in obstetric practice are more selective for GR. Similarly, there may be differences in local tissue concentration governed by differences in transport in blood (binding to and cellular release from CBG), ability to cross physiological barriers (e.g. the blood–brain barrier) and metabolism of endogenous and synthetic glucocorticoids [39, 40].

14.4 11β-Hydroxysteroid Dehydrogenase Type 2 and the Feto-placental Glucocorticoid Barrier

Although glucocorticoids are highly lipophilic molecules and should readily cross the placenta, fetal glucocorticoid levels are normally much lower than in maternal circulation [41]. This is thought to be mediated by placental 11β-hydroxysteroid dehydrogenase-2 (11β-HSD2, an NAD-dependent 11β-dehydrogenase), which catalyses the conversion of active glucocorticoids (cortisol in humans, corticosterone in rats) to their inactive 11-keto metabolites (cortisone and 11-dehydrocorticosterone, respectively) [42]. 11β-HSD2 is located at the interface between maternal and fetal circulations in the syncytiotrophoblast in humans [21, 43] and the labyrinthine zone in rodents [44, 45], where it acts as a "barrier" preventing maternal glucocorticoids from accessing the fetus (Fig. 14.1) [46–48]. However, 10–20% of maternal cortisol can cross the placenta to the fetus and in rodents the peak of the circadian rhythm of plasma corticosterone penetrates the 11β-HSD2 barrier to an appreciable extent [49]. In guinea pigs, a decrease in placental 11β-HSD2 at term is associated with increased transfer of maternal cortisol to the fetus [50], which is presumably necessary for normal developmental processes. Similar late gestational falls in placental 11β-HSD2 activity are seen in mice and nearer to term in rats. However in primates including humans, 11β-HSD2 activity rises towards term, presumably because the fetal adrenals contribute more to the endogenous glucocorticoid surge that prepares the fetus for extrauterine life. Additionally, within a species, the efficiency of placental 11β-HSD2 near term varies considerably [51, 52].

Thus, reduction in placental 11β-HSD2 may result in overexposure of the fetus to maternal glucocorticoids, which has been proposed as a mechanism for the programming of later disease risk [8]. In humans, mutations of the gene encoding 11β-HSD2 are associated with significant reductions in birth weight [53], and 11β-HSD2 nullizygosity lowers birth weight in mice congenic on the C57Bl/6 strain background

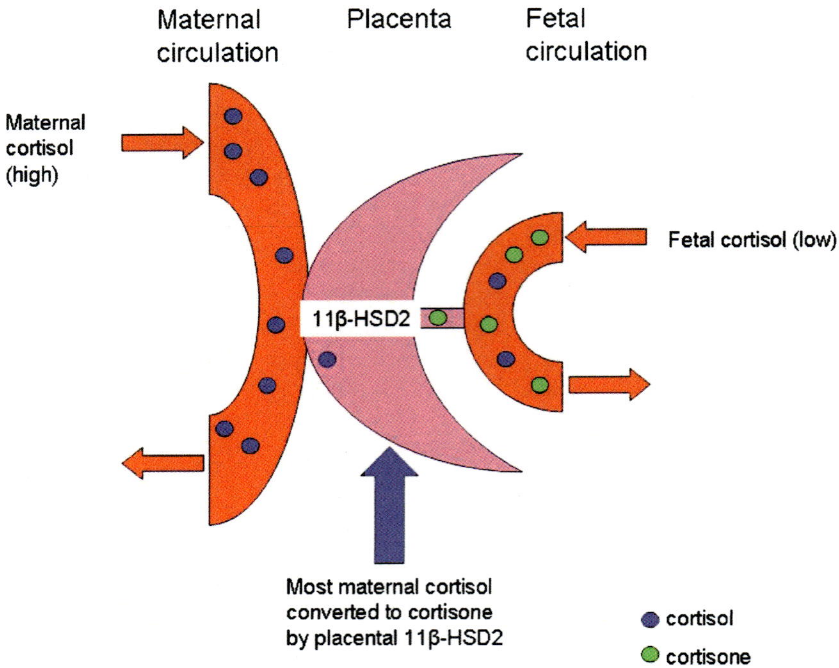

Fig. 14.1 Feto-placental barrier to glucocorticoids. Maternal glucocorticoids are inactivated by the enzyme 11β-HSD2 in the placenta which acts as a barrier preventing most maternal glucocorticoids from accessing the developing fetus

[54]. In terms of natural variation, in rodents lower placental 11β-HSD2 activity associates with the smallest fetuses [51], a finding which has been reproduced in humans in some [52, 55–57] but not all [58, 59] studies. The expression and/or activity of placental 11β-HSD2 may be affected by several key maternal environmental factors. The precise molecular bases for its control have yet to be fully delineated, although recent evidence suggests that epigenetic mechanisms such as DNA methylation may play a role in modulating its expression [60, 61]. In vitro "placental" cell 11β-HSD2 is regulated by glucocorticoids [62], catecholamines acting via adrenergic receptors [63], components of tobacco smoke [64], various inflammatory signals [65, 66] progesterone, estrogen, and nitric oxide [67]. In vivo, placental 11β-HSD2 activity is downregulated by stress, illness, inflammation, infection, and hypoxia [68–70]. Intriguingly, in nutritional models of programming, maternal protein restriction in rodents reduces the activity of 11β-HSD2 in the placenta [71], suggesting that 11β-HSD2 activity is influenced by maternal environmental factors. Other environmental insults such as maternal malnutrition may also operate through glucocorticoids in exerting their programming effects. In support of this notion, the programming of hypertension by maternal protein restriction during pregnancy in the rat can be prevented by the inhibition of maternal corticosterone biosynthesis

during pregnancy [72]. Conversely, glucocorticoid treatment in rodents associates with reduced food intake and impaired weight gain [73, 74], providing further support for an interrelationship between these hypotheses.

14.5 Glucocorticoid Programming

Fetal glucocorticoid load can be increased by a number of means. Synthetic glucocorticoids such as dexamethasone and betamethasone are poor substrates for 11β-HSD2 and will readily cross the placenta following maternal administration. Fetal glucocorticoid exposure can also be increased by inhibiting feto-placental 11β-HSD2 by liquorice or its derivatives such as carbenoxolone [42]. Maternal stress leads to a large number of cardiovascular and endocrine changes in the mother, including increases in plasma ACTH, β-endorphin, glucocorticoid, and catecholamine concentrations and the levels of glucocorticoids associated with such physiological stress may overcome the placental 11β-HSD2 barrier. Maternal stress also reduces placental 11β-HSD2 in some models [68]. These strategies have been employed in a number of animal models, which show that prenatal glucocorticoid excess has persistent effects throughout the lifespan. Prenatal dexamethasone,

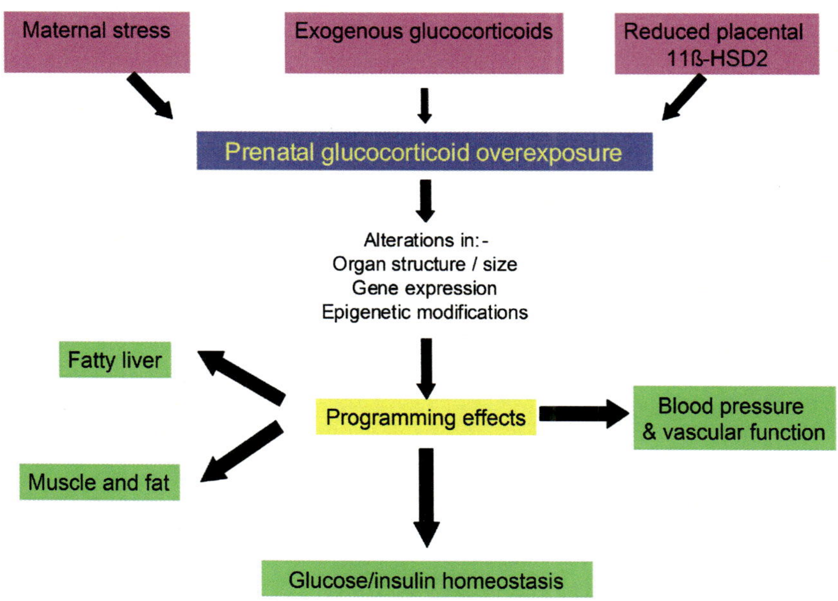

Fig. 14.2 Glucocorticoids in fetal programming. Prenatal overexposure to glucocorticoids as a consequence of maternal stress, exogenous glucocorticoids, or decreased placental levels of the enzyme 11β-HSD2 are associated with programming effects on blood pressure and vascular function and glucose/insulin homeostasis, increased susceptibility to the development of a fatty liver and effects on muscle and adipocyte development and function

maternal stress, or 11β-HSD2 inhibition are associated with programming of higher adult blood pressure, glucose, and insulin levels in rats, sheep, and other species (Fig. 14.2) [33, 51, 73, 75–82] including non-human primates [83, 84].

That glucocorticoid effects can be mediated directly on the fetus and its placenta rather than indirectly via alterations in maternal food intake or biology has been demonstrated using a 11β-HSD2 knockout mouse model. "Heterozygote" crosses of 11β-HSD2$^{+/-}$ mice results in the presence of wild-type, heterozygous, and null offspring in the same pregnancy and in this model, birth weight follows the feto-placental genotype so that 11β-HSD2 null offspring have the lowest birth weight [54]. Heterozygote offspring show birth weights intermediate between their wild type and 11β-HSD2$^{-/-}$ homozygous littermates, suggesting that variation of feto-placental 11β-HSD2 determines fetal growth and presumably programming. Indeed, because maternal glucocorticoid levels are much higher (2- to 10-fold higher) than those of the fetus, subtle changes in placental 11β-HSD2 activity may have profound effects on fetal glucocorticoid exposure [46, 48].

14.6 Programming of Cardiovascular and Metabolic Systems

14.6.1 Programming of Blood Pressure and Vascular Function

Cortisol elevates blood pressure in fetal and neonatal sheep when infused directly in utero [85, 86] and the administration of betamethasone to pregnant baboons elevates fetal blood pressure [87]. In rats, antenatal glucocorticoid overexposure is associated with a persistent elevation in arterial blood pressure in adulthood in both male and female offspring [51, 73, 74, 80]. Intriguingly, in one rat model, detailed study revealed that while prenatal dexamethasone programmed stress-induced hypertension, blood pressure was lower in the offspring when undisturbed [88]. Programmed effects of prenatal glucocorticoid excess on blood pressure are also found to persist into adulthood in sheep [76, 79, 89, 90] and in a non-human primate model [83]. The timing of glucocorticoid exposure appears to be important in the programming of hypertension; exposure to glucocorticoids during the final week of pregnancy is sufficient to produce permanent adult hypertension in the rat [80]; indeed recent studies suggest that exposure to excess glucocorticoid for just 2 days at this time is sufficient to programme altered renal development and hypertension in the absence of altered fetal growth [91]. In contrast, in sheep, such effects are seen after glucocorticoid exposure earlier in gestation [75, 77, 92]. The reason for such differences is unclear but may reflect the complex species-specific patterns of expression of glucocorticoid receptors and the isoenzymes of 11β-HSD [42], which regulate maternal glucocorticoid transfer to the fetus and modulate glucocorticoid action in individual tissues, and/or differences in down-stream processes that can affect glucocorticoid-induced maturational effects in particular cells. In rats, maternal administration of carbenoxolone, a potent inhibitor of 11β-HSD, also leads to reduced birth weight and elevated blood pressure in the adult offspring [81]. The programming effects of carbenoxolone require the presence of maternal glucocorticoids, as the offspring of adrenalectomised pregnant rats are protected from carbenoxolone actions upon birth weight and adult hypertension [81].

Glucocorticoid programming of blood pressure is likely to involve a number of processes. Prenatal glucocorticoid overexposure is associated with an irreversible reduction in nephron number in rodents [93–95] and sheep [96], although not in marmosets [97]. Additionally, in rats, prenatal dexamethasone exposure is associated with increased renal glucocorticoid sensitivity, with increased renal expression of GR, decreased renal expression of 11β-HSD2, elevated renal Na/K-ATPase-α1 [98], and with altered proximal tubule and thick ascending limb transport [99, 100]. Rats exposed to glucocorticoids prenatally also show altered activity of the renin–angiotensin–aldosterone system [98, 101] and increased expression of the angiotensin type 1 and 2 receptors and angiotensin-converting enzyme [102, 103].

Glucocorticoid programming is associated with alterations in vascular responsivity to vasoconstrictors in rats [88, 104], with altered aortic vasodilatation in mice [105] and with enhancement of endothelin-induced vasoconstriction and attenuation of endothelium-dependent vasorelaxation in sheep [106]. Prenatal glucocorticoid exposure alters reactivity of the coronary arteries in the newborn lamb prior to the development of systemic hypertension [107]. Additionally, the offspring have altered cardiac noradrenergic innervation and sympathetic activity of baroreceptor response [25, 102]. Changes in expression of several other genes in the heart have been reported, including glucose transporter 1, Akt/protein kinase B, specific uncoupling proteins, peroxisome proliferator-activated receptor (PPAR)-gamma, and calreticulin [108, 109]. Overexpression of cardiac calreticulin is known to cause cardiac dysfunction and death [109]. Thus, increased coronary heart disease deaths in individuals born with low birth weight may reflect programmed primary cardiac dysfunction as well as the increased prevalence of cardiovascular risk factors such as hypertension.

14.6.2 Programming of Glucose and Insulin Homeostasis

Prenatal glucocorticoid overexposure in rats as a result of 11β-HSD2 inhibition or maternal dexamethasone administration programs permanent hyperglycemia and hyperinsulinemia in adulthood [33, 82, 110]. As with programming of blood pressure, the last third of gestation appears to be an important "window" during which glucocorticoid exposure results in programming effects. Exposure in early gestation or during the neonatal period does not appear to produce the same long-lasting changes in blood glucose and insulin levels [33, 111]. Additionally, the effects of carbenoxolone, an 11β-HSD2 inhibitor, on birth weight and adult glucose metabolism can be prevented by maternal adrenalectomy, confirming that they are dependent on maternal glucocorticoids [82]. Increasing endogenous glucocorticoid production through prenatal stress (which presumably overwhelms the activity of 11β-HSD2 and may downregulate the enzyme as well) is thought to have similar persisting effects [112, 113].

Maternal glucocorticoid administration has an effect on cord glucose and insulin levels in the ovine fetus [114] and on glucose homeostasis in the adult offspring. Intriguingly, in sheep, antenatal glucocorticoid exposure with or without fetal growth restriction altered glucose metabolism [92]; maternal but not fetal injections of betamethasone-restricted fetal growth [34], although offspring of both groups had altered glucose metabolism postnatally [92] suggesting that programming relates to fetal exposure to excess glucocorticoids in utero, rather than intrauterine growth retardation per se. The molecular mechanisms through which prenatal supraphysiological levels of glucocorticoids program hyperglycemia have not been fully determined, but may involve derangements in several target organs. In particular, these effects may relate to altered structure or function of the endocrine pancreas and/or insulin-sensitive target tissues. At least in sheep, the observed programming effects may be dependent on the type of glucocorticoid used [115]. Programming effects of prenatal glucocorticoid overexposure on glucose–insulin homeostasis have also been reported in non-human primate models; as prenatal dexamethasone overexposure is associated with the development of impaired glucose tolerance and hyperinsulinemia in the African vervet monkey *Chlorocebus aethiops* [83].

In terms of mechanism, glucocorticoids regulate expression of critical hepatic metabolic enzymes, notably phosphoenolpyruvate carboxykinase (PEPCK), which develops in late gestation and catalyses a rate-limiting step in gluconeogenesis. In rats, in utero exposure to dexamethasone induces lifelong elevations in PEPCK mRNA and enzyme activity, selectively within the periportal region of the hepatic acinus, the site of gluconeogenesis [33]. PEPCK is the rate-limiting enzyme of gluconeogenesis [116] and transgenic mice with overexpression of hepatic PEPCK have impaired glucose tolerance [117]. In addition, over-expression of PEPCK in a rat hepatoma cell line impairs suppression of gluconeogenesis by insulin [118]. It has therefore been proposed that the increase in PEPCK in programmed animals may therefore be of functional significance in the pathogenesis of hyperglycemia following prenatal exposure to glucocorticoids [33]. PEPCK expression is normally regulated at the level of gene expression by distinct hepatocyte-enriched nuclear transcription activators that bind their cognate DNA motifs in the PEPCK gene promoter [119]. These include members of the hepatocyte nuclear factor family, such as (HNF)1, HNF3, HNF4, and HNF6; members of the CCAAT/enhancer binding protein (C/EBP) family; and GR itself. Intriguingly, livers of dexamethasone-programmed rats showed increased expression some of these key transcription factors, notably GR [33, 120] and HNF4α [121] in the liver, suggesting that the increase in hepatic PEPCK expression may be secondary to the alterations in these transcription factors. Increased hepatic GR expression is also seen in other models of in utero programming of hyperglycemia such as maternal protein restriction or uterine artery ligation [122]. This suggests that changes in transcription factors such as GR may provide a common mechanism through which intrauterine environmental insults might lead to persistent derangements in metabolic control.

Data from human and animal studies suggest that the microsomal enzyme 11β-HSD-1, which catalyses the reverse reaction, of regeneration of active glucocorticoids (cortisol, corticosterone) from their inactive forms (cortisone, 11-dehydrocortisone), may play an important role in the development of the metabolic syndrome in association with obesity by increasing local tissue glucocorticoid concentrations [123, 124]. Very recently, in a marmoset model, prenatal glucocorticoid programming was shown to result in increased expression of 11β-HSD1 in liver (increasing intrahepatic glucocorticoid concentrations), which is evident before the development of obesity or the metabolic syndrome [84]. Since glucocorticoids regulate a number of pathways controlling hepatic glucose and lipid metabolism [125], this has potential importance for prenatal programming of the metabolic syndrome. In support of this, prenatal dexamethasone is associated with enhanced hepatic PEPCK activity, suggestive of increased hepatic glucose output [84].

14.6.3 Programming of the Pancreas

Relatively little is known about the effects of prenatal exposure to glucocorticoids on the development of the endocrine pancreas. Glucocorticoid signalling is important in pancreatic development [126], and glucocorticoids have been shown to impair β-cell development in rats [127]. Prenatal undernutrition also causes marked restriction of fetal β-cell growth and impairs glucose-stimulated insulin secretion in adult rat offspring. In vitro, isolated pancreatic islets have decreased insulin content and show impaired secretory response to glucose and arginine [128]. Again, this effect appears to be dependent on maternal/fetal corticosterone, as preventing the increase in corticosterone in food-restricted dams restores β-cell mass. Indeed, fetal pancreatic insulin content correlates inversely with fetal corticosterone levels [127]. Reduced pancreatic β-cell mass is also impaired in the vervet model of prenatal dexamethasone overexposure [83]. The mechanisms by which glucocorticoids modulate pancreatic development are not fully understood, but in vitro data suggest that this may involve interaction with other transcription factors that control proliferation and/or differentiation of the pancreas [129]. Additionally, in the adult pancreas, glucocorticoids directly inhibit insulin secretion. Thus, elevated local and/or systemic glucocorticoid levels could lead to impaired β-cell function and contribute to hyperglycemia. This is indeed seen in the marmoset model of prenatal glucocorticoid overexposure in which pancreatic 11β-HSD1 expression is increased [84], and in the glucocorticoid-programmed rat and vervet monkey which show elevated basal and/or stress-induced circulating glucocorticoid concentrations [33, 83]. Finally, glucocorticoids influence the expression of insulin-like growth factor (IGF)-2, a key peptide growth factor in pancreatic development, in addition to the IGF receptor and several IGF-binding proteins [130].

14.6.4 Fatty Liver

Non-alcoholic fatty liver disease (NAFLD) is currently the most common form of chronic liver disease in children and adults [131] and is considered to be the hepatic manifestation of the metabolic syndrome [132]. Although NAFLD is strongly associated with obesity and insulin resistance [132–134], it is not clear why certain individuals are more susceptible to the development of NAFLD than others [135]. We have recently reported that prenatal glucocorticoid overexposure in rats is associated with the development of fatty liver when animals are maintained on a high-fat diet following weaning, in association with altered expression of genes important in lipid metabolism, particularly in adipose tissue depots [136]. Similar findings have been reported in other animal models of programming using prenatal undernutrition or exposure to a high-fat diet prenatally [137, 138] suggesting that fatty liver may be a common consequence of exposure to an "adverse environment" prenatally, particularly when combined with postnatal obesity. In humans, little is known of the relationship between the early life environment and liver fat content; however, recent data suggest that there may also be an influence of the prenatal environment on liver function [139].

14.6.5 Programming of Muscle and Fat

Prenatal glucocorticoid overexposure may also program long-term insulin resistance and hyperglycemia by altering expression of the glucoregulatory genes in tissues involved in insulin-sensitive glucose disposal, such as skeletal muscle. These may include changes in the glucose transporters, hormone receptors, and other intracellular signalling proteins. Prenatal dexamethasone treatment has been shown to program alterations in the expression of genes that regulate glucose uptake and fuel metabolism including GR, the glucose transporter slc2a4, uncoupling protein 3, PPARδ, and PPARγ coactivator-1α in adult skeletal muscle [110, 120].

Antenatal dexamethasone exposure in rats is also associated with alterations in offspring fat metabolism. Adult offspring of rat dams exposed to dexamethasone during gestation have increased intra-abdominal fat depots, with a parallel increase in leptin levels [140]. Moreover, in utero exposure to dexamethasone causes a marked increase in GR expression and attenuated fatty acid uptake in adult rats, selectively in visceral adipose tissue, which may contribute to both adipose and hepatic insulin resistance [120]. Maternal nutrient restriction during pregnancy has also been associated with increased adipose tissue GR expression and obesity in sheep [141–143]. In the marmoset, prenatal glucocorticoid overexposure programs increased 11β-HSD1 expression in subcutaneous fat, as well as liver. In obese humans and in monogenically obese rodents, 11β-HSD1 expression and activity are increased in adipose depots [123, 124] and transgenic overexpression of 11β-HSD1 selectively in adipose tissue causes visceral obesity and the metabolic syndrome [144]. Thus, long-term upregulation of 11β-HSD1 in adipose tissue may represent a novel mechanism for the fetal programming of adult obesity and the metabolic syndrome.

14.7 Evidence for Glucocorticoid Programming in Humans

The effects of prenatal glucocorticoid exposure observed in animal models including non-human primates could have huge implications if extrapolated to the human fetus. Glucocorticoids are used as immunosuppressants to control various maternal conditions such as connective tissue disorders [145] and are used extensively in obstetric practice, primarily to accelerate lung maturation in cases of threatened preterm labour [146] which may occur in up to 10% of pregnancies. While there is no doubt that such synthetic glucocorticoids enhance lung maturation and reduce mortality in preterm infants [147], in recent times 98% of British obstetric departments prescribed repeated courses of antenatal glucocorticoids [148], although there is little evidence for the safety and efficacy of such a regime [149]. In addition, women at risk of bearing fetuses at risk of congenital adrenal hyperplasia (CAH) may receive low-dose dexamethasone from the first trimester to suppress fetal adrenal androgen overproduction. Birth weight in such infants has been reported as normal [150, 151]; however, programming effects of antenatal glucocorticoids are seen in animal models in the absence of any reduction in birth weight, notably in non-human primate models [83, 84, 92].

The long-term effects of fetal glucocorticoid exposure in humans have been poorly investigated, mainly because these studies have been small, and duration of follow-up thus far short [152]. In one randomised controlled trial in which blood pressure was recorded in 81 individuals aged 20 years, mean systolic blood pressure was lower in those exposed to antenatal glucocorticoid treatment than in controls [153]. In contrast, in a non-randomised cohort of 177 adolescents aged 14 years, those exposed to glucocorticoid treatment had higher mean systolic and diastolic blood pressure than did those exposed to placebo [154]. In a recent study, a higher cortisol:cortisone ratio in umbilical venous cord blood (which may reflect reduced placental 11β-HSD2 activity) was associated with higher systolic blood pressure at age 3 years [155]. Antenatal glucocorticoid administration to preterm infants was associated with a reduction in glomerular filtration rate at the age of 19 years [156] suggesting that prenatal glucocorticoids may indeed have programming effects on the kidney and on blood pressure in humans.

In terms of glucose–insulin homeostasis, one study found that a single course of antenatal betamethasone was found to influence the maternal–fetal insulin–IGF–GH axis, particularly fetal IGF-2 levels, without measurable anthropometric changes at birth, although the implications of this beyond the neonatal period remain to be determined [157]. Nevertheless, in a recent double-blind, placebo-controlled, randomised trial of antenatal betamethasone for the prevention of neonatal respiratory distress syndrome, 534 individuals were followed up over 30 years. Although antenatal exposure to betamethasone did not significantly affect lipid profile, prevalence of diabetes or cardiovascular disease [158], betamethasone-exposed participants in this study did show evidence of increased insulin resistance. This might signify raised risk of diabetes and cardiovascular disease as this cohort ages [158].

Based upon findings in the prenatal dexamethasone-exposed rat model of low birth weight and adult hypercorticosteronaemia, recent studies have examined the relationship between birth weight and HPA function in adult humans. As in other animals, the human HPA axis appears to be programmed by the early life environment. Programming of the HPA axis appears to occur in disparate populations [159] and may precede overt adult disease [5], at least in a socially disadvantaged South African population. Higher plasma and urinary glucocorticoid levels are found in children and adults who were of lower birth weight [160, 161]. In children, low birth weight is associated with altered adrenocortical responses to stress in boys and altered basal adrenocortical activity in girls [162] and in adulthood, HPA responses to ACTH stimulation are exaggerated in those of low birth weight [5, 163], reflecting the stress axis biology elucidated in animal models. Furthermore, this HPA activation is associated with higher blood pressure, insulin resistance, glucose intolerance, and hyperlipidemia [163].

14.8 Mechanisms of Early Life Programming

As discussed throughout this review, there are a number of mechanisms which may underpin the programming effects of prenatal glucocorticoid overexposure. These include alterations in organ size or cell number, permanent changes in gene expression, and alterations in target organ responsiveness. Additionally, there has been much recent interest in the role of epigenetic changes in the early life origins of disease. The term "epigenetic" was originally coined by Conrad Waddington to describe how genotypes give rise to phenotypes during development [164]; however, more recently it has been used to describe changes in gene function that are not explained by changes in DNA sequence and which may be mitotically and/or meiotically heritable. Epigenetic modifications include DNA methylation, histone modifications, and small non-coding RNAs and the role of these modifications in early life programming and obesity will be discussed in detail in Chapters 6, 7, and 8 of this volume. In the dexamethasone-programmed rat, the phenotype of low birth weight and elevated hepatic PEPCK activity is transmitted to a second generation through both male and female lines [11]; transmission of the phenotype through the male line strongly suggests a role for epigenetic modifications in this model.

14.9 Conclusions and Implications for Human Health

Thus, there is accumulating data in humans, as in rodents, suggesting that prenatal glucocorticoid overexposure programs an adverse adult cardiovascular and metabolic phenotype, and these effects appear to be transmitted to a second generation. Whether this is an unusual or a common mechanism to explain the link between low birth weight/size at birth and adult disorders is the subject of ongoing studies, however, the similarities between the programmed phenotypes observed in the different models suggest that there may be common mechanisms underpinning the effects of exposure to environmental factors acting in early development. Early life programming may represent an adaptive response made by an organism in order to prepare it for an "expected" future environment; however, these effects may be deleterious when there is a mismatch between the predicted and the actual environment [165]. In the current climate, certainly in developed countries, in which high-calorie food is plentiful and exercise may be limited, this mismatch has clear implications for public health.

Although many animal programming studies have used a single insult, e.g. fetal glucocorticoid overexposure to investigate the mechanisms underpinning programming effects, in reality a developing fetus is likely to be exposed to multiple different agents or maternal lifestyle risk factors which may impact on development, so that multimodal challenges within the "expected" range may be more important than major changes in a single parameter. We have recently shown how a combination of different, but clinically relevant, fetal exposures interact to disrupt male reproductive development in an animal model of programming using fetal glucocorticoid overexposure in combination with dibutyl phthalate, a compound widely used in solvents and personal care products [166]. Given the widespread exposure of humans (and developing infants) to these and other environmental chemicals and their potential impact in combination with maternal diet or lifestyle factors, studies are required to address the effects of combinations of exposures on human health including obesity risk.

Epidemiological studies in humans suggest that there may be intergenerational effects on birth weight, cardiovascular risk factors, and type 2 diabetes [10, 167] and such effects have also been documented in animal models including with prenatal glucocorticoid overexposure [11, 168–175]. Importantly, a common phenotype in programmed animal models and in humans is altered body composition and a predisposition to the development of obesity and it is well documented that maternal obesity during pregnancy is associated with an increased risk of obesity and metabolic disease in offspring [176–179]. The implications for public health are profound, suggesting that exposure to an "insult" in early life may lead to an intergenerational cycle of effects including an increased risk of obesity in subsequent generations, and which may exacerbate the current obesity epidemic [180].

References

1. Ravelli AC, van der Meulen JH, Michels RP, et al. Glucose tolerance in adults after prenatal exposure to famine. Lancet. 1998;351(9097):173–7.
2. Barker DJP. In utero programming of chronic disease. Clin Sci. 1998;95:115–28.
3. Barker DJ, Hales CN, Fall CH, Osmond C, Phipps K, Clark PM. Type 2 (non-insulin-dependent) diabetes mellitus, hypertension and hyperlipidaemia (syndrome X): relation to reduced fetal growth. Diabetologia. 1993;36(1):62–7.
4. Barker DJ, Osmond C, Golding J, Kuh D, Wadsworth ME. Growth in utero, blood pressure in childhood and adult life, and mortality from cardiovascular disease. Br Med J. 1989;298(6673):564–7.
5. Levitt NS, Lambert EV, Woods D, Hales CN, Andrew R, Seckl JR. Impaired glucose tolerance and elevated blood pressure in low birth weight, nonobese, young South African adults: early programming of cortisol axis. J Clin Endocrinol Metab. 2000;85(12):4611–8.
6. Barker DJ, Gluckman PD, Godfrey KM, Harding JE, Owens JA, Robinson JS. Fetal nutrition and cardiovascular disease in adult life. Lancet. 1993;341(8850):938–41.
7. Yajnik CS, Fall CH, Vaidya U, et al. Fetal growth and glucose and insulin metabolism in four-year-old Indian children. Diab Med. 1995;12(4):330–6.

8. Edwards CR, Benediktsson R, Lindsay RS, Seckl JR. Dysfunction of placental glucocorticoid barrier: a link between the fetal environment and adult hypertension? Lancet. 1993;341(8841):355–7.
9. Seckl JR. Physiologic programming of the fetus. Clin Perinatol. 1998;25(4):939–62.
10. Drake AJ, Walker BR. The intergenerational effects of fetal programming: non-genomic mechanisms for the inheritance of low birth weight and cardiovascular risk. J Endocrinol. 2004;180:1–16.
11. Drake AJ, Walker BR, Seckl JR. Intergenerational consequences of fetal programming by in utero exposure to glucocorticoids in rats. Am J Physiol. 2005;288(1):R34–8.
12. Hales CN, Barker DJP. Type 2 (non-insulin-dependent) diabetes mellitus: the thrifty phenotype hypothesis. Diabetologia. 1992;35(7):595–601.
13. Arai Y, Gorski RA. Critical exposure time for androgenization of the developing hypothalamus in the female rat. Endocrinology. 1968;82(5):1010–4.
14. Gustafsson JA, Mode A, Norstedt G, Skett P. Sex steroid induced changes in hepatic enzymes. Ann Rev Physiol. 1983;45:51–60.
15. Yamamoto KR. Steroid receptor regulated transcription of specific genes and gene networks. Ann Rev Genet. 1985;19(1):209–52.
16. Sheppard KE. Corticosteroid receptors, 11 beta hydroxysteroid dehydrogenase and the heart. Vitam Horm. 2003;66:77–112.
17. Karst H, Berger S, Turiault M, Tronche F, Schutz G, Joels M. Mineralocorticoid receptors are indispensable for nongenomic modulation of hippocampal glutamate transmission by corticosterone. Proc Natl Acad Sci USA. 2005;102(52):19204–7.
18. Howlett TA, Rees LH, Besser GM. Cushing's syndrome. Clin Endocrinol Metab. 1985;14:911–45.
19. Cole TJ, Blendy JA, Monaghan AP, Schmid W, Aguzzi A, Schutz G. Molecular genetic analysis of glucocorticoid signalling during mouse development. Steroids. 1995;60(1):93–6.
20. Speirs HJ, Seckl JR, Brown RW. Ontogeny of glucocorticoid receptor and 11beta-hydroxysteroid dehydrogenase type-1 gene expression identifies potential critical periods of glucocorticoid susceptibility during development. J Endocrinol. 2004;181(1):105–16.
21. Brown RW, Diaz R, Robson AC, et al. The ontogeny of 11 beta-hydroxysteroid dehydrogenase type 2 and mineralocorticoid receptor gene expression reveal intricate control of glucocorticoid action in development. Endocrinology. 1996;137(2):794–7.
22. Sun K, Yang K, Challis JR. Differential expression of 11 beta-hydroxysteroid dehydrogenase types 1 and 2 in human placenta and fetal membranes. J Clin Endocrinol Metab. 1997;82(1):300–5.
23. Condon J, Gosden C, Gardener D, et al. Expression of type 2 11beta-hydroxysteroid dehydrogenase and corticosteroid hormone receptors in early human fetal life. J Clin Endocrinol Metab. 1998;83(12):4490–7.
24. Costa A, Rocci MP, Arisio R, et al. Glucocorticoid receptors immunoreactivity in tissue of human embryos. J Endocr Invest. 1996;19:92–8.
25. Bian X, Seidler FJ, Slotkin TA. Fetal dexamethasone exposure interferes with establishment of cardiac noradrenergic innervation and sympathetic activity. Teratology. 1993;47(2):109–17.
26. Bian XP, Seidler FJ, Slotkin TA. Promotional role for glucocorticoids in the development of intracellular signalling: enhanced cardiac and renal adenylate cyclase reactivity to beta-adrenergic and non-adrenergic stimuli after low-dose fetal dexamethasone exposure. J Dev Physiol. 1992;17(6):289–97.
27. Celsi G, Kistner A, Eklof AC, Ceccatelli S, Aizman R, Jacobson SH. Inhibition of renal growth by prenatal dexamethsaone and the programming of blood pressure in the offspring. J Am Soc Nephrol. 1997;8:A1360–A1360.
28. Ballard PL. Glucocorticoids and differentiation. In: Rousseau GG, editor. Glucocorticoid hormone action (Monographs in endocrinology). Berlin: Springer; 1979. pp. 493–7.
29. Fowden AL. Endocrine regulation of fetal growth. Reprod Fertil Dev. 1995;7:351–63.

30. Ward RM. Pharmacologic enhancement of fetal lung maturation. Clin Perinatol. 1994;21(3):523–42.
31. Reinisch JM, Simon NG, Karow WG, Gandelman R. Prenatal exposure to prednisone in humans and animals retards intrauterine growth. Science. 1978;202(4366):436–8.
32. Ikegami M, Jobe AH, Newnham J, Polk DH, Willet KE, Sly P. Repetitive prenatal glucocorticoids improve lung function and decrease growth in preterm lambs. Am J Respir Crit Care Med. 1997;156(1):178–84.
33. Nyirenda MJ, Lindsay RS, Kenyon CJ, Burchell A, Seckl JR. Glucocorticoid exposure in late gestation permanently programs rat hepatic phosphoenolpyruvate carboxykinase and glucocorticoid receptor expression and causes glucose intolerance in adult offspring. J Clin Invest. 1998;101(10):2174–81.
34. Newnham JP, Evans SF, Godfrey M, Huang W, Ikegami M, Jobe A. Maternal but not fetal, administration of corticosteroids restricts fetal growth. J Matern Fetal Med. 1999;8(3):81–7.
35. French NP, Hagan R, Evans SF, Godfrey M, Newnham JP. Repeated antenatal corticosteroids: size at birth and subsequent development. Am J Obstet Gynecol. 1999;180(1 Pt 1):114–21.
36. Bloom SL, Sheffield JS, McIntire DD, Leveno KJ. Antenatal dexamethasone and decreased birth weight. Obstet Gynecol. 2001;97(4):485–90.
37. Goland RS, Jozak S, Warren WB, Conwell IM, Stark RI, Tropper PJ. Elevated levels of umbilical cord plasma corticotropin-releasing hormone in growth-retarded fetuses. J Clin Endocrinol Metab. 1993;77(5):1174–9.
38. Goland RS, Tropper PJ, Warren WB, Stark RI, Jozak SM, Conwell IM. Concentrations of corticotrophin-releasing hormone in the umbilical-cord blood of pregnancies complicated by pre-eclampsia. Reprod Fertil Dev. 1995;7(5):1227–30.
39. McCabe L, Marash D, Li A, Matthews SG. Repeated antenatal glucocorticoid treatment decreases hypothalamic corticotropin releasing hormone mRNA but not corticosteroid receptor mRNA expression in the fetal guinea-pig brain. J Neuroendocrinol. 2001;13(5):425–31.
40. Rashid S, Lewis GF. The mechanisms of differential glucocorticoid and mineralocorticoid action in the brain and peripheral tissues. Clin Biochem. 2005;38:401–9.
41. Campbell AL, Murphy BE. The maternal-fetal cortisol gradient during pregnancy and at delivery. J Clin Endocrinol Metab. 1977;45:435–40.
42. Seckl JR. Glucocorticoids, feto-placental 11 beta-hydroxysteroid dehydrogenase type 2, and the early life origins of adult disease. Steroids. 1997;62(1):89–94.
43. Brown RW, Chapman KE, Kotelevtsev Y, et al. Cloning and production of antisera to human placental 11 beta-hydroxysteroid dehydrogenase type 2. Biochem J. 1996;313(Pt 3): 1007–17.
44. Waddell BJ, Atkinson HC. Production rate, metabolic clearance rate and uterine extraction of corticosterone during rat pregnancy. J Endocrinol. 1994;143(1):183–90.
45. Waddell BJ, Benediktsson R, Brown RW, Seckl JR. Tissue-specific messenger ribonucleic acid expression of 11beta-hydroxysteroid dehydrogenase types 1 and 2 and the glucocorticoid receptor within rat placenta suggests exquisite local control of glucocorticoid action. Endocrinology. 1998;139(4):1517–23.
46. Lopez Bernal A, Craft IL. Corticosteroid metabolism in vitro by human placenta, fetal membranes and decidua in early and late gestation. Placenta. 1981;2(4):279–85.
47. Benediktsson R, Calder AA, Edwards CR, Seckl JR. Placental 11 beta-hydroxysteroid dehydrogenase: a key regulator of fetal glucocorticoid exposure. Clin Endocrinol. 1997;46(2):161–6.
48. Bernal AL, Flint AP, Anderson AB, Turnbull AC. 11 beta-hydroxysteroid dehydrogenase activity in human placenta and decidua. J Steroid Biochem. 1980;13(9):1081–7.
49. Venihaki M, Carrigan A, Dikkes P, Majzoub JA. Circadian rise in maternal glucocorticoid prevents pulmonary dysplasia in fetal mice with adrenal insufficiency. Proc Natl Acad Sci USA. 2000;97(13):7336–41.

50. Sampath-Kumar R, Matthews SG, Yang K. 11beta-hydroxysteroid dehydrogenase type 2 is the predominant isozyme in the guinea pig placenta: decreases in messenger ribonucleic acid and activity at term. Biol Reprod. 1998;59(6):1378–84.
51. Benediktsson R, Lindsay RS, Noble J, Seckl JR, Edwards CR. Glucocorticoid exposure in utero: new model for adult hypertension. Lancet. 1993;341(8841):339–41.
52. Stewart PM, Rogerson FM, Mason JI. Type 2 11 beta-hydroxysteroid dehydrogenase messenger ribonucleic acid and activity in human placenta and fetal membranes: its relationship to birth weight and putative role in fetal adrenal steroidogenesis. J Clin Endocrinol Metab. 1995;80(3):885–90.
53. Dave-Sharma S, Wilson RC, Harbison MD, et al. Examination of genotype and phenotype relationships in 14 patients with apparent mineralocorticoid excess. J Clin Endocrinol Metab. 1998;83(7):2244–54.
54. Holmes MC, Abrahamsen CT, French KL, Paterson JM, Mullins JJ, Seckl JR. The mother or the fetus? 11beta-hydroxysteroid dehydrogenase type 2 null mice provide evidence for direct fetal programming of behavior by endogenous glucocorticoids. J Neurosci. 2006;26(14):3840–4.
55. McTernan CL, Draper N, Nicholson H, et al. Reduced Placental 11beta-Hydroxysteroid dehydrogenase type 2 mRNA levels in human pregnancies complicated by intrauterine growth restriction: An analysis of possible mechanisms. J Clin Endocrinol Metab. 2001;86(10):4979–83.
56. Shams M, Kilby MD, Somerset DA, et al. 11Beta-hydroxysteroid dehydrogenase type 2 in human pregnancy and reduced expression in intrauterine growth restriction. Hum Reprod. 1998;13(4):799–804.
57. Murphy VE, Zakar T, Smith R, Giles WB, Gibson PG, Clifton VL. Reduced 11beta-hydroxysteroid dehydrogenase type 2 activity is associated with decreased birth weight centile in pregnancies complicated by asthma. J Clin Endocrinol Metab. 2002;87(4):1660–8.
58. Rogerson FM, Kayes K, White PC. No correlation in human placenta between activity or mRNA for the K (type 2) isozyme of 11beta-hydroxysteroid dehydrogenase and fetal or placental weight. Tenth Int Congr Endocrinol Abstr. 1996;P1–231:193.
59. Rogerson FM, Kayes KM, White PC. Variation in placental type 2 11beta-hydroxysteroid dehydrogenase activity is not related to birth weight or placental weight. Mol Cell Endocrinol. 1997;128(1–2):103–9.
60. Alikhani-Koopaei R, Fouladkou F, Frey FJ, Frey BM. Epigenetic regulation of 11beta-hydroxysteroid dehydrogenase type 2 expression. J Clin Invest. 2004;114(8):1146–57.
61. Friso S, Pizzolo F, Choi S-W, et al. Epigenetic control of 11 beta-hydroxysteroid dehydrogenase 2 gene promoter is related to human hypertension. Atherosclerosis. 2008;119:323–7.
62. van Beek JP, Guan H, Julan L, Yang K. Glucocorticoids stimulate the expression of 11beta-hydroxysteroid dehydrogenase type 2 in cultured human placental trophoblast cells. J Clin Endocrinol Metab. 2004;89(11):5614–21.
63. Sarkar S, Tsai S-W, Nguyen TT, Plevyak M, Padbury JF, Rubin LP. Inhibition of placental 11beta -hydroxysteroid dehydrogenase type 2 by catecholamines via alpha -adrenergic signaling. Am J Physiol. 2001;281(6):R1966–R74.
64. Yang K, Julan L, Rubio F, Sharma A, Guan H. Cadmium reduces 11beta-hydroxysteroid dehydrogenase type 2 activity and expression in human placental trophoblast cells. Am J Physiol. 2006;290(1):E135–E42.
65. Julan L, Guan H, van Beek JP, Yang K. Peroxisome proliferator-activated receptor delta suppresses 11beta-hydroxysteroid dehydrogenase type 2 gene expression in human placental trophoblast cells. Endocrinology. 2005;146(3):1482–90.
66. Hardy DB, Pereria LE, Yang K. Prostaglandins leukotriene b4 are potent inhibitors of 11beta-hydroxysteroid dehydrogenase type 2 activity in human choriocarcinoma jeg-3 cells. Biol Reprod. 1999;61(1):40–5.
67. Pepe GJ, Albrecht ED. Actions of placental and fetal adrenal steroid hormones in primate pregnancy. Endocr Rev. 1995;16(5):608–48.

68. Mairesse J, Lesage J, Breton C, et al. Maternal stress alters endocrine function of the feto-placental unit in rats. Am J Physiol. 2007;292(6):E1526–E33.
69. Hardy DB, The YangK. Expression of 11beta-hydroxysteroid dehydrogenase type 2 is induced during trophoblast differentiation: effects of hypoxia. J Clin Endocrinol Metab. 2002;87(8):3696–701.
70. Welberg LAM, Thrivikraman KV, Plotsky PM. Chronic maternal stress inhibits the capacity to up-regulate placental 11beta-hydroxysteroid dehydrogenase type 2 activity. J Endocrinol. 2005;186(3):R7–R12.
71. Langley-Evans SC, Phillips GJ, Benediktsson R, et al. Protein intake in pregnancy, placental glucocorticoid metabolism and the programming of hypertension in the rat. Placenta. 1996;17(2–3):169–72.
72. Langley-Evans SC. Hypertension induced by foetal exposure to a maternal low-protein diet, in the rat, is prevented by pharmacological blockade of maternal glucocorticoid synthesis. J Hypertens. 1997;15(5):537–44.
73. Sugden MC, Langdown ML, Munns MJ, Holness MJ. Maternal glucocorticoid treatment modulates placental leptin and leptin receptor expression and materno-fetal leptin physiology during late pregnancy, and elicits hypertension associated with hyperleptinemia in the early-growth-retarded adult offspring. Eur J Endocrinol. 2001;145(4):529–39.
74. Woods LL, Weeks DA. Prenatal programming of adult blood pressure: role of maternal corticosteroids. Am J Physiol Regul Integr Comp Physiol. 2005;289(4):R955–R62.
75. Gatford KL, Wintour EM, De Blasio MJ, Owens JA, Dodic M. Differential timing for programming of glucose homoeostasis, sensitivity to insulin and blood pressure by in utero exposure to dexamethasone in sheep. Clin Sci. 2000;98(5):553–60.
76. Dodic M, Abouantoun T, O'Connor A, Wintour EM, Moritz KM. Programming effects of short prenatal exposure to dexamethasone in sheep. Hypertension. 2002;40(5):729–34.
77. Dodic M, May CN, Wintour EM, Coghlan JP. An early prenatal exposure to excess glucocorticoid leads to hypertensive offspring in sheep. Clin Sci. 1998;94(2):149–55.
78. Dodic M, Peers A, Coghlan JP, et al. Altered cardiovascular haemodynamics and baroreceptor-heart rate reflex in adult sheep after prenatal exposure to dexamethasone. Clin Sci. 1999;97(1):103–9.
79. Jensen EC, Gallaher BW, Breier BH, Harding JE. The effect of a chronic maternal cortisol infusion on the late-gestation fetal sheep. J Endocrinol. 2002;174(1):27–36.
80. Levitt NS, Lindsay RS, Holmes MC, Seckl JR. Dexamethasone in the last week of pregnancy attenuates hippocampal glucocorticoid receptor gene expression and elevates blood pressure in the adult offspring in the rat. Neuroendocrinology. 1996;64(6):412–8.
81. Lindsay RS, Lindsay RM, Edwards CR, Seckl JR. Inhibition of 11-beta-hydroxysteroid dehydrogenase in pregnant rats and the programming of blood pressure in the offspring. Hypertension. 1996;27(6):1200–4.
82. Lindsay RS, Lindsay RM, Waddell BJ, Seckl JR. Prenatal glucocorticoid exposure leads to offspring hyperglycemia in the rat: studies with the 11 beta-hydroxysteroid dehydrogenase inhibitor carbenoxolone. Diabetologia. 1996;39(11):1299–305.
83. de Vries A, Holmes MC, Heijnis A, et al. Prenatal dexamethasone exposure induces changes in nonhuman primate offspring cardiometabolic and hypothalamic-pituitary-adrenal axis function. J Clin Invest. 2007;117(4):1058–67.
84. Nyirenda MJ, Carter R, Tang JI, et al. Prenatal programming of metabolic syndrome in the common marmoset is associated with increased expression of 11beta-hydroxysteroid dehydrogenase type 1. Diabetes. 2009;58(12):2873–9.
85. Tangalakis K, Lumbers ER, Moritz KM, Towstoless MK, Wintour EM. Effect of cortisol on blood pressure and vascular reactivity in the ovine fetus. Exp Physiol. 1992;77(5): 709–17.
86. Berry LM, Polk DH, Ikegami M, Jobe AH, Padbury JF, Ervin MG. Preterm newborn lamb renal and cardiovascular responses after fetal or maternal antenatal betamethasone. Am J Physiol. 1997;272(6 Pt 2):R1972–9.

87. Koenen SV, Mecenas CA, Smith GS, Jenkins S, Nathanielsz PW. Effects of maternal betamethasone administration on fetal and maternal blood pressure and heart rate in the baboon at 0.7 of gestation. Am J Obstet Gynecol. 2002;186(4):812–7.
88. O'Regan D, Kenyon CJ, Seckl JR, Holmes MC. Prenatal dexamethasone 'programmes' hypotension, but stress-induced hypertension in adult offspring. J Endocrinol. 2008;196(2):343–52.
89. Dodic M, Samuel C, Moritz K, et al. Impaired cardiac functional reserve and left ventricular hypertrophy in adult sheep after prenatal dexamethasone exposure. Circ Res. 2001;89(7):623–9.
90. Dodic M, Hantzis V, Duncan J, et al. Programming effects of short prenatal exposure to cortisol. FASEB J. 2002;16(9):1017–26.
91. Singh RR, Cullen-McEwen LA, Kett MM, et al. Prenatal corticosterone exposure results in altered AT1/AT2, nephron deficit and hypertension in the rat offspring. J Physiol. 2007;579(2):503–13.
92. Moss TJ, Sloboda DM, Gurrin LC, Harding R, Challis JR, Newnham JP. Programming effects in sheep of prenatal growth restriction and glucocorticoid exposure. Am J Physiol Regul Integr Comp Physiol. 2001;281(3):R960–R70.
93. Ortiz LA, Quan A, Weinberg A, Baum M. Effect of prenatal dexamethasone on rat renal development. Kidney Int. 2001;59(5):1663–9.
94. Ortiz LA, Quan A, Zarzar F, Weinberg A, Baum M. Prenatal dexamethasone programs hypertension and renal injury in the rat. Hypertension. 2003;41(2):328–34.
95. Dickinson H, Walker DW, Wintour EM, Moritz K. Maternal dexamethasone treatment at midgestation reduces nephron number and alters renal gene expression in the fetal spiny mouse. Am J Physiol. 2007;292(1):R453–R61.
96. Wintour EM, Moritz KM, Johnson K, Ricardo S, Samuel CS, Dodic M. Reduced nephron number in adult sheep, hypertensive as a result of prenatal glucocorticoid treatment. J Physiol. 2003;549(3):929–35.
97. Bramlage CP, Schlumbohm C, Pryce CR, et al. Prenatal dexamethasone exposure does not alter blood pressure and nephron number in the young adult marmoset monkey. Hypertension. 2009;54(5):1115–22.
98. Wyrwoll CS, Mark PJ, Waddell BJ. Developmental programming of renal glucocorticoid sensitivity and the renin-angiotensin system. Hypertension. 2007;50(3):579–84.
99. Dagan A, Gattineni J, Cook V, Baum M. Prenatal programming of rat proximal tubule Na^+/H^+ exchanger by dexamethasone. Am J Physiol. 2007;292(3):R1230–5.
100. Dagan A, Habib S, Gattineni J, Dwarakanath V, Baum M. Prenatal programming of rat thick ascending limb chloride transport by low-protein diet and dexamethasone. Am J Physiol. 2009;297(1):R93–9.
101. O'Regan D, Kenyon CJ, Seckl JR, Holmes MC. Glucocorticoid exposure in late gestation in the rat permanently programs gender-specific differences in adult cardiovascular and metabolic physiology. Am J Physiol. 2004;287(5):E863–E70.
102. Wintour EM, Johnson K, Koukoulas I, Moritz K, Tersteeg M, Dodic M. Programming the cardiovascular system, kidney and the brain - a review. Placenta. 2003;24 Suppl A:S65–S71.
103. Zimmermann H, Gardner DS, Jellyman JK, Fowden AL, Giussani DA, Forhead AJ. Effect of dexamethasone on pulmonary and renal angiotensin-converting enzyme concentration in fetal sheep during late gestation. Am J Obstet Gynecol. 2003;189(5):1467–71.
104. Hadoke PW, Lindsay R, Seckl JR, Walker BR, Kenyon C. Altered vascular contractility in adult female rats with hypertension programmed by prenatal glucocorticoid exposure. J Endocrinol. 2006;188:435–42.
105. Roghair RD, Segar JL, Kilpatrick RA, Segar EM, Scholz TD, Lamb FS. Murine aortic reactivity is programmed equally by maternal low protein diet or late gestation dexamethasone. J Matern Fetal Neonatal Med. 2007;20(11):833–41.

106. Molnar J, Howe DC, Nijland MJM, Nathanielsz PW. Prenatal dexamethasone leads to both endothelial dysfunction and vasodilatory compensation in sheep. J Physiol. 2003;547(1): 61–6.
107. Roghair RD, Segar JL, Sharma RV, et al. Newborn lamb coronary artery reactivity is programmed by early gestation dexamethasone before the onset of systemic hypertension. Am J Physiol. 2005;289(4):R1169–R76.
108. Langdown ML, Holness MJ, Sugden MC. Early growth retardation induced by excessive exposure to glucocorticoids in utero selectively increases cardiac GLUT1 protein expression and Akt/protein kinase B activity in adulthood. J Endocrinol. 2001;169(1):11–22.
109. Langdown ML, Holness MJ, Sugden MC. Effects of prenatal glucocorticoid exposure on cardiac calreticulin and calsequestrin protein expression during early development and in adulthood. Biochem J. 2003;371(1):61–9.
110. Wyrwoll CS, Mark PJ, Mori TA, Waddell BJ. Developmental programming of adult hyperinsulinemia, increased proinflammatory cytokine production, and altered skeletal muscle expression of SLC2A4 (GLUT4) and uncoupling protein 3. J Endocrinol. 2008;198(3): 571–9.
111. Nyirenda MJ, Welberg LA, Seckl JR. Programming hyperglycaemia in the rat through prenatal exposure to glucocorticoids-fetal effect or maternal influence? J Endocrinol. 2001;170(3):653–60.
112. Lesage J, Del-Favero F, Leonhardt M, et al. Prenatal stress induces intrauterine growth restriction and programs glucose intolerance and feeding behaviour disturbances in the aged rat. J Endocrinol. 2004;181:291–6.
113. Avishai-Eliner S, Brunson KL, Sandman CA, Baram TZ. Stressed-out, or in (utero)? Trends Neurosci. 2002;25(10):518–24.
114. Sloboda DM, Newnham JP, Challis JRG. Repeated maternal glucocorticoid administration and the developing liver in fetal sheep. J Endocrinol. 2002;175:535–43.
115. De Blasio MJ, Dodic M, Jefferies AJ, Moritz KM, Wintour EM, Owens JA. Maternal exposure to dexamethasone or cortisol in early pregnancy differentially alters insulin secretion and glucose homeostasis in adult male sheep offspring. Am J Physiol. 2007;293(1): E75–E82.
116. Pilkis SJ, Granner DK. Molecular physiology of regulation of hepatic gluconeogenesis and glycolysis. Ann Rev Physiol. 1992;54:885–909.
117. Valera A, Pujol A, Pelegrin M, Bosch F. Transgenic mice overexpressing phosphoenolpyruvate carboxykinase develop non-insulin-dependent diabetes mellitus. Proc Natl Acad Sci USA. 1994;91(19):9151–4.
118. Rosella G, Zajac JD, Kaczmarczyk SJ, Andrikopoulos S, Proietto J. Impaired suppression of gluconeogenesis induced by overexpression of a noninsulin-responsive phosphoenolpyruvate carboxykinase gene. Mol Endocrinol. 1993;7(11):1456–62.
119. Xanthopoulos KG, Mirkovitch J. Gene regulation in rodent hepatocytes during development, differentiation and disease. Eur J Biochem. 1993;216(2):353–60.
120. Cleasby M, Kelly PA, Walker BR, Seckl JR. Programming of rat muscle and fat metabolism by in utero over-exposure to glucocorticoids. Endocrinology. 2003;144: 999–1007.
121. Nyirenda MJ, Dean S, Lyons V, Chapman KE, Seckl JR. Prenatal programming of hepatocyte nuclear factor 4α in the rat: a key mechanism in the 'foetal origins of hyperglycaemia'? Diabetologia. 2006;V49(6):1412–20.
122. Fowden AL, Forhead AJ. Endocrine mechanisms of intrauterine programming. Reproduction. 2004;127(5):515–26.
123. Livingstone DE, Jones GC, Smith K, et al. Understanding the role of glucocorticoids in obesity: tissue-specific alterations of corticosterone metabolism in obese Zucker rats. Endocrinology. 2000;141(2):560–3.
124. Rask E, Olsson T, Soderberg S, et al. Tissue-specific dysregulation of cortisol metabolism in human obesity. J Clin Endocrinol Metab. 2001;86(3):1418–21.

125. Macfarlane DP, Forbes S, Walker BR. Glucocorticoids and fatty acid metabolism in humans: fuelling fat redistribution in the metabolic syndrome. J Endocrinol. 2008;197(2):189–204.
126. Gesina E, Blondeau B, Milet A, et al. Glucocorticoid signalling affects pancreatic development through both direct and indirect mechanisms. Diabetologia. 2006;49:2939–47.
127. Blondeau B, Lesage J, Czernichow P, Dupouy JP, Breant B. Glucocorticoids impair fetal beta-cell development in rats. Am J Physiol Endocrinol Metab. 2001;281(3):E592–9.
128. Garofano A, Czernichow P, Breant B. Beta-cell mass and proliferation following late fetal and early postnatal malnutrition in the rat. Diabetologia. 1998;41(9):1114–20.
129. Gesina E, Tronche F, Herrera P, et al. Dissecting the role of glucocorticoids on pancreas development. Diabetes. 2004;53:2322–9.
130. Hill DJ, Duvillie B. Pancreatic development and adult diabetes. Pediatr Res. 2000;48(3):269–74.
131. Nobili V, Day C. Childhood NAFLD: a ticking time-bomb? Gut. 2009;58(11):1442.
132. Marchesini G, Brizi M, Bianchi G, et al. Nonalcoholic fatty liver disease: a feature of the metabolic syndrome. Diabetes. 2001;50(8):1844–50.
133. Marceau P, Biron S, Hould FS, et al. Liver pathology and the metabolic syndrome X in severe obesity. J Clin Endocrinol Metab. 1999;84(5):1513–7.
134. Pagano G, Pacini G, Musso G, et al. Nonalcoholic steatohepatitis, insulin resistance, and metabolic syndrome: further evidence for an etiologic association. Hepatology. 2002;35(2):367–72.
135. Anderson N, Borlak J. Molecular mechanisms and therapeutic targets in steatosis and steatohepatitis. Pharmacol Rev. 2008;60:311–57.
136. Drake AJ, Raubenheimer PJ, Kerrigan D, McInnes KJ, Seckl JR, Walker AJ. Prenatal dexamethasone programs expression of genes in liver and adipose tissue and increased hepatic lipid accumulation but not obesity on a high fat diet. Endocrinology. 2010;151(4): 1581–1587.
137. Bruce KD, Cagampang FR, Argenton M, et al. Maternal high-fat feeding primes steatohepatitis in adult mice offspring, involving mitochondrial dysfunction and altered lipogenesis gene expression. Hepatology. 2009;50(6):1796–808.
138. Magee TR, Han G, Cherian B, Khorram O, Ross MG, Desai M. Down-regulation of transcription factor peroxisome proliferator-activated receptor in programmed hepatic lipid dysregulation and inflammation in intrauterine growth-restricted offspring. Am J Obstet Gynecol. 2008;199(3):271.e1–5.
139. Fraser A, Ebrahim S, Davey Smith G, Lawlor DA. The associations between birthweight and adult markers of liver damage and function. Paediatr Perinat Epidemiol. 2008;22(1): 12–21.
140. Dahlgren J, Nilsson C, Jennische E, et al. Prenatal cytokine exposure results in obesity and gender-specific programming. Am J Physiol. 2001;281(2):E326–E34.
141. Whorwood CB, Firth KM, Budge H, Symonds ME. Maternal undernutrition during early to midgestation programs tissue-specific alterations in the expression of the glucocorticoid receptor, 11beta-hydroxysteroid dehydrogenase isoforms, and type 1 angiotensin ii receptor in neonatal sheep. Endocrinology. 2001;142(7):2854–64.
142. Gnanalingham MG, Mostyn A, Symonds ME, Stephenson T. Ontogeny and nutritional programming of adiposity in sheep: potential role of glucocorticoid action and uncoupling protein-2. Am J Physiol. 2005;289(5):R1407–R15.
143. Bispham J, Gopalakrishnan GS, Dandrea J, et al. Maternal endocrine adaptation throughout pregnancy to nutritional manipulation: consequences for maternal plasma leptin and cortisol and the programming of fetal adipose tissue development. Endocrinology. 2003;144(8):3575–85.
144. Masuzaki H, Paterson J, Shinyama H, et al. A transgenic model of visceral obesity and the metabolic syndrome. Science. 2001;294(5549):2166–70.
145. Rayburn WF. Glucocorticoid therapy for rheumatic diseases: maternal, fetal, and breastfeeding considerations. Am J Reprod Immunol. 1992;28:138–40.

146. Kattner E, Metze B, Waiss E, Obladen M. Accelerated lung maturation following maternal steroid treatment in infants born before 30 weeks gestation. J Perinat Med. 1992;20:449–57.
147. Crowley P. Prophylactic corticosteroids for preterm birth. Cochrane Database Syst Rev. 2000;2:CD000065.
148. Brocklehurst P, Gates S, McKenzie-McHarg K, Alfirevic Z, Chamberlain G. Are we prescribing multiple courses of antenatal corticosteroids? A survey of practice in the UK. Br J Obstet Gynaecol. 1999;106(9):977–9.
149. Whitelaw A, Thoresen M. Antenatal steroids and the developing brain. Arch Dis Child Fetal Neonatal Ed. 2000;83(2):F154–7.
150. Forest MG, David M, Morel Y. Prenatal diagnosis and treatment of 21-hydroxylase deficiency. J Steroid Biochem Mol Biol. 1993;45(1–3):75–82.
151. Mercado AB, Wilson RC, Cheng KC, Wei JQ, New MI. Prenatal treatment and diagnosis of congenital adrenal hyperplasia owing to steroid 21-hydroxylase deficiency. J Clin Endocrinol Metab. 1995;80(7):2014–20.
152. Aghajafari F, Murphy K, Willan A, et al. Multiple courses of antenatal corticosteroids: A systematic review and meta-analysis. Am J Obstet Gynecol. 2001;185:1073–80.
153. Dessens AB, Haas HS-d, Koppe JG. Twenty-year follow-up of antenatal corticosteroid treatment. Pediatrics. 2000;105(6):e77.
154. Doyle LW, Ford GW, Davis NM, Callanan C. Antenatal corticosteroid therapy and blood pressure at 14 years of age in preterm children. Clin Sci. 2000;98(2):137–42.
155. Huh S, Andrew R, Rich-Edwards J, Kleinman K, Seckl J, Gillman M. Association between umbilical cord glucocorticoids and blood pressure at age 3 years. BMC Med. 2008; 6(1):25.
156. Finken MJJ, Keijzer-Veen MG, Dekker FW, et al. Antenatal glucocorticoid treatment is not associated with long-term metabolic risks in individuals born before 32 weeks of gestation. Arch Dis Child Fetal Neonatal Ed. 2008;93(6):F442–7.
157. Ahmad I, Beharry KDA, Valencia AM, et al. Influence of a single course of antenatal betamethasone on the maternal-fetal insulin-IGF-GH axis in singleton pregnancies. Growth Horm IGF Res. 2006;16(4):267–75.
158. Dalziel SR, Walker NK, Parag V, et al. Cardiovascular risk factors after antenatal exposure to betamethasone: 30-year follow-up of a randomised controlled trial. Lancet. 2005;365(9474):1856–62.
159. Phillips DI, Walker BR, Reynolds RM, et al. Low birth weight predicts elevated plasma cortisol concentrations in adults from 3 populations. Hypertension. 2000;35(6):1301–6.
160. Clark PM, Hindmarsh PC, Shiell AW, Law CM, Honour JW, Barker DJ. Size at birth and adrenocortical function in childhood. Clin Endocrinol. 1996;45(6):721–6.
161. Phillips DI, Barker DJ, Fall CH, et al. Elevated plasma cortisol concentrations: a link between low birth weight and the insulin resistance syndrome? J Clin Endocrinol Metab. 1998;83(3):757–60.
162. Jones A, Godfrey KM, Wood P, Osmond C, Goulden P, Phillips DIW. Fetal growth and the adrenocortical response to psychological stress. J Clin Endocrinol Metab. 2006;91(5): 1868–71.
163. Reynolds RM, Walker BR, Syddall HE, et al. Altered control of cortisol secretion in adult men with low birth weight and cardiovascular risk factors. J Clin Endocrinol Metab. 2001;86(1):245–50.
164. Waddington CH. The strategy of the genes. London: Allen and Unwin; 1957.
165. Gluckman PD, Hanson MA. Living with the past: evolution, development, and patterns of disease. Science. 2004;305(5691):1733–6.
166. Drake AJ, van den Driesche S, Scott HM, Hutchison GR, Seckl JR, Sharpe RM. Glucocorticoids amplify dibutyl phthalate-induced disruption of testosterone production and male reproductive development. Endocrinology. 2009;150(11):5055–64.
167. Drake AJ, Liu L. Intergenerational transmission of programmed effects: public health consequences. Trends in Endocrinology and Metabolism 2010;21(4):206–213.

168. Burdge GC, Slater-Jefferies JL, Torrens C, Phillips ES, Hanson MA, Lillycrop KA. Dietary protein restriction of pregnant rats in the F0 generation induces altered methylation of hepatic gene promoters in the adult male offspring in the F1 and F2 generations. Br J Nutr. 2007;97:435–9.
169. Harrison M, Langley-Evans SC. Intergenerational programming of impaired nephrogenesis and hypertension in rats following maternal protein restriction during pregnancy. Br J Nutr. 2009;101(07):1020–30.
170. Anway MD, Cupp AS, Uzumcu M, Skinner MK. Epigenetic transgenerational actions of endocrine disruptors and male fertility. Science. 2005;308(5727):1466–9.
171. Zambrano E, Martinez-Samayoa PM, Bautista CJ, et al. Sex differences in transgenerational alterations of growth and metabolism in progeny (F2) of female offspring (F1) of rats fed a low protein diet during pregnancy and lactation. J Physiol. 2005;566(1):225–36.
172. Francis D, Diorio J, Liu D, Meaney MJ. Nongenomic transmission across generations of maternal behavior and stress responses in the rat. Science. 1999;286(5442):1155–8.
173. Anderson CM, Lopez F, Zimmer A, Benoit JN. Placental insufficiency leads to developmental hypertension and mesenteric artery dysfunction in two generations of Sprague-Dawley rat offspring. Biol Reprod. 2006;74(3):538–44.
174. Jimenez-Chillaron JC, Isganaitis E, Charalambous M, et al. Intergenerational transmission of glucose intolerance and obesity by in utero undernutrition in mice. Diabetes. 2009;58(2):460–8.
175. Benyshek DC, Johnston CS, Martin JF. Glucose metabolism is altered in the adequately-nourished grand-offspring (F3 generation) of rats malnourished during gestation and perinatal life. Diabetologia. 2006;49:1117–9.
176. Samuelsson A-M, Matthews PA, Argenton M, et al. Diet-induced obesity in female mice leads to offspring hyperphagia, adiposity, hypertension, and insulin resistance: a novel murine model of developmental programming. Hypertension. 2008;51(2):383–92.
177. Armitage JA, Taylor PD, Poston L. Experimental models of developmental programming: consequences of exposure to an energy rich diet during development. J Physiol. 2005;565(1):3–8.
178. Khan IY, Dekou V, Douglas G, et al. A high-fat diet during rat pregnancy or suckling induces cardiovascular dysfunction in adult offspring. Am J Physiol Regul Integr Comp Physiol. 2005;288(1):R127–R33.
179. Taylor PD, Poston L. Developmental programming of obesity in mammals. Exp Physiol. 2007;92(2):287–98.
180. Classen TJ. Measures of the intergenerational transmission of body mass index between mothers and their children in the United States, 1981–2004. Econ Hum Biol. 2010;8(1): 30–43.

Chapter 15
Hypothalamic Fetal Programming of Energy Homeostasis

Clement C. Cheung and Holly A. Ingraham

15.1 Introduction

Prenatal events have now been recognized as an important influence for the development of adult traits. In particular, an unfavorable in utero environment predisposes the fetus to a higher risk of disease acquisition later in life. This observation was best represented by the seminal epidemiological work of Barker and colleagues in the late 1980s when they reported the association between adult diseases, such as coronary heart disease and T2DM, with poor fetal growth parameters, such as low birthweight (LBW) [1–4]. This has been elaborated as the "Barker hypothesis," which states that adult diseases "originate through adaptations that the fetus makes when it is undernourished." Recent research that links a variety of diseases to LBW has now expanded the Barker hypothesis to the concept of "Developmental Origins of Health and Disease" (DOHaD). Numerous clinical and epidemiological studies have since validated the basic tenets of this hypothesis [5]. These studies have invariably used birthweight, or a combination of birthweight and gestational age, as surrogate markers for alteration of prenatal events. However, epidemiological studies are unable to elucidate the underlying mechanisms that link abnormal birthweight to fetal programming. In order to test this hypothesis and define the basic mechanisms of fetal programming, various experimental paradigms have recreated both low or high birthweight in animal models. Indeed, experimental rodent models recapitulate observations from human epidemiological studies. In this chapter, we will summarize several commonly used animal models and examine the hypothalamus as a potential target site that responds to adverse maternal nutritional status and directly affects fetal programming.

C.C. Cheung (✉)
Departments of Pediatrics, University of California, San Francisco, CA, USA; Department of Cellular and Molecular Pharmacology, University of California, San Francisco, CA, USA
e-mail: clement.cheung@ucsf.edu

R.H. Lustig (ed.), *Obesity Before Birth*, Endocrine Updates 30,
DOI 10.1007/978-1-4419-7034-3_15, © Springer Science+Business Media, LLC 2011

15.2 Prenatal Programming and Obesity

15.2.1 Epidemiological Studies

15.2.1.1 Human Maternal Undernutrition

Epidemiological studies show that LBW and premature birth, both proxies of an adverse in utero environment, are linked to postnatal obesity and metabolic abnormalities. Barker et al. first studied a cohort of British men and women born in Hertfordshire and showed that their risk of cardiovascular disease and metabolic syndrome was inversely correlated with their birthweight [2, 4]. Similar observations have been made between LBW parameters and coronary heart disease in men in Finland and women in the USA [6, 7]. Other supporting evidence comes from the Dutch famine and Leningrad famine studies where the cohorts experienced different duration of malnutrition across development. Dutch men and women who were in utero during the famine but raised in a well-nourished environment showed impaired glucose tolerance and signs of insulin resistance as adults [8, 9]. On the contrary, Leningrad men and women did not exhibit significant metabolic alterations if their malnutrition in utero continued after birth [10]. These two studies led to the idea that adult disease occurs when the fetal and postnatal environments are inconsistent, such that adaptation by the fetus becomes deleterious when confronted with this new postnatal environment. The DOHaD hypothesis also emphasizes that fetal adaptations are developmentally regulated. The highest adult obesity rate in the Dutch cohort studies was seen in those that were exposed to famine during the first half of pregnancy, whereas lower obesity rates were observed in those that were exposed during the last trimester [9].

Another epidemiological example is premature birth, in which LBW predicts metabolic abnormalities and other diseases in the adult. Preterm infants have an increased risk of adult cardiovascular disease [11] and develop increased insulin resistance early in childhood that persists into young adulthood [12, 13]. Premature birth may be indicative of poor maternal growth and a suboptimal in utero environment, which can disrupt normal fetal development of metabolic and appetite control. Clinical and epidemiological studies suggest any unfavorable conditions, such as maternal undernutrition, during in utero development that precipitate prematurity may shape the fetus in ways that alter fetal physiology and increase susceptibility to metabolic problems later in life. Emerging evidence shows that prematurity, in itself, even with normal weight for gestational age, is associated with diabetes and cardiovascular problems later in life [14, 15]. Abnormal birthweight may simply be one of several endpoints of an adverse of unfavorable in utero condition.

15.2.1.2 Human Maternal Overnutrition

Recent epidemiological studies have suggested a U-shaped relationship between birthweight and adult obesity and metabolic problems [16–18]. A common observation is that maternal obesity is linked to neonatal macrosomia and the subsequent increase in obesity (see Chapter Chapter 10) [19–21]. Excessive nutrients in the maternal environment likely program the fetus to have an increased propensity for metabolic problems. Maternal obesity frequently is confounded by other co-morbid factors, such as gestational diabetes mellitus (GDM). In fact, retrospective studies in the Pima Indians showed that obesity in the offspring was related to maternal glycemic control, with a higher prevalence of obesity occurring in children born to mothers with GDM (see Chapter 9) [22, 23]. Even with normal birthweight, an association between GDM and the development of adult obesity in the offspring is observed [22, 23]. As such, whereas both maternal weight and birthweight are surrogate markers linking maternal overnutrition to the development of obesity later in life, "perceived" maternal overnutrition due to GDM remains a risk factor despite normal maternal weight or birthweight.

15.2.2 Animal Studies

Epidemiological observations and clinical studies on human subjects provide the foundation for the DOHaD hypothesis [5]. However, understanding the basic mechanisms of DOHaD requires the use of non-human experimental paradigms. To this end, different animal models have been used to recreate conditions of prenatal undernutrition or overnutrition. All of these models seek to perturb birthweight. More importantly, in these animal models, experimentally induced abnormal birthweight is associated with abnormal metabolic profiles later in life, thus recapitulating observations in human epidemiological studies. These experimental animal models provide a starting point to begin defining the molecular mechanisms underlying DOHaD. Several species have been used in these studies, including mice, rats, sheep, and non-human primates. Rodent species are a popular choice due to their relatively short life spans and the ease of prenatal manipulation. Despite some species differences, rodent species, like non-rodent species, possess adaptive responses to maximize fetal survival. In the following sections we will focus on rodent studies because they are both extensive and experimentally diverse. Several common experimental models will be highlighted to illustrate how each is used to study DOHaD.

15.3 Models to Induce Prenatal Maternal Undernutrition

15.3.1 Caloric Restriction

To produce newborns that are underweight or show intrauterine growth retardation (IUGR), several studies have imposed total caloric restriction by limiting food availability during pregnancy (see Chapter 11). Animals with LBW subsequently exhibit abnormal metabolic profiles during adulthood. The offspring of rats fed 50% less calories than controls during the first 2 weeks of pregnancy are slightly smaller and gained significantly more weight when fed a normal diet later in life. In addition, male rats gained more weight than controls when placed on a high-fat diet [24]. Furthermore, it has been shown that a 50% maternal food restriction paradigm also reduces β-cell mass of offspring at birth, thus rendering the animals glucose intolerant in later life [25, 26]. In another study, mice fed 50% less calories than controls during the second half of pregnancy gave birth to smaller pups with severe glucose intolerance noted by 6 months, and basal hypersecretion of insulin observed as early as 2 months [27]. Thus, these studies show that the postnatal catch-up growth following LBW is accompanied by an increased risk of glucose intolerance. On the other hand, when caloric restriction (50%) is imposed in the lactating dam, the resulting LBW pups do not exhibit either catch-up growth or glucose intolerance [28]. Mice that exhibited no catch-up growth also exhibited reduced adiposity at weaning.

15.3.2 Protein Restriction

In addition to the caloric restriction model, another model that has been extensively used to induce IUGR is the low-protein model, which is particularly popular in understanding the role of IUGR in kidney development [18]. In this model, the experimental maternal diet consists of only 5–10% of protein as compared to the 15–20% protein found in the normal diet. Many studies have shown that a low-protein diet during pregnancy results in low fetal weight, which is accompanied by pancreatic under-development, impaired β-cell function, and decreased insulin production [29, 30]. This programming effect can be seen even if exposure to a low-protein diet is limited to the final trimester of pregnancy [31]. Furthermore, as observed with the maternal caloric restriction model, a low-protein diet in utero exhibits a similar catch-up growth effect [27, 28]. For example, Ozanne et al. showed that LBW pups exposed to a maternal low-protein diet are able to catch up in weight when suckled by a normal mother and culled to half the normal litter size [32, 33]. After exposure to low-protein diet in utero, rats placed on a highly palatable diet achieve catch-up growth and go on to become more obese with higher fasting leptin levels than control rats exposed to a normal prenatal environment [32, 33]. Although these studies illustrate that restriction of a selected macronutrient (e.g., protein) does exert clear fetal programming effects on metabolic profiles of offspring, the metabolic effects observed in a total caloric restriction model are far more robust [34].

15.4 Models to Induce Prenatal Maternal Overnutrition

15.4.1 High-Fat Diet

Maternal diet-induced obesity is commonly used as an animal model to study the impacts of maternal overnutrition on the energy homeostasis of the offspring [35]. The majority of these models utilize a high-fat diet that is imposed several weeks before gestation and continues during both pregnancy and lactation (see Chapter 9). Because the exposure period to the high-fat diet in some models encompasses both the prenatal and postnatal period, it is sometimes difficult to assess the prenatal fetal programming effect versus the lactational effect. By measuring birthweight, which is not influenced by the postnatal maternal nutritional condition [36–43], no clear consensus has emerged on the impact of a maternal high-fat diet and the birthweight of offspring. The majority of studies report no difference in litter birthweight between obese dams and control dams, regardless of whether the high-fat diet was administered prior to pregnancy [40–43] or during gestation [36]. Conflicting studies report both an increase and decrease in pup birthweight born to obese dams [37–39]. Confounding factors leading to these diverse results might include the composition and duration of the high-fat diet. Nonetheless, these results seem to support the notion that birthweight is only one of many surrogate markers to assess the impact of adverse events in utero. Lack of changes in birthweight does not necessarily preclude the programming effects of maternal overnutrition on fetal and postnatal physiology. Indeed, earlier studies showed that when female rats were given a high-fat diet commencing at weaning until the end of pregnancy, their offspring showed similar birthweight to controls, but were hyperinsulinemic, with increased pancreatic insulin content at birth, and obesity and glucose intolerance in adulthood [44]. A postnatal high-carbohydrate diet can further worsen the offspring's metabolic profiles (see Chapter 13) [43]. These results are supported by another study that also showed decreased plasma leptin levels in pups born to obese dams [40].

In experiments that specifically isolate the prenatal period from the postnatal lactational period, Shankar et al. used an intragastric feeding model to provide an obesogenic liquid diet for 3 weeks prior to mating; their model induced a 21% weight gain in female rats at the time of conception relative to those that were fed intragastrically with a regular diet [42]. Both the obese and lean females received a normal diet during pregnancy. At birth, all pups were cross-fostered to normal dams limiting their exposure to an obesogenic environment to the prenatal period only. All pups had comparable weight at birth and weaning; however, when male offspring were challenged to a high-fat diet post-weaning, those that were born to obese dams gained significantly more weight than those born to lean dams. On a regular diet, offspring of obese compared to lean dams exhibited comparable body weights, but had higher body fat content, with increased serum leptin, insulin, and resistin, and decreased serum adiponectin, when normalized to percent fat [42]. Oral glucose tolerance testing showed that the offspring of the obese dams had worsened insulin resistance independent of the post-weaning diet. Adipocyte hypertrophy was observed in offspring of obese dams and was further exacerbated by an obese diet.

A study by Chang et al. further demonstrates the long-term programming effects of an in utero maternal high-fat diet [36]. Dams that were maintained on a high-fat diet during pregnancy exclusively gave birth to pups of comparable birthweight to controls, but had higher body weight and percent body fat at day 70 of life as well as higher serum triglycerides, leptin, and insulin levels. More significant is the observation that this prenatal exposure to a high-fat diet stimulated proliferation and migration of neuronal precursor cells in the embryonic hypothalamus that eventually differentiate to become orexigenic peptide neurons [36].

15.4.2 Gestational Diabetes Mellitus (GDM)

GDM in humans often results in either abnormally large or small birthweight. In rodents, GDM can be induced with streptozotocin (STZ), which destroys pancreatic β-cells in a dose-dependent manner. Low-dose STZ administered during pregnancy results in mild GDM with offspring exhibiting macrosomia and high birthweight [45]. At birth, these mildly obese pups display higher pancreatic insulin content and have elevated plasma insulin to maintain normal euglycemia [45]. Both male and female offspring have accelerated postnatal growth. By 10 weeks of age, they show glucose intolerance and insulin resistance, as revealed by hyperinsulinemic-euglycemic clamp [45, 46]. Female pups develop GDM during their pregnancy and give rise to a third generation of pups with increased birthweight suggesting a potential epigenetic mechanism in promoting this trans-generational phenomenon [46]. Of note, high-dose STZ induces severe GDM in mothers, and pups with LBW also show abnormal β-cell physiology and develop GDM themselves [18].

15.5 Central Mechanisms for Fetal Programming

15.5.1 Perinatal Hypothalamic Controls of Energy Homeostasis

The hypothalamus controls food intake and regulates body weight and is critical for maintaining energy homeostasis. As such, it may be a potential site for fetal programming effects of maternal undernutrition and overnutrition. In order to formulate the possible role of the hypothalamus in fetal programming, it is essential to understand the components and development of the hypothalamic neurocircuitry that governs energy homeostasis. Hypothalamic nuclei form connections with each other and with other regions of the brain to regulate energy homeostasis. The mediobasal hypothalamus contains two nuclei that are thought to be satiety centers of the brain – the arcuate nucleus (ARC) and the ventromedial nucleus (VMN). The ARC, in particular, is one of the most-studied hypothalamic nuclei and has been shown to play a critical role in the control of appetite, food intake, and glucose homeostasis [47, 48]. Peripheral metabolic signals, such as leptin and insulin, interact in a cell-type-specific manner with the orexigenic neuropeptide (NPY)/agouti-related peptide (AgRP) neurons, and the proopiomelanocortin (POMC) neurons, with the anorexigenic α-melanocyte stimulating hormone (α-MSH) as its major cleavage peptide product [49, 50]. Further interactions occur with neural inputs coming from other hypothalamic nuclei as well as extrahypothalamic brain regions. Major neural afferent signals into the ARC include the dorsomedial hypothalamic nucleus (DMN), the lateral hypothalamic area (LHA), and the brainstem. The integrated information is relayed through efferent fibers from the ARC to areas such as the paraventricular nucleus (PVN), which express melanocortin-4 receptors (MC4R) that bind its natural agonist, α-MSH, and its antagonist, AgRP, or back to the DMN and the brainstem. Please see Chapter 3 for a complete discussion of ARC physiology. The importance of hypothalamic neurocircuitry in regulating adult energy homeostasis is well established based on studies from naturally occurring mutants, genetically engineered animals, and other experimental manipulations (see Chapter 3). However, the role of this circuitry in perinatal energy homeostasis is still poorly understood.

During development of the rat, the ARC is believed to form between embryonic days (E)12 and E17 with peak development at E15 [51]. NPY immunoreactivity (NPY-ir) in the hypothalamus is first seen at E13 and ARC NPY-ir cell bodies and fiber staining are detectable around E16 [52]. NPY-ir is detected in the ARC early on, but remains relatively low in the first postnatal week, then rises in intensity starting at postnatal days (P)10–11 [53]. Furthermore, NPY-ir fibers are found in DMH and PVN around P5–10 and increase in intensity around P15 [53]. Consistent with the expression profile of the NPY peptide, NPY transcripts are expressed at P0 and increase progressively until peaking at P16 [54]. Adult hypothalamic NPY transcripts are localized exclusively to the ARC, in contrast to the much broader expression earlier in development, which includes DMN, PVN, and the lateral hypothalamus [54]. The role of ARC NPY in energy homeostasis during the perinatal period has not been fully explored but limited evidence suggests that NPY neurons in the neonatal ARC might be unimportant for feeding behavior [55].

AgRP, which is expressed only in the hypothalamus and colocalizes with NPY neurons, mimics the developmental expression pattern observed for NPY. AgRP mRNA expression is low at birth and gradually increases throughout the second and third postnatal week [53, 56]. AgRP-ir is also detected at low levels in the ARC at P0 but begins to rise at P5 and peaks at P21. This temporal pattern of AgRP-ir has also been observed for other hypothalamic regions, with expression observed at P5–P10 in the PVN and at P10–P15 in the DMN and LHA [53, 56].

The hypothalamic anorexigenic system develops in a similar manner as the orexigenic system. POMC mRNA can be detected as early as E10.5 in the presumptive ARC [57]. POMC-ir is first detected at E12 but α-MSH-ir is not seen until E16 [58]. Postnatally, POMC mRNA remains low but begins to increase between P5–10 and P21 in the ARC [59]. Immunostaining of α-MSH can be found in the ARC as early as the first postnatal week [60]; however, these positive signals may originate from extra-hypothalamic sites rather than being produced locally in the ARC [61]. Whether α-MSH participates during the postnatal period to control feeding remains controversial [62]. Indeed, while one group has shown that α-MSH may induce weight gain early on [63], another group has reported the opposite effect [64].

There is a temporal appearance of NPY- and AgRP-ir in hypothalamic nuclei including the PVN, LHA, and DMN. This developmental pattern mimics the development of ARC projections to these hypothalamic nuclei which occur by P6 for the

DMN, by P10 for the PVN, and by P12 for the LHA [62]. Development of ARC projections to these nuclei also coincides with the appearance of leptin-induced c-Fos activity in these different hypothalamic areas [62]. These results suggest that leptin may play a role in the development of hypothalamic neurocircuitry.

15.5.2 Perinatal Leptin

Leptin has long been known as an adipocyte-derived satiety signal based on extensive research in adult animals in which peripheral or central administration of leptin leads to hypophagia, increased metabolic rate, and weight loss [47, 48]. However, the physiological role of leptin in neonatal animals is a topic of active investigation. Leptin receptor (LepR) mRNA is expressed in the hypothalamic ependymal layer at E18, ARC at E21, and DMN at P3 [65]. Postnatally, LepR and the leptin-signaling long form of LepR (LepRb) transcripts in the hypothalamus increase beginning at the second postnatal week [65–68]. LepR expression in cerebral vessels also exhibits a developmental pattern, and as such may impact leptin transport into the brain during postnatal growth [69]. Although the hypothalamic expression of LepR and LepRb starts at the late embryonic stage, responsiveness to leptin rodent species can be variable during the prenatal and postnatal periods. Indeed, when embryonic ARC neurons are cultured they are unresponsive to leptin, despite the fact that these cells possess the components for leptin signaling, including signal transducer and activator of transcription-3 (STAT3) and components of the mitogen-associated protein kinase pathway [66]. The postnatal hypothalamus appears to be responsive to leptin as demonstrated by an increase in the suppressor of cytokine signaling 3 (SOCS3), an intracellular marker of leptin action. One study showed SOCS3 activation with an intraperitoneal leptin injection (3 μg/g) as early as P4 [67]. Using an acute leptin injection in P10 rats, others observed activation of SOCS3 and POMC and inhibition of NPY in the hypothalamus or rostral ARC [70]. Leptin likely acts directly on ARC neurons because intraperitoneal leptin administration leads to c-Fos induction in the ARC of P6 rats [62]. Surprisingly, the normal leptin-induced hypophagia seen in adults is not observed in offspring at P3, P5, or P8 [70], even though these animals can respond to α-MSH administration [63]. This dissociation between leptin signaling and leptin's expected function leads to speculation that the action of leptin during perinatal development may be different from that of the adult [70]. Indeed, there is emerging data on the role of leptin as a neurotrophic agent [71].

It is well established that plasma leptin exhibits a developmental pattern in neonates [72–75]. Depending on the study, postnatal circulating leptin levels peak around the second week of life: P10 in rats [72, 74] and P7–16 in mice [73, 75]. The rise in plasma leptin coincides with the development of hypothalamic circuitry [62], leading to the speculation that neonatal leptin may influence the formation and maturation of hypothalamic neuronal projections. Indeed, *ob/ob* mice that are deficient in leptin show abnormal neuronal projections from ARC to the PVN, DMN, and

LHA; ARC fiber projections to the PVN are re-established after leptin replacement between P4 and P12 (10 mg/kg) [62]. Interestingly, this effect of leptin is specific to the ARC and occurs only during development. Non-leptin-sensitive pathways in *ob/ob* mice developed normally and leptin replacement in adults was ineffective in normalizing these ARC to PVN projections. Furthermore, ARC explants develop neurite outgrowth upon leptin exposure, suggesting that leptin may act directly on ARC neurons as a neurotrophic factor [71].

A misplaced leptin surge has been linked to the development of maladapted hypothalamic response to maternal undernutrition. In neonatal male mice, a relatively mild maternal caloric restriction of 30% advances both the onset and amplitude of the leptin surge, which correlates with increased weight gain, leptin resistance, and glucose intolerance when animals are placed on a high-fat diet during adulthood [75]. Altering the timing of the leptin surge also disrupts the metabolic profiles of normal mice born to a normal female. Indeed, administering exogenous leptin during P5.5–P10.5 to normal mice resulted in metabolic abnormalities at the adult stage [75]. Moreover, susceptibility to a high-fat diet in adults born from severely food-restricted dams is reversed by neonatal leptin treatment between the ages of P3 and P13 [76]. Although this study did not determine if the neonatal leptin profile was altered with the severe maternal food restriction, these results suggest that a normal postnatal leptin surge is critical for normal energy homeostasis. Consistent with this hypothesis is the worsened obesity and leptin resistance on a high-fat diet during adulthood when the leptin surge is blocked with a leptin antagonist given between P2 and P13 [77]. Collectively, these data imply that the neonatal leptin surge is needed for normal hypothalamic development, and any reduction in the normal postnatal surge, such as perinatal undernutrition, would thus alter these developmental pathways [72]. Interestingly, a follow-up study in male offspring demonstrated sexual dimorphism of the leptin surge [78], underscoring the potential importance of sex steroids on fetal programming effects.

The source for leptin that contributes to the neonatal surge is currently unknown. While serum leptin correlates tightly with body adiposity in adult, such a relationship is questionable during perinatal development. Fetal and neonatal leptin is likely of non-adipocyte origin. Leptin in the fetus may come from the placenta, which is known to express both leptin and LepR, as well as from the mother [79]. Excess glucocorticoid administration to the mother can reduce transplacental passage of leptin to the fetus [79]. It is reasonable to suggest that unfavorable nutritional status may also affect maternal leptin transfer to the developing fetus. Indeed, it has been shown that leptin administration to pregnant rats fed on a low-protein diet, and during the subsequent lactation period, can prevent their female offspring from developing high-fat diet-induced weight gain and glucose intolerance [80]. This study did not differentiate the effects of prenatal versus postnatal leptin administration; therefore, it is unclear if and how leptin in the prenatal stage exerts similar effects on programming, as shown for the postnatal surge. Finally, neonatal leptin may also come from the stomach [81] or from maternal breast milk, and then absorbed into the offspring circulation to shape metabolic fate [82].

15.6 Abnormal Hypothalamic Regulation of Fetal Programming

15.6.1 Fetal Hypothalamic Alterations in Maternal Overnutrition

Effects of perinatal overnutrition on the offspring's hypothalamic gene expression have been studied extensively for a limited number of hypothalamic gene markers. Analysis of the postnatal lactational period suggests that pre-weaning overnutrition leads to early upregulation in orexigenic gene expression and downregulation in anorexigenic gene expression [35]. These gene changes may program for the development of hyperphagia and obesity later in life. However, a unifying theme as to the precise genetic changes of *prenatal* overnutrition on the hypothalamic appetite regulatory system has yet to be established. Variations in experimental observations are often noted between studies and may result from different methodologies, such as whole hypothalamus dissection versus hypothalamic nuclei microdissection, the macronutrient content of a high-fat diet versus control diet, the duration of the maternal high-fat diet exposure, and the time point of gene expression analyses (Table 15.1). In one study, rat dams exposed to a high-fat diet (34% energy as fat) for 5 weeks prior to mating gave birth to normal weight male pups with decreased transcripts of NPY, mTOR, POMC, MC4R and components of the leptin signaling pathway including LepRb and STAT3 [40]. Hypoleptinemia was associated with these hypothalamic gene changes, but the drop in both NPY and POMC was surprising. In contrast to this study, another study carried out with a high-fat diet (60% energy as fat) for 10 weeks prior to pregnancy showed elevated hypothalamic gene expression levels in AgRP, NPY, POMC, MC4R, LepRb, STAT3, and IR-β in the E21 fetus [38], with decreased protein levels of hypothalamic STAT3 and IRS-2. Interestingly, these E21 fetuses of high-fat diet-fed mothers appeared hyperleptinemic and hyperinsulinemic [38, 44]. These studies show that the metabolic hormonal milieu during development, such as leptin and insulin, may result in hypothalamic gene changes [38, 40]. The functional implication of such genetic changes cannot be easily deduced because the physiological actions of hypothalamic neuropeptides during the perinatal period may differ from that of the adult. For instance, there is evidence that the perinatal POMC system may serve an orexigenic function to maximize weight gain [63].

Changes in hypothalamic gene expression at P0 for five orexigenic neuropeptides – galanin, enkephalin, and dynorphin in the PVN and orexin and MCH in the perifornical lateral hypothalamus (PFLH) – underscore the diversity of these appetite-regulating hypothalamic neuropeptides following a prenatal high-fat diet. For example, in the ARC, galanin mRNA decreased along with the two other orexigenic neuropeptides, NPY and AgRP [36]. The five orexigenic neuropeptide genes in the PVN and PFLH remained elevated through P15 when the dams continued on high-fat diet. Even as late as P70, offspring born to obese dams had elevated galanin mRNA and peptide levels in the PVN, at a time when they exhibited elevated body weight, caloric intake, and serum leptin, insulin, and triglyceride levels. Further evidence for the importance of the PVN and PFLH orexigenic neuropeptide

Table 15.1 Changes in birthweight and selective hypothalamic genes/neuropeptides from various fetal programming animal models

Treatment	Duration	Species	Birthweight	Source	NPY	POMC	LepRb	Reference
Maternal overnutrition								
High-fat diet								
60%	Weaning–P21	Rat	↔ (E21)	Hypo. (E21)	↑	↑	↑	[38]
50%	E6–P15	Rat	↔ (P0)	ARC (P21)	↓	n.a.	n.a.	[36]
45%	Weaning–P21	Rat	↓ (P0)	n.a.	n.a.	n.a.	n.a.	[39]
34%	5 weeks prior*–P21	Rat	↑ (P1)	Hypo. (P19)	(↓)	↑	↓	[37]
34%	5 weeks prior*–P21	Rat	↔ (P1)	Hypo. (P1)	↓	↓	↓	[40]
Maternal undernutrition								
Caloric restriction								
30%	E1–E21	Rat	↓ (P0)	Hypo. (4 months, baseline)	↔	↔	↓	[87]
				Hypo. (4 months, fasting)	↓	↑	↔	[87]
50%	E14–P21	Rat	↓ (P0)	Hypo. (P4)	(↓)	(↓)	n.a.	[72]
				Hypo. (P14)	↔	↓	n.a.	[72]
50%	E10–P21	Rat	↓ (P1)	Hypo. (P1)	n.a.	n.a.	↑	[85]
70%	E10–E18	Mouse	↓ (E18)	PVN (9 weeks)	↑	n.a.	↓ (LepRa)	[75]
Protein restriction								
10%	E0–P21	Rat	↓ (P0)	PVN (P20)	↑	n.a.	n.a.	[83]
9%	E0–E12	Mouse	n.a.	Hypo. (E12)	↑	↑	↑	[84]
8%	E0–E21	Rat	↓ (P0)	Hypo. (P22)	↑	n.a.	n.a.	[90]

Arrows indicate changes compared to the control; % in caloric restriction represents % of food intake relative to the control; % in high-fat diet and protein restriction represents the percentage of energy derived from the macronutrient in the experimental diet

ARC arcuate nucleus, *E* embryonic day, *Hypo* hypothalamus, *m* month, *n.a.* data not available, *P* postnatal day, *PVN* paraventricular nucleus, *prior to mating, (↓) a decreasing trend, ↔ no change

system comes from observations that density of neurons that express these neuropeptides in the PVN and PFLH were significantly elevated in the offspring of obese dams as early as P0 [36]. These authors further showed that a high-fat diet in utero increased circulating lipids that could stimulate neurogenesis of the developing hypothalamus, in particular, the orexigenic neurons in the PVN and PFLH [36]. Taken together, these studies do show that exposure to a high-fat diet in utero alters hypothalamic gene expression in the offspring, although the details are still to be sorted out.

15.6.2 Fetal Hypothalamic Alterations in Maternal Undernutrition

Whereas the transcriptional effects of maternal overnutrition in offspring hypothalami have been well studied, the impact of maternal undernutrition needs further investigation. As with overnutrition studies, results from maternal undernutrition can vary due to the type, duration, and severity of the restriction the rodent species used, and the age of the offspring when metabolic and hypothalamic parameters are studied (Table 15.1).

Early studies on hypothalamic regulation of maternal undernutrition focused primarily on the perinatal rather than the prenatal period. In female rats kept on a low protein diet (10%) throughout gestation and lactation, offspring had LBW and at weaning showed a decrease in plasma insulin level, which was accompanied by an elevation in NPY levels in the PVN and the LHA [83]. No changes were observed in the ARC NPY or in plasma leptin level. In fact, mouse fetuses from dams receiving a low-protein diet exhibited elevated hypothalamic mRNA expressions of NPY, AgRP, POMC, and LepRb as early as E12 [84]. In the caloric restriction model, there are altered hypothalamic gene expressions in the IUGR pups that are consistent with their attenuated response to anorexigenic agents [72, 85, 86]. As discussed in the previous section, 50% maternal food restriction during the perinatal period of the rat, from E14 to time of weaning at P21, resulted in IUGR offspring in which their postnatal leptin surge was attenuated and shifted earlier from P10 to P7 [72]. Concomitant with these changes, they also observed decreased POMC mRNA at P14 and decreased POMC neuronal projections to the PVN in the IUGR pups. Paradoxically, neither NPY mRNA levels in the ARC nor NPY projections to the PVN changed (Table 15.1) [72]. In a study led by Desai et al., in which a maternal food restriction model of 50% was imposed from E10 to P21 in the rat, IUGR pups at P1 showed an increase in hypothalamic LepRb mRNA and total STAT3 protein but a decrease in phosphorylated STAT3 (see Chapter 11). The apparent leptin resistance in these IUGR animals is further supported by their reduced response to leptin and other anorexigenic agents at 6 weeks of age [85]. In addition to leptin resistance as a potential mechanism for the late-onset obesity, IUGR animals also show enhanced response to orexigenic hormones, as evidenced by an increase in ghrelin-evoked overall excitatory electrophysiological response in hypothalamic slices of IUGR animals [86].

In the study by Yura et al., which specifically focused on the mouse prenatal period, maternal caloric restriction of 30% beginning at E10.5 led to IUGR pups that experienced a premature rise in leptin levels at P8 instead of the normal P16. The offspring were more susceptible to high-fat diet-induced obesity later in life and exhibited decreased responsiveness to leptin, possibly due to impaired leptin transport across the blood-brain barrier [75]. The hypothalamus of the IUGR animals at 10 weeks of age showed elevated NPY and CART projections to the PVN, which could be mimicked by neonatal exogenous administration of leptin (Table 15.1) [75]. A similar study in rats by Breton et al. [87] yielded dramatically different results. There, using a similar 70% food restriction imposed during the entire pregnancy, the resulting IUGR pups did not exhibit catch-up growth and showed impaired glucose tolerance and abnormal hypothalamic response to fasting at 4 months of age [87]. Moreover, as adults, their body weight remained smaller, which was accompanied by a decrease in hypothalamic LepRb mRNA and an increase in hypothalamic insulin receptor mRNA levels. Fasting for 48 h normalized these receptor mRNA levels to that of the control. Unlike the previous study by Yura et al., there was no difference in hypothalamic POMC and NPY mRNA between IUGR and normal adults; however, upon fasting, IUGR adults displayed a rise in POMC mRNA levels [87]. These apparent discrepancies highlight the difficulty in generalizing how prenatal and perinatal maternal undernutrition alter developmental pathways in the hypothalamus (Table 15.1).

The Barker hypothesis emphasizes that adult diseases occur when the fetal programming effects of undernutrition maladapt to the postnatal environment that is rich in nutrition. As such, the timing of catch-up growth may determine whether an IUGR animal exhibits late-onset obesity or metabolic dysfunction [28, 88]. Early catch-up growth has been linked to unfavorable metabolic profiles later in life [28, 89, 90]. IUGR pups paired with lactating mothers that were on a normal diet showed early catch-up growth whereas those paired with a low-protein diet showed late catch-up growth. At the time of weaning, late catch-up growth animals showed a favorable metabolic profile, with low insulin, glucose, and triglyceride in light of hyperphagia and elevated NPY and AgRP mRNA levels [90]. When the two groups were challenged in adulthood with a 48-h fast, followed by 2-h refeeding, no difference was reported between groups in body weight, hypothalamic NPY, AgRP, POMC, or CART mRNA levels. However, in support of results by others [75], the early catch-up growth rats showed a significantly elevated leptin level prior to weaning [90], and an attenuated hypothalamic response to exogenous leptin at P5 [89], suggestive of leptin resistance. Unknown at this point is how the underlying hypothalamic changes at birth contribute to the differential responses in early and late catch-up growth. A possible mechanism may involve the hypothalamic POMC system. The POMC promoter has been shown to be selectively methylated by early overfeeding [91] and some CpG islands in POMC gene were found to be over-methylated in the early catch-up animals and under-methylated in late catch-up animals [89]. As such, fetal programming of undernutrition may be mediated in part by epigenetic changes in ARC POMC neurons.

Fetal programming effects of maternal undernutrition may involve fundamental alterations in the development of the hypothalamus and its neurocircuitry. This may involve changes in developmental genes rather than the traditional hypothalamic neuropeptide genes, such as POMC, AgRP, and NPY. Recent studies show that prenatal low-protein diet suppressed the expression levels of many developmental genes in the hypothalamus as early as P0, including those that are involved in cellular development, such as members of the BMP family; cell cycle proliferation, such as cyclin D1; and synaptogenesis, such as Syn1 and Syp [89]. Furthermore, differential expression of these developmental genes in response to early versus late catch-up growth is observed [89], thus underscoring the possibility that perinatal nutritional status can directly impact development of the hypothalamus. In fact, in the caloric restriction model, IUGR pups showed increased brain-derived neurotrophic factor in the hypothalamus at E21, in support of the notion that maternal undernutrition alters fetal hypothalamic genes involved in development [92]. This model shares similar observations with the prenatal overnutrition model [36] in that maternal caloric restriction also resulted in hypothalamic neuronal proliferation, based on increased BrDU incorporation in the median eminence, PVN, ARC, and VMH [92]. As such, fetal nutritional programming can be a manifestation of altered hypothalamic wiring and development that results in long-lasting effects.

15.7 Conclusions

Consistent with the DOHaD hypothesis, epidemiological studies provide ample evidence that prenatal nutritional conditions can predispose offspring for metabolic abnormalities later in life. Experimental gestational models using rodent species have shown that suboptimal maternal nutritional status (either overnutrition or undernutrition) can program the fetus and alter the in utero development of the offspring, resulting in abnormal birthweight or abnormal postnatal growth. Specific environmental conditions after birth can exert metabolic strains on the programmed offspring, leading to maladaptation and adverse metabolic consequences. Although the molecular mechanisms that govern fetal programming are poorly understood, recent studies have shown that the hypothalamus may be one target that adapts to prenatal nutritional status and responds by changing gene expression and circuitry. Specifically, changes in the maternal nutritional environment are clearly associated with alterations in hypothalamic orexigenic and anorexigenic neuropeptides expression. Similarly, changes in hypothalamic neuronal proliferation and projections would also change in favor of an orexigenic environment. Such changes in both neuronal proliferation and gene expression are likely to form the mechanistic basis by which the fetus adapts to the perceived unfavorable environment. These factors coupled to the timing and magnitude of the postnatal leptin profile would then be predicted to change the development of the postnatal hypothalamic neurocircuitry. When offspring are presented with challenges that deviate from the norm, such as early catch-up growth due to caloric abundance, the hypothalamic wiring may become maladaptive, leading to the development of obesity and metabolic dysfunction. A clear understanding of the molecular mechanisms underlying fetal programming will facilitate the development of therapeutic agents and shape changes in clinical paradigms and public policy. In so doing, the goal will be to institute preventive measures early in life to improve global health and lessen the economic burdens of metabolic diseases.

References

1. Barker DJ, Bull AR, Osmond C, Simmonds SJ. Fetal and placental size and risk of hypertension in adult life. BMJ. Aug 4 1990;301(6746):259–62.
2. Barker DJ, Hales CN, Fall CH, Osmond C, Phipps K, Clark PM. Type 2 (non-insulin-dependent) diabetes mellitus, hypertension and hyperlipidaemia (syndrome X): relation to reduced fetal growth. Diabetologia. Jan 1993;36(1):62–7.
3. Barker DJ, Osmond C, Golding J, Kuh D, Wadsworth ME. Growth in utero, blood pressure in childhood and adult life, and mortality from cardiovascular disease. BMJ. Mar 4 1989;298(6673):564–7.
4. Barker DJ, Winter PD, Osmond C, Margetts B, Simmonds SJ. Weight in infancy and death from ischaemic heart disease. Lancet. Sep 9 1989;2(8663):577–80.
5. Newnham JP, Ross MG. Early life origins of human health and disease. Basel: Karger; 2009.
6. Eriksson JG, Forsen T, Tuomilehto J, Winter PD, Osmond C, Barker DJ. Catch-up growth in childhood and death from coronary heart disease: longitudinal study. BMJ. Feb 13 1999;318(7181):427–31.
7. Rich-Edwards JW, Stampfer MJ, Manson JE, et al. Birth weight and risk of cardiovascular disease in a cohort of women followed up since 1976. BMJ. Aug 16 1997;315(7105):396–400.
8. Ravelli AC, van der Meulen JH, Michels RP, et al. Glucose tolerance in adults after prenatal exposure to famine. Lancet. Jan 17 1998;351(9097):173–7.
9. Ravelli GP, Stein ZA, Susser MW. Obesity in young men after famine exposure in utero and early infancy. N Engl J Med. Aug 12 1976;295(7):349–53.
10. Stanner SA, Bulmer K, Andres C, et al. Does malnutrition in utero determine diabetes and coronary heart disease in adulthood? Results from the Leningrad siege study, a cross sectional study. BMJ. Nov 22 1997;315(7119):1342–8.
11. Irving RJ, Belton NR, Elton RA, Walker BR. Adult cardiovascular risk factors in premature babies. Lancet. Jun 17 2000;355(9221):2135–6.
12. Hofman PL, Regan F, Jackson WE, et al. Premature birth and later insulin resistance. N Engl J Med. Nov 18 2004;351(21):2179–86.
13. Hovi P, Andersson S, Eriksson JG, et al. Glucose regulation in young adults with very low birth weight. N Engl J Med. May 17 2007;356(20):2053–63.
14. Kaijser M, Bonamy AK, Akre O, et al. Perinatal risk factors for diabetes in later life. Diabetes. Mar 2009;58(3):523–6.
15. Rotteveel J, van Weissenbruch MM, Twisk JW. Delemarre-Van de Waal HA. Infant and childhood growth patterns, insulin sensitivity, and blood pressure in prematurely born young adults. Pediatrics. Aug 2008;122(2):313–21.
16. Gluckman PD, Hanson MA. Developmental and epigenetic pathways to obesity: an evolutionary-developmental perspective. Int J Obes (Lond). Dec 2008;32 Suppl 7: S62–S71.
17. Gluckman PD, Hanson MA, Cooper C, Thornburg KL. Effect of in utero and early-life conditions on adult health and disease. N Engl J Med. Jul 3 2008;359(1):61–73.
18. McMillen IC, Robinson JS. Developmental origins of the metabolic syndrome: prediction, plasticity, and programming. Physiol Rev. Apr 2005;85(2):571–633.

19. Maffeis C, Micciolo R, Must A, Zaffanello M, Pinelli L. Parental and perinatal factors associated with childhood obesity in north-east Italy. Int J Obes Relat Metab Disord. May 1994;18(5):301–5.
20. Parsons TJ, Power C, Manor O. Fetal and early life growth and body mass index from birth to early adulthood in 1958 British cohort: longitudinal study. BMJ. Dec 8 2001;323(7325): 1331–5.
21. Rugholm S, Baker JL, Olsen LW, Schack-Nielsen L, Bua J, Sorensen TI. Stability of the association between birth weight and childhood overweight during the development of the obesity epidemic. Obes Res. Dec 2005;13(12):2187–94.
22. Hillier TA, Pedula KL, Schmidt MM, Mullen JA, Charles MA, Pettitt DJ. Childhood obesity and metabolic imprinting: the ongoing effects of maternal hyperglycemia. Diabetes Care. Sep 2007;30(9):2287–92.
23. Pettitt DJ, Baird HR, Aleck KA, Bennett PH, Knowler WC. Excessive obesity in offspring of Pima Indian women with diabetes during pregnancy. N Engl J Med. Feb 3 1983;308(5):242–5.
24. Jones AP, Simson EL, Friedman MI. Gestational undernutrition and the development of obesity in rats. J Nutr. Aug 1984;114(8):1484–92.
25. Garofano A, Czernichow P, Breant B. Beta-cell mass and proliferation following late fetal and early postnatal malnutrition in the rat. Diabetologia. Sep 1998;41(9):1114–20.
26. Shahkhalili Y, Moulin J, Zbinden I, Aprikian O, Mace K. Comparison of two models of intrauterine growth restriction for early catch-up growth and later development of glucose intolerance and obesity in rats. Am J Physiol Regul Integr Comp Physiol. Jan 2010;298(1):R141–6.
27. Jimenez-Chillaron JC, Hernandez-Valencia M, Reamer C, et al. Beta-cell secretory dysfunction in the pathogenesis of low birth weight-associated diabetes: a murine model. Diabetes. Mar 2005;54(3):702–11.
28. Jimenez-Chillaron JC, Hernandez-Valencia M, Lightner A, et al. Reductions in caloric intake and early postnatal growth prevent glucose intolerance and obesity associated with low birthweight. Diabetologia. Aug 2006;49(8):1974–84.
29. Dahri S, Snoeck A, Reusens-Billen B, Remacle C, Hoet JJ. Islet function in offspring of mothers on low-protein diet during gestation. Diabetes. Dec 1991;40 Suppl 2:115–20.
30. Petrik J, Reusens B, Arany E, et al. A low protein diet alters the balance of islet cell replication and apoptosis in the fetal and neonatal rat and is associated with a reduced pancreatic expression of insulin-like growth factor-II. Endocrinology. Oct 1999;140(10):4861–73.
31. Bertin E, Gangnerau MN, Bellon G, Bailbe D. Arbelot De Vacqueur A, Portha B. Development of beta-cell mass in fetuses of rats deprived of protein and/or energy in last trimester of pregnancy. Am J Physiol Regul Integr Comp Physiol. Sep 2002;283(3): R623–R30.
32. Cripps RL, Martin-Gronert MS, Archer ZA, Hales CN, Mercer JG, Ozanne SE. Programming of hypothalamic neuropeptide gene expression in rats by maternal dietary protein content during pregnancy and lactation. Clin Sci (Lond). Jul 2009;117(2):85–93.
33. Ozanne SE, Lewis R, Jennings BJ, Hales CN. Early programming of weight gain in mice prevents the induction of obesity by a highly palatable diet. Clin Sci (Lond). Feb 2004;106(2):141–5.
34. Bieswal F, Ahn MT, Reusens B, et al. The importance of catch-up growth after early malnutrition for the programming of obesity in male rat. Obesity (Silver Spring). Aug 2006;14(8):1330–43.
35. Plagemann A. Perinatal programming and functional teratogenesis: impact on body weight regulation and obesity. Physiol Behav. Dec 15 2005;86(5):661–8.
36. Chang GQ, Gaysinskaya V, Karatayev O, Leibowitz SF. Maternal high-fat diet and fetal programming: increased proliferation of hypothalamic peptide-producing neurons that increase risk for overeating and obesity. J Neurosci. Nov 12 2008;28(46):12107–19.
37. Chen H, Morris MJ. Differential responses of orexigenic neuropeptides to fasting in offspring of obese mothers. Obesity (Silver Spring). Jul 2009;17(7):1356–62.

38. Gupta A, Srinivasan M, Thamadilok S, Patel MS. Hypothalamic alterations in fetuses of high fat diet-fed obese female rats. J Endocrinol. Mar 2009;200(3):293–300.
39. Howie GJ, Sloboda DM, Kamal T, Vickers MH. Maternal nutritional history predicts obesity in adult offspring independent of postnatal diet. J Physiol. Feb 15 2009;587(Pt 4):905–15.
40. Morris MJ, Chen H. Established maternal obesity in the rat reprograms hypothalamic appetite regulators and leptin signaling at birth. Int J Obes (Lond). Jan 2009;33(1):115–22.
41. Page KC, Malik RE, Ripple JA, Anday EK. Maternal and postweaning diet interaction alters hypothalamic gene expression and modulates response to a high-fat diet in male offspring. Am J Physiol Regul Integr Comp Physiol. Oct 2009;297(4):R1049–R57.
42. Shankar K, Harrell A, Liu X, Gilchrist JM, Ronis MJ, Badger TM. Maternal obesity at conception programs obesity in the offspring. Am J Physiol Regul Integr Comp Physiol. Feb 2008;294(2):R528–R38.
43. Srinivasan M, Katewa SD, Palaniyappan A, Pandya JD, Patel MS. Maternal high-fat diet consumption results in fetal malprogramming predisposing to the onset of metabolic syndrome-like phenotype in adulthood. Am J Physiol Endocrinol Metab. Oct 2006;291(4):E792–9.
44. Srinivasan M, Aalinkeel R, Song F, et al. Maternal hyperinsulinemia predisposes rat fetuses for hyperinsulinemia, and adult-onset obesity and maternal mild food restriction reverses this phenotype. Am J Physiol Endocrinol Metab. Jan 2006;290(1):E129–E34.
45. Oh W, Gelardi NL, Cha CJ. Maternal hyperglycemia in pregnant rats: its effect on growth and carbohydrate metabolism in the offspring. Metabolism. Dec 1988;37(12):1146–51.
46. Oh W, Gelardi NL, Cha CJ. The cross-generation effect of neonatal macrosomia in rat pups of streptozotocin-induced diabetes. Pediatr Res. Jun 1991;29(6):606–10.
47. Elmquist JK, Coppari R, Balthasar N, Ichinose M, Lowell BB. Identifying hypothalamic pathways controlling food intake, body weight, and glucose homeostasis. J Comp Neurol. Dec 5 2005;493(1):63–71.
48. Schwartz MW, Woods SC, Porte D Jr., Seeley RJ, Baskin DG. Central nervous system control of food intake. Nature. Apr 6 2000;404(6778):661–71.
49. Mayer CM, Belsham DD. Insulin directly regulates NPY and AgRP gene expression via the MAPK MEK/ERK signal transduction pathway in mHypoE-46 hypothalamic neurons. Mol Cell Endocrinol. Aug 13 2009;307(1–2):99–108.
50. Williams KW, Margatho LO, Lee CE, et al. Segregation of acute leptin and insulin effects in distinct populations of arcuate proopiomelanocortin neurons. J Neurosci. Feb 17 2010;30(7):2472–9.
51. Markakis EA. Development of the neuroendocrine hypothalamus. Front Neuroendocrinol. Jul 2002;23(3):257–91.
52. Woodhams PL, Allen YS, McGovern J, et al. Immunohistochemical analysis of the early ontogeny of the neuropeptide Y system in rat brain. Neuroscience. May 1985;15(1):173–202.
53. Grove KL, Allen S, Grayson BE, Smith MS. Postnatal development of the hypothalamic neuropeptide Y system. Neuroscience. 2003;116(2):393–406.
54. Singer LK, Kuper J, Brogan RS, Smith MS, Grove KL. Novel expression of hypothalamic neuropeptide Y during postnatal development in the rat. Neuroreport. Apr 7 2000;11(5): 1075–80.
55. Luquet S, Perez FA, Hnasko TS, Palmiter RD. NPY/AgRP neurons are essential for feeding in adult mice but can be ablated in neonates. Science. Oct 2005;310(5748):683–5.
56. Nilsson I, Johansen JE, Schalling M, Hokfelt T, Fetissov SO. Maturation of the hypothalamic arcuate agouti-related protein system during postnatal development in the mouse. Brain Res Dev Brain Res. Mar 31 2005;155(2):147–54.
57. Elkabes S, Loh YP, Nieburgs A, Wray S. Prenatal ontogenesis of pro-opiomelanocortin in the mouse central nervous system and pituitary gland: an in situ hybridization and immunocytochemical study. Brain Res Dev Brain Res. Mar 1 1989;46(1):85–95.
58. Khachaturian H, Alessi NE, Munfakh N, Watson SJ. Ontogeny of opioid and related peptides in the rat CNS and pituitary: an immunocytochemical study. Life Sci. 1983;33 Suppl 1:61–4.

59. Ahima RS, Hileman SM. Postnatal regulation of hypothalamic neuropeptide expression by leptin: implications for energy balance and body weight regulation. Regul Pept. Aug 25 2000;92(1–3):1–7.
60. Grayson BE, Kievit P, Smith MS, Grove KL. Critical determinants of hypothalamic appetitive neuropeptide development and expression: species considerations. Front Neuroendocrinol. Jan 2010;31(1):16–31.
61. Grove KL, Smith MS. Ontogeny of the hypothalamic neuropeptide Y system. Physiol Behav. Jun 2003;79(1):47–63.
62. Bouret SG, Draper SJ, Simerly RB. Formation of projection pathways from the arcuate nucleus of the hypothalamus to hypothalamic regions implicated in the neural control of feeding behavior in mice. J Neurosci. Mar 17 2004;24(11):2797–805.
63. Mauri A, Melis MR, Deiana P, Loviselli A, Volpe A, Argiolas A. Melanocortins and opioids modulate early postnatal growth in rats. Regul Pept. Sep 22 1995;59(1):59–66.
64. Glavas MM, Joachim SE, Draper SJ, Smith MS, Grove KL. Melanocortinergic activation by melanotan II inhibits feeding and increases uncoupling protein 1 messenger ribonucleic acid in the developing rat. Endocrinology. Jul 2007;148(7):3279–87.
65. Carlo AS, Meyerhof W, Williams LM. Early developmental expression of leptin receptor gene and [125I]leptin binding in the rat forebrain. J Chem Neuroanat. May 2007;33(3): 155–63.
66. Carlo AS, Pyrski M, Loudes C, et al. Leptin sensitivity in the developing rat hypothalamus. Endocrinology. Dec 2007;148(12):6073–82.
67. Cottrell EC, Cripps RL, Duncan JS, et al. Developmental changes in hypothalamic leptin receptor: relationship with the postnatal leptin surge and energy balance neuropeptides in the postnatal rat. Am J Physiol Regul Integr Comp Physiol. Mar 2009;296(3):R631–9.
68. Morash BA, Imran A, Wilkinson D, Ur E, Wilkinson M. Leptin receptors are developmentally regulated in rat pituitary and hypothalamus. Mol Cell Endocrinol. Nov 28 2003;210(1–2):1–8.
69. Pan W, Hsuchou H, Tu H, Kastin AJ. Developmental changes of leptin receptors in cerebral microvessels: unexpected relation to leptin transport. Endocrinology. Mar 2008;149(3): 877–85.
70. Proulx K, Richard D, Walker CD. Leptin regulates appetite-related neuropeptides in the hypothalamus of developing rats without affecting food intake. Endocrinology. Dec 2002;143(12):4683–92.
71. Bouret SG, Draper SJ, Simerly RB. Trophic action of leptin on hypothalamic neurons that regulate feeding. Science. Apr 2 2004;304(5667):108–10.
72. Delahaye F, Breton C, Risold PY, et al. Maternal perinatal undernutrition drastically reduces postnatal leptin surge and affects the development of arcuate nucleus proopiomelanocortin neurons in neonatal male rat pups. Endocrinology. Feb 2008;149(2):470–5.
73. Devaskar SU, Ollesch C, Rajakumar RA, Rajakumar PA. Developmental changes in ob gene expression and circulating leptin peptide concentrations. Biochem Biophys Res Commun. Sep 8 1997;238(1):44–7.
74. Smith JT, Waddell BJ. Developmental changes in plasma leptin and hypothalamic leptin receptor expression in the rat: peripubertal changes and the emergence of sex differences. J Endocrinol. Mar 2003;176(3):313–9.
75. Yura S, Itoh H, Sagawa N, et al. Role of premature leptin surge in obesity resulting from intrauterine undernutrition. Cell Metab. Jun 2005;1(6):371–8.
76. Vickers MH, Gluckman PD, Coveny AH, et al. Neonatal leptin treatment reverses developmental programming. Endocrinology. Oct 2005;146(10):4211–6.
77. Attig L, Solomon G, Ferezou J, et al. Early postnatal leptin blockage leads to a long-term leptin resistance and susceptibility to diet-induced obesity in rats. Int J Obes (Lond). Jul 2008;32(7):1153–60.
78. Vickers MH, Gluckman PD, Coveny AH, et al. The effect of neonatal leptin treatment on postnatal weight gain in male rats is dependent on maternal nutritional status during pregnancy. Endocrinology. Apr 2008;149(4):1906–13.

79. Smith JT, Waddell BJ. Leptin distribution and metabolism in the pregnant rat: transplacental leptin passage increases in late gestation but is reduced by excess glucocorticoids. Endocrinology. Jul 2003;144(7):3024–30.
80. Stocker CJ, Wargent E, O'Dowd J, et al. Prevention of diet-induced obesity and impaired glucose tolerance in rats following administration of leptin to their mothers. Am J Physiol Regul Integr Comp Physiol. May 2007;292(5):R1810–8.
81. Bado A, Levasseur S, Attoub S, et al. The stomach is a source of leptin. Nature. Aug 20 1998;394(6695):790–3.
82. Sanchez J, Priego T, Palou M, Tobaruela A, Palou A, Pico C. Oral supplementation with physiological doses of leptin during lactation in rats improves insulin sensitivity and affects food preferences later in life. Endocrinology. Feb 2008;149(2):733–40.
83. Plagemann A, Waas T, Harder T, Rittel F, Ziska T, Rohde W. Hypothalamic neuropeptide Y levels in weaning offspring of low-protein malnourished mother rats. Neuropeptides. Feb 2000;34(1):1–6.
84. Terroni PL, Anthony FW, Hanson MA, Cagampang FR. Expression of agouti-related peptide, neuropeptide Y, pro-opiomelanocortin and the leptin receptor isoforms in fetal mouse brain from pregnant dams on a protein-restricted diet. Brain Res Mol Brain Res. Oct 31 2005;140 (1–2):111–5.
85. Desai M, Gayle D, Han G, Ross MG. Programmed hyperphagia due to reduced anorexigenic mechanisms in intrauterine growth-restricted offspring. Reprod Sci. May 2007;14(4):329–37.
86. Yousheng J, Nguyen T, Desai M, Ross MG. Programmed alterations in hypothalamic neuronal orexigenic responses to ghrelin following gestational nutrient restriction. Reprod Sci. Sep 2008;15(7):702–9.
87. Breton C, Lukaszewski MA, Risold PY, et al. Maternal prenatal undernutrition alters the response of POMC neurons to energy status variation in adult male rat offspring. Am J Physiol Endocrinol Metab. Mar 2009;296(3):E462–E72.
88. Isganaitis E, Jimenez-Chillaron J, Woo M, et al. Accelerated postnatal growth increases lipogenic gene expression and adipocyte size in low-birth weight mice. Diabetes. May 2009;58(5):1192–200.
89. Coupe B, Amarger V, Grit I, Benani A, Parnet P. Nutritional programming affects hypothalamic organization and early response to leptin. Endocrinology. Feb 2010;151(2):702–13.
90. Coupe B, Grit I, Darmaun D, Parnet P. The timing of "catch-up growth" affects metabolism and appetite regulation in male rats born with intrauterine growth restriction. Am J Physiol Regul Integr Comp Physiol. Sep 2009;297(3):R813–R24.
91. Plagemann A, Harder T, Brunn M, et al. Hypothalamic proopiomelanocortin promoter methylation becomes altered by early overfeeding: an epigenetic model of obesity and the metabolic syndrome. J Physiol. Oct 15 2009;587(Pt 20):4963–76.
92. Coupe B, Dutriez-Casteloot I, Breton C, et al. Perinatal undernutrition modifies cell proliferation and brain-derived neurotrophic factor levels during critical time-windows for hypothalamic and hippocampal development in the male rat. J Neuroendocrinol. Jan 2009;21(1):40–8.

Chapter 16
Adipocyte Development and Experimental Obesity

Elvira Isganaitis and Mary-Elizabeth Patti

16.1 Introduction

Childhood obesity rates have reached epidemic levels worldwide, particularly in industrialized countries. Thus, prevention of childhood obesity has become a major public policy imperative in North America [1]. However, the multifaceted nature of the obesity epidemic has complicated efforts to address this public health challenge. Obesity stems from a fundamental mismatch between energy supply and energy demand. This mismatch can be modulated by both genetic and environmental factors affecting nutrition, macronutrient selection, appetite, activity, and energy expenditure. In addition, insulin, leptin, thyroxine, cortisol, growth hormone, and other hormonal signals can further modulate obesity risk by altering systemic energy balance and metabolism or through direct effects in diverse tissues, including brain, skeletal muscle, and adipose tissue.

In this chapter, we will focus on adipose tissue biology, given its central role not only as a fat storage depot for excessive calories but also as a key mediator of systemic inflammation and secretion of regulatory adipocytokines. At a molecular level, adipose phenotypes are regulated by complex networks affecting both adipocyte differentiation (adipogenesis) and lipid accumulation (lipogenesis) [2–4]. The emerging understanding of the role of brown adipose tissue (BAT) in thermogenic energy expenditure suggests that regulators of brown adipocyte differentiation and function may further shape obesity risk in humans [4, 5]. Thus, working knowledge of the developmental and signaling events that regulate adipose tissue growth is a prerequisite to developing targeted preventive strategies to meet the growing childhood obesity epidemic. We will review the transcriptional and hormonal control of adipose tissue growth and function, provide an overview of the embryology

E. Isganaitis (✉)
Division of Cellular and Molecular Physiology, Joslin Diabetes Center Harvard Medical School, Boston, MA, USA
e-mail: elvira.isganaitis@joslin.harvard.edu

R.H. Lustig (ed.), *Obesity Before Birth*, Endocrine Updates 30,
DOI 10.1007/978-1-4419-7034-3_16,

of white and brown adipose tissue, and discuss how disruptions in the prenatal environment can affect adipocyte differentiation, growth, and function in both human infants and experimental models.

16.2 Mechanisms of Adipose Tissue Growth and Function

16.2.1 Hyperplasia Versus Hypertrophy

Adipose tissue growth results from two interrelated processes: (a) hyperplasia, the differentiation of fibroblast-like mesenchymal precursors into mature adipocytes through a process termed "adipogenesis," and (b) hypertrophy, in which lipid synthesis (lipogenesis) and lipid uptake lead to increased adipocyte size. Adipogenesis is considered the dominant process during early life, as the number of adipocyte cells in the human body increases during prenatal and early postnatal life and is established by late childhood or adolescence [6]. Later expansion of adipose tissue throughout adulthood occurs mostly via adipocyte hypertrophy; consistent with this, there is a strong correlation between adipocyte diameter and adult BMI [7]. However, recent studies examining incorporation of atmospheric ^{14}C derived from Cold War era nuclear bomb tests into adipocyte DNA have suggested that a small amount of adipogenesis continues to occur throughout the life span, accounting for annual turnover of about 10% of the total adipocyte population. This low rate of production of new adipocytes appears to remain stable throughout adulthood and is not influenced by BMI, diet, or weight change [7].

Adipogenesis is a multistage process (Fig. 16.1) that begins with the proliferation of mesenchymal stem cells that have the ability to both self-renew and differentiate along multiple lineages (myocyte, osteocyte, or white/brown adipocyte). Some of these mesenchymal precursors become committed preadipocytes, cells which are morphologically similar to fibroblasts but fated to differentiate exclusively along the adipocyte lineage. These preadipocytes then go through several rounds of mitosis before undergoing growth arrest due to contact inhibition. Growth-arrested preadipocytes remain responsive to several types of hormonal signals (e.g.,

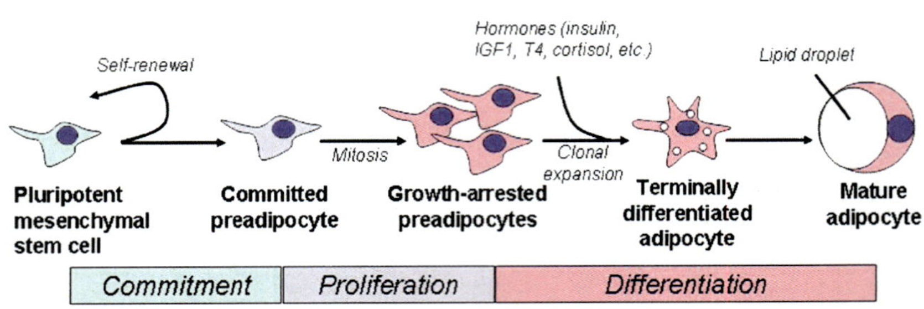

Fig. 16.1 Adipogenesis in white adipose tissue

insulin, glucocorticoids, IGF-1, and thyroxine), which can trigger further rounds of mitotic clonal expansion and differentiation. This period of mitotic clonal expansion is characterized by upregulation of CCAAT/enhancer-binding proteins (C/EBP-β and C/EBP-δ), leucine zipper transcription factors which together with peroxisome proliferator-activated receptor gamma (PPAR-γ) initiate the adipogenic program (Table 16.1), and subsequent induction of genes involved in lipogenesis (e.g., fatty acid synthase, SREBP-1, and acetyl CoA carboxylase (Acc1)), carbohydrate metabolism (e.g., Glut4), and adipokine secretion. The mature adipocyte is characterized at a transcriptional level by high levels of expression of PPAR-γ, aP2, C/EBP-α, and C/EBP-β. As a result of ongoing lipogenesis and lipid uptake, the terminally differentiated adipocyte acquires lipid droplets that coalesce and eventually occupy the majority of the cell, giving the mature adipocyte its characteristic "signet-ring" shape. Most data describing the canonical adipogenic program have been derived from in vitro studies of the murine 3T3-L1 preadipocyte line [8], with validation in a host of murine models.

Table 16.1 Summary of genes involved in adipocyte differentiation

Process	Gene	Function
Commitment of mesenchymal stem cells to preadipocyte lineage	Wnt10a, Wnt5b, and β-catenin	– Organ morphogenesis [14] – Inhibition of Wnt induces adipogenesis in preadipocytes and myocytes [13]
	BMP2, BMP4, BMP7	– Organ morphogenesis – Commitment to white preadipocyte fate (BMP2, 4) [11] – Commitment to brown preadipocyte fate (BMP7) [12]
	Ebf1	– Early B-cell factor [17]
	Acid-labile subunit (ALS)	– Regulates IGFBP [16]
	RARβ	– Retinoic acid receptor [15]
	Zfp423	– Regulates PPARγ via BMP signaling [200]
Mitotic clonal expansion	D-type cyclins, Cdk4	– Early G1 phase of mitosis – Influence differentiation via PPAR-γ [201]
	E2F factors	– G1 to S transition [202]
	Rev-erbα	– Clock protein, regulates circadian rhythm – Required for mitotic clonal expansion, but at high levels can inhibit differentiation [203]

Table 16.1 (continued)

Process	Gene	Function
Promoters of adipocyte differentiation	PPAR-γ	– Nuclear receptor; ligand of thiazolidinedione antidiabetic drugs; endogenous ligand unknown – Required for adipogenesis [204] and function [205] – Dominant negative mutations in humans cause lipodystrophy
	C/EBP-β, C/EBP-δ	– Ablation causes significant reduction in WAT [206]
	C/EBP-α	– Transcriptionally active in mature adipocytes; role in insulin-dependent glucose uptake [206]
	Klf4, Klf5, Klf6, Klf15	– Zinc-finger transcription factors [207]
	Ebf1	– Activates PPARγ and CEBP α[17]
	Insulin	– Peptide hormone [206]
	IGF1	– Peptide hormone [206]
	TR	– Thyroid hormone receptor [206]
	Dio2	– Thyroid hormone deiodinase; converts T4 to the active T3 [206]
	Schnurri	– Interacts with SMAD1/4 to activate PPARγ [208]
	Retsat	– Retinol saturase [209]
Inhibitors of differentiation	Adipose (Adp)	– Corepressor; interacts with HDAC3, H2B, and H4 to reduce PPAR-γ activity [210]
	Klf2	– Zinc-finger transcription factor [207]
	Pref1/Dlk1	– Imprinted gene encoding an EGF-like factor [211] – High expression in preadipocytes; downregulated during differentiation
	NCoR1, 2 (SMRT)	– Nuclear receptor corepressor [212]
	Sirt1, Sirt2	– Nuclear receptor corepressor ([213], [214])
	Hedgehog (Hh)	– Interacts with GATA2 to divert mesenchymal precursors from preadipocyte fate [215]

Table 16.1 (continued)

Process	Gene	Function
	RIP140	– Nuclear receptor corepressor [216]
	GATA2/3	– Represses PPARγ transcription to inhibit terminal differentiation [206]
	IRF3, IRF4	– Interferon regulatory factors [206]
	p53	– Tumor suppressor [206]
	Myostatin	– Activation of TGFβ/Smad signaling, downregulation of PPARγ [217]
	TNFα	– Proinflammatory cytokine; inhibits late adipogenesis via ERK1/2 [38]
Lipogenesis	SREBP1c	– Master regulator of lipid metabolism [218]
	ChREBP	– Carbohydrate-responsive regulation of lipid metabolism [219]
	Lpin1	– Upregulates PPARγ and lipid accumulation [220] – Deficiency causes lipodystrophy
	Glut1 and Glut4	– Glucose transporters, provide substrate for lipogenesis [18]
	Dgat1	– Mediates triglyceride synthesis [221]

By contrast, relatively little is known about the earliest stages of adipogenesis, during which pluripotent mesenchymal stem cells become committed preadipocytes. For decades, a major challenge in adipocyte biology was the lack of clear markers to identify and track preadipocytes, which are difficult to discriminate from other types of mesenchymal stem cells and fibroblasts in a complex tissue in vivo. The recent identification of unique surface markers ($CD29^+$:$CD34^+$:Sca-1^+:$CD24^+$) which characterize mesenchymal precursor cells able to differentiate into adipocytes has allowed efficient cell sorting and should facilitate the study of the early stages of adipogenesis [9]. Indeed, such precursors have been identified in adipose depots, but also (unexpectedly) in the vascular tissue [10]. Moreover, work using the pluripotent C3H10T1/2 stem cell line has highlighted the role of several members of the bone morphogenetic protein (BMP) family in commitment of pluripotent precursors to the adipocyte lineage. Notably, BMP2 and BMP4 have been linked to white preadipocyte development [11], while BMP7 has been linked to brown preadipocyte fate [12]. Other cellular messengers including Wnt, Ebf-1, IGFBP-1, and retinoic acid signaling have also been implicated in mesenchymal cell differentiation toward the preadipocyte fate [13–17].

16.2.2 Adipocyte Hypertrophy and Lipogenesis

Cellular enlargement or hypertrophy occurs through the accumulation of triglyceride (TG) within the adipocyte, either via uptake of fatty acids from circulating chylomicrons or VLDL particles or through de novo lipogenesis (fatty acid and TG synthesis). These processes allow adipose tissue to store prodigious amounts of energy, accounting for 10–15 kg of body weight in a lean young adult and representing over 130,000 kcal, or 200 meals [18]. These energy stores can be mobilized through lipolysis (i.e., breakdown of TG into glycerol and fatty acids) during short- and long-term fasting. Thus, the relative balance between lipid uptake, de novo lipogenesis, and lipolysis determines adipocyte size; each of these processes is strongly influenced by nutritional and hormonal conditions.

The majority of fatty acids used for adipocyte TG synthesis are derived from plasma TG; fatty acid entry into the adipocyte requires the action of lipoprotein lipase (LPL) to hydrolyze fatty acids from the glycerol backbone. LPL expression and activity in adipose tissue are increased in the fed state and stimulated by insulin [19]. Adipose VLDL-receptor expression aids in adipocyte lipid uptake by binding to ApoE-rich lipoprotein particles (e.g., VLDL and chylomicrons) and bringing them in close proximity to LPL on the adipocyte surface; thus, VLDL-receptor-deficient mice are resistant to high-fat diet-induced obesity [20]. Because fatty acids cannot passively diffuse into adipocytes, their uptake is further regulated by transporters including CD36/FAT, fatty acid transport protein (FATP), and fatty-acid-binding protein (FABPpm). CD36/FAT normally shuttles between an intracellular pool and the plasma membrane. Increased CD36/FAT at the plasma membrane could potentially contribute to lipid accumulation in adipocytes, as observed in obese, leptin-resistant Zucker rats [21].

Stable isotope studies in humans suggest that de novo lipogenesis of fatty acids creates <4 g of fatty acids/day, with the liver and adipose tissue contributing similarly to the total fatty acid pool (i.e., 1–2 g/day), an amount dwarfed by the ~80 g typically derived from the diet [18]. The regulation of lipogenesis in adipose tissue has not been as well characterized as in liver, where it is stimulated by glucose and insulin and inhibited by glucagon and polyunsaturated fatty acids (PUFA). At a transcriptional level, the effects of insulin and glucose to activate fatty acid synthase (FAS) are mediated by sterol regulatory element-binding protein 1c (SREBP-1c) and carbohydrate response element-binding protein (ChREBP), whereas the inhibitory effects of PUFA are mediated by LXRα. While SREBP-1c, ChREBP, and LXRα are expressed in adipose tissue, it is not clear whether they are regulated in a similar fashion as in liver. For example, high-carbohydrate feeding increases lipogenic gene expression two- to threefold in liver but not in adipose tissue; conversely, high-fat feeding reduces lipogenic gene expression in liver but not in adipose [22, 23]. Upon completion of fatty acid synthesis and glyceroneogenesis, fatty acids are esterified to glycerol-3-phosphate to form TG via the sequential actions of glycerol-3-phosphate acyltransferase (GPAT) to monoglycerides (MG), 1-acylglycerol-3-phosphate acyltransferases (AGPATs) to dlglycerides (DG), lipin, and diacylglycerol acyltransferase (DGAT) to TG [18]. Not surprisingly, fatty acid and TG synthesis pathways require robust mitochondrial function [24].

16.2.3 Adipocyte Lipolysis

The rate of adipose tissue lipolysis – the hydrolysis of TG into glycerol and free fatty acids – is a key determinant of adipocyte size and adipose mass. Hormone-sensitive lipase (HSL), discovered in 1960 and so named because of its tight regulation by insulin and catecholamines, was long presumed to be the rate-limiting enzyme for adipose tissue lipolysis [25, 26]. However, with the discovery that transgenic mice lacking HSL have only minor impairment in lipolysis (despite large adipocytes), it became clear that additional enzymes must also contribute to adipose tissue lipolysis [27]. Adipose triglyceride lipase (ATGL) was identified in 2004 as a second triglyceride hydrolase which accounts for HSL-independent lipolytic activity in adipocytes [28]. ATGL has a high affinity for TG, while HSL can hydrolyze TG, DG, and MG, though it has the highest affinity for DG [29]. Both HSL and ATGL are tightly regulated by hormonal and nutritional status. During fasting or starvation, HSL and ATGL hydrolyze TG to release FA and glycerol for energy generation by other tissues. Catecholamines and β-adrenergic receptor agonists acting through the second messenger cAMP [30] are the classic triggers of adipose tissue lipolysis, but additional signaling pathways including growth hormone (GH) [31], AMP-activated protein kinase [32], MAP kinase [33], extracellular-signal-regulated kinase (ERK) [34], atrial natriuretic peptides (ANP) [35], thyrotropin (which may be a particularly important stimulator of lipolysis in the immediate postnatal period) ([36], [37]), and cytokine signaling [38] are also potent mediators of lipolysis. Conversely, insulin is a strong inhibitor of lipolysis [39].

16.3 Endocrinology of Adipose Tissue

For many years, adipose tissue was viewed as an energy storage depot. However, the pioneering discovery of leptin in 1994 brought a radical reconceptualization of the role of adipose tissue as an active endocrine tissue [40]. Adipose tissue secretion of leptin is a key effector of adipose-CNS feedback loops regulating appetite, satiety, and energy expenditure. Leptin levels are proportional to total white adipose tissue mass (except in the setting of leptin resistance); leptin deficiency causes obesity and hyperphagia in *ob/ob* mice and in rare cases in humans (see Chapter 3) [41]. Many other metabolically important adipose-secreted factors were identified following the discovery of leptin. Adiponectin, identified in 1996 using mRNA differential display screening, is highly abundant in the circulation and its levels tend to inversely correlate with total body fat stores, although some have described a direct correlation with subcutaneous adipose mass [42]. Adiponectin increases insulin sensitivity [43] and stimulates lipid oxidation in multiple tissues [44, 45] via cell-surface adiponectin receptors. Visfatin (NAMPT), described in 2005, is another adipocyte-secreted factor linked to insulin sensitivity; while these effects were initially believed to be mediated by insulin-like effects [46], subsequent data supported that visfatin effects were likely mediated by NAD biosynthesis [47], potentially contributing to sirtuin-1 (SIRT1)-dependent pathway activity [48]. Visfatin levels are correlated with visceral fat mass and BMI, but not with plasma leptin, suggesting that these adipokines have distinct modes of regulation or that different types of adipocytes might be responsible for their secretion [49].

Many additional adipocyte-secreted factors appear to contribute to insulin resistance and are mostly proinflammatory. These include resistin (secreted by adipocytes in mice but by adipose tissue resident macrophages in humans) [50], interleukin-6 (IL-6) [51], and retinol-binding protein-4 (RBP-4) [52, 53]. Resident adipose tissue macrophages also secrete several proinflammatory cytokines that influence systemic insulin resistance, including tumor necrosis factor-alpha (TNF-α), monocyte chemoattractant protein-1 (MCP-1), and plasminogen activation inhibitor-1 (PAI-1) [54]. Interestingly, macrophages residing in adipose tissue of lean mice have a secretory profile distinct from macrophages residing in adipose tissue of high-fat diet-fed mice [55]; for example, macrophages in lean animals tend to secrete the anti-inflammatory cytokine IL-10 [55], which may contribute to a more favorable metabolic and inflammatory profile. Similarly, differences in populations of T-regulatory (T(reg)) cells within adipose tissue, as demonstrated by reductions in CD4(+) Foxp3(+) T(reg) cells in obese rodents [56], could contribute to differences in adipose tissue inflammatory secretion patterns.

16.4 Prenatal Development of Adipose Tissue Depots

16.4.1 White Adipose Tissue

The time course of white adipose tissue (WAT) development varies across species. In humans, adipose tissue growth begins during the second trimester of gestation. Similar patterns are observed in nonhuman primates, sheep, cattle, pigs, rabbits, and guinea pigs, which have significant white adipose tissue stores detectable by light microscopy as newborns [57]. Notably, rats and mice still have no detectable white adipose tissue at birth, but undergo white adipose tissue expansion during the early postnatal period [57].

In humans, the first WAT depots make their appearance at approximately 14 weeks gestation. Based on autopsy studies in 488 genetically normal fetuses obtained at gestational ages ranging from 1 to 42 weeks, Poissonnet et al. established a chronology of prenatal WAT development [58]. Fat pads in the head and neck appear first (14–14.5 weeks), followed by the trunk and abdominal cavity, while those in the lower limbs develop last (16.5 weeks). The earliest sites of WAT development are those with the greatest vascular supply. At a cellular level, WAT depots initially are comprised of clusters of preadipocytes – mesenchymal cells with a distinct stellate shape – adjacent to blood vessels. One to 4 weeks after making their first appearance, preadipocytes begin to accumulate small intracellular lipid vacuoles. These lipid droplets then coalesce, eventually yielding the typical unilocular morphology of a mature white adipocyte. The majority of adipocytes have formed by the end of the second trimester, but the cells remain small. Adipose depots undergo a period of rapid expansion, driven largely by TG synthesis within adipocytes, during the third trimester. Indeed, the capacity for de novo lipogenesis of fatty acids from glucose increases during the last trimester of gestation [59]. The total fat mass has been estimated to increase from 1–2% during the second trimester to 10–28% for a 3–4.5 kg newborn, or an average body fat percentage of 16% in term infants [57, 60].

This WAT expansion is strongly influenced by prenatal nutrition. A prominent example of this is seen in infants of diabetic mothers, who are exposed to high ambient glucose concentrations; glucose and insulin secretory responses are likely to contribute to excess adiposity and high birth weight [61]. While fetal adipose tissue development is generally proportional to the maternal nutrient supply, apparently paradoxical effects have been noted in experimental models. For example, in sheep, nutrient restriction during the first half of gestation (coinciding with implantation and initial placental growth) results in accelerated WAT accretion during the latter half of gestation, after nutrient supply has been restored [62]. Of note, adipose tissue develops identically in male and female fetuses, suggesting that differences in fat distribution between men and women are driven by hormonal differences arising later in life [58].

16.4.2 Brown Adipose Tissue

Humans and other mammals have substantial brown adipose tissue (BAT) depots at birth, accounting for approximately 2% of the weight of a newborn term infant [63]. Such BAT is essential for adaptation to postnatal life, allowing for maintenance of body temperature in the cooler ex utero environment via nonshivering thermogenesis. Indeed, BAT is able to generate 300 times more calories per gram of tissue than any other organ in the human body [64]. Given this robust heat production, achieved via the action of UCP1 to uncouple mitochondrial respiration, BAT depends on a dense vascular supply, extensive sympathetic innervation, and abundant mitochondria, which impart its typical "brown" color [65].

BAT first makes an appearance by the 20th week of gestation, with expression of UCP1 in some depots. Postmortem studies suggest that BAT development is complete by 35 weeks gestation, with minimal growth between 35 weeks and term [66]. Small-for-gestational-age (SGA) fetuses have similar BAT development and depot size as non-growth-restricted fetuses [66]. UCP1 expression is highly sensitive to nutritional cues during pregnancy, with higher levels seen with increases in maternal nutrient supply or obesity [57] and downregulation of UCP1 and reduced adipose tissue mass seen with maternal nutrient restriction [64]. In addition, fetal levels of thyroid hormone, catecholamines, leptin, and prolactin and abundance of their respective receptors and signaling proteins also influence UCP1 expression and BAT thermogenic capacity [67–69]. At term, labor and parturition further stimulate these endocrine signaling pathways (particularly thyroid and catecholamines) to maximally activate BAT thermogenesis. Further stimulation of BAT thermogenic capacity may be achieved through the action of thyroid hormone deiodinases, which activate thyroxine (T4) to tri-iodothyronine (T3) intracellularly. In lambs and rodents, BAT deiodinase activity increases throughout gestation and peaks several days after birth, amplifying thermogenic capacity [70, 71]. Reduced BAT activation has been described with preterm delivery and cesarian section [72]. The traditional view that BAT is only metabolically active in small mammals and during the early postnatal period in humans was challenged recently by the description of metabolically active BAT depots in adults [5, 73], with discrete BAT depots in the supraclavicular region, paraspinal areas of the back, and suprarenal region [65]. In addition, small numbers of brown adipocytes can also be found within visceral fat and skeletal muscle, potentially contributing to strain-dependent differences in energy expenditure and sensitivity to diet-induced obesity in mice [74].

16.4.3 Developmental Origins of WAT Versus BAT

Recent studies have challenged the concept that BAT and WAT originate from common precursors (i.e., preadipocytes). BAT can also arise from a distinct mesenchymal lineage having more transcriptional signatures in common with myogenic than adipogenic precursors [75]. In addition, Spiegelman et al. have suggested that brown adipocytes may undergo transdifferentiation from myoblasts through the transcription factor PRDM16 [76]. Given that such studies were carried out in mouse and in vitro models, it remains unclear whether BAT in humans also arises from myogenic lineages. Transforming growth factor beta (TGF-β) and BMP7 signaling have also been implicated in the molecular regulation of BAT differentiation through pathways distinct from WAT differentiation [12, 77].

16.4.4 Body Fat Distribution

Obesity is a well-established risk factor for diabetes, cardiovascular disease, several forms of cancer, and premature mortality [78]. Beyond total adipose tissue mass, the *distribution* of body fat is also a key determinant of disease risk, even among individuals with normal BMI [79]. In individuals with the so-called apple-shaped obesity, excess body fat is centrally or abdominally distributed, reflecting fat within the omentum and surrounding the intra-abdominal organs. Such central obesity, measured clinically by a high waist:hip ratio, is more common in men and among Asian ethnic groups and is a strong risk factor for metabolic syndrome, hyper-cholesterolemia, diabetes, and cardiovascular disease ([80, 81]). On the other hand, individuals with "pear-shaped" obesity concentrate adipose tissue in the gluteal and femoral regions, a pattern common in women and quantified by high thigh circumference or low waist:hip ratio. The pear-shaped/peripheral fat distribution does not significantly increase risk of chronic disease, likely because the excess adipose tissue is comprised of subcutaneous rather than visceral fat. Indeed, increased subcutaneous fat may have metabolic benefits, including a reduced risk of insulin resistance, diabetes, and dyslipidemia [82–84]. Transplantation of subcutaneous fat improves insulin sensitivity in mice, regardless of whether it is implanted into the abdominal cavity or the subcutaneous area, suggesting that subcutaneous fat has cell-autonomous properties to improve metabolism [85].

The developmental processes that give rise to interindividual differences in fat distribution are still not well understood. Body composition studies in twins indicate that fat distribution is a highly heritable trait, and that genetic influences account for 30–70% of interindividual variability in body fat distribution (see Chapter 2) [86]. Distinct patterns of body fat distribution are also seen in individuals with heritable lipodystrophy syndromes, further illustrating the role of genetics in body composition. Several lipodystrophy-associated genes including *Lmna*, *PPARγ*, *Cav1*, *BSCL2*, *AGPAT2*, and *Akt2* play a role in adipogenesis, lipogenesis, and/or droplet formation (see Chapter 8) [87]. Developmental genes have also been implicated in fat distribution. Visceral adipocytes and adipocyte precursors express higher levels of the embryonic patterning gene *HoxA5*, whereas subcutaneous adipocytes and preadipocytes have higher expression of *HoxA10*, *HoxC9*, *Shox2*, and *En1* [88]. In addition, some developmental genes (*Tbx15*, *Glyp4*, and *HoxA5*) correlate closely with BMI and abdominal obesity (waist:hip ratio), although the relevance of these genes to adipocyte development and biology is still unclear [89].

16.5 The Prenatal Nutritional Environment, Body Composition, and Obesity Risk

16.5.1 Prenatal Undernutrition, Low Birth Weight, and Adiposity

Over the past two decades, environmental and nutritional stressors acting during critical developmental windows have been recognized as important determinants of body composition and obesity risk (Fig. 16.2) [90–93]. Low birth weight (LBW) is a biomarker reflecting prenatal nutrition, the intrauterine environment (placental function, hypoxia, infection), and genetics (see Fig. 16.3). Studies among the survivors of the Dutch famine of WWII also documented an increased risk of obesity in young men whose mothers had suffered severe undernutrition during pregnancy, further highlighting the role of the prenatal nutritional environment in offspring disease risk [94]. In follow-up studies done in middle age, women (but not men) whose mothers had been exposed to famine during pregnancy had increased central obesity and higher BMI [95]. Obesity risk was greatest in individuals whose mothers were exposed to famine around the time of conception or during the first trimester of pregnancy, whereas exposure to famine in mid- or late gestation did not affect obesity risk or fat distribution, but did reduce birth weight and increase diabetes risk [96–103]. Some of the variability likely stems from differences in methodology; many studies documenting a link between LBW and later adiposity have only found associations after adjusting for current weight or BMI [100, 102–104]. By contrast,

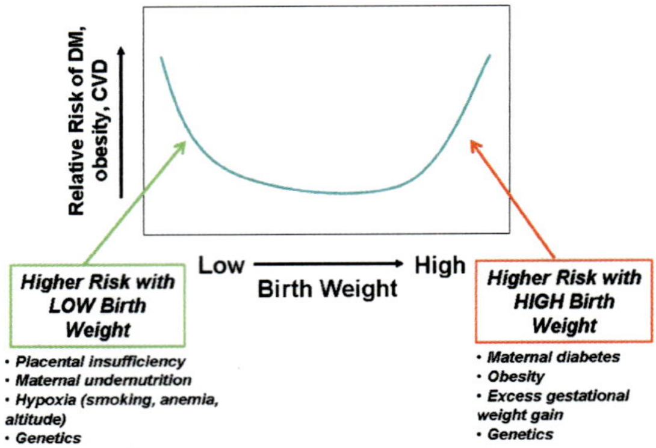

Fig. 16.2 Both low birth weight and high birth weight (markers of prenatal growth and nutrition) are associated with long-term metabolic disease risk for offspring

associations between LBW and measures of central adiposity (skinfold thickness, waist:hip ratio) have been fairly consistent across populations [91, 100, 102, 103, 105–111], although some groups have failed to detect an association [112–115]. The link between LBW and reduced muscle mass during infancy, childhood, and adulthood has been even more reproducible than associations with obesity or central adiposity (reviewed in [116]).

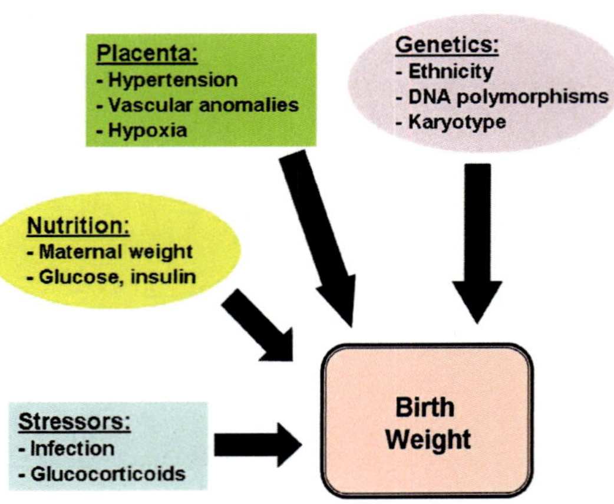

Fig. 16.3 Low birth weight is a biomarker reflecting the prenatal environment, nutrition, and genetics

16.5.2 Role of Accelerated Postnatal Growth ("Catch-Up Growth")

Mechanisms underpinning the association between LBW and later changes in body composition remain incompletely understood. However, postnatal growth patterns appear to be a key contributor to risk. Indeed, LBW infants typically undergo accelerated postnatal growth with upward crossing of percentiles. Catch-up growth during infancy and early childhood. Catch-up growth has been associated with risk of obesity, increased fat mass, metabolic syndrome, and diabetes, even when considered independently from birth weight [117–120]. Similarly, in a mouse model of prenatal undernutrition with modulation of postnatal growth, prevention of catch-up growth prevented glucose intolerance and obesity in LBW mice (Fig. 16.4). Adipose tissue accretion is more pronounced than increases in lean mass during catch-up growth; thus, some groups have used the term "catch-up fat" to reflect this phenomenon [121, 122].

Several hormonal and metabolic alterations may contribute to increased fat accumulation in LBW infants with catch-up growth, including lower TSH, higher blood glucose, and lower serum cortisol:cortisone ratio as compared with LBW children without catch-up growth [123, 124]. Moreover, a study of LBW infants at age 1 year showed defective postprandial ghrelin suppression in infants who had undergone catch-up growth, potentially contributing to alterations in appetite and satiety [125]. Increased insulin signaling may also promote adipose tissue growth; indeed, LBW infants may have increased insulin sensitivity in early life, but go on to develop insulin resistance with time, as early as age 1 year [123]. The role of the growth hormone axis in catch-up growth is less clear. Some studies have reported increased postnatal IGF-1 secretion in LBW children with catch-up growth [124]; others have noted resistance to the effects of GH and IGF-1, potentially mediated through increases in IGF-binding protein-1 (IGFBP-1), a negative regulator of IGF-1 bioactivity [126, 127]. Still, the phenotypic similarities between GH

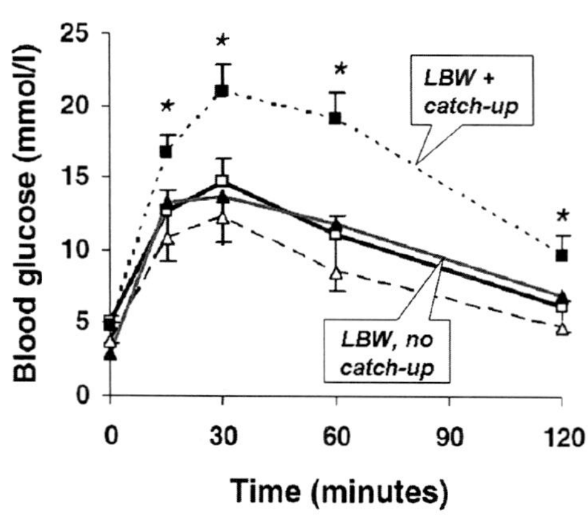

Fig. 16.4 Prevention of postnatal catch-up growth normalizes glucose tolerance in prenatally undernourished low birth weight (LBW) mice. Graph shows glucose excursion following 2 mg/kg intraperitoneal injection of glucose in 6-month-old male mice, $n = 6$/group; *denotes $p < 0.05$ versus controls by ANOVA. Open squares, controls; open triangles, normal birth weight with reduced postnatal growth; filled squares, LBW with catch-up growth; filled triangles, LBW with reduced postnatal growth. From [222]

deficiency and prenatal undernutrition, including reduced lean body mass, central obesity, and cardiovascular disease, suggest that reduced GH action could contribute to LBW-associated complications. Consistent with this, GH and IGF-1 treatment of prenatally undernourished rodents can protect against the subsequent development of obesity and hypertension [128, 129], and GH treatment of SGA children can result in lasting improvements in muscle and adipose mass [130].

16.6 Prenatal Undernutrition, LBW, and Adipocyte Biology

Given the links between LBW, altered body composition, and accelerated postnatal adipose tissue growth, several research groups have examined whether alterations in adipocyte function may contribute to developmentally programmed obesity risk. Abnormalities in adipogenesis, lipogenesis, hormone signaling, and adipokine secretion have been described in adipose tissue in both LBW humans and experimental animal models of suboptimal prenatal nutrition.

16.6.1 Adipogenesis, Lipogenesis, and Lipolysis in SGA Humans

No published studies have directly examined ex vivo differentiation capacity of mesenchymal precursors or preadipocytes isolated from SGA individuals. However, the fact that polymorphisms in PPARγ2 (a critical regulator of adipocyte differentiation, reviewed above) are linked to birth weight and to features of the metabolic syndrome supports the hypothesis that differences in PPARγ2 activity could contribute to abnormal adipogenesis and/or adipose metabolic functionality in SGA individuals [131]. Additional studies will be required to better define the role, if any, of altered adipogenesis in LBW-associated phenotypes in humans.

Studies evaluating whether alterations in lipogenic or lipolytic capacity contribute to obesity in SGA infants have yielded conflicting results, particularly at very early time points. Stable isotope studies using [2–13C]glycerol and [6,6-2H2]glucose in SGA newborns within the first 48 h of life have shown both increased and reduced lipolysis [132, 133]. Similarly, free fatty acid levels as a surrogate measure of lipolysis have been shown to be either increased [134] or unchanged in SGA infants [135]. However, studies carried out later in childhood and in early adulthood have been more consistent, demonstrating increased basal and catecholamine-stimulated lipolysis [136, 137]. Such increases in lipolysis may be a reflection of increased white adipose tissue mass in SGA individuals and/or the subsequent development of adipose tissue insulin resistance. Limited data are available concerning rates of adipocyte lipogenesis in SGA individuals. In an analysis of adipocyte size in Pima Indians, individuals with a history of SGA tended to have larger adipocytes, potentially consistent with increased lipogenesis or lipid uptake [137].

16.6.2 Adipogenesis, Lipolysis, and Lipogenesis in Experimental Models

Given the limitations of clinical research in human children, experimental animal models are critical for our understanding of mechanisms mediating prenatal nutrition-associated adipose phenotypes, including the role of adipogenesis.

Low-protein feeding of rats during gestation is a widely used model of prenatal undernutrition in which pregnant dams are fed a protein-reduced diet (8% of total calories as protein vs. 20% of total calories in controls); prenatally undernourished offspring develop progressive glucose intolerance, visceral obesity, and premature mortality, replicating phenotypes observed in SGA humans [138]. In a study of the transcriptional regulation of adipose tissue growth in this model, Guan et al. noted that several genes involved in adipocyte differentiation and extracellular matrix remodeling were upregulated in low-protein-exposed offspring, suggesting increased adipogenesis [139]. Studies of ex vivo differentiation capacity of primary preadipocytes failed to detect differences between prenatally undernourished and control offspring in early life (i.e., age 1 day or at weaning), but did show increased rates of preadipocyte proliferation in adulthood when obese was already established [140, 141]. However, when prenatally undernourished offspring were allowed to undergo accelerated postnatal catch-up growth (i.e., by culling litters from eight to four pups per nursing dam), alterations in adipogenesis were exaggerated, with increased preadipocyte proliferation and expression of cyclin D1 notable even in 28-day-old weanling pups [142]. These data suggest that the postnatal growth rate is a key determinant of obesity risk in prenatally undernourished rodents, similar to the synergistic effects of SGA and catch-up growth in determining risk of chronic disease in humans.

Studies of adipose tissue development using distinct models of prenatal growth restriction have also pointed to increased adipogenic capacity as a contributor to obesity risk. In a rodent model of prenatal undernutrition induced through 50% calorie restriction of pregnant dams, visceral fat from offspring pups had significant upregulation of PPARγ and its heterodimerizing partner RXRα [143]. Similarly, using an ovine model of poor prenatal growth achieved through maternal food restriction, expression of PPARγ was increased in visceral fat of prenatally growth-restricted lambs [144] [132–137].

Data from experimental models of prenatal undernutrition have provided evidence for alterations in both lipolytic and lipogenic function of adipocytes. Similar to some of the published observations in SGA individuals, adipocytes from prenatally protein-restricted rats have increased catecholamine-stimulated lipolysis, and resistance to insulin-mediated inhibition of lipolysis [145], most prominent in intra-abdominal adipose depots [146].

Large (hypertrophic) adipocytes are a consistent phenotype observed in prenatally undernourished offspring. In a rat model of IUGR (50% food restriction of pregnant dams), size of visceral adipocytes was increased in early life (3 weeks) and throughout adulthood, in parallel with increased expression of genes involved in fatty acid uptake (LPL) and synthesis (FAS) [143]. Increased visceral adipose

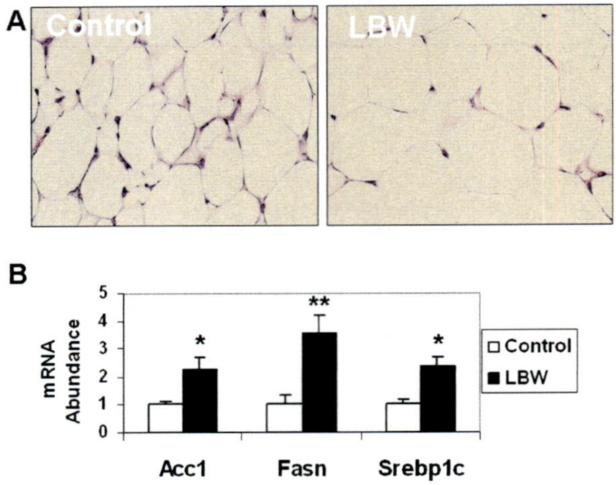

Fig. 16.5 Prenatal undernutrition results in adipocyte hypertrophy and increased lipogenic gene expression. (**a**) Prenatally undernourished LBW mice have marked adipocyte hypertrophy compared to controls at age 3 weeks, corresponding to the end of the lactation period. (**b**) Adipose tissue gene expression (by RT-PCR) shows marked upregulation of lipogenic genes in LBW mice as compared to controls. Males, age 3 weeks, $n = 6$/group. $^{*}p < 0.05$, $^{**}p < 0.01$. Adapted from [148]

tissue expression of lipogenic genes has also been observed in LBW lambs [147]. Similarly, in our mouse model of prenatal food restriction, adipocyte size was significantly increased in undernourished offspring, with upregulation of several lipogenic genes (*FASN*, *SREBP-1c*, *ACC1*) (see Fig. 16.5), even in the absence of measurable differences in food intake or insulin levels [148]. Interestingly, adipocyte morphology and gene expression were normalized by prevention of postnatal catch-up growth, again reinforcing the concept that early postnatal growth rates are key determinants of LBW-associated phenotypes.

16.7 Hormone Signaling in SGA-Associated Obesity and Experimental Models

Several hormonal axes, including insulin, cortisol, catecholamines, and IGF-1/growth hormone signaling, may contribute to differences in adipocyte development and function following prenatal undernutrition. Indeed, alterations in each of these hormonal axes have been described in SGA individuals (discussed in preceding chapters). Given the important role these hormones are known to play in adipocyte biology, many groups have examined whether these signals might contribute to excess adipose tissue growth in SGA individuals or in animal models of prenatal undernutrition.

Both reductions and increases in insulin signaling have been demonstrated in SGA individuals. SGA infants are more insulin sensitive than AGA infants early in life [123], but go on to develop insulin resistance with time, as early as age 1 year. Longitudinal increases in fasting insulin levels in SGA infants are closely related to catch-up weight gain during the first 3 years of life [149]. In a study of primary preadipocytes cultured from prepubertal children, expression of several insulin signaling proteins including insulin receptor, Akt, and Erk was decreased in adipocytes from SGA compared with AGA children, pointing to insulin resistance [150]. Similarly, young adults with a history of SGA had reduced expression of insulin signaling proteins including PI3 kinase, Akt, PKC, and Glut4 in fat and muscle [151–153]. Together, these data support the hypothesis that tissue-specific insulin sensitivity varies over time. The early postnatal window of increased insulin sensitivity in SGA infants may promote adipogenesis and "catch-up fat," with a subsequent transition to peripheral insulin resistance. Although this theory has not been tested directly in humans, such patterns have been observed in mouse models of LBW, in which rapid postnatal catch-up growth is associated with early insulin sensitivity and hypersecretion, followed by obesity, progressive β-cell dysfunction, and T2DM [154]. Similarly in prenatally undernourished rats, catch-up growth is associated with increased insulin-stimulated glucose uptake in adipocytes [145] but lower glucose uptake by muscle [155].

Altered glucocorticoid signaling has also attracted interest as a potential mediator of obesity in SGA individuals, given its important role in stress responses and the phenotypic similarities between the central obesity and glucose intolerance seen in cortisol excess states (e.g., Cushing's syndrome) and following prenatal undernutrition. Indeed, administration of high-dose glucocorticoids (e.g., dexamethasone) during gestation in rodents and sheep leads to offspring phenotypes similar to those seen with prenatal undernutrition, including LBW, visceral obesity, hypertension, and glucose intolerance [156]. Moreover, several groups have described alterations in glucocorticoid signaling in SGA individuals (see Chapter 14). At the level of the adipocyte, glucocorticoid signaling is dependent on expression of the glucocorticoid receptor (GR) and on the activity of the enzymes 11β-hydroxysteroid dehydrogenase-1 (11βHSD1) and type 2 (11βHSD2), which activate cortisone to the more potent cortisol and inactivate cortisol to cortisone, respectively. Patients with visceral adiposity have increased GR and 11βHSD1 and reduced 11βHSD2 expression ([157, 158]). Metabolite patterns, including elevated cortisol to cortisone ratios, similarly suggest increased 11βHSD1 activity and/or reduced 11βHSD2 activity in SGA children [159]. In an ovine model of developmental programming induced through prenatal glucocorticoid treatment, visceral fat mass in the offspring was correlated with increased expression of GR and 11βHSD1 [160].

SGA infants have alterations in sympathetic innervation and signaling, which have been hypothesized to contribute to the risk of hypertension (see Chapter 12) [161, 162]. Intriguingly, the Trp64Arg polymorphism in the β_3-adrenergic receptor has been linked to insulin sensitivity in SGA children, further suggesting the importance of adrenergic signaling in prenatal undernutrition-associated phenotypes [163]. At the level of the adipocyte, increased sensitivity to catecholamine signaling may contribute to increased lipolysis in SGA individuals [136]. On the other hand, reduced catecholamine signaling could reduce BAT thermogenesis, which could reduce resting energy expenditure and increase risk of weight gain. While BAT function has not been directly evaluated in SGA humans, a sheep model of prenatal growth restriction via umbilical artery ligation demonstrated reductions in BAT norepinephrine content, which would be expected to reduce thermogenic capacity [164].

The GH/IGF-1 axis is another key hormonal determinant of body composition which has been implicated in phenotypes associated with prenatal undernutrition. The phenotypic similarities between GH deficiency states and SGA-associated complications (e.g., central obesity, paucity of lean mass, and cardiovascular risk), together with the observation that GH treatment of SGA children improves body composition and metabolic risk, have spurred interest in the role of GH/IGF-1 in SGA-associated obesity. While some studies on the role of GH/IGF-1 signaling in SGA have been equivocal, several groups have noted resistance to the effects of GH and IGF1, potentially mediated through increases in IGF binding protein-1 (IGFBP-1), a negative regulator of IGF-1 bioactivity ([165, 166]). Similarly, IGF-1 exposure of preadipocytes isolated from prepubertal children with a history of SGA resulted in reduced IGF-1 receptor phosphorylation and activation of downstream signaling as compared to controls, pointing to defects in IGF-1 signaling [150].

16.8 Adipokines in SGA-Associated Obesity and Experimental Models

At birth, SGA infants have lower leptin levels than AGA and LGA infants, likely reflecting lower WAT stores [167, 168]. By childhood and adulthood, however, most studies demonstrate increased leptin levels in SGA individuals, likely reflecting their increased fat mass [169]. In several experimental models of IUGR (including maternal protein restriction, prenatal glucocorticoid treatment, and uterine artery ligation), prenatally stressed offspring develop hyperleptinemia in the early postnatal period, suggesting dysregulation of the adipoinsular feedback system and early onset of leptin resistance (see Chapter 1) [170–172]. In support of this concept, anorexic responses to central leptin infusions are reduced in low-protein-exposed offspring. However, it remains unclear from these data whether excess adiposity is driving both increased leptin and leptin resistance or whether leptin resistance is a primary defect [173].

Somewhat counterintuitively, adiponectin levels are reduced in SGA newborns despite their decreased body weight [174–176]. This is contrary to patterns in adults and in animal models of obesity, in which adiponectin levels are inversely related to body weight. Thus, these data imply potential early alterations in adipocyte function leading to reduced adiponectin secretion. This relative decrease in circulating adiponectin persists into later childhood and early adulthood [177–180], with even lower adiponectin levels seen in SGA individuals with catch-up growth [181, 182] and with greater insulin resistance [127, 183]. In turn, low levels of adiponectin could provide a potential mechanism for the association between LBW, catch-up growth, and risk of diabetes. However, some studies have failed to document a correlation between adiponectin levels and indices of insulin resistance in individuals with a history of SGA [177, 182], suggesting that differences in adiponectin secretion may not fully account for "developmental programming." Experimental models will be required to test whether alterations in adiponectin levels and/or action contribute mechanistically to obesity and its associated metabolic phenotypes. Visfatin, another putative adipokine linked to improved insulin action [184], is not altered in SGA children [179], and is thus unlikely to play a role in developmentally programmed metabolic phenotypes.

Adipose tissue secretion of proinflammatory adipokines is another potential contributor to insulin resistance and diabetes risk in SGA individuals; however, the evidence for this is still limited. Most published studies have examined plasma or cord blood levels of cytokines in individuals belonging to different birth weight categories. Some groups have described increased IL-6, TNF-α, and C-reactive protein in cord blood from SGA infants [185]. However, such data do not indicate whether such differences are due to increased inflammation in adipose tissue, inflammation in other organs, or potential infectious processes (e.g., congenital infections) which may have also contributed to IUGR. Other studies of SGA infants have found reductions in cord blood IL-6 [186]. Genetic polymorphisms in TNFα have been linked to both birth weight and insulin resistance (as assessed by fasting insulin-to-glucose ratios) [187]. However, in a study of prepubertal SGA children, plasma TNFα levels were not altered as a function of birth weight or insulin resistance [188]. Plasma levels of resistin, an adipokine correlated with insulin resistance, is reduced in short SGA individuals [189]. Taken together, these data do not suggest that increased systemic inflammation plays a major role in predisposing SGA individuals to insulin resistance during early life. Indeed, studies of global gene expression in rodent models of prenatal undernutrition have shown significant downregulation of genes associated with inflammation in visceral fat [139], an interesting observation which stands in contrast to both human and experimental models of obesity (e.g., high-fat diet feeding, *ob/ob*, *db/db*), in which adipose tissue inflammation is a hallmark [190].

16.9 Future Directions: Potential Role of Epigenetic and Developmental Mechanisms in Prenatal Undernutrition-Associated Obesity

Epigenetics refers to changes in gene expression caused by factors other than the primary DNA sequence. Examples of epigenetic regulation include DNA methylation, histone modifications (e.g., acetylation and methylation), and regulatory microRNAs. Since epigenetic regulation can be modulated by nutrition during prenatal life (see Chapter 8) [191], epigenetic mechanisms have been proposed as mediators of lasting changes in tissue structure, function, and gene expression during suboptimal developmental environments. Such mechanisms have been identified in many metabolically important tissues that contribute to developmental programming, including (a) histone modifications and DNA methylation at the promoter for *Pdx-1*, a regulator of pancreatic development and function [192], (b) histone modifications leading to reduced expression of glucose transporter-4 (GLUT4) in muscle [193], and (c) histone modifications and reductions in DNA methylation at the GR promoter in liver [194, 195].

How epigenetic regulation might contribute to accelerated adipose tissue growth following prenatal undernutrition has not yet been elucidated. This is surprising given that epigenetic mechanisms are known to be important for adipose tissue development. For example, imprinting, the epigenetic process in which alleles are activated/silenced depending on their parent of origin, affects adipose tissue expression of several genes known to regulate adipose differentiation, including *Pref-1*, *Peg-1*, and *Necdin* [3, 4, 196]. Intriguingly, *Pref-1* expression is reduced in WAT from prenatally undernourished mice [197]. Moreover, targeted inactivation of the H3K4 histone methyltransferase MLL3 results in reduced white adipose mass, while knockout of the H3 acetylation inhibitor JDP2 results in obesity [198, 199]. Indirect evidence supporting a role for epigenetic mechanisms in the pathogenesis of LBW-associated obesity has come from the observations by our lab and others that phenotypes associated with intrauterine undernutrition (LBW, glucose intolerance) can be transmitted, via the paternal line, to subsequent generations, even in the absence of nutritional or other experimental modifications during the subsequent pregnancies [197].

Even more broadly, alterations in the nutritional or metabolic environment during key developmental periods, including intrauterine and early postnatal life, may alter developmental trajectories. For example, could alterations in nutrition and tissue/cellular metabolism during critical stages affect stem cell proliferation, function, or lineage specification? Thus, further studies directly examining whether epigenetic or developmental mechanisms contribute to alterations in adipose tissue development and/or function in experimental models and humans are likely to identify additional novel mechanisms mediating developmentally programmed obesity risk.

16.10 Conclusions

The current obesity epidemic can be conceptualized not only as the product of the excessive energy intake and inadequate energy expenditure that characterize the Western lifestyle but also as the culmination of a complex choreography of molecular events that are initiated during prenatal and early postnatal life, which shape adipocyte fate and function throughout life. As schematized in Fig. 16.6, disruptions to the prenatal environment including undernutrition, overnutrition, placental insufficiency, and other stressors can perturb critical events in adipocyte development, leading to both intrinsic adipocyte dysfunction and alterations in the adipose tissue and systemic metabolic environment, associated with changes in body fat

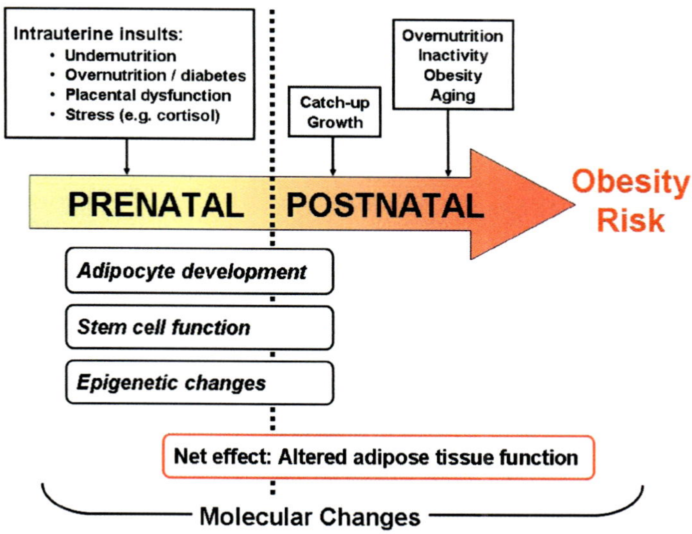

Fig. 16.6 Risk factors for and potential molecular mediators of obesity following exposure to abnormal prenatal environments. Adapted from [223]

distribution, lipolysis, lipogenesis, and adipokine secretion. At a mechanistic level, these changes in adipocyte physiology result from altered hormonal signaling and changes in gene expression, likely mediated through a series of disruptions in epigenetic regulation and altered developmental trajectories. The full characterization of such mechanisms will be a critical and fruitful area for investigation and hopefully for identification of potential novel therapies to reverse metabolic defects in LBW individuals.

Acknowledgments We gratefully acknowledge research grant support from the American Diabetes Association (research grant and mentored postdoctoral fellowship awards to MEP and EI), the Graetz Foundation (to MEP), the Lawson-Wilkins Pediatric Endocrine Society (to EI), and Canadian Institutes of Health Research (to EI).

References

1. Wojcicki JM, Heyman MB. Let's move – childhood obesity prevention from pregnancy and infancy onward. N Engl J Med. 2010;362(16):1457–9.
2. Gregoire FM, Smas CM, Sul HS. Understanding adipocyte differentiation. Physiol Rev. 1998;78(3):783–809.
3. Takahashi M, Kamei Y, Ezaki . O. Mest/Peg1 imprinted gene enlarges adipocytes and is a marker of adipocyte size. Am J Physiol Endocrinol Metab. 2005;288(1):E117–E24.
4. Tseng YH, Butte AJ, Kokkotou E, et al. Prediction of preadipocyte differentiation by gene expression reveals role of insulin receptor substrates and necdin. Nat Cell Biol. 2005;7(6):601–11.
5. Cypess AM, Lehman S, Williams G, et al. Identification and importance of brown adipose tissue in adult humans. N Engl J Med. 2009;360(15):1509–17.

6. Knittle JL, Timmers K, Ginsberg-Fellner F, Brown RE, Katz DP. The growth of adipose tissue in children and adolescents. Cross-sectional and longitudinal studies of adipose cell number and size. J Clin Invest. 1979;63(2):239–46.
7. Spalding KL, Arner E, Westermark PO, et al. Dynamics of fat cell turnover in humans. Nature. 2008;453(7196):783–7.
8. Green H, Kehinde O. An established preadipose cell line and its differentiation in culture. II. Factors affecting the adipose conversion. Cell. 1975;5(1):19–27.
9. Rodeheffer MS, Birsoy K, Friedman JM. Identification of white adipocyte progenitor cells in vivo. Cell. 2008;135(2):240–9.
10. Tang W, Zeve D, Suh JM, et al. White fat progenitor cells reside in the adipose vasculature. Science. 2008;322(5901):583–6.
11. Huang H, Song TJ, Li X, et al. BMP signaling pathway is required for commitment of C3H10T1/2 pluripotent stem cells to the adipocyte lineage. Proc Natl Acad Sci USA. 2009;106(31):12670–5.
12. Tseng YH, Kokkotou E, Schulz TJ, et al. New role of bone morphogenetic protein 7 in brown adipogenesis and energy expenditure. Nature. 2008;454(7207):1000–4.
13. Arango NA, Szotek PP, Manganaro TF, et al. Conditional deletion of beta-catenin in the mesenchyme of the developing mouse uterus results in a switch to adipogenesis in the myometrium. Dev Biol. 2005;288(1):276–83.
14. Ross SE, Hemati N, Longo KA, et al. Inhibition of adipogenesis by Wnt signaling. Science. 2000;289(5481):950–3.
15. Monteiro MC, Wdziekonski B, Villageois P, et al. Commitment of mouse embryonic stem cells to the adipocyte lineage requires retinoic acid receptor beta and active GSK3. Stem Cells Dev. 2009;18(3):457–63.
16. Fritton JC, Kawashima Y, Mejia W, et al. The insulin-like growth factor-1 binding protein acid-labile subunit alters mesenchymal stromal cell fate. J Biol Chem. 2010;285(7):4709–14.
17. Akerblad P, Lind U, Liberg D, Bamberg K, Sigvardsson M. Early B-cell factor (O/E-1) is a promoter of adipogenesis and involved in control of genes important for terminal adipocyte differentiation. Mol Cell Biol. 2002;22(22):8015–25.
18. Large V, Peroni O, Letexier D, Ray H, Beylot M. Metabolism of lipids in human white adipocyte. Diabetes Metab. 2004;30(4):294–309.
19. Mead JR, Irvine SA, Ramji DP. Lipoprotein lipase: structure, function, regulation, and role in disease. J Mol Med. 2002;80(12):753–69.
20. Goudriaan JR, Tacken PJ, Dahlmans VE, et al. Protection from obesity in mice lacking the VLDL receptor. Arterioscler Thromb Vasc Biol. 2001;21(9):1488–93.
21. Luiken JJ, Arumugam Y, Dyck DJ, et al. Increased rates of fatty acid uptake and plasmalemmal fatty acid transporters in obese Zucker rats. J Biol Chem. 2001;276(44):40567–73.
22. Letexier D, Pinteur C, Large V, Frering V, Beylot M. Comparison of the expression and activity of the lipogenic pathway in human and rat adipose tissue. J Lipid Res. 2003;44(11):2127–34.
23. Diraison F, Dusserre E, Vidal H, Sothier M, Beylot M. Increased hepatic lipogenesis but decreased expression of lipogenic gene in adipose tissue in human obesity. Am J Physiol Endocrinol Metab. 2002;282(1):E46–E51.
24. De Pauw A, Tejerina S, Raes M, Keijer J, Arnould T. Mitochondrial (dys)function in adipocyte (de)differentiation and systemic metabolic alterations. Am J Pathol. 2009;175(3):927–39.
25. Hollenberg CH, Raben MS, Astwood EB. The lipolytic response to corticotropin. Endocrinology. 1961;68:589–98.
26. Vaughan M, Berger JE, Steinberg D. Hormone-sensitive lipase and monoglyceride lipase activities in adipose tissue. J Biol Chem. 1964;239:401–9.
27. Osuga J, Ishibashi S, Oka T, et al. Targeted disruption of hormone-sensitive lipase results in male sterility and adipocyte hypertrophy, but not in obesity. Proc Natl Acad Sci USA. 2000;97(2):787–92.

28. Zimmermann R, Strauss JG, Haemmerle G, et al. Fat mobilization in adipose tissue is promoted by adipose triglyceride lipase. Science. 2004;306(5700):1383–6.
29. Zimmermann R, Lass A, Haemmerle G, Zechner R. Fate of fat: the role of adipose triglyceride lipase in lipolysis. Biochim Biophys Acta. 2009;1791(6):494–500.
30. Steinberg D, Huttunen JK. The role of cyclic AMP in activation of hormone-sensitive lipase of adipose tissue. Adv Cyclic Nucleotide Res. 1972;1:47–62.
31. Goodman HM, Kostyo JL. Altered profiles of biological activity of growth hormone fragments on adipocyte metabolism. Endocrinology. 1981;108(2):553–8.
32. Rossmeisl M, Flachs P, Brauner P, et al. Role of energy charge and AMP-activated protein kinase in adipocytes in the control of body fat stores. Int J Obes Relat Metab Disord. 2004;28 Suppl 4:S38–S44.
33. Soeder K, Snedden S, Cao W, et al. The β_3-adrenergic receptor activates mitogen-activated protein kinase in adipocytes through a G_i-dependent mechanism. JBC. 1999;274(17): 12017–22.
34. Juan CC, Chang CL, Lai YH, Ho LT. Endothelin-1 induces lipolysis in 3T3-L1 adipocytes. Am J Physiol Endocrinol Metab. 2005;288(6):E1146–E52.
35. Sengenes C, Berlan M, De Glisezinski I, Lafontan M, Galitzky J. Natriuretic peptides: a new lipolytic pathway in human adipocytes. FASEB J. 2000;14(10):1345–51.
36. Gagnon A, Antunes TT, Ly T, et al. Thyroid-stimulating hormone stimulates lipolysis in adipocytes in culture and raises serum free fatty acid levels in vivo. Metabolism. 2010;59(4):547–53.
37. Marcus C, Ehren H, Bolme P, Arner P. Regulation of lipolysis during the neonatal period. Importance of thyrotropin. J Clin Invest. 1988;82(5):1793–7.
38. Cawthorn WP, Sethi JK. TNF-alpha and adipocyte biology. FEBS Lett. 2008;582(1):117–31.
39. Moskowitz J, Fain JN. Hormonal regulation of lipolysis and phosphorylase activity in human fat cells. J Clin Invest. 1969;48(10):1802–8.
40. Zhang Y, Proenca R, Maffei M, et al. Positional cloning of the mouse obese gene and its human homologue. Nature. 1994;372(6505):425–32.
41. Montague CT, Farooqi IS, Whitehead JP, et al. Congenital leptin deficiency is associated with severe early onset obesity in humans. Nature. 1997;387:903–8.
42. Hu E, Liang P, Spiegelman BM. AdipoQ is a novel adipose-specific gene dysregulated in obesity. JBC. 1996;271(18):10697–703.
43. Yamauchi T, Kamon J, Waki H, et al. The fat-derived hormone adiponectin reverses insulin resistance associated with both lipoatrophy and obesity. Nat Med. 2001;7(8):941–6.
44. Yamauchi T, Kamon J, Minokoshi Y, et al. Adiponectin stimulates glucose utilization and fatty-acid oxidation by activating AMP-activated protein kinase. Nat Med. 2002;8(11):1288–95.
45. Civitarese AE, Ukropcova B, Carling S, et al. Role of adiponectin in human skeletal muscle bioenergetics. Cell Metab. 2006;4(1):75–87.
46. Fukuhara A, Matsuda M, Nishizawa M, et al. Visfatin: a protein secreted by visceral fat that mimics the effects of insulin. Science. 2005;307(5708):426–30.
47. Revollo JR, Korner A, Mills KF, et al. Nampt/PBEF/Visfatin regulates insulin secretion in beta cells as a systemic NAD biosynthetic enzyme. Cell Metab. 2007;6(5):363–75.
48. Nakahata Y, Sahar S, Astarita G, Kaluzova M, Sassone-Corsi P. Circadian control of the NAD+ salvage pathway by CLOCK-SIRT1. Science. 2009;324(5927):654–7.
49. Berndt J, Kloting N, Kralisch S, et al. Plasma visfatin concentrations and fat depot-specific mRNA expression in humans. Diabetes. 2005;54(10):2911–6.
50. Steppan CM, Bailey ST, Bhat S, et al. The hormone resistin links obesity to diabetes. Nature. 2001;409(6818):307–12.
51. Mohamed-Ali V, Goodrick S, Rawesh A, et al. Subcutaneous adipose tissue releases interleukin-6, but not tumor necrosis factor-alpha, in vivo. J Clin Endocrinol Metab. 1997;82(12):4196–200.
52. Yang Q, Graham TE, Mody N, et al. Serum retinol binding protein 4 contributes to insulin resistance in obesity and type 2 diabetes. Nature. 2005;436(7049):356–62.

53. Graham TE, Yang Q, Bluher M, et al. Retinol-binding protein 4 and insulin resistance in lean, obese, and diabetic subjects. N Engl J Med. 2006;354(24):2552–63.
54. Galic S, Oakhill JS, Steinberg GR. Adipose tissue as an endocrine organ. Mol Cell Endocrinol. 2010;316(2):129–39.
55. Lumeng CN, Bodzin JL, Saltiel AR. Obesity induces a phenotypic switch in adipose tissue macrophage polarization. J Clin Invest. 2007;117(1):175–84.
56. Feuerer M, Herrero L, Cipolletta D, et al. Lean, but not obese, fat is enriched for a unique population of regulatory T cells that affect metabolic parameters. Nat Med. 2009;15(8): 930–9.
57. Kiess W, Petzold S, Topfer M, et al. Adipocytes and adipose tissue. Best Pract Res Clin Endocrinol Metab. 2008;22(1):135–53.
58. Poissonnet CM, Burdi AR, Garn SM. The chronology of adipose tissue appearance and distribution in the human fetus. Early Hum Dev. 1984;10(1–2):1–11.
59. Andersen GE, Christensen NC, Petersen MB, Johansen KB. Fatty acid composition of subcutaneous adipose tissue in mother-infant pairs. Acta Paediatr Scand. 1987;76(1):87–90.
60. Widdowson EM, Spray CM. Chemical development in utero. Arch Dis Child. 1951;26(127):205–14.
61. Whitelaw A. Subcutaneous fat in newborn infants of diabetic mothers: an indication of quality of diabetic control. Lancet. 1977;1(8001):15–8.
62. Bispham J, Gopalakrishnan GS, Dandrea J, et al. Maternal endocrine adaptation throughout pregnancy to nutritional manipulation: consequences for maternal plasma leptin and cortisol and the programming of fetal adipose tissue development. Endocrinology. 2003;144(8):3575–85.
63. Symonds ME, Lomax MA. Maternal and environmental influences on thermoregulation in the neonate. Proc Nutr Soc. 1992;51(2):165–72.
64. Symonds ME, Mostyn A, Pearce S, Budge H, Stephenson T. Endocrine and nutritional regulation of fetal adipose tissue development. J Endocrinol. 2003;179(3):293–9.
65. Au-Yong IT, Thorn N, Ganatra R, Perkins AC, Symonds ME. Brown adipose tissue and seasonal variation in humans. Diabetes. 2009;58(11):2583–7.
66. Moragas A, Toran N. Prenatal development of brown adipose tissue in man. A morphometric and biomathematical study. Biol Neonate. 1983;43(1–2):80–5.
67. Cannon B, Nedergaard J. Adrenergic regulation of brown adipocyte differentiation. Biochem Soc Trans. 1996;24(2):407–12.
68. Schermer SJ, Bird JA, Lomax MA, Shepherd DA, Symonds ME. Effect of fetal thyroidectomy on brown adipose tissue and thermoregulation in newborn lambs. Reprod Fertil Dev. 1996;8(6):995–1002.
69. Stephenson T, Budge H, Mostyn A, et al. Fetal and neonatal adipose maturation: a primary site of cytokine and cytokine-receptor action. Biochem. Soc Trans. 2001;29(Pt 2):80–5.
70. Wu SY, Kim JK, Chopra IJ, Murata Y, Fisher DA. Postnatal changes in lambs of two pathways for thyroxine 5′-monodeiodination in brown adipose tissue. Am J Physiol. 1991;261(2 Pt 1):E257–E61.
71. Iglesias R, Fernandez JA, Mampel T, Obregon MJ, Villarroya F. Iodothyronine 5′-deiodinase activity in rat brown adipose tissue during development. Biochim Biophys Acta. 1987;923(2):233–40.
72. Clarke L, Heasman L, Firth K, Symonds ME. Influence of route of delivery and ambient temperature on thermoregulation in newborn lambs. Am J Physiol. 1997;272(6 Pt 2): R1931–9.
73. Virtanen KA, Lidell ME, Orava J, et al. Functional brown adipose tissue in healthy adults. N Engl J Med. 2009;360(15):1518–25.
74. Almind K, Manieri M, Sivitz WI, Cinti S, Kahn CR. Ectopic brown adipose tissue in muscle provides a mechanism for differences in risk of metabolic syndrome in mice. Proc Natl Acad Sci USA. 2007;104(7):2366–71.

75. Timmons JA, Wennmalm K, Larsson O, et al. Myogenic gene expression signature establishes that brown and white adipocytes originate from distinct cell lineages. Proc Natl Acad Sci USA. 2007;104(11):4401–6.
76. Seale P, Bjork B, Yang W, et al. PRDM16 controls a brown fat/skeletal muscle switch. Nature. 2008;454(7207):961–7.
77. Teruel T, Valverde AM, Benito M, Lorenzo M. Transforming growth factor beta 1 induces differentiation-specific gene expression in fetal rat brown adipocytes. FEBS Lett. 1995;364(2):193–7.
78. Olshansky SJ, Passaro DJ, Hershow RC, et al. A potential decline in life expectancy in the United States in the 21st century. N Engl J Med. 2005;352(11):1138–45.
79. Oliveira A, Rodriguez-Artalejo F, Severo M, Lopes C. Indices of central and peripheral body fat: association with non-fatal acute myocardial infarction. Int J Obes (Lond). 2010;34(4):733–41.
80. Klein S, Allison DB, Heymsfield SB, et al. Waist circumference and cardiometabolic risk: a consensus statement from Shaping America's Health: Association for Weight Management and Obesity Prevention; NAASO, the Obesity Society; the American Society for Nutrition; and the American Diabetes Association. Obesity (Silver Spring). 2007;15(5):1061–7.
81. Carey VJ, Walters EE, Colditz GA, et al. Body fat distribution and risk of non-insulin-dependent diabetes mellitus in women. The Nurses' Health Study. Am J Epidemiol. Apr 1 1997;145:614–9.
82. Snijder MB, Dekker JM, Visser M, et al. Associations of hip and thigh circumferences independent of waist circumference with the incidence of type 2 diabetes: the Hoorn Study. Am J Clin Nutr. 2003;77(5):1192–7.
83. Misra A, Garg A, Abate N, et al. Relationship of anterior and posterior subcutaneous abdominal fat to insulin sensitivity in nondiabetic men. Obes Res. 1997;5(2):93–9.
84. Tanko LB, Bagger YZ, Alexandersen P, Larsen PJ, Christiansen C. Peripheral adiposity exhibits an independent dominant antiatherogenic effect in elderly women. Circulation. 2003;107(12):1626–31.
85. Tran TT, Yamamoto Y, Gesta S, Kahn CR. Beneficial effects of subcutaneous fat transplantation on metabolism. Cell Metab. 2008;7(5):410–20.
86. Nelson TL, Vogler GP, Pedersen NL, Hong Y, Miles TP. Genetic and environmental influences on body fat distribution, fasting insulin levels and CVD: are the influences shared? Twin Res. 2000;3(1):43–50.
87. Garg A, Agarwal AK. Lipodystrophies: disorders of adipose tissue biology. Biochim Biophys Acta. 2009;1791(6):507–13.
88. Vohl MC, Sladek R, Robitaille J, et al. A survey of genes differentially expressed in subcutaneous and visceral adipose tissue in men. Obes Res. 2004;12(8):1217–22.
89. Gesta S, Bluher M, Yamamoto Y, et al. Evidence for a role of developmental genes in the origin of obesity and body fat distribution. Proc Natl Acad Sci USA. 2006;103(17):6676–81.
90. Gluckman PD, Hanson MA, Cooper C, Thornburg KL. Effect of in utero and early-life conditions on adult health and disease. N Engl J Med. 2008;359(1):61–73.
91. Law CM, Barker DJ, Osmond C, Fall CH, Simmonds SJ. Early growth and abdominal fatness in adult life. J Epidemiol Community Health. 1992;46(3):184–6.
92. Barker DJ, Osmond C, Golding J, Kuh D, Wadsworth ME. Growth in utero, blood pressure in childhood and adult life, and mortality from cardiovascular disease. BMJ. 1989;298(6673):564–7.
93. Barker DJ, Hales CN, Fall CH, et al. Type 2 (non-insulin-dependent) diabetes mellitus, hypertension and hyperlipidaemia (syndrome X): relation to reduced fetal growth. Diabetologia. 1993;36(1):62–7.
94. Ravelli GP, Stein ZA, Susser MW. Obesity in young men after famine exposure in utero and early infancy. N Engl J Med. 1976;295(7):349–53.
95. Ravelli AC, Der Meulen JH, Osmond C, Barker DJ, Bleker OP. Obesity at the age of 50 year in men and women exposed to famine prenatally. Am J Clin Nutr. 1999;70(5):811–6.

96. Stein AD, Zybert PA, van de BM, Lumey LH. Intrauterine famine exposure and body proportions at birth: the Dutch Hunger Winter. Int J Epidemiol. 2004;33(4):831–6.
97. Stein AD, Kahn HS, Rundle A, et al. Anthropometric measures in middle age after exposure to famine during gestation: evidence from the Dutch famine. Am J Clin Nutr. 2007;85(3):869–76.
98. Ravelli ACJ, van der Meulen JHP, Michels RPJ, et al. Glucose tolerance in adults after prenatal exposure to famine. Lancet. 1998;351:173–7.
99. Frisancho AR, Klayman JE, Matos J. Newborn body compositon and its relationship to linear growth. Am J Clin Nutr. 1977;30(5):704–11.
100. Garnett SP, Cowell CT, Baur LA, et al. Abdominal fat and birth size in healthy prepubertal children. Int. J Obes Relat Metab Disord. 2001;25(11):1667–73.
101. Frisancho AR. Prenatal compared with parental origins of adolescent fatness. Am J Clin Nutr. 2000;72(5):1186–90.
102. Loos RJ, Beunen G, Fagard R, Derom C, Vlietinck R. Birth weight and body composition in young adult men – a prospective twin study. Int J Obes Relat Metab Disord. 2001;25(10):1537–45.
103. Loos RJ, Beunen G, Fagard R, Derom C, Vlietinck R. Birth weight and body composition in young women: a prospective twin study. Am J Clin Nutr. 2002;75(4):676–82.
104. Kensara OA, Wootton SA, Phillips DI, et al. Fetal programming of body composition: relation between birth weight and body composition measured with dual-energy X-ray absorptiometry and anthropometric methods in older Englishmen. Am J Clin Nutr. 2005;82(5):980–7.
105. Okosun IS, Liao Y, Rotimi CN, Dever GE, Cooper RS. Impact of birth weight on ethnic variations in subcutaneous and central adiposity in American children aged 5–11 years. A study from the Third National Health and Nutrition Examination Survey. Int J Obes Relat Metab Disord. 2000;24(4):479–84.
106. Bavdekar A, Yajnik CS, Fall CH, et al. Insulin resistance syndrome in 8-year-old Indian children: small at birth, big at 8, or both?. Diabetes. 1999;48(12):2422–9.
107. Labayen I, Moreno LA, Blay MG, et al. Early programming of body composition and fat distribution in adolescents. J Nutr. 2006;136(1):147–52.
108. Malina RM, Katzmarzyk PT, Beunen G. Birth weight and its relationship to size attained and relative fat distribution at 7 to 12 years of age. Obes Res. 1996;4(4):385–90.
109. Barker M, Robinson S, Osmond C, Barker DJ. Birth weight and body fat distribution in adolescent girls. Arch Dis Child. 1997;77(5):381–3.
110. Sachdev HS, Fall CH, Osmond C, et al. Anthropometric indicators of body composition in young adults: relation to size at birth and serial measurements of body mass index in childhood in the New Delhi birth cohort. Am J Clin Nutr. 2005;82(2):456–66.
111. Gunnarsdottir I, Birgisdottir BE, Benediktsson R, Gudnason V, Thorsdottir I. Association between size at birth, truncal fat and obesity in adult life and its contribution to blood pressure and coronary heart disease; study in a high birth weight population. Eur J Clin Nutr. 2004;58(5):812–8.
112. Rogers IS, Ness AR, Steer CD, et al. Associations of size at birth and dual-energy X-ray absorptiometry measures of lean and fat mass at 9–10 year of age. Am J Clin Nutr. 2006;84(4):739–47.
113. Matthes JW, Lewis PA, Davies DP, Bethel JA. Body size and subcutaneous fat patterning in adolescence. Arch Dis Child. 1996;75(6):521–3.
114. Euser AM, Finken MJ, Keijzer-Veen MG, et al. Associations between prenatal and infancy weight gain and BMI, fat mass, and fat distribution in young adulthood: a prospective cohort study in males and females born very preterm. Am J Clin Nutr. 2005;81(2):480–7.
115. Sayer AA, Syddall HE, Dennison EM, et al. Birth weight, weight at 1 year of age, and body composition in older men: findings from the Hertfordshire Cohort Study. Am J Clin Nutr. 2004;80(1):199–203.
116. Wells JC, Chomtho S, Fewtrell MS. Programming of body composition by early growth and nutrition. Proc Nutr Soc. 2007;66(3):423–34.

117. Bhargava SK, Sachdev HS, Fall CH, et al. Relation of serial changes in childhood body-mass index to impaired glucose tolerance in young adulthood. N Engl J Med. 2004;350(9):865–75.
118. Ekelund U, Ong KK, Linne Y, et al. Association of weight gain in infancy and early childhood with metabolic risk in young adults. J Clin Endocrinol Metab. 2007;92(1):98–103.
119. Ekelund U, Ong K, Linne Y, et al. Upward weight percentile crossing in infancy and early childhood independently predicts fat mass in young adults: the Stockholm Weight Development Study (SWEDES). Am J Clin Nutr. 2006;83(2):324–30.
120. Fall CH, Sachdev HS, Osmond C, et al. Adult metabolic syndrome and impaired glucose tolerance are associated with different patterns of BMI gain during infancy: data from the New Delhi Birth Cohort. Diabetes Care. 2008;31(12):2349–56.
121. Dulloo AG, Girardier L. Adaptive changes in energy expenditure during refeeding following low-calorie intake: evidence for a specific metabolic component favoring fat storage. Am J Clin Nutr. 1990;52(3):415–20.
122. Harris PM. Changes in adipose tissue of the rat due to early undernutrition followed by rehabilitation. 1. Body composition and adipose tissue cellularity. Br J Nutr. 1980;43(1): 15–26.
123. Mericq V, Ong KK, Bazaes R, et al. Longitudinal changes in insulin sensitivity and secretion from birth to age three years in small- and appropriate-for-gestational-age children. Diabetologia. 2005;48(12):2609–14.
124. Iniguez G, Ong K, Bazaes R, et al. Longitudinal changes in insulin-like growth factor-I, insulin sensitivity, and secretion from birth to age three years in small-for-gestational-age children. J Clin Endocrinol Metab. 2006;91(11):4645–9.
125. Iniguez G, Ong K, Pena V, et al. Fasting and post-glucose ghrelin levels in SGA infants: relationships with size and weight gain at one year of age. J Clin Endocrinol Metab. 2002;87(12):5830–3.
126. Chatelain PG, Nicolino M, Claris O, Salle B, Chaussain J. Multiple hormone resistance in short children born with intrauterine growth retardation? Horm Res. 1998;49 Suppl 2:20–2.
127. Challa AS, Evagelidou EN, Cholevas VI, et al. Growth factors and adipocytokines in prepubertal children born small for gestational age: relation to insulin resistance. Diabetes Care. 2009;32(4):714–9.
128. Vickers MH, Ikenasio BA, Breier BH. IGF-I treatment reduces hyperphagia, obesity, and hypertension in metabolic disorders induced by fetal programming. Endocrinology. 2001;142(9):3964–73.
129. Vickers MH, Ikenasio BA, Breier BH. Adult growth hormone treatment reduces hypertension and obesity induced by an adverse prenatal environment. J Endocrinol. 2002;175(3):615–23.
130. Leger J, Garel C, Fjellestad-Paulsen A, Hassan M, Czernichow P. Human growth hormone treatment of short-stature children born small for gestational age: effect on muscle and adipose tissue mass during a 3-year treatment period and after 1 year's withdrawal. J Clin Endocrinol Metab. 1998;83(10):3512–6.
131. Eriksson J, Lindi V, Uusitupa M, et al. The effects of the Pro12Ala polymorphism of the PPARgamma-2 gene on lipid metabolism interact with body size at birth. Clin Genet. 2003;64(4):366–70.
132. Patel D, Kalhan S. Glycerol metabolism and triglyceride-fatty acid cycling in the human newborn: effect of maternal diabetes and intrauterine growth retardation. Pediatr Res. 1992;31(1):52–8.
133. Diderholm B, Ewald U, Ahlsson F, Gustafsson J. Energy substrate production in infants born small for gestational age. Acta Paediatr. 2007;96(1):29–34.
134. Bazaes RA, Salazar TE, Pittaluga E, et al. Glucose and lipid metabolism in small for gestational age infants at 48 hours of age. Pediatrics. 2003;111(4 Pt 1):804–9.
135. Christensen NC. Free fatty acids, glycerol and triglycerides during the first 24 hours in infants with a birth weight less than or equal to 2700 grams. Acta Paediatr Scand. 1981;70(4):485–90.

136. Boiko J, Jaquet D, Chevenne D, et al. In situ lipolytic regulation in subjects born small for gestational age. Int J Obes (Lond). 2005;29(6):565–70.
137. Stefan N, Weyer C, Levy-Marchal C, et al. Endogenous glucose production, insulin sensitivity, and insulin secretion in normal glucose-tolerant Pima Indians with low birth weight. Metabolism. 2004;53(7):904–11.
138. Ozanne SE, Nicholas HC. Poor fetal growth followed by rapid postnatal catch-up growth leads to premature death. Mech Ageing Dev. 2005;126(8):852–4.
139. Guan H, Arany E, van Beek JP, et al. Adipose tissue gene expression profiling reveals distinct molecular pathways that define visceral adiposity in offspring of maternal protein-restricted rats. Am J Physiol Endocrinol Metab. 2005;288(4):E663–E73.
140. Bieswal F, Hay SM, McKinnon C, et al. Prenatal protein restriction does not affect the proliferation and differentiation of rat preadipocytes. J Nutr. 2004;134(6):1493–9.
141. Zhang T, Guan H, Arany E, Hill DJ, Yang K. Maternal protein restriction permanently programs adipocyte growth and development in adult male rat offspring. J Cell Biochem. 2007;101(2):381–8.
142. Bol VV, Reusens BM, Remacle CA. Postnatal catch-up growth after fetal protein restriction programs proliferation of rat preadipocytes. Obesity (Silver Spring). 2008;16(12):2760–3.
143. Desai M, Guang H, Ferelli M, Kallichanda N, Lane RH. Programmed upregulation of adipogenic transcription factors in intrauterine growth-restricted offspring. Reprod Sci. 2008;15(8):785–96.
144. Duffield JA, Vuocolo T, Tellam R, et al. Intrauterine growth restriction and the sex specific programming of leptin and peroxisome proliferator activated receptor gamma (PPARgamma) mRNA expression in visceral fat in the lamb. Pediatr Res. 2009;66(1):59–65.
145. Ozanne SE, Dorling MW, Wang CL, Nave BT, Impaired PI. 3-kinase activation in adipocytes from early growth-restricted male rats. Am J Physiol Endocrinol Metab. 2001;280(3): E534–9.
146. Ozanne SE, Dorling MW, Wang CL, Petry CJ. Depot-specific effects of early growth retardation on adipocyte insulin action. Horm Metab Res. 2000;32(2):71–5.
147. Muhlhausler BS, Ritorto V, Schultz C, et al. Birth weight and gender determine expression of adipogenic, lipogenic and adipokine genes in perirenal adipose tissue in the young adult sheep. Domest Anim Endocrinol. 2008;35(1):46–57.
148. Isganaitis E, Jimenez-Chillaron J, Woo M, et al. Accelerated postnatal growth increases lipogenic gene expression and adipocyte size in low-birth weight mice. Diabetes. 2009;58(5):1192–200.
149. Colle E, Schiff D, Andrew G, Bauer CB, Fitzhardinge P. Insulin responses during catch-up growth of infants who were small for gestational age. Pediatrics. 1976;57(3):363–71.
150. Iniguez G, Ormazabal P, Lopez T, et al. IGF-IR/ERK content and response to IGF-I and insulin in adipocytes from small for gestational age children. Growth Horm IGF Res. 2009;19(3):256–61.
151. Jensen CB, Martin-Gronert MS, Storgaard H, et al. Altered PI3-kinase/Akt signalling in skeletal muscle of young men with low birth weight. PLoS One. 2008;3(11):e3738.
152. Ozanne SE, Jensen CB, Tingey KJ, et al. Decreased protein levels of key insulin signalling molecules in adipose tissue from young men with a low birthweight – potential link to increased risk of diabetes? Diabetologia. 2006;49(12):2993–9.
153. Ozanne SE, Jensen CB, Tingey KJ, et al. Low birthweight is associated with specific changes in muscle insulin-signalling protein expression. Diabetologia. 2005;48(3):547–52.
154. Jimenez-Chillaron JC, Hernandez-Valencia M, Reamer C, et al. Beta-cell secretory dysfunction in the pathogenesis of low birth weight-associated diabetes: a murine model. Diabetes. 2005;54(3):702–11.
155. Cettour-Rose P, Samec S, Russell AP, et al. Redistribution of glucose from skeletal muscle to adipose tissue during catch-up fat: a link between catch-up growth and later metabolic syndrome. Diabetes. 2005;54(3):751–6.
156. Seckl JR, Meaney MJ. Glucocorticoid programming. Ann N Y Acad Sci. 2004;1032:63–84.

157. Engeli S, Bohnke J, Feldpausch M, et al. Regulation of 11beta-HSD genes in human adipose tissue: influence of central obesity and weight loss. Obes Res. 2004;12(1):9–17.
158. Boullu-Ciocca S, Paulmyer-Lacroix O, Fina F, et al. Expression of the mRNAs coding for the glucocorticoid receptor isoforms in obesity. Obes Res. 2003;11(8):925–9.
159. Tenhola S, Turpeinen U, Halonen P, Hamalainen E, Voutilainen R. Association of serum lipid concentrations, insulin resistance index and catch-up growth with serum cortisol/cortisone ratio by liquid chromatography tandem mass spectrometry in children born small for gestational age. Pediatr Res. 2005;58(3):467–71.
160. Gnanalingham MG, Mostyn A, Symonds ME, Stephenson T. Ontogeny and nutritional programming of adiposity in sheep: potential role of glucocorticoid action and uncoupling protein-2. Am J Physiol Regul Integr Comp Physiol. 2005;289(5):R1407–R15.
161. Johansson S, Norman M, Legnevall L, et al. Increased catecholamines and heart rate in children with low birth weight: perinatal contributions to sympathoadrenal overactivity. J Intern Med. 2007;261(5):480–7.
162. Tenhola S, Martikainen A, Rahiala E, et al. Increased adrenocortical and adrenomedullary hormonal activity in 12-year-old children born small for gestational age. J Pediatr. 2002;141(4):477–82.
163. Wang X, Cui Y, Tong X, Ye H, Li S. Effects of the Trp64Arg polymorphism in the beta3-adrenergic receptor gene on insulin sensitivity in small for gestational age neonates. J Clin Endocrinol Metab. 2004;89(10):4981–5.
164. Oyama K, Padbury J, Martinez A, et al. Effects of fetal growth retardation on the development of central and peripheral catecholaminergic pathways in the sheep. J Dev Physiol. 1992;18(5):217–22.
165. van der KD, Deal C, de Kort S, et al. Insulin-like growth factor-binding protein-1: serum levels, promoter polymorphism, and associations with components of the metabolic syndrome in short subjects born small for gestational age. J Clin Endocrinol Metab. 2009;94(4): 1386–92.
166. Iwashita M, Sakai K, Kudo Y, Takeda Y. Phosphoisoforms of insulin-like growth factor binding protein-1 in appropriate-for-gestational-age and small-for-gestational-age fetuses. Growth Horm IGF. Res. 1998;8(6):487–93.
167. Harigaya A, Nagashima K, Nako Y, Morikawa A. Relationship between concentration of serum leptin and fetal growth. J Clin Endocrinol Metab. 1997;82(10):3281–4.
168. Marchini G, Fried G, Ostlund E, Hagenas L. Plasma leptin in infants: relations to birth weight and weight loss. Pediatrics. 1998;101(3 Pt 1):429–32.
169. Pulzer F, Haase U, Knupfer M, et al. Serum leptin in formerly small-for-gestational-age children during adolescence: relationship to gender, puberty, body composition, insulin sensitivity, creatinine, and serum uric acid. Metabolism. 2001;50(10):1141–6.
170. Vickers MH, Breier BH, Cutfield WS, Hofman PL, Gluckman PD. Fetal origins of hyperphagia, obesity, and hypertension and postnatal amplification by hypercaloric nutrition. Am J Physiol Endocrinol Metab. 2000;279(1):E83–7.
171. Sugden MC, Langdown ML, Munns MJ, Holness MJ. Maternal glucocorticoid treatment modulates placental leptin and leptin receptor expression and materno-fetal leptin physiology during late pregnancy, and elicits hypertension associated with hyperleptinaemia in the early-growth-retarded adult offspring. Eur J Endocrinol. 2001;145(4):529–39.
172. Nusken KD, Dotsch J, Rauh M, Rascher W, Schneider H. Uteroplacental insufficiency after bilateral uterine artery ligation in the rat: impact on postnatal glucose and lipid metabolism and evidence for metabolic programming of the offspring by sham operation. Endocrinology. 2008;149(3):1056–63.
173. Desai M, Gayle D, Han G, Ross MG. Programmed hyperphagia due to reduced anorexigenic mechanisms in intrauterine growth-restricted offspring. Reprod Sci. 2007;14(4): 329–37.
174. Sivan E, Mazaki-Tovi S, Pariente C, et al. Adiponectin in human cord blood: relation to fetal birth weight and gender. J Clin Endocrinol Metab. 2003;88(12):5656–60.

175. Laudes M, Oberhauser F, Bilkovski R, et al. Human fetal adiponectin and retinol-binding protein (RBP)-4 levels in relation to birth weight and maternal obesity. Exp Clin Endocrinol Diabetes. 2009;117(3):146–9.
176. Gohlke BC, Bartmann P, Fimmers R, et al. Fetal adiponectin and resistin in correlation with birth weight difference in monozygotic twins with discordant growth. Horm Res. 2008;69(1):37–44.
177. Jaquet D, Deghmoun S, Chevenne D, Czernichow P, Levy-Marchal C. Low serum adiponectin levels in subjects born small for gestational age: impact on insulin sensitivity. Int J Obes (Lond). 2006;30(1):83–7.
178. Tamakoshi K, Yatsuya H, Wada K, et al. Low birth weight is associated with reduced adiponectin concentration in adult. Ann Epidemiol. 2006;16(9):669–74.
179. Ibanez L, Lopez-Bermejo A, Suarez L, et al. Visceral adiposity without overweight in children born small for gestational age. J Clin Endocrinol Metab. 2008;93(6):2079–83.
180. Ibanez L, Lopez-Bermejo A, Diaz M, et al. High-molecular-weight adiponectin in children born small- or appropriate-for-gestational-age. J Pediatr. 2009;155(5):740–2.
181. Cianfarani S, Martinez C, Maiorana A, et al. Adiponectin levels are reduced in children born small for gestational age and are inversely related to postnatal catch-up growth. J Clin Endocrinol Metab. 2004;89(3):1346–51.
182. Iniguez G, Soto N, Avila A, et al. Adiponectin levels in the first two years of life in a prospective cohort: relations with weight gain, leptin levels and insulin sensitivity. J Clin Endocrinol Metab. 2004;89(11):5500–3.
183. Tenhola S, Todorova B, Jaaskelainen J, et al. Serum glucocorticoids and adiponectin associate with insulin resistance in children born small for gestational age. Eur J Endocrinol. 2010;162(3):551–7.
184. Araki S, Dobashi K, Kubo K, et al. Plasma visfatin concentration as a surrogate marker for visceral fat accumulation in obese children. Obesity (Silver Spring). 2008;16(2):384–8.
185. Amarilyo G, Oren A, Mimouni FB, et al. Increased cord serum inflammatory markers in small-for-gestational-age neonates. J Perinatol. 2010.
186. Martos-Moreno GA, Barrios V, Sáenz de Pipaón M, et al. Influence of prematurity and growth restriction on the adipokine profile, IGF1, and ghrelin levels in cord blood: relationship with glucose metabolism. Eur J Endocrinol. 2009;161(3):381–9.
187. Casano-Sancho P, Lopez-Bermejo A, Fernandez-Real JM, et al. The tumour necrosis factor (TNF)-alpha-308GA promoter polymorphism is related to prenatal growth and postnatal insulin resistance. Clin Endocrinol (Oxf). 2006;64(2):129–35.
188. Jefferies CA, Hofman PL, Keelan JA, Robinson EM, Cutfield WS. Insulin resistance is not due to persistently elevated serum tumor necrosis-alpha levels in small for gestational age, premature, or twin children. Pediatr Diabetes. 2004;5(1):20–5.
189. Willemsen RH, van Dijk M, de Rijke YB, et al. Effect of growth hormone therapy on serum adiponectin and resistin levels in short, small-for-gestational-age children and associations with cardiovascular risk parameters. J Clin Endocrinol Metab. 2007;92(1):117–23.
190. Murano I, Barbatelli G, Parisani V, et al. Dead adipocytes, detected as crown-like structures, are prevalent in visceral fat depots of genetically obese mice. J Lipid Res. 2008;49(7): 1562–8.
191. Waterland RA, Jirtle RL. Transposable elements: targets for early nutritional effects on epigenetic gene regulation. Mol Cell Biol. 2003;23(15):5293–300.
192. Park JH, Stoffers DA, Nicholls RD, Simmons RA. Development of type 2 diabetes following intrauterine growth retardation in rats is associated with progressive epigenetic silencing of Pdx1. J Clin Invest. 2008;118(6):2316–24.
193. Raychaudhuri N, Raychaudhuri S, Thamotharan M, Devaskar SU. Histone code modifications repress glucose transporter 4 expression in the intrauterine growth-restricted offspring. J Biol Chem. 2008;283(20):13611–26.
194. Lillycrop KA, Phillips ES, Jackson AA, Hanson MA, Burdge GC. Dietary protein restriction of pregnant rats induces and folic acid supplementation prevents epigenetic modification of hepatic gene expression in the offspring. J Nutr. 2005;135(6):1382–6.

195. Lillycrop KA, Phillips ES, Torrens C, et al. Feeding pregnant rats a protein-restricted diet persistently alters the methylation of specific cytosines in the hepatic PPAR alpha promoter of the offspring. Br J Nutr. 2008;100(2):278–82.
196. Moon YS, Smas CM, Lee K, et al. Mice lacking paternally expressed Pref-1/Dlk1 display growth retardation and accelerated adiposity. Mol Cell Biol. 2002;22(15):5585–92.
197. Jimenez-Chillaron JC, Isganaitis E, Charalambous M, et al. Intergenerational transmission of glucose intolerance and obesity by in utero undernutrition in mice. Diabetes. 2009;58(2):460–8.
198. Lee J, Saha PK, Yang QH, et al. Targeted inactivation of MLL3 histone H3-Lys-4 methyltransferase activity in the mouse reveals vital roles for MLL3 in adipogenesis. Proc Natl Acad Sci USA. 2008;105(49):19229–34.
199. Nakade K, Pan J, Yoshiki A, et al. JDP2 suppresses adipocyte differentiation by regulating histone acetylation. Cell Death Differ. 2007;14(8):1398–405.
200. Gupta RK, Arany Z, Seale P, et al. Transcriptional control of preadipocyte determination by Zfp423. Nature. 2010;464(7288):619–23.
201. Abella A, Dubus P, Malumbres M, et al. Cdk4 promotes adipogenesis through PPARgamma activation. Cell Metab. 2005;2(4):239–49.
202. Fajas L, Landsberg RL, Huss-Garcia Y, et al. E2Fs regulate adipocyte differentiation. Dev Cell. 2002;3(1):39–49.
203. Fontaine C, Staels B. The orphan nuclear receptor Rev-erbalpha: a transcriptional link between circadian rhythmicity and cardiometabolic disease. Curr Opin Lipidol. 2007;18(2):141–6.
204. Lehrke M, Lazar MA. The many faces of PPARgamma. Cell. 2005;123(6):993–9.
205. Tontonoz P, Spiegelman BM. Fat and beyond: the diverse biology of PPARgamma. Annu Rev Biochem. 2008;77:289–312.
206. Lefterova MI, Zhang Y, Steger DJ, et al. PPARgamma and C/EBP factors orchestrate adipocyte biology via adjacent binding on a genome-wide scale. Genes Dev. 2008;22(21):2941–52.
207. Brey CW, Nelder MP, Hailemariam T, Gaugler R, Hashmi S. Kruppel-like family of transcription factors: an emerging new frontier in fat biology. Int J Biol Sci. 2009;5(6):622–36.
208. Jin W, Takagi T, Kanesashi SN, et al. Schnurri-2 controls BMP-dependent adipogenesis via interaction with Smad proteins. Dev Cell. 2006;10(4):461–71.
209. Moise AR, Lobo GP, Erokwu B, et al. Increased adiposity in the retinol saturase-knockout mouse. FASEB J. 2010;24(4):1261–70.
210. Suh JM, Zeve D, McKay R, et al. Adipose is a conserved dosage-sensitive antiobesity gene. Cell Metab. 2007;6(3):195–207.
211. Sul HS. Minireview: Pref-1: role in adipogenesis and esenchymal cell fate. Mol Endocrinol. 2009;23(11):1717–25.
212. Yu C, Markan K, Temple KA, et al. The nuclear receptor corepressors NCoR and SMRT decrease peroxisome proliferator-activated receptor gamma transcriptional activity and repress 3T3-L1 adipogenesis. J Biol Chem. 2005;280(14):13600–5.
213. Picard F, Kurtev M, Chung N, et al. Sirt1 promotes fat mobilization in white adipocytes by repressing PPAR-gamma. Nature. 2004;429(6993):771–6.
214. Jing E, Gesta S, Kahn CR. SIRT2 regulates adipocyte differentiation through FoxO1 acetylation/deacetylation. Cell Metab. 2007;6(2):105–14.
215. Suh JM, Gao X, McKay J, et al. Hedgehog signaling plays a conserved role in inhibiting fat formation. Cell Metab. 2006;3(1):25–34.
216. Leonardsson G, Steel JH, Christian M, et al. Nuclear receptor corepressor RIP140 regulates fat accumulation. Proc Natl Acad Sci USA. 2004;101(22):8437–42.
217. Guo W, Flanagan J, Jasuja R, et al. The effects of myostatin on adipogenic differentiation of human bone marrow-derived mesenchymal stem cells are mediated through cross-communication between Smad3 and Wnt/beta-catenin signaling pathways. J Biol Chem. 2008;283(14):9136–45.

218. Kim JB, Spiegelman BM. ADD1/SREBP1 promotes adipocyte differentiation and gene expression linked to fatty acid metabolism. Genes Dev. 1996;10:1096–107.
219. Postic C, Dentin R, Denechaud PD, Girard J. ChREBP, a transcriptional regulator of glucose and lipid metabolism. Annu Rev Nutr. 2007;27:179–92.
220. Phan J, Reue K. Lipin, a lipodystrophy and obesity gene. Cell Metab. 2005;1(1):73–83.
221. Beylot M, Peroni O, Diraison F, Large V. In vivo studies of intrahepatic metabolic pathways. Diab Metab. 1997;23(3):251–7.
222. Jimenez-Chillaron JC, Hernandez-Valencia M, Lightner A, et al. Reductions in caloric intake and early postnatal growth prevent glucose intolerance and obesity associated with low birthweight. Diabetologia. 2006;49(8):1974–84.
223. Woo M, Patti ME. Diabetes risk begins in utero. Cell Metab. 2008;8(1):5–7.

Part IV
Environmental Obesogens

Chapter 17
The Obesogen Hypothesis of Obesity: Overview and Human Evidence

Jerrold J. Heindel

17.1 Introduction

Obesity has reached alarming levels in the United States, especially in children. Data from NHANES surveys (1976–1980 and 2003–2006) show that the prevalence of obesity has increased for children aged 2–5 years (5.0–12.4%), for those aged 6–11 years (6.5–17.0%), and for those aged 12–19 years (5.0–17.6%) [1]. In addition, the prevalence of overweight infants under 6 months has increased by 73% between 1980 and 2001, from 3.4 to 5.9% [2]. Addressing the obesity epidemic is going to require serious consideration of both traditional (i.e., diet and exercise) and nontraditional risk factors, including the role of endocrine-disrupting chemicals (EDCs) and other environmental chemicals.

There is no doubt that obesity, like every complex disease, will have both a genetic and an environmental component. Thus, it will not be possible to understand the etiology of complex diseases such as obesity without understanding both these genetic and environmental components and how they interact. However, until recently, the focus has been on understanding the genetics of obesity and on trying to reduce weight in overweight and obese people. It is clear that this approach has not fared well; despite tremendous time and effort, few genes have been identified [3]. Furthermore, it is not possible to change your genetic background. Lastly, people lose weight but tend to gain it back, even while on weight loss pharmacotherapy [4]. The focus on intervention has been costly in terms of both human health and potential and puts a tremendous burden on our health care system.

A proactive approach that prevents weight gain and obesity would be better for the American public, government, and our health care system. Recent "epidemics" of chronic diseases like diabetes, childhood asthma, ADHD, and obesity must have an environmental trigger, since genetic modifications cannot account for such large

J.J. Heindel (✉)
Division of Extramural Research and Training, National Institute of Environmental Health Sciences, Research Triangle Park, NC, USA
e-mail: heindelj@niehs.nih.gov

R.H. Lustig (ed.), *Obesity Before Birth*, Endocrine Updates 30,
DOI 10.1007/978-1-4419-7034-3_17,

increases over such a short time. Thus, focusing on the environment, which can be changed, is a promising approach.

17.2 "Developmental Origins of Health and Disease" Paradigm

There has recently been a major paradigm shift in relation to the onset of disease. It is now becoming clear that diseases that show up later in life may actually have their origin during development (in utero and first few years of life). This new paradigm is called the "Developmental Origins of Health and Disease (DoHaD)" [5]. This concept was first used in the field of nutrition, where epidemiologic studies found that low birth weight (LBW) babies resulting from poor nutrition of their mothers had latent appearance of disease in adult life, including increased susceptibility to noncommunicable diseases such as coronary heart disease, obesity, type 2 diabetes mellitus (T2DM), osteoporosis, and metabolic dysfunction. These studies represent some examples in the literature that have led to a substantial research effort focusing on perinatal influences and subsequent chronic disease [6, 7]. Indeed, there is a large literature examining the developmental basis of obesity in humans, particularly focusing on altered nutrition [8].

Maternal factors such as obesity during pregnancy and gestational diabetes mellitus are both well-recognized risk factors for increased birth weight and increased adiposity and insulin resistance later in childhood [9, 10]. A large number of epidemiological studies have demonstrated a direct relationship between birth weight and BMI later in life. These data support the seeming paradox of increased adult adiposity associated with both ends of the birth weight spectrum: higher BMI with higher birth weight and increased central adiposity with LBW [11]. Thus, infants who experience fetal undernutrition are also more likely to develop hyperlipidemia, central obesity, and insulin resistance in childhood which then puts them at greater risk of developing cardiovascular diseases and T2DM in adulthood, especially if LBW is followed by rapid weight gain during childhood [9, 10]. Collectively, there is a large literature in humans demonstrating that childhood obesity and other metabolic traits associated with the development of cardiometabolic disease in adulthood can stem from the maternal environment (especially altered maternal nutrition) independent of the behavior of the child.

The fact that the prevalence of overweight infants under 6 months has increased markedly between 1980 and 2001 [2] points to a role for developmental programming in the obesity epidemic. There are also human data indicating that feeding during the first week of life can be an important determinant of subsequent weight gain. Stettler et al. [12] showed that weight gain in the first week of life in formula-fed infants was associated with overweight status 2–3 decades later. Other studies have shown that weight gain during the first few months of life is related to overweight in adulthood [13]. Thus, it is clear that nutrition during the developmental period in utero and in the first few months to years of life is important in determining metabolic status later in life.

17.3 Environmental Toxicants

Animal studies have long documented that the in utero developmental period is a sensitive window for perturbation; not just for nutrition factors, but also for environmental chemicals. Indeed, supporting evidence for the developmental basis of disease concept developed independently in the field of environmental toxicology, where it was recognized that between 2 and 5% of all live births have major developmental abnormalities. Up to 40% of these defects have been estimated to result from maternal exposures to harmful environmental agents that impact the intrauterine environment. Depending on agent, timing, and dose, environmental chemicals can cause death, malformations, LBW, or functional changes [14–16]. These toxicant-induced functional changes most likely result from altered gene expression or protein regulation associated with abnormal cell proliferation and differentiation involved in interactions between various cell types and the establishment of cell lineages. These changes may lead to abnormal morphological and/or functional characteristics of the tissues, organs, and systems. These functional changes are not detected by measuring birth weight or length. Sophisticated analyses of molecular changes at the cellular level are needed to detect these subtle changes. In addition, the latency between exposure and detection of the disease/dysfunction that results from the functional change may be many years or even decades. The end result of these functional changes due to environmental agent exposure during development is an animal that is sensitized, rendering it more susceptible to diseases later in life.

The "Developmental Origins of Health and Disease" paradigm which focuses on environmental chemical exposures includes the following features that are not only important for the paradigm in general but also for obesity as the disease endpoint:

- Time-specific (vulnerable window) and tissue-specific effects can occur.
- The initiating in utero environmental insult can act alone or in concert with other environmental stressors. That is, there could be an in utero exposure that would lead by itself to pathophysiology later in life or there could be in utero exposure combined with a neonatal exposure (same or different environmental stressor(s)) or adult exposure that could trigger or exacerbate the pathophysiology. There are now animal data supporting this two-hit model.
- The pathophysiology can manifest as (a) occurrence of a disease that otherwise would not have happened; (b) an increase in risk for a disease that would normally be of lower prevalence; and (c) either an earlier onset of a disease that would have occurred anyway or an exacerbation of such a disease.
- The pathophysiology can have a variable latent period, from neonatal onset, to early childhood, to puberty, to early adulthood, or to late adulthood depending on the environmental stressor, time of exposure, and tissue/organ affected.
- The environmental exposure can lead to aberrant developmental programming that permanently alters gland, organ, or system potential. These states of altered potential or compromised function are likely to result from epigenetic changes, e.g., altered gene expression due to effects on imprinting, and the underlying methylation-related protein–DNA relationships associated with chromatin

remodeling or changes in protein structure and function. The end result is an individual that is sensitized such that it will be more susceptible to certain diseases later in life.

- Exposure of one individual to an environmental stressor (environmental chemical, nutritional, or combinations) may have little effect, whereas another individual will develop overt disease or dysfunctions due to differences in genetic background (including genetic polymorphisms).
- The effect of environmental chemical exposures can be transgenerational, affecting future generations presumably via alterations of epigenetic marks across generations.
- Extrapolation of risk from environmental exposures can be difficult because effects need not follow a monotonic dose–response relationship. Low-dose effects of environmental chemicals may not be the same as the effects that occur at higher doses. Also, environmental toxicant effects may have entirely different effects on the embryo, fetus, or perinatal organism as compared with the adult.
- Effects of in utero exposure to environmental toxicants or nutritional changes can occur in the absence of reduced birth weight or body length. The lack of a specific easily measurable biomarker like birth weight makes it more difficult to assess developmental effects. Thus, new more sensitive biomarkers of exposure are needed.

17.4 The Obesogen Hypothesis of Obesity

The above discussion provides data to support the concept that susceptibility to obesity, like many other diseases, starts during development. It also introduces the importance of the role of environmental chemical exposures in the etiology of many complex diseases.

Conventional wisdom holds that obesity is primarily the result of overeating and failing to exercise sufficiently to burn the excess calories consumed. While it is self-evident that fat cannot be accumulated without a higher caloric intake than expenditure, recent research in a number of laboratories around the world has identified chemicals that themselves promote weight gain and adiposity. An emerging literature now implicates developmental exposure to endocrine-disrupting chemicals (EDCs) in the developmental programming of obesity via altered control of adipose tissue development, control of food intake, metabolism, insulin sensitivity, and lipid metabolism [17, 18].

Scientists have coined the term "obesogens" for chemicals that promote weight gain and obesity. Obesogens can promote obesity by increasing the number of fat cells (and fat storage into existing fat cells), by changing the amount of calories burned at rest, by altering energy balance to favor storage of calories, and by altering the mechanisms through which the body regulates appetite and satiety. In other words, obesogens alter developmental programming resulting in an altered "set point" or sensitivity for developing obesity later in life. The prediction is that developmental exposure to obesogens will result in increased weight gain per unit of food consumed and also possibly less weight loss per amount of exercise, e.g., an altered set point for gaining weight [17–19].

Examples of obesogens include several estrogenic chemicals (e.g., genistein, diethylstilbestrol, bisphenol A), perfluorooctanoic acid (PFOA), smoking/nicotine, tributyltin, phthalates, fructose, monosodium glutamate, and certain organophosphate pesticides. In addition, other environmental chemicals have been associated with development of diabetes in humans, including arsenic, cadmium, dioxin, polychlorinated biphenyls (PCBs), and other types of halogenated organic compounds [20–24]. The animal data supporting the obesogen hypothesis will be presented in Chapters 18 and 19.

The mechanisms proposed for the effects of obesogen exposure during development on obesity later in life are alterations in the epigenetic system, which is developing at the time of the obesogen exposure. Epigenetic programming during fetal and infant life determines how the genes we inherit at conception function throughout the remainder of our lives [25]. Each individual's unique epigenetic program determines how all of the body's hormonal regulatory systems come together to control the metabolic processes involved in body weight control, from appetite to storage of fat in fat cells. Epigenetic regulation of gene expression includes methylation of CpG islands, presumably in the gene promoter region, which results in repression of gene expression, and the covalent modifications of the tails of histone proteins which package the DNA. Changes in histone modifications are complex and can result in either an opening of the histone cores (which favors gene expression) or tightly packed chromatin structure (which inhibits gene expression). These marks are laid down during development when tissues are forming and are heritable during cell division, particularly mitosis, and are involved in controlling tissue differentiation. Although generally stable, environmental chemicals and nutritional alterations can cause changes in epigenetic marks, especially during development [26, 27]. Obesogen alterations in epigenetic programming results in altered gene expression leading to functional changes in the various components of the energy homeostasis system including brain, muscle, GI tract, pancreas, liver, and adipose tissue. An important aspect of the obesogen hypothesis is that it might be possible to measure alterations in epigenetic marks (DNA methylation and/or chromatin remodeling) as biomarkers of obesogen exposure.

The obesogen hypothesis of obesity makes two important points. First, susceptibility to obesity starts during development (in utero and the first few years of life). Second, susceptibility to obesity is due in part to the influence of endocrine-disrupting chemicals that alter developmental programming and thus the set point for gaining weight later in life. The important conclusion from research on obesogens is that the origins of obesity lie not only in traditional risk factors such as diet and exercise but also in the interplay between genes and the fetal and early postnatal environment. Environmental obesogen exposure is a previously unsuspected risk factor that exacerbates the effects of diet and exercise to promote the development of obesity.

As noted by Newbold et al. [19], public health risks can no longer be based on the assumption that overweight and obesity are just personal choices involving the quantity and kind of foods we eat combined with inactivity, but rather complex events including exposure to obesogens during development that may be contributing to the obesity epidemic.

Importantly, the obesogen hypothesis of obesity changes the focus from genetics to environment as a major cause of obesity. It shifts the argument away from treatment (which has not been successful) to prevention and from adulthood to development (in utero and early childhood) as the time for susceptibility for obesity, and thus as the time to focus preventive efforts. This emerging hypothesis offers hope that the obesity epidemic can be controlled, since it is possible to prevent or reduce environmental exposures.

17.5 Human Data Supporting the Obesogen Hypothesis of Obesity

Thus far, there have been few studies investigating the association between developmental exposure to environmental toxicants and weight gain later in life. The reasons are several fold. First, the field of developmental origins of obesity is quite new. Second, it is difficult to get accurate exposure assessments during development. Third, it is difficult to follow children for long periods of time to assess the development of obesity. The few published studies focus on developmental exposures and increased weight gain in the first few years of life. While important to prove the concept, it will be critical to assess the long-term effects of developmental exposures to obesogens along with improved measures of actual exposures throughout in utero development and the first few years of life.

17.5.1 Smoking

Smoking during pregnancy is proof of principle for the obesogen hypothesis in humans. Maternal smoking during pregnancy has been reported to reduce both birth weight and crown to heel length. However, children of smoking mothers often show catch-up growth before 1 year of age and then continue to gain weight over the next years. In addition, smoking during pregnancy seems to influence obesity later in life independently of its effects on LBW, indicating complex effects of smoking on both fetal development and susceptibility to weight gain [28]. Oken et al. [29] ran a meta-analysis of smoking during pregnancy and overweight in over 84,000 children from 16 separate epidemiology studies. The pooled odds ratio (OR) was 1.5 (95% CI: 1.36–1.65), indicating a role for smoking during pregnancy in the etiology of childhood obesity. It is not clear which trimester is most sensitive to the effects of smoking on obesity later in life; however, it has been reported that smoking during early pregnancy had the biggest effect on overweight children, with an OR of 1.52 and for obese children with an OR of 2.22 at school entry age in Bavaria [30]. Verulst showed that children of smoking mothers had higher BMI by 1 year of age

[31], and in separate studies, increased BMI was also apparent at 6. 5 years [32], at 8 years [33], and even at 33 years of age [34]. Syme et al. [35] recently showed that adolescents in late puberty exposed prenatally to smoking demonstrated higher quantities of both subcutaneous fat (26%) and intra-abdominal fat (33%). Overall, while the weight gain in children from maternal smoking is small, the effect is consistent and persistent and thus indicates in utero priming of obesity risk by maternal smoking. Maternal smoking thus contributes to the overall increase in weight gain both across the United States, especially in the non-Hispanic, White, and Black communities [36], and around the world [29].

The biological mechanisms mediating the effects of maternal smoking and increased weight gain in children are thought to be due to altered prenatal programming of insulin, leptin, and glucocorticoid resistance [37]. While it is clear that human studies cannot develop causal relationships, the relationship between maternal smoking and childhood obesity fits the major epidemiologic criteria of temporal relationship, biological plausibility, consistency, as well as dose–response relationship, strength of association, and coherence [37]. Furthermore, the human studies have been replicated in animal studies, where causal relationships have been shown. Thus, the association between maternal smoking and childhood obesity is about as strong as can be determined from epidemiologic data.

17.5.2 Persistent Organic Pollutants

Verhulst et al. [31] showed in a longitudinal study that prenatal exposure to DDE and PCBs, measured in cord blood, was associated with increased BMI during early childhood. Mothers' smoking synergized with the effect of these exposures alone on weight gain. This study confirmed an earlier study by Hertz-Picciotto et al. [38] that showed that prenatal PCBs were associated with increased growth in 5-year-old boys. The organochlorine hexachlorobenzene, a currently banned persistent pesticide, has also been linked to weight gain. Children with the highest hexachlorobenzene levels in their cord blood were heavier and had a higher BMI (OR 2.02) at age 6 years than did children with lower levels [32]. This association was independent of socioeconomic status, maternal education, parity, maternal obesity, and birth weight. All of these studies have measured chemicals that persist for long periods in the body; thus, a single measurement of their levels can be used to determine exposure.

These data show that developmental exposures to environmental toxicants can indeed alter the weight gain of infants and children, presumably via passage through the placenta and altering gene expression in various tissues that control food intake, metabolism, and fat cell number. From these few studies, it is not yet clear what the site of action of these environmental chemicals may be. It is also not clear if the effects will indeed last a lifetime, as is the case in animal studies.

The human literature on obesogens is limited at this time. This is due to the fact that these studies are expensive and that most chemicals are not persistent and thus one measurement will not be sufficient to define exposure in utero and/or during the first few years of life. To move forward, improved exposure assessment will be needed in order to link exposure levels during pregnancy and the first years of life to obesity, not only in childhood but throughout adult life.

17.6 Adult Exposures to Environmental Agents and Obesity

While the focus of this review is on the developmental origins of obesity, it is also clear that adult exposures can also contribute to obesity. In addition, if adult exposures to specific obesogens can lead to weight gain, it is likely that developmental exposures to the same compounds will have an even more profound effect. Thus, it becomes important to assess the effects of developmental exposure to these obesogens on childhood and adult weight gain.

17.6.1 Fructose

Fructose, by virtue of its metabolic effects, can be designated as an endocrine disruptor. It has been shown to be taken up by liver, which is solely responsible for its metabolism, by an active transport system and is phosphorylated by fructokinase. Isocaloric administration of fructose to adults causes accumulation of intra-abdominal fat along with insulin resistance [39, 40]. There are also data supporting fructose as a cause of the increasing trend of nonalcoholic fatty liver disease (NAFLD) in humans [41]. Lastly, fructose also causes hyperlipidemia which reduces leptin transport across the blood–brain barrier, contributing to leptin resistance and thus interfering with appetite control [42]. There are currently no studies examining the effects of fructose during development on obesity in children. However, there is ubiquitous exposure during pregnancy. If the effects shown in adults are confirmed during development, it would indicate fructose as a significant contributor to the developmental basis of obesity in humans. The examination of the possible role of fructose during development on the programming of "obesity" is critically needed.

17.6.2 Monosodium Glutamate (MSG)

Monosodium glutamate is a food additive used as a flavoring agent to enhance taste. It is considered "generally regarded as safe" (GRAS) for humans by the Food and Drug Administration. Consumption has increased worldwide over the past few decades. Neonatal administration of MSG in animal models results in obesity due to hypothalamic excitotoxic neuronal death, with resultant alterations of the neuroendocrine system controlling feeding behavior [43]. In humans, there is also a comprehensive cross-sectional study showing that people who consumed an average of 0.33 g/day had an increased prevalence of overweight [44]. Since exposure is ubiquitous, there is a great need to examine the effect of exposures during pregnancy on weight gain in human offspring.

17.6.3 Phthalates

Phthalates are a ubiquitous class of compounds commonly used as softeners in plastics like polyvinyl chloride (plasticizers). Several phthalate esters have animal toxicity, including reproductive toxicity and obesity [45]. There is one cross-sectional study linking urinary phthalate metabolites and BMI and waist circumference in adults [46]. It showed that there was a positive correlation between BMI and waist circumference for urinary levels of six phthalate metabolites, with a bigger effect in males aged 20–59 than in older males or females. There are no human studies or animal studies that have examined developmental exposures to low-dose phthalates and weight gain later in life. However, in animals, phthalates have been shown to activate PPAR-gamma, which helps differentiate preadipocytes to adipocytes and plays an important role in fat cell development [45]. Thus, it seems logical to design both human and animal studies to examine developmental exposures to a variety of phthalates and to assess exposure to weight gain in early childhood and into adulthood.

17.7 Recommendations

1. Validate the obesogen hypothesis in humans using environmental exposures during development that have been shown to cause weight gain in rodent models, including bisphenol A, diethylstilbestrol, genestein (soy phytoestrogens), organochlorine pesticides, tributyltin, and perfluorooctanoic acid.
2. Examine the effects of fructose, high-fructose corn syrup, and monosodium glutamate in epidemiologic studies focusing on developmental exposures and childhood and lifetime increased weight gain and obesity.
3. Examine the interaction of altered nutrition with environmental chemical exposures during development in the etiology of obesity later in life.
4. Examine the effect of mixtures of chemical exposures during development on obesity later in life in humans using bioinformatic analyses to define which environmental chemicals in the mixture are responsible for the weight gain.
5. Integrate scientists studying the role of developmental nutrition and weight gain later in life with scientists examining the role of developmental environmental exposures and weight gain later in life.
6. Understand the mechanisms whereby developmental exposures to altered nutrition or environmental toxicants can cause weight gain years and decades later long after exposures are dissipated. Initially, focus on epigenetics and epigenetic marks.

References

1. NHANES Data on the Prevalence of Overweight Among Children and Adolescents: United States. 2003–2006. CDC National Center for Health Statistics, Health E-Stat.
2. Kim J, Peterson KE, Scanlon KS, Fitzmaurice GM, Must A, Oken E, Rifas-Shiman SL, Rich-Edwards JW, Gillman MW. Trends in overweight from 1980 through 2001 among preschool-aged children enrolled in a health maintenance organization. Obesity. 2006;14:1107–2.
3. Loos RJF. Recent progress in the genetics of common obesity. Br J Clin Pharm. 2009;68: 811–29.
4. Hill AJ. Does dieting make you fat? Br J Nutr. 2004;92:S15–8.
5. Wadhwa PD, Buss C, Entringer S, Swanson JM. Developmental origins of health and disease: brief history of the approach and current focus on epigenetic mechanisms. Semin Reprod Med. 2009;27:358–68.
6. Barker DJ. The origins of the developmental origins theory. J Intern Med. 2007;261:412–7.
7. Gluckman PD, Hanson MA, Pinal C. The developmental origins of adult disease. Matern Child Nutr. 2005;1(3):130–41.
8. Gluckman PD, Hanson MA, Beedle AS, Raubenheimer D. Fetal and neonatal pathways to obesity. Front Horm Res. 2008;36:61–72.
9. Fall C. Maternal nutrition: effects on health in the next generation. Indian J Med Res. 2009;130:593–9.
10. Wright CS, Rifas-Shiman SL, Rich-Edwards JW, Taveras EM, Gillman MW, Oken E. Intrauterine exposure to gestational diabetes, childhood adiposity, and blood pressure. Am J Hypertens. 2009;22:215–20.
11. Oken E, Gillman MW. Fetal origins of obesity. Obes Res. 2003;11:496–506.
12. Stettler N, Stallings VA, Troxel AB, Zhao J, Schinnar R, Nelson SE, Ziegler EE, Strom SJ. Weight gain in the first week of life and overweight in adulthood: a cohort study of European American subjects fed infant formula. Circulation. 2005;111:1897–903.
13. Stettler N. Nature and strength of epidemiological evidence for origins of childhood and adulthood obesity in the first year of life. Int J Obes. 2007;31:1035–43.
14. Newbold RR, Heindel JJ. Developmental exposures and implications for early and latent disease. In: Woodruff TJ, Janssen SJ, Guillette LJ and Giudice LC editors. Environmental impacts on reproductive health and fertility. Cambridge University Press; New York, NY 2010. pp. 92–102.
15. Newbold RR, Heindel JJ. Developmental origins of health and disease: the importance of environmental exposures. In: Newnham JP and Ross MD editors. Early life origins of human health and disease. Karger Press, Basel, Switzerland 2009. pp. 41–50.
16. Grandjean P. PPTOX prenatal programming and toxicity. Basic Clin Pharmacol Toxicol. 2008;102(2):1–273.
17. Grun F, Blumberg B. Minireview: the case for obesogens. Mol Endocrinol. 2009;23:1127–34.
18. Heindel JJ, vom Saal FS. Role of nutrition and environmental endocrine disrupting chemicals during the perinatal period on the aetiology of obesity. Mol Cell Endocrinol. 2009;304:90–6.
19. Newbold R, Padilla-Banks E, Jefferson W. Molecular and cellular endocrinology. Mol Cell Endocrinol. 2009;304:84–9.
20. Edwards JR, Prozialeck WC. Cadmium, diabetes and chronic kidney disease. Toxicol Appl Pharmacol. 2009;238:289–93.
21. Longnecker MP, Daniels JL. Environmental contaminants as etiologic factors for diabetes. Environ Health Perspect. 2001;109 Suppl 6:871–6.
22. Tseng CH. The potential biological mechanisms of arsenic-induced diabetes mellitus. Toxicol Appl Pharmacol. 2004;197:67–83.
23. Schwartz GG, Il'yasova D, Ivanova A. Urinary cadmium, impaired fasting glucose, and diabetes in the NHANES III. Diabetes Care. 2003;26:468–70.
24. Uemura H, Arisawa K, Hiyoshi M, Kitayama A, Takami H, Sawachika F, Dakeshita S, Nii K, Satoh H, Sumiyoshi Y, Morinaga K, Kodama K, Suzuki T, Nagai M, Suzuki T. Prevalence

of metabolic syndrome associated with body burden levels of dioxin and related compounds among Japan's general population. Environ Health Perspect. 2009;117:568–73.
25. Pozharny Y, Lambertini L, Clunie G, Ferrara L, Lee M-J. Epigenetics in women's health care. Mt Sinai J Med. 2010;77:225–35.
26. Bollati V, Baccarelli A. Environmental epigenetics. Heredity. 2010;105(1):105–12. Feb 24 2010; [Epub ahead of print].
27. Heijmans BT, Tobi EW, Lumey LH, Slagboom PE. The epigenome, archive of the prenatal environment. Epigenetics. 2009;4:1–6.
28. van der Meulen Jan. Commentary: maternal smoking during pregnancy and obesity in the offspring. Int J Epidemiol. 2002;31:420–1.
29. Oken E, Levitan E, Gillman M. Maternal smoking during pregnancy and child overweight: systematic review and meta-analysis. Int J Obes. 2008;32:201–10.
30. Toschke AM, Montgomery SM, Pfeiffer U, von Kries R. Early intrauterine exposure to tobacco-inhaled products and obesity. Am J Epidemiol. 2003;158:1068–74.
31. Verhulst SL, Nelen V, Hond ED, Kiippen G, Beunckens C, Vael C, Schoeters G, Desager K. Intrauterine exposure to environmental pollutants and body mass index during the first 3 years of life. Environ Health Perspect. 2009;117:122–6.
32. Smink A, Ribas-Fito N, Garcia R, Torrent M, Mendez MA, Grimalt JO, Sunyer J. Exposure to hexachlorobenzene during pregnancy increases the risk of overweight in children aged 6 years. Acta Paediatr. 2008;97:1465–9.
33. Chen A, Pennell M, Klebanoff M, et al. Maternal smoking during pregnancy in relation to child overweight: follow-up to age 8 years. Int J Epidemiol. 2006;35:121–30.
34. Power C, Jefferis B. Fetal environment and subsequent obesity: a study of material smoking. Int J Epidemiol. 2002;31:413–9.
35. Syme C, Abrahamowicz M, Mahboubi A, et al. Prenatal exposure to maternal cigarette smoking and accumulation of intra-abdominal fat during adolescence. Obesity. 2009;18(5): 1021–5.
36. Sharma AJ, Cogswell ME, Li R. Dose-response associations between maternal smoking during pregnancy and subsequent childhood obesity: effect modification by maternal race/ethnicity in a low-income US cohort. Am J Epidemiol. 2008;168(9):995–1007.
37. Huang JS, Lee TA, Lu MC. Prenatal programming of childhood overweight and obesity. Matern Child Health. 2007;11:461–73.
38. Hertz-Picciotto I, Charles MJ, James RA, Keller JA, Willman E, Teplin S. In utero polychlorinated biphenyl exposures in relation to fetal and early childhood growth. Epidemiology. 2005;16:648–56.
39. Perez-Pozo SE, Schold J, Nakagawa T, Sanchez-Lozada LG, Johnson RJ, Lillo JL. Excessive fructose intake induces the features of metabolic syndrome in health adult men: role of uric acid in the hypertensive response. Int J Obes. 2010;34:454–61.
40. Bantle JP. Dietary fructose and metabolic syndrome and diabetes. J Nutr. 2009;139:1263S–8S.
41. Lim JS, Mietus-Snyder M, Valente A, Schwarz JM, Lustig RH. The role of fructose in the pathogenesis of NAFLD and the metabolic syndrome. Nat Rev Gastroenterol Hepatol. 2010;7(5):251–64 [April 6 ahead of print].
42. Banks WA, Coon AB, Robinson SM, Moinuddin A, Shultz JM, Nakaoke R, et al. Triglycerides induce leptin resistance at the blood-brain barrier. Diabetes. 2004;53:1253–60.
43. Dawson R. Developmental and sex-specific effects of low dose neonatal monosodium glutamate administration on mediobasal hypothalamic chemistry. Neuroendocrinology. 1986;42:158–66.
44. He K, Daviglus ML, Dyer AR, Van Horn L, Garside D, Zhu L, Guo D, Wu Y, Shou B, Stamler J. INTERMAP Cooperative Research Group Association of monosodium glutamate intake with overweight in Chinese adults: the INTERMAP study. Obesity. 2008;16:1875–80.
45. Desvergne B, Feige JN, Casals-Sasas C. PPAR-mediated activity of phthalates: a link to the obesity epidemic?. Mol Cell Endo. 2009;304:43–8.
46. Hatch E, Nelson J, Stahlhut R, et al. Association of endocrine disruptors and obesity: perspectives from epidemiological studies. Int J Andrology. Jan 22 2010;33(2):324–32.

Chapter 18
Perinatal Exposure to Endocrine Disrupting Chemicals with Estrogenic Activity and the Development of Obesity

Retha R. Newbold

18.1 Introduction

Obesity, defined as a body mass index (BMI) greater than 30, has been identified as a significant public health threat [1, 2]. Over the past 2–3 decades, the prevalence of obesity has risen dramatically in wealthy industrialized countries and also in poorer underdeveloped nations where it often coexists with undernutrition [3, 4]. In 2008, the Centers for Disease Control (CDC) reported that obesity had reached epidemic and alarming proportions, with more than 60% of US adults being either obese or overweight [5]. Similar statistics have been reported for many European countries, the Middle East, Australia, and China. The reasons for this sharp increase in overweight/obesity are not well understood but multiple factors including infection, high-fructose diets, genetics/epigenetics, increased maternal age, sleep debt, use of certain pharmaceuticals, and the built environment have all been proposed to play a role [6].

Obesity is a problem for all ages, but it is of particular concern for children since most obese and overweight children grow up to be obese adults, predisposing them to a lifetime of adverse health consequences. Unfortunately, the number of children and adolescents who are overweight, or at risk for being overweight, has risen even faster than that reported in adults [7]. Although a recent report suggests that the increase in obesity prevalence appears to have finally leveled off in the past few years, there is still no indication of any decreases in prevalence [8]. Since obesity is such a challenge to treat effectively once it is established, prevention is of upmost importance.

Obesity is a complex disease, affecting virtually all ages, races, sexes, and socioeconomic groups and with serious social and psychological repercussions.

R.R. Newbold (✉)
National Institute of Environmental Health Sciences (NIEHS), National Institutes of Health (NIH), Research Triangle Park, NC 27709, USA
e-mail: newbold1@niehs.nih.gov; newboldretha@hotmail.com

The author is now retired but the research was conducted while employed by NIEHS.

R.H. Lustig (ed.), *Obesity Before Birth*, Endocrine Updates 30,
DOI 10.1007/978-1-4419-7034-3_18, © Springer Science+Business Media, LLC 2011

Further, obesity and overweight are major contributors to the global burden of chronic diseases including type 2 diabetes mellitus (T2DM), hyperinsulinemia and insulin resistance, coronary heart disease, high blood pressure, stroke, gout, fatty liver disease, asthma and pulmonary problems, gallbladder disease, kidney disease, reproductive problems, osteoarthritis, and some forms of cancer [9–11]. Many of these illnesses are being reported in obese children. Consequently, health professionals warn that our current generation of children may be the first in history to experience a shorter life expectancy than their parents due to the impact of obesity-related diseases.

The etiology of obesity is unknown, but is most likely caused by a complicated interaction between genetic, behavioral, and environmental factors. The most common assumptions are thought to be overeating high-caloric fatty diets combined with a sedentary lifestyle which is imposed on a background of genetic predisposition for the disease. Although much interest has centered on these factors with a specific focus on incorporating healthy foods in our diets and more exercise in our lifestyle, prevention of obesity remains elusive.

Recent evidence points to the contribution of endocrine-disrupting chemicals (EDCs) to the high prevalence of obesity. EDCs are chemicals, synthetic or naturally occurring, that mimic or interfere with the production or activity of hormones of the endocrine system leading to adverse health effects. There is particular concern about EDCs that have estrogenic activity, are lipophilic, and are resistant to metabolism. These compounds are known to bioaccumulate because they can be stored in body fat and then readily transferred via the placenta to the fetus or via lactation to the neonate.

Exposure to environmental estrogens, especially in utero and during early neonatal development, can interfere with the normal function of the endocrine system by affecting the balance of hormones that regulate vital body functions, including growth, stress response, sex development, gender behavior, ability to reproduce, production and utilization of insulin, and metabolic rate. Recent advances in research confirm that EDCs can disrupt the gene-controlled, normal signaling systems that determine every aspect of embryonic and fetal development. Although EDCs may have numerous hormonal activities, including estrogenic, antiestrogenic, androgenic, antiandrogenic, progestestational, antithyroid, only chemicals with estrogenic activity will be discussed in this review.

18.2 The Developmental Origins of Adult Disease

Exposure to EDCs is of utmost concern for the developing fetus or infant [12–15]. The developing fetus and neonate are particularly sensitive to perturbation by EDCs because the placenta does not completely protect the unborn fetus from its external environment, and the organism undergoes periods of extremely rapid cell division and differentiation in utero, resulting in cells that could differentiate abnormally and pass altered programming on to subsequent generations. In many cases, this prenatal programming is irreversible, while adult exposure is usually reversible and disappears after exposure ceases. Further, the developing organism lacks the protective mechanisms that are available to the adult, such as DNA repair mechanisms, a fully competent immune system, detoxifying enzymes, liver metabolism, and a mature blood/brain barrier [12]. Also, the developing fetus and neonate have increased metabolic rates as compared to adults, which in some cases make them more sensitive to chemical toxicity. It is now well established in the fields of nutrition and endocrine disruption that developmental exposure to environmental chemicals can interfere with complex differentiating endocrine signaling pathways and cause adverse consequences later in life [16, 17]. The well-known reproductive tract toxicity of diethylstilbestrol (DES) is one of the best examples of adverse consequences of EDCs (for review, see [12, 18]). The concept of the "developmental origins of adult disease" [19], as the term implies, suggests there is a lag time between time of exposure and manifestation of disease. In other words, the effects of developmental exposure may not be readily apparent until much later in life.

Another key concept in endocrine disruption is that there may be nontraditional dose–response curves, such as an inverted "U" or even multiple "U"-shaped curves [20], making it impossible to predict responses in the low-dose environmental exposure range based on knowledge of exposures in the high-dose range. Further, because of the increased sensitivity of differentiating tissues, chemicals can exert effects at levels previously thought to be too low to be toxic. Although these concepts have been well accepted for hormones and neurotransmitters, they are just emerging as issues for EDCs.

Transgenerational effects may also be seen following developmental exposure to EDCs where not only the exposed individual, but also subsequent generations are affected. This idea implies that the mechanisms of transmission occur through the germ line through genetic and/or epigenetic events. In the case of epigenetic changes, effects are not due to genetic damage, but a modification of factors that regulate gene expression such as DNA methylation and/or histone acetylation. Thus far, studies have mainly focused on epigenetic changes in reproductive tract tissues [21–26]; however, similar effects can conceivably occur in other differentiating endocrine-responsive tissues. This area of epigenetic research and programming by EDCs is an exciting new field of study that may revolutionize how we view the "developmental basis of adult disease" suggesting that our susceptibility for disease may be programmed prior to or during fetal life.

Recently, EDCs have been shown to influence adipocyte development [15, 27–32]. These environmental chemicals have been termed "obesogens," referring to the idea that they inappropriately regulate lipid metabolism and adipogenesis to promote obesity [33]. Obesogens are discussed in more detail in Chapters 17 and 19. In vitro studies have described the disruptive effects of EDCs on normal adipocyte development and on homeostatic control over adipogenesis and early energy balance [33, 34]. Further, numerous experimental animal studies also describe an association of obesity and developmental exposure to numerous EDCs. Although uncertainties remain about the full extent of health consequences that follow exposure to EDCs (especially low-dose exposures experienced by the general population), we are just beginning to understand the complexities and interactions of endocrine signaling in adipocytes and their role in energy homeostasis.

18.3 Experimental Evidence for Involvement of Environmental Estrogens in Obesity

Although a relationship between EDCs and obesity had been proposed previously, Baillie-Hamilton published a landmark paper in 2002 postulating a role for chemical toxins in the etiology of obesity by showing that the obesity epidemic coincided with the marked increase of industrial chemicals in the environment over the past 40 years [27]. She further speculated that the current obesity epidemic could not be explained solely by increases in food intake and/or decreases in physical activity. She cited numerous studies where chemicals including pesticides, organophosphates, polychlorinated biphenyls, polybrominated biphenyls, phthalates, bisphenol A, heavy metals, and some solvents caused weight gain and proposed that these chemicals were interfering with energy homeostasis by altering weight-controlling hormones, altering sensitivity to neurotransmitters, or altering activity of the sympathetic nervous system [27]. It is interesting that in a few of the cited studies, the chemicals were actually designed to have growth-promoting properties such as with DES, which was widely used by the livestock industry specifically for this role [35].

In the past several years, an increasing number of studies have been designed to address the effects of EDC exposure on weight gain and loss. Numerous studies have shown that exposure to numerous environmental estrogens during critical periods of differentiation, at low dosage, can alter developmental programming, resulting in obesity in the offspring.

Performing studies on the role of environmental estrogens on development requires the maintenance of estrogen-free baseline condition. The type of diet used in experimental animal studies is known to play an important role in the attainment of puberty, body weight gain, and timing of developmental endpoints [36]. We used NIH 31 lab chow because it was relatively low in phytoestrogen content and had no measureable estrogenic activity. Another animal husbandry issue that had to be considered was the type of bedding. We used hardwood chip bedding with no estrogenic activity rather than corncob bedding which is often contaminated with mycotoxins which exert estrogenic potency.

18.4 Diethylstilbestrol (DES)

DES, a potent synthetic nonsteroidal estrogen, was first synthesized in 1938. Soon after, it became widely used by clinicians to treat numerous medical conditions and by researchers to study effects of estrogens in experimental paradigms. In addition, it was used as a feed supplement to fatten sheep and cattle, and to improve their feed efficiency. Thus, the effects of DES on energy balance and metabolism were known early on in animals, but the mechanisms were not well understood.

DES became widely prescribed to pregnant women from the 1940s through the 1970s as it was assumed that its estrogenic potency would prevent threatened miscarriages. It is estimated that a range of 2–8 million pregnancies worldwide were exposed to DES. Today, it is well documented that prenatal DES treatment resulted in a low but nonetheless significant increase in neoplastic lesions in the reproductive tract and a high incidence of benign reproductive lesions in both the male and female offspring exposed during prenatal life. Exposure to DES was a clear example that prenatal exposure could lead to adult disease; in this case reproductive disease. To study the mechanisms involved in DES toxicity, we developed experimental mouse models of perinatal (prenatal or neonatal) DES exposure [37], where outbred mice were treated with DES on prenatal days 9–16 of gestation (the period of major organogenesis in the mouse) [38] or neonatal days 1–5 [39, 40] (a period of cellular differentiation of the reproductive tract and a critical period of immune, behavioral, and adipocyte differentiation). These prenatal and neonatal DES animal models have successfully duplicated, and in some cases predicted, many of the reproductive alterations (structural, function, cellular, and molecular) observed in similarly DES-exposed humans [40]. Further, these models have also shown multigenerational transmission of disease patterns. It is assumed that epigenetic mechanisms are responsible for the transmission of these effects [41].

Although our initial focus was on reproductive tract abnormalities and subfertility/infertility, we subsequently examined the relationship of perinatal DES treatment with the development of obesity later in life. We wanted to determine if DES was an "obesogen" as well as a reproductive toxicant, and if so, what were its molecular targets and the mechanisms through which it might act. For our first obesity experiments, mice were treated with DES on prenatal days 9–16. High prenatal DES doses (10–100 μg/kg maternal weight) resulted in offspring with lower birth weight compared to controls; however, these offspring experienced a "catch-up period" during neonatal and juvenile life so that by weaning they were similar to controls. By adulthood, the prenatal DES mice were much larger than controls. Low prenatal DES exposure had no effect on weight at birth but still caused obesity later in life [30]. (Doses greater than 100 μg/kg maternal body weight decreased pup numbers and increased malformations such that weight was dependent on the health of the animal [38].)

Subsequent mechanistic studies followed and involved treating female mice neonatally, instead of prenatally, with DES on days 1–5; this time period corresponds to an active period of cell differentiation in many tissues, including immune, behavioral, and adipocyte differentiation, and neural networks important in endocrine signaling. A low dose of DES at 1 μg/kg/day did not affect female pup body weight during treatment, but did induce a significant increase in body weight in adults by 4–6 months of age (male mice treated as neonates did not demonstrate an increase in body weight under the conditions of study) [29]. Similar to high prenatal DES doses, high neonatal DES (1 mg/kg/day) caused a significant decrease in body weight during treatment, but it was followed by "catch-up" growth around puberty

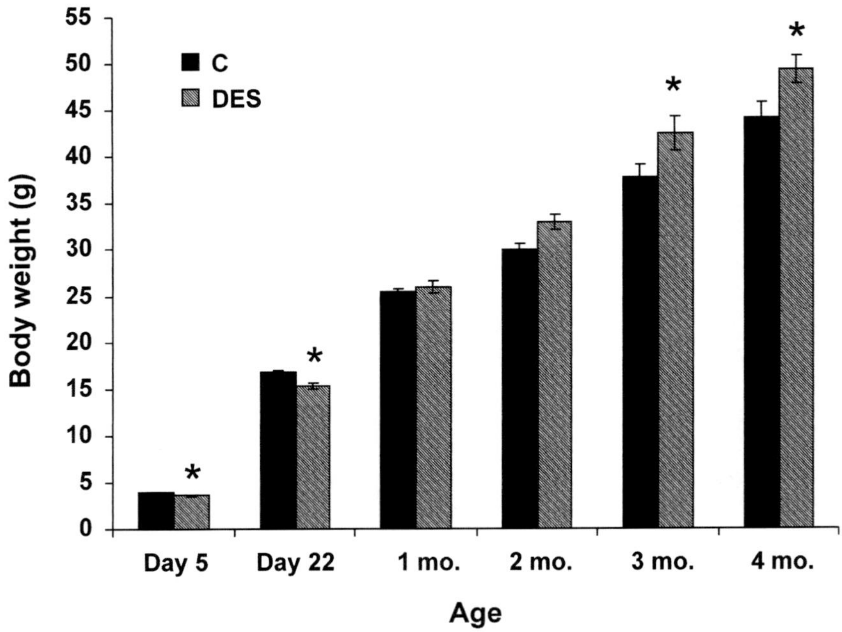

Fig. 18.1 Body weight of control and DES-treated mice. Body weight (in grams) plotted on the *y* axis was measured at various ages indicated on the *x* axis. Mice treated neonatally with DES (1,000 μg/kg/day = 1 mg/kg/day) high dose caused significantly lower body weights during treatment which ended on day 5; lower weight continued until day 22 of life as compared to controls (C). By ~1 month, DES mice caught up to controls and by 2 months they surpassed controls and ultimately gained a significantly higher body weight compared to controls at 3–4 months. Numbers are the mean ± S.E.M.; asterisk (*) denotes significance using ANOVA followed by Dunnett's test ($p < 0.05$). Data were published in [42]

(~1 month) and then finally resulted in a significant increase in body weight of the DES-treated mice compared to controls after ~2 months of age (Fig. 18.1) [42]. This "catch-up" in weight in DES-treated animals is reminiscent of the "thrifty phenotype," a well-known phenomenon in the field of nutrition, which was described in human infants who received poor nutrition during fetal life but later had "catch-up" growth that resulted in overweight and obesity later in life [43]. Further studies indicated that the increase in body weight in neonatal DES-exposed mice was associated with an increase in percent body fat as determined by mouse densitometry [31, 32]. Figure 18.2a is a representative photograph of control and DES-treated mice, which illustrates the size differences between the two groups. Figure 18.2b shows images of control and DES mice that were generated by Piximus densitometry, again showing the size differences between the groups [42]. Note the enhanced abdominal circumferences in the DES mouse, which is reported in humans to be a risk factor in cardiovascular disease associated with obesity and metabolic syndrome.

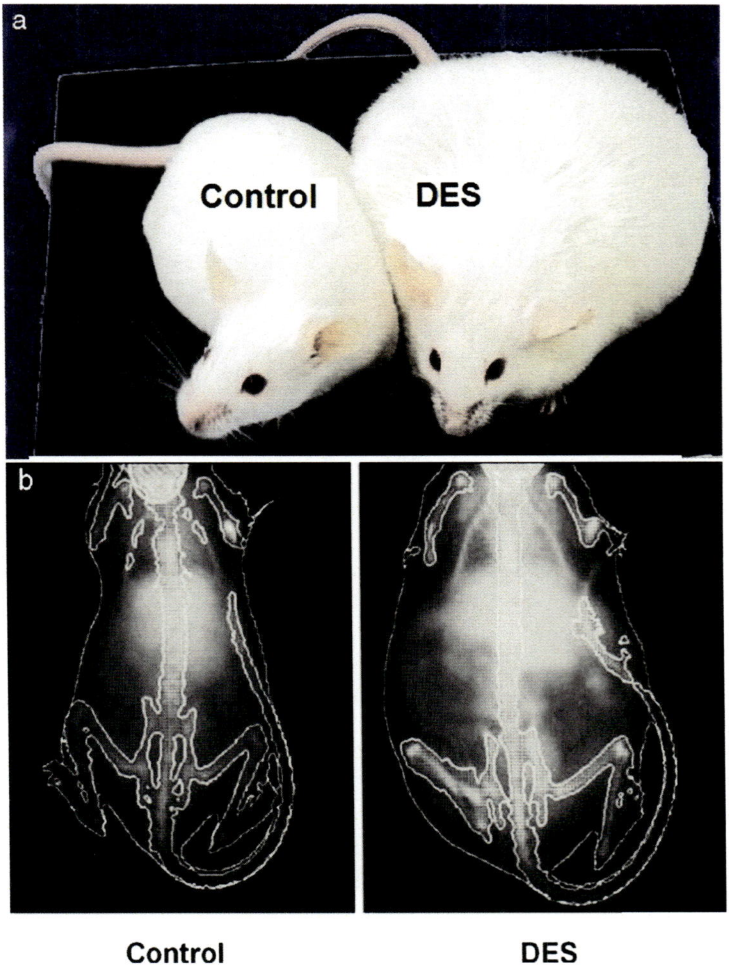

Fig. 18.2 Representative photograph of control and DES-treated mice. (**a**) Photo shows the difference in body size between the two groups. (**b**) Images of control and DES-treated mice as generated by Piximus densitometry. Note the enlarged abdominal circumference in the DES mice [42]

To determine if DES was a unique estrogen in causing its effects on weight gain, we treated neonatal mice on days 1–5 with other estrogenic compounds such as 2-hydroxyestradiol (20 mg/kg/day) or 4-hydroxyestradiol (0.1 mg/kg/day), doses that are approximately equal in estrogenic activity to low-dose DES. These compounds also caused a significant increase in body weight at 4 months of age, indicating DES is not the only estrogen capable of causing overweight and obesity [30].

Increased body weight in both low and high DES-treated mice compared to controls was observed throughout adulthood; however, by 18 months of age, statistical differences in body weight between DES-treated mice and controls were difficult to show because individual animal variability within groups increased as they aged, due to the altered health status of the DES animals. We concluded that since various doses of DES resulted in obesity whether or not pups were underweight during treatment, most likely multiple pathways were involved in programming for obesity by environmental estrogens.

Since densitometry images of DES-treated mice suggested excessive abdominal fat [44], specific fat pads were weighed to determine fat pad changes throughout the mouse. Weights of inguinal, parametrial, gonadal, and retroperitoneal fat pads were all increased in DES-treated mice as compared to controls at 6–8 months of age, suggesting a potential impact on cardiovascular disease following developmental exposure to DES. Brown fat pad weights were not significantly altered in these animals [30].

Examination of DES-treated mice (1 mg/kg/day) and controls at 2 months of age, prior to onset of obesity, showed elevated serum levels of leptin, adiponectin, IL-6, and triglycerides, suggesting these endpoints may be important early markers of subsequent adult disease. Elevated levels of leptin are not surprising, considering the increased number and size of the adipocytes in the DES-treated mice, but the increase in adiponectin was not expected since low levels usually correlate with diabetes. This may indicate insensitivity to these hormones and/or a loss of the negative feedback mechanisms that regulate adipogenesis, but additional study is needed to determine the mechanisms involved. At 6 months of age, insulin and all of the serum markers except triglycerides were found to be significantly elevated as compared to controls [32].

Glucose levels were also measured in DES (1 mg/kg/day) and control mice at 2 months of age prior to the development of obesity [32]. Interestingly, 25% of the DES-treated mice had significantly higher glucose levels and slower glucose clearance rate [32]. Additional glucose measurements in older mice may help determine if a higher percentage of mice are affected with age, and if higher and sustained levels of glucose can be demonstrated. To date, our data suggest that obesity observed in perinatal DES-treated mice will be associated with the development of diabetes, similar to the association of obesity with diabetes in humans. Further, other studies from our laboratory support a role for altered glucose metabolism since we have shown a high prevalence of islet cell hyperplasia in the pancreas of mice exposed to DES or other environmental estrogens, including BPA and genistein (unpublished).

Since the balance between activity levels and food intake contributes to obesity, ambulatory activity was measured in DES-treated (1 mg/kg/day) and control mice at 2 months of age before a difference in body weight could be detected. Overall, no statistical difference could be shown in activity between groups, although the DES group showed slightly less movement as compared to controls; however, this was not sufficient to explain the enhanced weight gain in DES-treated mice as they aged [32]. Feed consumption was also measured; DES-treated mice consumed approximately 3 g/day more than controls over the course of the experiment but the amounts were not statistically different between the groups [32]. Taken into account both the marginal decrease in activity and the small increase in food intake in DES-treated mice as compared to controls, it is unlikely these two measurements can solely explain the development of obesity in DES-treated mice.

Since a recent study described a role for developmental genes in the origins of obesity and body fat distribution in mice and humans [45], we determined whether exposure to EDCs with estrogenic activity altered gene expression involved in programming adipocytes during development. Several genes were implicated in altering adipocyte differentiation and function (*Hoxa5*, *Gpc4*, and *Tbx15*) and fat cell distribution (*Thbd*, *Nr2f1*, and *Sfrp2*). We investigated changes in gene expression by microarray analysis in uterine samples from DES-treated mice (1 mg/kg/day) compared to controls at postnatal day 19. Genes involved in adipocyte differentiation were not different in the uterus following neonatal DES exposure; however, genes involved in fat distribution were altered. *Thbd* and *Nr2f1* were significantly downregulated, while *Sfrp2* was significantly upregulated in DES-treated uteri compared to controls [46]. These findings support the idea that environmental estrogens may play a role in regulating the expression of obesity-related genes in development. The identification of genes and molecular mechanisms responsive to EDCs in promoting obesity is an exciting area of new research.

Other investigators have also reported similar associations between perinatal DES exposure and development of obesity later in life [47]. Nikaido et al. treated pregnant mice with DES on days 15–19 with 0.5 or 10 μg/kg. By 16 weeks of age, all the female DES offspring treated with 10 μg/kg were heavier than corresponding controls.

18.5 Bisphenol A

Bisphenol A (BPA), a component of polycarbonate plastics and epoxy resins, is currently receiving much attention from the public, governmental regulatory agencies, and industry advocates due to its high production volume (>800 million kilograms annually in the USA alone) and widespread human exposure [48]. BPA is used in the manufacture of numerous products and has been shown to leach from the linings of food cans [49], polycarbonate baby bottles and other beverage containers [50], and dental sealants and composites [51], suggesting that humans are routinely exposed to this chemical through numerous sources and routes of exposure. Further indication of human exposure is shown by studies reporting measurable BPA levels in human urine [52]; serum [53]; breast milk [54]; and maternal and fetal plasma, amniotic fluid, and placental tissues [55, 56]. BPA is also halogenated (brominated or chlorinated) to produce flame retardants; tetrabromobisphenol A (TBBPA) is most commonly used, with >60,000 tons produced annually [57, 58]. Studies report that levels of brominated flame retardants are increasing in the serum of adults, and its level in infants and children is even higher [59].

BPA is often described as a "weak" estrogen; however, an emerging number of cellular and molecular studies find that it has potential for many other biological activities at low but environmentally relevant exposure levels. In addition to binding to the nuclear estrogen receptor (ER) alpha and ER beta, BPA interacts with a variety of other cellular targets including binding to a nonclassical membrane-bound form of the ER (ncmER), a recently identified orphan nuclear receptor termed estrogen-related receptor gamma (ERR gamma), a seven-transmembrane estrogen receptor called GPR30, and the aryl hydrocarbon receptor (AhR). Interactions with ncmER and ERR gamma are especially noteworthy because BPA binds to these receptors with high affinity. BPA has also been shown to act as an androgen receptor antagonist and to interact with thyroid hormone receptors (for review, see [60]).

Experimental animal studies have reported that very low doses of BPA in the range of human exposures can exert effects if administered during development. An increasing number of "low-dose" studies have suggested that perinatal BPA exposure is associated with a variety of abnormalities in the male and female reproductive tissues and mammary gland tissues (for review of low-dose BPA effects, see [61, 62]. Studies showing an association of BPA with obesity have received less attention; however, data from both mice and rats have shown increased body weights in animals that were exposed to low doses of BPA during prenatal or neonatal development [47, 63–69]. The later study suggests this increase in body weight is sex specific but timing and dose may also contribute to the complexity of these findings since other studies reported effects in both males and females. Interestingly, a recent paper reports similar increases in body weights of pups obtained from moms fed BPA in their diets during pregnancy; the doses were low and considered "ecologically relevant" at 1 μg/kg diet (1 ppb BPA) [70]. Thus, regardless of route of exposure, low doses of BPA appear to cause weight gain in pups. In contrast, Ryan et al. report that the differences in body weight observed at weaning disappear as the mice age [70]. This may be due to palatability of the diet, which was changed at weaning since both control and BPA mice did not continue to gain weight on the new diets. Taken together, these experimental studies on BPA point out the sensitivity of the developmental period to disruption by EDCs, but they also suggest the complexity of the mechanisms involved in the development of obesity.

In vitro studies with BPA provide additional evidence for a role in the development of obesity and further suggest specific targets; BPA causes 3T3-L1 cells (mouse fibroblast cells that can differentiate into adipocytes) to increase differentiation [71], and in combination with insulin, BPA accelerates adipocyte formation [72, 73]. Other in vitro studies also show that low doses of BPA, similar to DES, impair calcium signaling in pancreatic alpha-cells, disrupt beta-cell function, and cause insulin resistance [74, 75]. Low environmentally relevant doses of BPA have also been reported to inhibit adiponectin and stimulate the release of inflammatory adipokines such as interleukin-6 (IL-6) and tumor necrosis factor alpha (TNF-α) from human adipose tissue, suggesting that BPA is involved in obesity and the related metabolic syndrome [76, 77]. Further, other studies have linked BPA exposure to disruption of pancreatic beta-cell function and blood glucose homeostasis in mice [78], suggesting changes consistent with metabolic syndrome.

Epidemiologic studies also support an association between BPA and obesity and insulin resistance. BPA was detected at high levels in both nonobese and obese women with polycystic ovarian syndrome (PCOS) as compared with nonobese normal women, suggesting possible involvement of BPA in PCOS [79].

18.6 Phytoestrogens

In recent years, efforts to implement healthier eating lifestyles have resulted in an increased consumption of soy products and soy supplements, which has as a result increased human exposure to phytoestrogens. Ironically, although phytoestrogens are considered by some as a preventive factor for obesity, they may instead play a role in causing the disease. Genistein and daidzein are two of the most abundant phytoestrogens in the human diet. Because of its estrogenic activity, genistein has been proposed to play a role in health maintenance by improving lipid and carbohydrate homeostasis. Recent studies have shown that genistein at pharmacologically high doses does indeed inhibit adipose deposition, but at low doses similar to that found in Western and Eastern diets (such as in soy milk or food supplements), genistein induced adipose tissue deposition, especially in males [80]. Further, this increase in adipose tissue deposition by genistein was correlated with mild peripheral insulin resistance. Similar to our findings with DES, genistein caused abnormal programming of factors involved in weight homeostasis, but it did not affect absolute food consumption [80]. Thus, genistein can affect adipose tissue deposition, and its effects may be dose dependent and gender specific, but further research is clearly needed.

Developmental exposure to numerous other naturally estrogenic substances has exhibited increased body weight, including resveratrol found in grapes and red wine and zearalenone, a mycotoxin synthesized by *Fusarium* mold and present in "moldy" grains, especially corn [47]. Phytoestrogens and mycoestrogens, both singly or in combination with other chemicals, may have multiple pathways of action and are likely involved in adipogeneis and energy metabolism. Whether they have beneficial or harmful effects or cause no effects in humans remains to be determined, but the outcome likely depends on dosage and timing of exposure.

Epidemiologic studies also support the idea that phytoestrogens may contribute to overweight babies who are fed soy-based infant formula [81] (for review on effects of soy formula, see [82]).

18.7 Other EDCs

An overview of the toxicology literature suggests that exposure to many other EDCs can cause weight gain, including pesticides. For example, organochlorines such as DDT, endrin, lindane, and hexachlorobenzene; organophosphates; carbamates; polychlorinated biphenyls; polybrominated biphenols which are used as fire retardants; other plastic components such as phthalates; perfluoroctanoic acid (PFOA); heavy metals such as cadmium, lead, and arsenic; and solvents have all been associated phenomenologically with weight gain (for review, see [27]). Many of these chemicals are discussed in Chapter 19. The weight gain associated with these chemicals tends to occur at low levels of exposure, rather than at high doses, where most toxicity studies tend to be conducted. Further, many pharmaceuticals also play a role in altered weight homeostasis and/or altered hormone levels; in fact, many prescribed drugs (including those commonly used in oncology, cardiology, immunology, and psychiatry) have the unwanted side effects of weight gain [27]. While these medicines are normally prescribed for adults where their effects on weight gain would most likely be reversible, the possible irreversible impact on the unborn fetus and young child due to inadvertent contamination cannot be underestimated.

18.8 Proposed Modes of Action

EDCs likely cause their effects through a variety of mechanisms. However, the most commonly proposed mechanism involves direct binding to nuclear receptors, such as estrogen receptor α inducing agonist activity. Alternatively, they could act as nuclear receptor antagonists. EDCs could also act indirectly, for example, they could disrupt hormone levels by inhibiting aromatase activity such as the P450 family members CYP19 and CYP3A1 which convert testosterone to estradiol, or by activating expression of various P450 enzymes. Finally, another mechanism that has been proposed is altering neuronal synapse formation [83] which could affect release of brain-produced substances that bind to nuclear receptors which then may alter central energy regulation. These proposed mechanisms may be altered singly or in combination. Further, the exact target tissue is unknown, but multiple target sites appear likely, including adipocytes, brain, liver, stomach, pancreas, as discussed in other chapters in this volume. The mechanism of how EDCs cause their effects on weight homeostasis and energy balance is an important area of future research.

18.9 Conclusions

The data included in this review support the idea that brief exposure early in development to environmental chemicals with estrogenic activity increases body weight gain with age and alters markers predictive of obesity and metabolic disease in experimental animals. Furthermore, human epidemiologic studies, discussed in more detail in Chapter 17, are at least consistent with the findings in experimental animals and show a link between exposure to environmental estrogens and the development of obesity [27, 28]. Lastly, the use of soy-based infant formula containing the estrogenic component genistein has been positively associated with obesity later in life [81]. Using the DES animal model as an important research tool to study "obesogens," the mechanisms involved in altered weight homeostasis (direct and/or endocrine feedback loops, i.e., ghrelin, leptin, etc.) by environmental estrogens can be elucidated [29–32]. In addition, this animal model may shed light on areas of prevention. Public health risks can no longer be based on the assumption that overweight and obesity are just personal choices involving increased food intake combined with inactivity, but rather that complex events including exposure to environmental chemicals during development may be contributing to our current obesity epidemic.

References

1. Ogden CL, Yanovski SZ, Carroll MD, Flegal KM. The epidemiology of obesity. Gastroenterology. May 2007;132(6):2087–102.
2. Oken E, Gillman MW. Fetal origins of obesity. Obes Res. 2003;11:496–506.
3. Caballero B. The global epidemic of obesity: an overview. Epidemiol Rev. 2007;29:1–5.
4. Cunningham E. Where can I find obesity statistics?. J Am Diet Assoc. Apr 2010;110(4):656.
5. Centers for Disease Control and Prevention. Report on overweight and obesity. http://www.cdc.gov/nccdphp/dnpa/obesity: 2008. Accessed April 28, 2010.
6. McAllister EJ, Dhurandhar NV, Keith SW, et al. Ten putative contributors to the obesity epidemic. Crit Rev Food Sci Nutr. Nov 2009;49(10):868–913.
7. Ogden CL, Flegal KM, Carroll MD, Johnson CL. Prevalence and trends in overweight among US children and adolescents, 1999–2000. JAMA. Oct 9 2002;288(14):1728–32.
8. Flegal KM, Carroll MD, Ogden CL, Curtin LR. Prevalence and trends in obesity among US adults, 1999–2008. JAMA. Jan 20 2010;303(3):235–41.
9. Collins S. Overview of clinical perspectives and mechanisms of obesity. Birth Defects Res A Clin Mol Teratol. Jul 2005;73(7):470–1.
10. Mokdad AH, Ford ES, Bowman BA, et al. Prevalence of obesity, diabetes, and obesity-related health risk factors, 2001. JAMA. Jan 1 2003;289(1):76–9.
11. Mokdad AH, Serdula MK, Dietz WH, Bowman BA, Marks JS, Koplan JP. The spread of the obesity epidemic in the United States, 1991–1998. JAMA. Oct 27 1999;282(16):1519–22.
12. Bern B. The fragile fetus vol. XXI. Princeton, NJ: Princeton Scientific; 1992.
13. Heindel JJ. Role of exposure to environmental chemicals in the developmental basis of disease and dysfunction. Reprod Toxicol. Apr–May 2007;23(3):257–9.
14. Heindel JJ. Animal models for probing the developmental basis of disease and dysfunction paradigm. Basic Clin Pharmacol Toxicol. Feb 2008;102(2):76–81.
15. Heindel JJ, Levin E. Developmental origins and environmental influences–Introduction. NIEHS symposium. Birth Defects Res A Clin Mol Teratol. Jul 2005;73(7):469.
16. Gluckman PD, Hanson MA. The developmental origins of the metabolic syndrome. Trends Endocrinol Metab. May–Jun 2004;15(4):183–7.
17. Colborn T, Dumanoski D, Myers JP. Our stolen future. New York, NY: Penguin Books; 1996.
18. NIH. DES Research Update, NIH Publication No. 00-4722. Bethesda, MD: NTH; 1999.
19. Barker DJ, Eriksson JG, Forsen T, Osmond C. Fetal origins of adult disease: strength of effects and biological basis. Int J Epidemiol. Dec 2002;31(6):1235–9.
20. vom Saal FS, Akingbemi BT, Belcher SM, et al. Chapel Hill bisphenol A expert panel consensus statement: integration of mechanisms, effects in animals and potential to impact human health at current levels of exposure. Reprod Toxicol. Aug–Sep 2007;24(2):131–8.
21. Anway MD, Cupp AS, Uzumcu M, Skinner MK. Epigenetic transgenerational actions of endocrine disruptors and male fertility. Science. Jun 3 2005;308(5727):1466–9.
22. Anway MD, Skinner MK. Epigenetic programming of the germ line: effects of endocrine disruptors on the development of transgenerational disease. Reprod Biomed Online. Jan 2008;16(1):23–5.
23. Newbold RR, Padilla-Banks E, Jefferson WN. Adverse effects of the model environmental estrogen diethylstilbestrol are transmitted to subsequent generations. Endocrinology. Jun 2006;147 6 Suppl:S11–7.
24. Skinner MK, Anway MD. Epigenetic transgenerational actions of vinclozolin on the development of disease and cancer. Crit Rev Oncog. Aug 2007;13(1):75–82.

25. Skinner MK, Anway MD, Savenkova MI, Gore AC, Crews D. Transgenerational epigenetic programming of the brain transcriptome and anxiety behavior. PLoS One. 2008;3(11):e3745.
26. Tang WY, Newbold R, Mardilovich K, et al. Persistent hypomethylation in the promoter of nucleosomal binding protein 1 (Nsbp1) correlates with overexpression of Nsbp1 in mouse uteri neonatally exposed to diethylstilbestrol or genistein. Endocrinology. Dec 2008;149(12):5922–31.
27. Baillie-Hamilton PF. Chemical toxins: a hypothesis to explain the global obesity epidemic. J Altern Complement Med. Apr 2002;8(2):185–92.
28. Heindel JJ. Endocrine disruptors and the obesity epidemic. Toxicol Sci. Dec 2003;76(2): 247–9.
29. Newbold RR, Padilla-Banks E, Jefferson WN, Heindel JJ. Effects of endocrine disruptors on obesity. Int J Androl. Apr 2008;31(2):201–8.
30. Newbold RR, Padilla-Banks E, Snyder RJ, Jefferson WN. Developmental exposure to estrogenic compounds and obesity. Birth Defects Res A Clin Mol Teratol. Jul 2005;73(7): 478–80.
31. Newbold RR, Padilla-Banks E, Snyder RJ, Jefferson WN. Perinatal exposure to environmental estrogens and the development of obesity. Mol Nutr Food Res. Jul 2007;51(7):912–7.
32. Newbold RR, Padilla-Banks E, Snyder RJ, Phillips TM, Jefferson WN. Developmental exposure to endocrine disruptors and the obesity epidemic. Reprod Toxicol. Apr–May 2007;23(3):290–6.
33. Grun F, Blumberg B. Environmental obesogens: organotins and endocrine disruption via nuclear receptor signaling. Endocrinology. Jun 2006;147 6 Suppl:S50–5.
34. Grun F, Watanabe H, Zamanian Z, et al. Endocrine-disrupting organotin compounds are potent inducers of adipogenesis in vertebrates. Mol Endocrinol. Sep 2006;20(9):2141–55.
35. Raun A, Preston R. History of diethylstilbestrol use in livestock. http://www.asas.org/oldsite/Bios/Raunhist.pdf: 2002.
36. Thigpen JE, Setchell KD, Ahlmark KB, et al. Phytoestrogen content of purified, open- and closed-formula laboratory animal diets. Lab Anim Sci. 1999;49(5):530–6.
37. Newbold RR. Cellular and molecular effects of developmental exposure to diethylstilbestrol: implications for other environmental estrogens. Environ Health Perspect. 1995;103(7):83–7.
38. McLachlan JA, Newbold RR, Bullock BC. Long-term effects on the female mouse genital tract associated with prenatal exposure to diethylstilbestrol. Cancer Res. 1980;40:3988–99.
39. Newbold RR, Bullock BC, McLachlan JA. Uterine adenocarcinoma in mice following developmental treatment with estrogens: a model for hormonal carcinogenesis. Cancer Res. 1990;50(23):7677–81.
40. Newbold R. Lessons learned from perinatal exposure to diethylstilbestrol (DES). Toxicol Appl Pharmacol. 2004;199:142–50.
41. Newbold RR, McLachlan JA. Transplacental hormonal carcinogenesis: diethylstilbestrol as an example. In: Huff J, Boyd J, Barrett JC, editors. Cellular and molecular mechanisms of hormonal carcinogenesis: environmental influences. New York, NY: Wiley-Liss; 1996. pp. 131–47.
42. Newbold RR, Padilla-Banks E, Jefferson WN. Environmental estrogens and obesity. Mol Cell Endocrinol. May 25 2009;304(1-2):84–9.
43. Gluckman PD, Hanson MA, Pinal C. The developmental origins of adult disease. Matern Child Nutr. Jul 2005;1(3):130–41.
44. Gillum RF. The association of the ratio of waist to hip girth with blood pressure, serum cholesterol and serum uric acid in children and youths aged 6–17 years. J Chronic Dis. 1987;40(5):413–20.
45. Gesta S, Bluher M, Yamamoto Y, et al. Evidence for a role of developmental genes in the origin of obesity and body fat distribution. Proc Natl Acad Sci USA. Apr 25 2006;103(17):6676–81.
46. Newbold RR, Jefferson WN, Grissom SF, Padilla-Banks E, Snyder RJ, Lobenhofer EK. Developmental exposure to diethylstilbestrol alters uterine gene expression that may be associated with uterine neoplasia later in life. Mol Carcinog. Sep 2007;46(9):783–96.

47. Nikaido Y, Yoshizawa K, Danbara N, et al. Effects of maternal xenoestrogen exposure on development of the reproductive tract and mammary gland in female CD-1 mouse offspring. Reprod Toxicol. Aug–Sep 2004;18(6):803–11.
48. Zoeller RT, Bansal R, Parris C. Bisphenol-A, an environmental contaminant that acts as a thyroid hormone receptor antagonist in vitro, increases serum thyroxine, and alters RC3/neurogranin expression in the developing rat brain. Endocrinology. Feb 2005;146(2):607–12.
49. Brotons JA, Olea-Serrano MF, Villalobos M, Olea N. Xenoestrogens released from lacquer coating in food cans. Environ Health Perspect. 1994;1994(103):608–12.
50. Biles JE, McNeal TP, Begley TH, Hollifield HC. Determination of bisphenol-A in reusable polycarbonate food-contact plastics and migration to food simulating liquids. J Agric Food Chem. 1997;45:3541–4.
51. Olea N, Pulgar R, Perez P, et al. Estrogenicity of resin-based composites and sealants used in dentistry. Environ Health Perspect. Mar 1996;104(3):298–305.
52. Calafat AM, Ye X, Wong LY, Reidy JA, Needham LL. Exposure of the U.S. population to bisphenol A and 4-tertiary-octylphenol: 2003-2004. Environ Health Perspect. Jan 2008;116(1):39–44.
53. Takeuchi T, Tsutsumi O. Serum bisphenol a concentrations showed gender differences, possibly linked to androgen levels. Biochem Biophys Res Commun. Feb 15 2002;291(1):76–8.
54. Ye X, Kuklenyik Z, Needham LL, Calafat AM. Measuring environmental phenols and chlorinated organic chemicals in breast milk using automated on-line column-switching-high performance liquid chromatography-isotope dilution tandem mass spectrometry. J Chromatogr B Analyt Technol Biomed Life Sci. Feb 2 2006;831(1–2):110–5.
55. Padmanabhan V, Siefert K, Ransom S, et al. Maternal bisphenol-A levels at delivery: a looming problem? J Perinatol. Apr 2008;28(4):258–63.
56. Schonfelder G, Flick B, Mayr E, Talsness C, Paul M, Chahoud I. In utero exposure to low doses of bisphenol A lead to long-term deleterious effects in the vagina. Neoplasia. Mar–Apr 2002;4(2):98–102.
57. WHO. TetrabromobisphenolA and derivatives:environmental health criteria no. 172. Geneva: World Health Organization; 1995.
58. European Union Updated European Risk Assessment Report 4,4'-Isopropylidenediphenol (Bisphenol A). Environment Addendum of February 2008 (to be read in conjunction withEU RAR of BPA published in 2003). http:ecb.jrc.it/documents/Existing-Chemicals/RISKASSESSMENT/ADDENDUM/bisphenola add 325.pdf; 2008. Accessed April 28, 2010.
59. Thomsen C, Lundanes E, Becher G. Brominated flame retardants in archived serum samples from Norway: a study on temporal trends and the role of age. Environ Sci Technol. Apr 1 2002;36(7):1414–8.
60. Wetherill YB, Akingbemi BT, Kanno J, et al. In vitro molecular mechanisms of bisphenol A action. Reprod Toxicol. Aug–Sep 2007;24(2):178–98.
61. NTP. CEHR Brief on bisphenol A. National toxicology program. Research Triangle Park, NC: NTP. 2008.
62. Richter CA, Birnbaum LS, Farabollini F, et al. In vivo effects of bisphenol A in laboratory rodent studies. Reprod Toxicol. Aug–Sep 2007;24(2):199–224.
63. Howdeshell KL, Hotchkiss AK, Thayer KA, Vandenbergh JG, vom Saal FS. Exposure to bisphenol A advances puberty. Nature. Oct 21 1999;401(6755):763–4.
64. Ashby J, Tinwell H, Haseman J. Lack of effects for low dose levels of bisphenol A and diethylstilbestrol on the prostate gland of CF1 mice exposed in utero. Regul Toxicol Pharmacol. Oct 1999;30(2 Pt 1):156–66.
65. Takai Y, Tsutsumi O, Ikezuki Y, et al. Preimplantation exposure to bisphenol A advances postnatal development. Reprod Toxicol. Jan–Feb 2001;15(1):71–4.
66. Honma S, Suzuki A, Buchanan DL, Katsu Y, Watanabe H, Iguchi T. Low dose effect of in utero exposure to bisphenol A and diethylstilbestrol on female mouse reproduction. Reprod Toxicol. Mar–Apr 2002;16(2):117–22.

67. Nikaido Y, Danbara N, Tsujita-Kyutoku M, Yuri T, Uehara N, Tsubura A. Effects of prepubertal exposure to xenoestrogen on development of estrogen target organs in female CD-1 mice. In Vivo. May–Jun 2005;19(3):487–94.
68. Rubin BS, Murray MK, Damassa DA, King JC, Soto AM. Perinatal exposure to low doses of bisphenol A affects body weight, patterns of estrous cyclicity, and plasma LH levels. Environ Health Perspect. Jul 2001;109(7):675–80.
69. Somm E, Schwitzgebel VM, Toulotte A, et al. Perinatal exposure to bisphenol a alters early adipogenesis in the rat. Environ Health Perspect. Oct 2009;117(10):1549–55.
70. Ryan KK, Haller AM, Sorrell JE, Woods SC, Jandacek RJ, Seeley RJ. Perinatal Exposure to Bisphenol-A and the Development of Metabolic Syndrome in CD-1 Mice. Endocrinology. June 2010;151(6):2603–12. Mar 29 2010. [e published].
71. Sakurai K, Kawazuma M, Adachi T, et al. Bisphenol A affects glucose transport in mouse 3T3-F442A adipocytes. Br J Pharmacol. Jan 2004;141(2):209–14.
72. Masuno H, Kidani T, Sekiya K, et al. Bisphenol A in combination with insulin can accelerate the conversion of 3T3-L1 fibroblasts to adipocytes. J Lipid Res. May 2002;43(5):676–84.
73. Masuno H, Iwanami J, Kidani T, Sakayama K, Honda K. Bisphenol a accelerates terminal differentiation of 3T3-L1 cells into adipocytes through the phosphatidylinositol 3-kinase pathway. Toxicol Sci. Apr 2005;84(2):319–27.
74. Alonso-Magdalena P, Laribi O, Ropero AB, et al. Low doses of bisphenol A and diethylstilbestrol impair Ca^{2+} signals in pancreatic alpha-cells through a nonclassical membrane estrogen receptor within intact islets of Langerhans. Environ Health Perspect. Aug 2005;113(8): 969–77.
75. Alonso-Magdalena P, Morimoto S, Ripoll C, Fuentes E, Nadal A. The estrogenic effect of bisphenol A disrupts pancreatic beta-cell function in vivo and induces insulin resistance. Environ Health Perspect. Jan 2006;114(1):106–12.
76. Ben-Jonathan N, Hugo ER, Brandebourg TD. Effects of bisphenol A on adipokine release from human adipose tissue: Implications for the metabolic syndrome. Mol Cell Endocrinol. May 25 2009;304(1–2):49–54.
77. Hugo ER, Brandebourg TD, Woo JG, Loftus J, Alexander JW, Ben-Jonathan N. Bisphenol A at environmentally relevant doses inhibits adiponectin release from human adipose tissue explants and adipocytes. Environ Health Perspect. Dec 2008;116(12):1642–7.
78. Ropero AB, Alonso-Magdalena P, Garcia-Garcia E, Ripoll C, Fuentes E, Nadal A. Bisphenol-A disruption of the endocrine pancreas and blood glucose homeostasis. Int J Androl. Apr 2008;31(2):194–200.
79. Takeuchi T, Tsutsumi O, Ikezuki Y, Takai Y, Taketani Y. Positive relationship between androgen and the endocrine disruptor, bisphenol A, in normal women and women with ovarian dysfunction. Endocr J. Apr 2004;51(2):165–9.
80. Penza M, Montani C, Romani A, et al. Genistein affects adipose tissue deposition in a dose-dependent and gender-specific manner. Endocrinology. Dec 2006;147(12):5740–51.
81. Stettler N, Stallings VA, Troxel AB, et al. Weight gain in the first week of life and overweight in adulthood: a cohort study of European American subjects fed infant formula. Circulation. Apr 19 2005;111(15):1897–903.
82. Rozman KK, Bhatia J, Calafat AM, et al. NTP-CERHR expert panel report on the reproductive and developmental toxicity of soy formula. Birth Defects Res B Dev Reprod Toxicol. Aug 2006;77(4):280–397.
83. Shinomiya N, Shinomiya M. Dichlorodiphenyltrichloroethane suppresses neurite outgrowth and induces apoptosis in PC12 pheochromocytoma cells. Toxicol Lett. Feb 3 2003;137(3):175–83.

Chapter 19
The Role of Environmental Obesogens in the Obesity Epidemic

Amanda Janesick and Bruce Blumberg

19.1 Introduction

Nearly 260 years ago, prenatal exposure to a particular toxin, ethanol, was observed to have deleterious effects to the developing fetus [1]. During Prohibition in the United States, behavioral problems exhibited by children of "immoderate" alcohol-consuming families were attributed to poor social upbringing [2]. By the 1970s, methodical investigation of infants born to alcoholic mothers firmly established a prenatal component contributing to the common display of behavioral and mental problems [3, 4]. Acceptance of fetal alcohol syndrome (FAS) was slow because alcoholics were considered to be morally corrupt, social deviants who bred the same type of people [2]. Today, however, FAS is considered a rather obvious illustration of developmental programming because the teratogenic effects of ethanol are often robust and quickly discernable. Unfortunately, the effects of environmental chemicals that contribute to obesity and metabolic disease are not quite as visible, especially early in life. Major consequences of obesity such as diabetes and heart disease occur much later in life, and even early childhood obesity is more conveniently ascribed to a general lack of dietary restraint and/or lack of exercise. Indeed, the same stigma that plagued the acceptance of FAS is likely to affect the recognition and public awareness of the "obesity before birth" argument.

The conventional wisdom is that people can budget their diets as they do their finances: calories eaten should not exceed calories expended, otherwise, the body will drift toward a positive energy balance [5]. Suppose, though, that metabolic set points are perturbed from the beginning of life. For example, babies born to mothers who smoke exhibit a classic trend: low birth weight, with increased risk of obesity and metabolic syndrome later in life [6]. This pattern is characterized in the Developmental Origins of Health and Disease (DOHaD) hypothesis, which was

A. Janesick (✉)
Department of Developmental and Cell Biology, University of California, Irvine, CA 92697-2300, USA
e-mail: ajanesic@uci.edu

R.H. Lustig (ed.), *Obesity Before Birth*, Endocrine Updates 30,
DOI 10.1007/978-1-4419-7034-3_19,

developed after epidemiologists noted that poor maternal nutrition was correlated with reduced perinatal growth followed by a deliberate progression of adult disease in offspring [7–9]. In simple terms, the fetus "anticipates" that it will be born into a nutrient-deprived environment and makes suitable adjustments to its metabolic program. If the environment turns out to be food rich, then the adult will not be able to cope [10]. Low birth weight can be the outcome of multiple environmental stressors (not all nutrient based) and is indicative of a trajectory toward cardiovascular disease, diabetes, and obesity [11–14]. During certain critical developmental time windows (e.g., periconception), with relatively low exposure to a stressor, the fetus might appear completely normal [15], yet subtle developmental cues still exist and will manifest themselves later in life. Most studies supporting the DOHaD hypothesis are primarily nutritional in nature, thus the potential of environmental toxins to modulate developmental pathways that control energy and metabolism is mostly unexplored. Whether the stressor is coming from the outside, or produced endogenously by the parent, virtually all identified compounds that induce obesity are endocrine disrupting chemicals (EDCs). Many are either direct ligands for hormone receptors or affect components in metabolic signaling pathways under hormonal control.

19.2 An Archetype for Prenatal Chemical Exposure Leading to Obesity (Obesogens): Tributyltin

"Obesogens" are chemical compounds that can promote obesity by increasing the number of fat cells (and fat storage into existing fat cells), by changing the amount of calories burned at rest, by altering energy balance to favor storage of calories, and by altering the mechanisms through which the body regulates appetite and satiety.

Organotins are a family of compounds that contain at least one Sn—C bond. Invented in the 1850s, these "organic bodies of tin" were less a discovery of the compounds themselves than an educational instrument that encouraged the development of organometallic chemistry and the concept of valence number [16]. Currently, organotins are prevalent in industry, used in fungicides, wood preservatives, and heat stabilizers in polyolefin plastics [17]. Organotins were once widely used as antifouling paints on boats in the 1960–1970s, and have since been regulated, but not completely phased out [18]. Because organotins are lipophilic, they readily bioaccumulate in bacteria, algae, and aquatic invertebrates [19]. Concern over the biological consequences of organotin exposure was first reported when the female gastropod mollusk, exposed to tributyltin (TBT), developed a sperm duct, seminal vesicle, and penis [20, 21]. Neurotoxic [22] and mitochondrial toxic [23, 24] effects were also observed. Reproductive effects were first observed in higher vertebrates when it was noted that exposure to TBT masculinized genetically female Japanese flounder [25]. Subsequently, it was found that *Xenopus laevis* tadpoles exposed to low levels of tributyltin exhibited ectopic fat cell production; a novel and unexpected finding [26]. TBT was thus identified as the first "obesogen."

In mice, a single, prenatal exposure to TBT during gestation, results in premature accumulation of fat in adipose tissues [26] (Fig. 19.1). In accord with nutritional experiments supporting the DOHaD hypothesis, the mice were born slightly underweight, but had already stored fat at the expense of total body mass [26]. By 6 months, the mice were significantly heavier, despite normal diet and exercise (unpublished). Histological sections of newborn liver, testis, mammary gland, and inguinal adipose tissue (which normally do not store lipids before feeding commences) all showed pronounced lipid accumulation in the pups born to TBT-treated mothers [26]. Hence, the tendency to store excess fat was already programmed before the mouse was born, simply due to a single exposure of TBT, at a dose equivalent to what humans might acquire, inadvertently, from their environment. TBT is one of few examples of an exogenous chemical that generates an obese phenotype in both sexes, solely due to in utero exposure. The mechanisms underlying why early life exposure to chemicals, like TBT, might increase a person's propensity toward obesity is the focus of this review.

19.3 Obesogens Acting on Estrogen/Androgen Metabolism

Estrogens in the adult are protective against android (abdominal) obesity and metabolic disease. The ovariectomized rat (a model for menopause in women and estrogen deficiency in men) has abdominal obesity, which is reversed upon treatment with estrogen [27, 28]. In 3T3-L1 preadipocytes constitutively expressing the estrogen receptor, triglyceride levels, and lipoprotein lipase expression are decreased [29]. Conversely, knockout of the estrogen receptor leads to increased white adipose depot size, central weight gain, and impaired glucose metabolism [30, 31]. The same phenotypes seen with estrogen insufficiency can also be simulated by the inhibition of aromatase, an enzyme that converts testosterone to estradiol. Aromatase knockout mice are obese and this phenotype is attributed to an estrogen deficit, as opposed to testosterone excess [32]. Metabolic disease, fatty liver, and abdominal obesity have also been demonstrated in a human case study where CYP19A1, the gene encoding aromatase, is rendered non-functional [33]. Interestingly, tributyltin (TBT) is an inhibitor of P450-mediated aromatase expression and/or action, in both fish and humans [34, 35]. The masculinization of female mollusks by TBT is thought to result from inhibition of aromatase; although there is also evidence that TBT acts through nuclear receptors to inhibit aromatase expression. Whether and to what degree TBT perturbs estrogen availability in mammals to affect adiposity is currently unknown.

Prenatal exposure to excess estrogen does not protect the fetus against obesity, despite the fact that estrogen promotes leanness in adults. The most prevalent model for studying prenatal estrogen exposure is the diethylstilbestrol (DES) mouse. DES is a synthetic estrogen that actually binds to the estrogen receptor two to three times stronger than does the natural ligand, 17β-estradiol [36]. When mice are treated prenatally with low-dose DES, they give birth to pups that are initially smaller, but

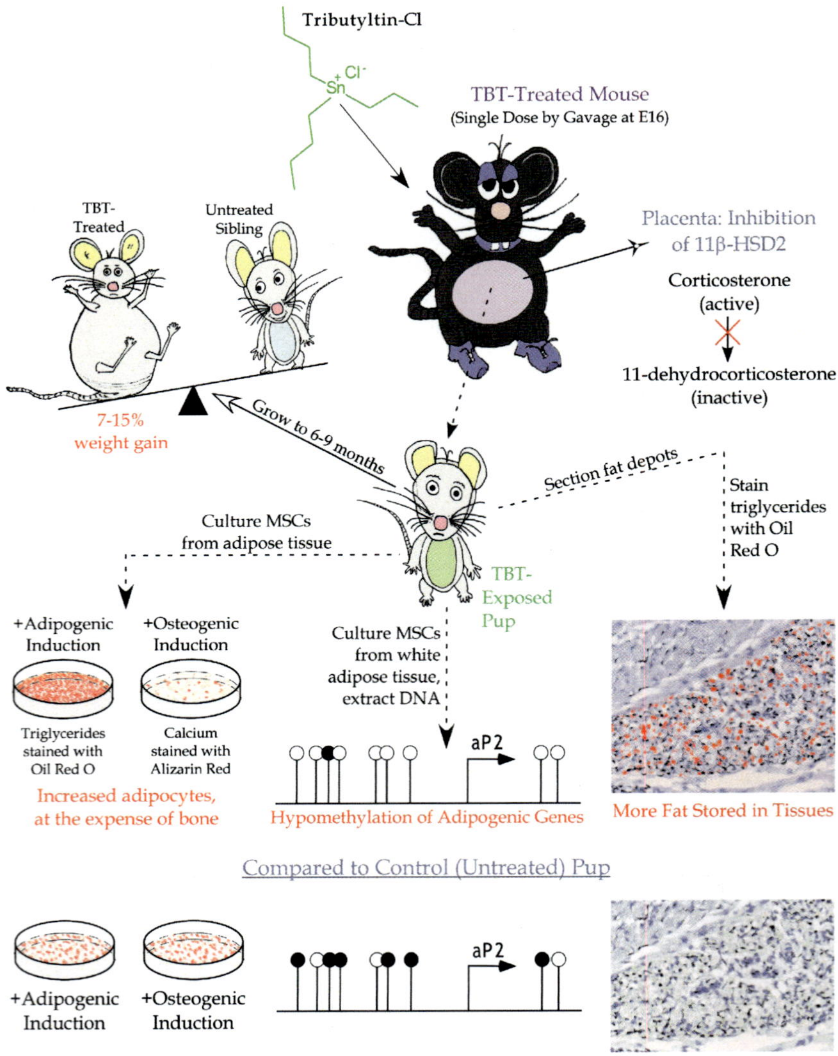

Fig. 19.1 Prenatal exposure to tributyltin (TBT) predisposes an organism to be obese. A single exposure to TBT at embryonic day 16 causes a host of changes in developing animals. TBT exposure alters the expression of 11β-HSD2 in the placenta, which could increase glucocorticoid levels. Prenatal TBT exposure produces pups that have already stored fat in tissues at birth, compared with control animals that do not. Multipotent stromal cells from exposed animals are predisposed to develop into adipocytes at the expense of bone cells. Promoters of some PPARγ target genes are undermethylated in MSCs from exposed animals compared to controls. This increased number of adipocytes may be important in the 7–15% weight gain seen in exposed animals from 6 to 9 months of age

become heavier later in life [37]. The environmental estrogen bisphenol-A (BPA), activates the estrogen receptor and is also an inverse antagonist (i.e., activator) of the estrogen-related receptor [38]. BPA treatment of pregnant dams results in smaller offspring that exhibit "catch-up" growth and are significantly heavier by 6 weeks of age [39]. Dichlorodiphenyl-dichloroethylene (DDE), the major metabolite of the pesticide DDT, is both an estrogen receptor activator and an anti-androgen [40, 41]. Mothers who lived along the Lake Michigan shoreline, exposed to high levels of DDT, were more likely to have a child that exhibited elevated BMI in adulthood [42]. One area of active study concerning the obesogenic effects of estrogen is the regulation of leptin and its receptor by estrogens [43]. High levels of maternal leptin are correlated with high fetal leptin [44] which is a precursor to weight gain later in life. The obesogenic effects of estrogenic chemicals are explored more fully in Chapter 17.

19.4 Obesogens Acting on Glucocorticoid Metabolism

Disruption of glucocorticoid homeostasis also contributes to the pathogenesis of obesity and metabolic syndrome. Obesity is linked to a general increase of positive feedback within the hypothalamic–pituitary–adrenocortical (HPA) axis, leading to an oversecretion of cortisol from the adrenal gland [45–49]. This does not necessarily translate to higher circulating cortisol levels in the blood; and for that reason, obesity is not associated with systemic hypercortisolism, as in the case of Cushing's syndrome. Rather, the hypercortisolism observed in obesity is intracellular and peripheral in nature, often characterized by the impaired ability to clear or inactivate cortisol in adipose tissue, particularly visceral adipose tissue [50]. Visceral adiposity is particularly dangerous since it is associated with all the major health consequences and mortality risk of obesity (reviewed in [51]). In addition, the visceral adipose tissue itself is populated with more glucocorticoid receptors (GRs) than subcutaneous tissue [52, 53]. Since glucocorticoids increase adipocyte proliferation and their differentiation from stromal cells, the presence of excess glucocorticoids or GRs will undoubtedly stimulate adipogenesis locally [54–56].

One popular hypothesis that links obesity to the HPA axis is the dysregulation of 11β-hydroxysteroid dehydrogenase type-1 (11βHSD1) (see Chapter 13). 11βHSD1 is expressed wherever the glucocorticoid receptor is found (i.e., ubiquitously) and primarily functions to convert the inactive cortisone (or 11-dehydrocorticosterone in rodents) into the active cortisol (or corticosterone in rodents) (reviewed in [57]). In humans, obesity and metabolic syndrome are associated with elevated 11βHSD1 [50, 58, 59]. The phenomenon is also observed in obese Zucker rats, where 11βHSD1 is increased specifically in omental adipose tissue [60]. Concomitantly, the Zucker rats showed decreased 11βHSD1 expression in the liver, which might lead to a compensatory effect whereby the HPA is stimulated to release more corticosterone [50]. The alternate dehydrogenase (11βHSD2) functions in the opposite direction; it converts active cortisol (or corticosterone) to inactive cortisone (or 11-dehydrocorticosterone) and is mostly expressed in the kidney, colon, salivary glands, and placenta, where mineralocorticoid receptors are present [61–63]. 11βHSD2 is expressed at low levels in adipose tissue and its reduction might be correlated with obesity [64, 65]. However, deficiency of 11βHSD2 at the kidney results primary in increased mineralocorticoid receptor activation, hypokalemia, and hypertension [66].

Excess glucocorticoid exposure during pregnancy is commonly associated with lower birth weights, but increased risk of cardiovascular disease, diabetes, and hypertension in the adult offspring (reviewed in [67]). Endogenous stimulation of glucocorticoid levels in the mother can potentially wreak havoc on fetal metabolism. In studies of maternal distress, where the mother's physiological state is negative or depressed, the mother produces more corticotropin-releasing hormone, which in turn leads to increased cortisol secretion, and reduced birth weight in the offspring (reviewed in [68]). Exogenous stimulation of glucocorticoid levels in the mother is also common. For example, ethanol exposure in guinea pigs led to elevated levels of cortisol in the mother (measured in the saliva) which was transmitted to fetal blood and amniotic fluid [69]. When pregnant rats were given the synthetic glucocorticoid dexamethasone, the birth weight of the offspring was reduced, followed by an increased risk for hypertension in adults [70]. Monkeys treated with dexamethasone during pregnancy had offspring that were normal at birth, but exhibited significant weight gain at 2 months of age [71]. These monkey infants grew to develop obesity and demonstrated all signs of metabolic syndrome (increased blood pressure, high total cholesterol, decreased HDL, and insulin resistance).

Recently, a study showed that increased cortisol production rates in adults were associated with visceral adiposity. Importantly, however, weight loss did not return cortisol production to normal [72]. Obesity was not the source of the elevated cortisol production rates; rather, a perturbed HPA axis was a predisposing mechanism for obesity. This mechanism might account in part for why people cannot lose weight effectively. In this view, any environmental toxin that perturbs the HPA axis in early life could also contribute to obesity and subsequent resistance to weight loss. There are many possible mechanisms by which xenobiotic chemicals can influence glucocorticoid metabolism to disrupt energy balance, appetite, and the stress response (reviewed in [73]). Given that 11βHSD1 catalyzes the conversion of inactive to active glucocorticoids, one possible way to disturb the HPA axis would be to render 11βHSD1 hyperactive. Adult rats given a daily dose of alcohol throughout the first 22 days of gestation gave birth to offspring that demonstrated a significant increase in 11βHSD1 activity, with a subsequent increase in serum cortisol, in both liver and adipose tissue [74]. Hence, it is no surprise that alcohol exposure in utero leads to an activated HPA axis [75] and is associated with glucose intolerance in the adult [76, 77].

Of course, the fetus is normally shielded against excess glucocorticoids because placental 11βHSD2 is highly expressed throughout pregnancy to reduce fetal cortisol exposure [78]. Prenatal inhibition of 11βHSD2 by carbenoxolone administration throughout pregnancy leads to reduced birth weight, anxious behavior, and increased secretion of corticotropin-releasing hormone in rats [79]. Cadmium, dithiocarbamates, and organotins all have the potential to reduce 11βHSD2 activity in the placenta [80–82]. Hence, one plausible mechanism for obesity in offspring from mothers exposed to tributyltin (TBT) is that placental 11βHSD2 activity is reduced. In fact, TBT is readily transferred from the mother and accumulates in the fetal placenta, liver, and brain [83]. Hence, the leaking of glucocorticoids to the fetus through the activation of 11βHSD1, or placental inhibition of 11βHSD2, is a potential mode of action for environmental chemicals. This is an attractive idea because the dehydrogenases function in the direct activation or inactivation of cortisol. However, due to the complexity of the HPA axis, there are many more avenues of endocrine disruption on glucocorticoid metabolism yet to be uncovered. For example, corticosteroid-binding globulin (CBG) activity is negatively correlated with BMI, waist-to-hip ratio, and insulin resistance in healthy adults [84]. Adipose tissue that is deficient in CBG cannot evacuate cortisol to the blood. In humans with CBG deficiency, preadipocytes readily proliferate and differentiate into adipocytes [85]. Hence, an EDC that lessened CBG activity might also lead to obesity in the adult.

19.5 Obesogens Acting on Peroxisome Proliferator-Activated Receptors

Unlike steroid receptors, which have long been associated with growth, metabolism, and reproductive development, the peroxisome proliferator-activated receptors (PPARs) were originally recognized because certain chemicals activated these receptors to increase peroxisome proliferation in rats [86, 87]. Recent research has focused on PPAR involvement in lipid metabolism and adipogenesis. PPARα is primarily expressed in the liver and is stimulated upon starvation [88], where free fatty acids, once liberated from adipose tissue and transported into the blood, are oxidized in the liver, resulting in ketone bodies that provide energy to muscular tissue and the brain (reviewed in [89]). Fatty acids are natural ligands for PPARα, although drugs such as fenofibrate and gemfibrozil (used to lower LDL levels) also increase PPARα activity [90]. PPARγ is primarily expressed in adipocytes [91] and upon activation, increases adipogenesis [92]. Thiazolidinediones (TZDs), which combat type 2 diabetes, are potent activators of PPARγ [93]. PPARα activation is thought to protect against obesity, whereas stimulation of PPARγ is obesogenic. Therefore, PPARγ has become a focus of many recent obesity-related studies. Nevertheless, chronic stimulation of PPARα leads to glucose intolerance, as well as deterioration of the heart muscle due to lipotoxicity [94–96]. Thus, while PPARα converts fat into energy, it can limit the uptake of glucose into tissues, leading to diabetes.

Like all PPARs, PPARγ forms a heterodimer with the retinoid-X receptor (RXR), a binding partner for multiple nuclear receptors. The ligand-binding pocket of PPARγ is large [97] and can accommodate various chemical structures [98]. PPARγ promiscuity is well demonstrated by the fact that tributyltin (TBT) has nanomolar affinity for PPARγ, yet its structure is highly dissimilar to fatty acids and TZDs

[26, 99]. Indeed, the mechanistic basis for TBT-promoted adipogenesis is most strongly supported by evidence that TBT is an agonist for PPARγ and RXR [100]. Competitive binding assays show that TBT has comparable affinity for RXR, as do synthetic RXR agonists [26]. TBT was actually a better activator of PPARγ even compared to TZDs such as troglitazone [26, 100]. The crystal structure of TBT along with the RXRα ligand-binding domain plus a coactivator fragment shows that TBT binds covalently to RXR [101], which means that it will not readily dissociate once attached. While there is no structural evidence for TBT association with PPARγ, the PPARγ antagonist, T0070907 [102], reduced TBT-stimulated adipogenesis, indicating that the obesogenic activity of TBT is likely mediated through activation of PPARγ [103].

Inappropriate stimulation of PPARs by EDCs is a potential factor underlying the etiology of many forms of obesity. This point is perhaps best made by pharmaceutical obesogens (TZDs) used to treat diabetes. Because TZDs are effective agonists of PPARγ, they promote weight gain in humans by increasing adipose tissue differentiation [104, 105], even as they improve insulin resistance and blood glucose. Since drugs aberrantly modulate PPARγ to stimulate adipogenesis, EDCs like TBT can do the same. However, TBT is not the most ubiquitous EDC to which humans are exposed. Some phthalates (see Chapter 16) are also PPARγ agonists [106] and stimulate the proliferation of adipocytes in the 3T3-L1 cell culture model [107]. Phthalate metabolites are associated with increased waist circumference in men [108], and therefore, are predicted to be obesogenic. Phthalates are ubiquitous organic chemicals that give plastics such as polyvinyl chloride (PVC) with more flexibility and durability. Since phthalates are not permanently bonded to PVC, they readily leach into food, from medical devices and materials used in construction and manufacturing. Phthalates are probably able to cross the feto-placental barrier, as demonstrated by a simulated human placental perfusion ex vivo model [109]. Identifying the role of phthalates as obesogens is an important topic for future research.

19.6 Epigenetics: The Gene–Environment Connection

Obesogens are predicted to influence the prenatal programming of obesity through epigenetic modification of gene activity; an attractive mechanism frequently invoked to explain complex environment–gene interactions [110]. There are more than 6,000 genes expected to influence body weight. Of these, about 10 times more genes favor the increase rather than decrease of weight [111]. Epigenetic modification of any of these genes theoretically could result in "developmental plasticity," which allows an organism to make rapid adaptations to changing environments by altering levels of gene expression via DNA methylation, modification of histone proteins, or alteration of mitochondrial function [112–114]. During development, the embryo undergoes genome-wide DNA demethylation and remethylation [115–117], which is coupled to corresponding changes in histone acetyl transferase activity

[118]. The first wave of methylation reprogramming occurs prior to the blastocyst stage and establishes which cells will commit to a particular lineage [119]. The second wave occurs during the development of the testes or ovaries, where the primordial germ cells incorporate sex-specific imprinting patterns [120]. During both of these time windows, an exogenous chemical can impose changes (in some cases permanent) in the methylation status of DNA.

Alterations in the methylation status of certain genes have been observed in offspring that experience malnutrition in the womb. Fetal liver derived from rats fed a low-protein diet showed promoter hypermethylation in the liver X-receptor (LXR) [121] and hypomethylation in PPARα [122]. The methylation-deficient status of PPARα was rescued by supplementing the low-protein diet with folic acid, a methyl donor [122]. These modifications could plausibly disturb normal lipid homeostasis and impair metabolism, perhaps leading to obesity. Chemical-induced alterations in DNA methylation status have also been observed for diethylstilbestrol (DES) [123] and the dioxin TCDD [124]. In preimplantation embryos, DNA methyltransferase activity was altered depending on whether the embryo was exposed to TCDD, DES, or polychlorinated biphenyl-153 (PCB153) [125]. Liver nuclear extracts derived from TBT-treated rats showed increased histone acetyl transferase activity [126]. Therefore, by affecting the levels of enzymes, such as DNA methyltransferase and histone acetyl transferase, which have broad impacts on gene regulation, these EDCs can conceivably transmogrify the entire epigenetic landscape. Hence, exposure to environmental chemicals has the potential to remodel the behavior of the myriad of genes that are connected to obesity.

The maternal programming of adipose tissue development is fundamentally concerned with epigenetic modifications that alter stem cell fate. Adipogenesis is a differentiation event in the mesodermal lineage wherein multipotent stromal cells (MSCs) or more restricted derivatives give rise to fat cells. MSCs have the potential to mature into various tissues including bone, muscle, cartilage, or adipose [127]. MSCs harvested from epididymal or ovarian fat pads of mice exposed to TBT in utero differentiate into significantly more fat cells, compared to controls [103]. Indeed, adipogenesis occurred at the expense of osteogenesis, suggesting that prenatal exposure to TBT biased the MSC population toward the adipogenic lineage [103]. TBT likely induces epigenetic changes within the MSC compartment that promote demethylation of adipogenic genes. It is currently controversial whether active demethylation of adipogenic genes (with a corresponding up-regulation in expression) is indicative of MSC differentiation into adipocytes. Recent evidence shows that in a population of pure adipose-derived MSCs, adipogenic genes are already hypomethylated in the MSCs, suggesting that MSCs are predisposed to adipogenesis [128]. Hence, an environmental chemical might augment the innate hypomethylated state of adipogenic genes or increase the methylation of other lineages, such that the MSC pool is biased prior to adipocyte differentiation. In support of this model, uninduced MSCs harvested from mice exposed to TBT in utero show decreased methylation in the promoter region of fatty acid-binding protein 4 (FABP4), a marker of adipocytes; suggesting that the MSC population has already been epigenetically modified to favor adipogenesis [103]. Future experiments will be required to identify what other genes are required to mediate the effects of prenatal TBT exposure in the MSC compartment, committing more MSCs to the adipogenic lineage.

About 40 years ago, in an effort to properly measure and define obesity, researchers postulated that the number of fat cells in the adult is fixed and that people gain or lose weight by filling or emptying these cells with fat [129, 130]. Recently, this hypothesis was proven correct, but with an important modification. The number of fat cells in an adult is essentially constant as had been supposed. However, in contrast to previous dogma, adipocytes are continually undergoing apoptosis [131] and being replenished [132]. Using the same [^{14}C]-labeling method employed to prove that adults have the capacity to produce new brain cells, researchers have shown that the life span of a fat cell is approximately 10 years in both obese and lean subjects [133]. During severe weight loss (e.g., gastric bypass), the number of fat cells remained constant, while cell volume decreased [133]. This suggests that obese individuals possess a pool of MSCs that is intrinsically biased toward replenishing fat cells, i.e., that obese individuals have a steady state level of adipocytes that may be higher than non-obese people. Such a bias could be regulated by epigenetic changes due to exposure to environmental cues experienced during critical developmental windows. Chemicals like TBT influence the number of MSCs committed toward the adipogenic fate by remodeling the chromatin, favoring the expression of genes that promote adipogenesis. Notwithstanding these recent advances, there is much yet to be learned about how epigenetic contributions modulate the prenatal programming of MSC fate and what role obesogens play in this process.

19.7 Conclusion

Prenatal exposure to obesogens is likely to be an underestimated contributor to the obesity epidemic. Although unhealthy food consumed in large portions together with insufficient physical activity are likely to be among the chief substrates of weight gain, rates of obesity have increased in infants [134], as well as children and adults. This suggests that obesity is being programmed prenatally or in early childhood. There is increasing evidence that supports the proposal that environmental chemicals may contribute to the prenatal programming of obesity (see Chapter 16). Prenatal exposure to tributyltin, a chemical for which the mechanism of action is known, predisposes organisms to obesity, suggesting that the DOHaD model is applicable to effects of chemical exposure, in addition to altered nutrition. There are numerous EDCs more prevalent in the environment than tributyltin that have been linked to metabolic disease and whose increased usage mirrors the rising trend of obesity. The metabolic pathways targeted by most of these chemicals remain to be determined and firm links between chemical exposure and obesity should be based on understanding the underlying mechanisms. Understanding how chemicals enter the body and are transferred to the developing fetus is still not well understood. Epigenetics and the regulation of the stem cell lineages will provide answers to the mechanistic questions regarding how obesogens disrupt the endocrine system. This will inform the development of therapeutics and perhaps even non-pharmacologic solutions to the obesity problem.

Lastly, an important policy issue raised by our work is that of personal responsibility. While it is undeniable that the balance of our food intake and activity is reflected in total body weight, it is equally true that obesity is a multifactorial disease with inputs from many different developmental pathways. Works in our laboratory and elsewhere have revealed critical roles for EDCs in body weight. A more complete understanding of how these pathways impact the body's homeostatic mechanisms for energy balance, adipocyte number, appetite, and satiety will allow future research to move forward without being limited by the simplistic model that caloric intake and exercise can be trivially balanced like a checkbook to achieve optimum weight.

Acknowledgments Work in the authors' laboratory was supported by a grant from the NIH R01 ES015849. A.J. is a pre-doctoral trainee of NSF IGERT DGE 0549479.

References

1. Fielding H. An enquiry into the causes of the late increase of robbers, etc. with some proposals for remedying this growing evil. London: A. Millar; 1751.
2. Warren KR, Hewitt BG. Fetal alcohol spectrum disorders: when science, medicine, public policy, and laws collide. Dev Disabil Res Rev. 2009;15(3):170–5.
3. Lemoine P, Harousseau H, Borteyru JP, Menuet JC. Children of alcoholic parents–observed anomalies: discussion of 127 cases. Arch Francaises De Pediatr. 1968;25:830–2.
4. Jones KL, Smith DW. Recognition of the fetal alcohol syndrome in early infancy. Lancet. Nov 3 1973;302(7836):999–1001.
5. Hill JO, Peters JC. Environmental contributions to the obesity epidemic. Science. May 29 1998;280(5368):1371–4.
6. Power C, Jefferis BJ. Fetal environment and subsequent obesity: a study of maternal smoking. Int J Epidemiol. Apr 2002;31(2):413–9.
7. Barker DJ, Osmond C. Infant mortality, childhood nutrition, and ischaemic heart disease in England and Wales. Lancet. May 10 1986;1(8489):1077–81.
8. Barker DJ, Osmond C. Low birth weight and hypertension. BMJ. Jul 9 1988;297(6641): 134–5.
9. Barker DJ, Osmond C, Golding J, Kuh D, Wadsworth ME. Growth in utero, blood pressure in childhood and adult life, and mortality from cardiovascular disease. BMJ. Mar 4 1989;298(6673):564–7.
10. Gluckman PD, Hanson MA, Beedle AS, Raubenheimer D. Fetal and neonatal pathways to obesity. Front Horm Res. 2008;36:61–72.
11. Ong KK, Dunger DB. Perinatal growth failure: the road to obesity, insulin resistance and cardiovascular disease in adults. Best Pract Res Clin Endocrinol Metab. Jun 2002;16(2): 191–207.
12. Ong KK, Ahmed ML, Emmett PM, Preece MA, Dunger DB. Association between postnatal catch-up growth and obesity in childhood: prospective cohort study. BMJ. Apr 8 2000;320(7240):967–71.
13. Barker D. Programming the baby. London: BMJ Publishing Group; 1994.
14. Ong KK. Size at birth, postnatal growth and risk of obesity. Horm Res. 2006;65 Suppl 3: 65–9.

15. Hanson MA, Gluckman PD. Developmental origins of health and disease: new insights. Basic Clin Pharmacol Toxicol. Feb 2008;102(2):90–3.
16. Nicholson JW. The early history of organotin chemistry. J Chem Educ. 1989;66(8):621–3.
17. Piver WT. Organotin compounds: industrial applications and biological investigation. Environ Health Perspect. Jun 1973;4:61–79.
18. Showalter S, Savarese J. Restrictions on the use of marine antifouling paints containing tributyltin and copper. 2004. http://nsglc.olemiss.edu/Advisory/Antifouling.pdf.
19. Hoch M. Organotin compounds in the environment – an overview. Appl Geochem. 2001;16(7–8):719–43.
20. Blaber SJM. The occurrence of a penis-like outgrowth behind the right tentacle in spent females of *Nucella lapillus*. Proc Malacol Soc Lond 1970;39:231–3.
21. Gibbs P, Bryan G. Reproductive failure in populations of the dog-whelk, *Nucella lapillus*, caused by imposex induced by tributyltin from antifouling paints. J Marine Biol Assoc UK. 1986;66:767–77.
22. Bryan GW, Gibbs PE, Hummerstone LG, Burt GR. Uptake and transformation of 14C-labelled tributyltin chloride by the dog-whelk, *Nucella lapillus*: importance of absorption from the diet. Marine Environ Res. 1989;28(1–4):241–5.
23. Snoeij NJ, Penninks AH, Seinen W. Biological activity of organotin compounds–an overview. Environ Res. Dec 1987;44(2):335–53.
24. Marinovich M, Viviani B, Galli CL. Reversibility of tributyltin-chloride-induced protein synthesis inhibition after ATP recovery in HEL-30 cells. Toxicol Lett. Aug 1990;52(3): 311–7.
25. Shimasaki Y, Kitano T, Oshima Y, Inoue S, Imada N, Honjo T. Tributyltin causes masculinization in fish. Environ Toxicol Chem. Jan 2003;22(1):141–4.
26. Grun F, Watanabe H, Zamanian Z, et al. Endocrine-disrupting organotin compounds are potent inducers of adipogenesis in vertebrates. Mol Endocrinol. Sep 2006;20(9):2141–55.
27. Wade GN, Gray JM, Bartness TJ. Gonadal influences on adiposity. Int J Obes. 1985;9 Suppl 1:83–92.
28. Laudenslager ML, Wilkinson CW, Carlisle HJ, Hammel HT. Energy balance in ovariectomized rats with and without estrogen replacement. Am J Physiol. May 1980;238(5): R400–5.
29. Homma H, Kurachi H, Nishio Y, et al. Estrogen suppresses transcription of lipoprotein lipase gene. Existence of a unique estrogen response element on the lipoprotein lipase promoter. J Biol Chem. Apr 14 2000;275(15):11404–11.
30. Heine PA, Taylor JA, Iwamoto GA, Lubahn DB, Cooke PS. Increased adipose tissue in male and female estrogen receptor-alpha knockout mice. Proc Natl Acad Sci USA. Nov 7 2000;97(23):12729–34.
31. Cooke PS, Heine PA, Taylor JA, Lubahn DB. The role of estrogen and estrogen receptor-alpha in male adipose tissue. Mol Cell Endocrinol. Jun 10 2001;178(1–2):147–54.
32. Jones ME, Thorburn AW, Britt KL, et al. Aromatase-deficient (ArKO) mice have a phenotype of increased adiposity. Proc Natl Acad Sci USA. Nov 7 2000;97(23):12735–40.
33. Maffei L, Rochira V, Zirilli L, et al. A novel compound heterozygous mutation of the aromatase gene in an adult man: reinforced evidence on the relationship between congenital oestrogen deficiency, adiposity and the metabolic syndrome. Clin Endocrinol (Oxf). Aug 2007;67(2):218–24.
34. Cooke GM. Effect of organotins on human aromatase activity in vitro. Toxicol Lett. Jan 25 2002;126(2):121–30.
35. Matthiessen P, Sumpter JP. Effects of estrogenic substances in the aquatic environment. EXS. 1998;86:319–35.
36. Korach KS, Sarver P, Chae K, McLachlan JA, McKinney JD. Estrogen receptor-binding activity of polychlorinated hydroxybiphenyls: conformationally restricted structural probes. Mol Pharmacol. Jan 1988;33(1):120–6.

37. Newbold RR, Padilla-Banks E, Snyder RJ, Jefferson WN. Developmental exposure to estrogenic compounds and obesity. Birth Defects Res A Clin Mol Teratol. Jul 2005;73(7):478–80.
38. Takayanagi S, Tokunaga T, Liu X, Okada H, Matsushima A, Shimohigashi Y. Endocrine disruptor bisphenol A strongly binds to human estrogen-related receptor gamma (ERRgamma) with high constitutive activity. Toxicol Lett. Dec 1 2006;167(2):95–105.
39. Cagampang F, Anthony F, Hanson M. P2-14 Developmental exposure to bisphenol-A leads to obesity and cardiovascular dysfunction in adult mouse offspring. Early Hum Dev. 2007;83 Suppl 1:S132–S133.
40. Kelce WR, Stone CR, Laws SC, Gray LE, Kemppainen JA, Wilson EM. Persistent DDT metabolite p,p'-DDE is a potent androgen receptor antagonist. Nature. Jun 15 1995;375(6532):581–5.
41. Kupfer D, Bulger WH. Studies on the mechanism of estrogenic actions of o,p'DDT: interactions with the estrogen receptor. Pestic Biochem Physiol. 1976;6(6):561–70.
42. Karmaus W, Osuch JR, Eneli I, et al. Maternal levels of dichlorodiphenyl-dichloroethylene (DDE) may increase weight and body mass index in adult female offspring. Occup Environ Med. Mar 2009;66(3):143–9.
43. Machinal F, Dieudonne MN, Leneveu MC, Pecquery R, Giudicelli Y. In vivo and in vitro ob gene expression and leptin secretion in rat adipocytes: evidence for a regional specific regulation by sex steroid hormones. Endocrinology. Apr 1999;140(4):1567–74.
44. Geary M, Pringle PJ, Persaud M, et al. Leptin concentrations in maternal serum and cord blood: relationship to maternal anthropometry and fetal growth. Br J Obstet Gynaecol. Oct 1999;106(10):1054–60.
45. Bjorntorp P. Neuroendocrine factors in obesity. J Endocrinol. Nov 1997;155(2):193–5.
46. Bjorntorp P, Rosmond R. Obesity and cortisol. Nutrition. Oct 2000;16(10):924–36.
47. Marin P, Darin N, Amemiya T, Andersson B, Jern S, Bjorntorp P. Cortisol secretion in relation to body fat distribution in obese premenopausal women. Metabolism. Aug 1992;41(8):882–6.
48. Björntorp P. Visceral obesity: a "civilization syndrome". Obes Res. 1993;1(3):206–22.
49. Chalew S, Nagel H, Shore S. The hypothalamic-pituitary-adrenal axis in obesity. Obes Res. Jul 1995;3(4):371–82.
50. Rask E, Olsson T, Soderberg S, et al. Tissue-specific dysregulation of cortisol metabolism in human obesity. J Clin Endocrinol Metab. Mar 2001;86(3):1418–21.
51. Wajchenberg BL. Subcutaneous and visceral adipose tissue: their relation to the metabolic syndrome. Endocr Rev. Dec 2000;21(6):697–738.
52. Rebuffe-Scrive M, Bronnegard M, Nilsson A, Eldh J, Gustafsson JA, Bjorntorp P. Steroid hormone receptors in human adipose tissues. J Clin Endocrinol Metab. Nov 1990;71(5):1215–9.
53. Rebuffe-Scrive M, Lundholm K, Bjorntorp P. Glucocorticoid hormone binding to human adipose tissue. Eur J Clin Invest. Oct 1985;15(5):267–71.
54. Hauner H, Entenmann G, Wabitsch M, et al. Promoting effect of glucocorticoids on the differentiation of human adipocyte precursor cells cultured in a chemically defined medium. J Clin Invest. Nov 1989;84(5):1663–70.
55. Bujalska IJ, Kumar S, Hewison M, Stewart PM. Differentiation of adipose stromal cells: the roles of glucocorticoids and 11beta-hydroxysteroid dehydrogenase. Endocrinology. Jul 1999;140(7):3188–96.
56. Bjorntorp P. Adipose tissue distribution and function. Int J Obes. Sep 1991;15 Suppl 2: 67–81.
57. Seckl JR, Morton NM, Chapman KE, Walker BR. Glucocorticoids and 11beta-hydroxysteroid dehydrogenase in adipose tissue. Recent Prog Horm Res. 2004;59: 359–93.
58. Wake DJ, Rask E, Livingstone DE, Soderberg S, Olsson T, Walker BR. Local and systemic impact of transcriptional up-regulation of 11beta-hydroxysteroid dehydrogenase type 1 in adipose tissue in human obesity. J Clin Endocrinol Metab. Aug 2003;88(8):3983–8.

59. Valsamakis G, Anwar A, Tomlinson JW, et al. 11beta-hydroxysteroid dehydrogenase type 1 activity in lean and obese males with type 2 diabetes mellitus. J Clin Endocrinol Metab. Sep 2004;89(9):4755–61.
60. Livingstone DE, Jones GC, Smith K, et al. Understanding the role of glucocorticoids in obesity: tissue-specific alterations of corticosterone metabolism in obese Zucker rats. Endocrinology. Feb 2000;141(2):560–3.
61. Krozowski Z, MaGuire JA, Stein-Oakley AN, Dowling J, Smith RE, Andrews RK. Immunohistochemical localization of the 11 beta-hydroxysteroid dehydrogenase type II enzyme in human kidney and placenta. J Clin Endocrinol Metab. Jul 1995;80(7): 2203–9.
62. Smith RE, Maguire JA, Stein-Oakley AN, et al. Localization of 11 beta-hydroxysteroid dehydrogenase type II in human epithelial tissues. J Clin Endocrinol Metab. Sep 1996;81(9):3244–8.
63. Hirasawa G, Sasano H, Takahashi K, et al. Colocalization of 11 beta-hydroxysteroid dehydrogenase type II and mineralocorticoid receptor in human epithelia. J Clin Endocrinol Metab. Nov 1997;82(11):3859–63.
64. Engeli S, Bohnke J, Feldpausch M, et al. Regulation of 11beta-HSD genes in human adipose tissue: influence of central obesity and weight loss. Obes Res. Jan 2004;12(1):9–17.
65. Milagro FI, Campion J, Martinez JA. 11-Beta hydroxysteroid dehydrogenase type 2 expression in white adipose tissue is strongly correlated with adiposity. J Steroid Biochem Mol Biol. Apr 2007;104(1–2):81–4.
66. Kotelevtsev Y, Brown RW, Fleming S, et al. Hypertension in mice lacking 11beta-hydroxysteroid dehydrogenase type 2. J Clin Invest. Mar 1999;103(5):683–9.
67. Seckl JR. Glucocorticoid programming of the fetus; adult phenotypes and molecular mechanisms. Mol Cell Endocrinol. Dec 20 2001;185(1–2):61–71.
68. Weinstock M. The potential influence of maternal stress hormones on development and mental health of the offspring. Brain Behav Immun. Jul 2005;19(4):296–308.
69. Iqbal U, Brien JF, Banjanin S, Andrews MH, Matthews SG, Reynolds JN. Chronic prenatal ethanol exposure alters glucocorticoid signalling in the hippocampus of the postnatal Guinea pig. J Neuroendocrinol. Sep 2005;17(9):600–8.
70. Benediktsson R, Lindsay RS, Noble J, Seckl JR, Edwards CR. Glucocorticoid exposure in utero: new model for adult hypertension. Lancet. Feb 6 1993;341(8841):339–41.
71. Schlumbohm C, Bramlage C, Strutz F, Armstrong V, Oellerich M, Fuchs E. Predictive value of maternal bodyweight, postnatal weight gain and prenatal dexamethasone overexposure for the development of obesity in adult marmoset monkeys. Exp Clin Endocrinol Diabetes. 2007;115(8).
72. Purnell JQ, Kahn SE, Samuels MH, Brandon D, Loriaux DL, Brunzell JD. Enhanced cortisol production rates, free cortisol, and 11beta-HSD-1 expression correlate with visceral fat and insulin resistance in men: effect of weight loss. Am J Physiol Endocrinol Metab. Feb 2009;296(2):E351–7.
73. Odermatt A, Gumy C. Glucocorticoid and mineralocorticoid action: why should we consider influences by environmental chemicals? Biochem Pharmacol. Nov 15 2008;76(10):1184–93.
74. Nammi S, Dembele K, Nyomba BL. Increased 11beta-hydroxysteroid dehydrogenase type-1 and hexose-6-phosphate dehydrogenase in liver and adipose tissue of rat offspring exposed to alcohol in utero. Am J Physiol Regul Integr Comp Physiol. Mar 2007;292(3):R1101–9.
75. Lee S, Schmidt D, Tilders F, Rivier C. Increased activity of the hypothalamic-pituitary-adrenal axis of rats exposed to alcohol in utero: role of altered pituitary and hypothalamic function. Mol Cell Neurosci. Oct 2000;16(4):515–28.
76. Chen L, Nyomba BL. Whole body insulin resistance in rat offspring of mothers consuming alcohol during pregnancy or lactation: comparing prenatal and postnatal exposure. J Appl Physiol. Jan 2004;96(1):167–72.
77. Chen L, Nyomba BL. Effects of prenatal alcohol exposure on glucose tolerance in the rat offspring. Metabolism. Apr 2003;52(4):454–62.

78. Edwards CR, Benediktsson R, Lindsay RS, Seckl JR. Dysfunction of placental glucocorticoid barrier: link between fetal environment and adult hypertension? Lancet. Feb 6 1993;341(8841):355–7.
79. Welberg LA, Seckl JR, Holmes MC. Inhibition of 11beta-hydroxysteroid dehydrogenase, the foeto-placental barrier to maternal glucocorticoids, permanently programs amygdala GR mRNA expression and anxiety-like behaviour in the offspring. Eur J Neurosci. Mar 2000;12(3):1047–54.
80. Yang K, Julan L, Rubio F, Sharma A, Guan H. Cadmium reduces 11 beta-hydroxysteroid dehydrogenase type 2 activity and expression in human placental trophoblast cells. Am J Physiol Endocrinol Metab. Jan 2006;290(1):E135–E42.
81. Atanasov AG, Nashev LG, Tam S, Baker ME, Odermatt A. Organotins disrupt the 11beta-hydroxysteroid dehydrogenase type 2-dependent local inactivation of glucocorticoids. Environ Health Perspect. Nov 2005;113(11):1600–6.
82. Atanasov AG, Tam S, Rocken JM, Baker ME, Odermatt A. Inhibition of 11 beta-hydroxysteroid dehydrogenase type 2 by dithiocarbamates. Biochem Biophys Res Commun. Aug 22 2003;308(2):257–62.
83. Cooke GM, Forsyth DS, Bondy GS, Tachon R, Tague B, Coady L. Organotin speciation and tissue distribution in rat dams, fetuses, and neonates following oral administration of tributyltin chloride. J Toxicol Environ Health A. 2008;71(6):384–95.
84. Fernandez-Real JM, Pugeat M, Grasa M, et al. Serum corticosteroid-binding globulin concentration and insulin resistance syndrome: a population study. J Clin Endocrinol Metab. Oct 2002;87(10):4686–90.
85. Joyner JM, Hutley LJ, Bachmann AW, Torpy DJ, Prins JB. Greater replication and differentiation of preadipocytes in inherited corticosteroid-binding globulin deficiency. Am J Physiol Endocrinol Metab. May 2003;284(5):E1049–E54.
86. Issemann I, Green S. Activation of a member of the steroid hormone receptor superfamily by peroxisome proliferators. Nature. Oct 18 1990;347(6294):645–50.
87. Lalwani ND, Reddy MK, Qureshi SA, Sirtori CR, Abiko Y, Reddy JK. Evaluation of selected hypolipidemic agents for the induction of peroxisomal enzymes and peroxisome proliferation in the rat liver. Hum Toxicol. Jan 1983;2(1):27–48.
88. Kersten S, Seydoux J, Peters JM, Gonzalez FJ, Desvergne B, Wahli W. Peroxisome proliferator-activated receptor alpha mediates the adaptive response to fasting. J Clin Invest. Jun 1999;103(11):1489–98.
89. Mandard S, Muller M, Kersten S. Peroxisome proliferator-activated receptor alpha target genes. Cell Mol Life Sci. Feb 2004;61(4):393–416.
90. Krey G, Braissant O, L'Horset F, et al. Fatty acids, eicosanoids, and hypolipidemic agents identified as ligands of peroxisome proliferator-activated receptors by coactivator-dependent receptor ligand assay. Mol Endocrinol. Jun 1997;11(6):779–91.
91. Kliewer SA, Xu HE, Lambert MH, Willson TM. Peroxisome proliferator-activated receptors: from genes to physiology. Recent Prog Horm Res. 2001;56:239–63.
92. Tontonoz P, Hu E, Spiegelman BM. Stimulation of adipogenesis in fibroblasts by PPAR gamma 2, a lipid-activated transcription factor. Cell. Dec 30 1994;79(7):1147–56.
93. Lehmann JM, Moore LB, Smith-Oliver TA, Wilkison WO, Willson TM, Kliewer SA. An antidiabetic thiazolidinedione is a high affinity ligand for peroxisome proliferator-activated receptor gamma (PPAR gamma). J Biol Chem. Jun 2 1995;270(22):12953–6.
94. Finck BN, Bernal-Mizrachi C, Han DH, et al. A potential link between muscle peroxisome proliferator- activated receptor-alpha signaling and obesity-related diabetes. Cell Metab. Feb 2005;1(2):133–44.
95. Finck BN, Han X, Courtois M, et al. A critical role for PPARa-mediated lipotoxicity in the pathogenesis of diabetic cardiomyopathy: modulation by dietary fat content. Proc Natl Acad Sci USA. Feb 4 2003;100(3):1226–31.
96. Finck BN, Lehman JJ, Leone TC, et al. The cardiac phenotype induced by PPARalpha overexpression mimics that caused by diabetes mellitus. J Clin Invest. Jan 2002;109(1):121–30.

97. Nolte RT, Wisely GB, Westin S, et al. Ligand binding and co-activator assembly of the peroxisome proliferator-activated receptor-gamma. Nature. Sep 10 1998;395(6698):137–43.
98. Maloney EK, Waxman DJ. trans-Activation of PPARalpha and PPARgamma by structurally diverse environmental chemicals. Toxicol Appl Pharmacol. Dec 1 1999;161(2):209–18.
99. Kanayama T, Kobayashi N, Mamiya S, Nakanishi T, Nishikawa J. Organotin compounds promote adipocyte differentiation as agonists of the peroxisome proliferator-activated receptor gamma/retinoid X receptor pathway. Mol Pharmacol. Mar 2005;67(3):766–74.
100. Grun F, Blumberg B. Environmental obesogens: organotins and endocrine disruption via nuclear receptor signaling. Endocrinology. Jun 2006;147 6 Suppl:S50–5.
101. le Maire A, Grimaldi M, Roecklin D, et al. Activation of RXR-PPAR heterodimers by organotin environmental endocrine disruptors. EMBO Rep. Apr 2009;10(4):367–73.
102. Lee G, Elwood F, McNally J, et al. T0070907, a selective ligand for peroxisome proliferator-activated receptor gamma, functions as an antagonist of biochemical and cellular activities. J Biol Chem. May 31 2002;277(22):19649–57.
103. Kirchner S, Kieu T, Chow C, Casey S, Blumberg B. Prenatal exposure to the environmental obesogen tributyltin predisposes multipotent stem cells to become adipocytes. Mol Endocrinol. Mar 2010;24(3):526–39.
104. Fonseca V, Foyt HL, Shen K, Whitcomb R. Long-term effects of troglitazone: open-label extension studies in type 2 diabetic patients. Diabetes Care. Mar 2000;23(3):354–9.
105. Shim WS, Do MY, Kim SK, et al. The long-term effects of rosiglitazone on serum lipid concentrations and body weight. Clin Endocrinol (Oxf). Oct 2006;65(4):453–9.
106. Hurst CH, Waxman DJ. Activation of PPARalpha and PPARgamma by environmental phthalate monoesters. Toxicol Sci. Aug 2003;74(2):297–308.
107. Feige JN, Gelman L, Rossi D, et al. The endocrine disruptor monoethyl-hexyl-phthalate is a selective peroxisome proliferator-activated receptor gamma modulator that promotes adipogenesis. J Biol Chem. Jun 29 2007;282(26):19152–66.
108. Stahlhut RW, van Wijgaarden E, Dye TD, Cook S, Swan SH. Concentrations of urinary phthalate metabolites are associated with increased waist circumferece and insulin resistance in adult U.S. males. Environ Health Perspect. 2007;115(6):876–82.
109. Mose T, Knudsen LE, Hedegaard M, Mortensen GK. Transplacental transfer of monomethyl phthalate and mono(2-ethylhexyl) phthalate in a human placenta perfusion system. Int J Toxicol. May–Jun 2007;26(3):221–9.
110. Dolinoy DC, Weidman JR, Jirtle RL. Epigenetic gene regulation: linking early developmental environment to adult disease. Reprod Toxicol. Apr–May 2007;23(3):297–307.
111. Reed D, Lawler M, Tordoff M. Reduced body weight is a common effect of gene knockout in mice. BMC Genet. 2008;9(1):4.
112. Godfrey KM, Lillycrop KA, Burdge GC, Gluckman PD, Hanson MA. Epigenetic mechanisms and the mismatch concept of the developmental origins of health and disease. Pediatr Res. May 2007;61(5 Pt 2):5R–10R.
113. Gluckman PD, Hanson MA. Living with the past: evolution, development, and patterns of disease. Science. Sep 17 2004;305(5691):1733–6.
114. Smiraglia DJ, Kulawiec M, Bistulfi GL, Gupta SG, Singh KK. A novel role for mitochondria in regulating epigenetic modification in the nucleus. Cancer Biol Ther. Aug 2008;7(8): 1182–90.
115. Reik W, Dean W, Walter J. Epigenetic reprogramming in mammalian development. Science. Aug 10 2001;293(5532):1089–93.
116. Anway MD, Skinner MK. Epigenetic transgenerational actions of endocrine disruptors. Endocrinology. Jun 2006;147 6 Suppl:S43–9.
117. Morgan HD, Santos F, Green K, Dean W, Reik W. Epigenetic reprogramming in mammals. Hum Mol Genet. Apr 15 2005;14 Spec No 1:R47–R58.
118. Vaissière T, Sawan C, Herceg Z. Epigenetic interplay between histone modifications and DNA methylation in gene silencing. Mutat Res/Rev Mutat Res. 2008;659(1–2):40–8.

119. Mayer W, Niveleau A, Walter J, Fundele R, Haaf T. Demethylation of the zygotic paternal genome. Nature. Feb 3 2000;403(6769):501–502.
120. Hajkova P, Erhardt S, Lane N, et al. Epigenetic reprogramming in mouse primordial germ cells. Mech Dev. Sep 2002;117(1–2):15–23.
121. van Straten EME, Bloks VW, Huijkman NCA, et al. The liver X-receptor gene promoter is hypermethylated in a mouse model of prenatal protein restriction. Am J Physiol Regul Integr Comp Physiol. Feb 1 2010;298(2):R275–R82.
122. Lillycrop KA, Phillips ES, Torrens C, Hanson MA, Jackson AA, Burdge GC. Feeding pregnant rats a protein-restricted diet persistently alters the methylation of specific cytosines in the hepatic PPARα Promoter of the offspring. Br J Nutr. 2008;100(02):278–82.
123. Li S, Washburn KA, Moore R, et al. Developmental exposure to diethylstilbestrol elicits demethylation of estrogen-responsive lactoferrin gene in mouse uterus. Cancer Res. Oct 1 1997;57(19):4356–9.
124. Wu Q, Ohsako S, Ishimura R, Suzuki JS, Tohyama C. Exposure of mouse preimplantation embryos to 2,3,7,8-tetrachlorodibenzo-p-dioxin (TCDD) alters the methylation status of imprinted genes H19 and Igf2. Biol Reprod. Jun 2004;70(6):1790–7.
125. Wu Q, Zhou ZJ, Ohsako S. Effect of environmental contaminants on DNA methyltransferase activity of mouse preimplantation embryos. Wei Sheng Yan Jiu. Jan 2006;35(1):30–2.
126. Osada S, Nishikawa J, Nakanishi T, Tanaka K, Nishihara T. Some organotin compounds enhance histone acetyltransferase activity. Toxicol Lett. Feb 15 2005;155(2):329–35.
127. Pittenger MF, Mackay AM, Beck SC, et al. Multilineage potential of adult human mesenchymal stem cells. Science. Apr 2 1999;284(5411):143–7.
128. Boquest AC, Noer A, Collas P. Epigenetic programming of mesenchymal stem cells from human adipose tissue. Stem Cell Rev. 2006;2(4):319–29.
129. Karam JH. Obesity: fat cells–not fat people. West J Med. Feb 1979;130(2):128–32.
130. Hirsch J, Han PW. Cellularity of rat adipose tissue: effects of growth, starvation, and obesity. J Lipid Res. Jan 1969;10(1):77–82.
131. Mader I, Wabitsch M, Debatin KM, Fischer-Posovszky P, Fulda S. Identification of a novel proapoptotic function of resveratrol in fat cells: SIRT1-independent sensitization to TRAIL-induced apoptosis. FASEB J. Jan 22 2010;24:1997–2009.
132. Muhlhausler B, Smith SR. Early-life origins of metabolic dysfunction: role of the adipocyte. Trends Endocrinol Metab. Mar 2009;20(2):51–7.
133. Spalding KL, Arner E, Westermark PO, et al. Dynamics of fat cell turnover in humans. Nature. Jun 5 2008;453(7196):783–7.
134. Kim J, Peterson KE, Scanlon KS, et al. Trends in overweight from 1980 through 2001 among preschool-aged children enrolled in a health maintenance organization. Obesity (Silver Spring). Jul 2006;14(7):1107–12.

Index

A
Adenylyl cyclase (ACIII), 81
Adipocyte, 173
adipogenesis
BMP, role in, 178
CAAT/enhancer-binding proteins (C/EBP), 177–178
chromatin remodeling and C/EBP transcription factors, 181–182
DNA methylation and gene expression, 184
histone methylation in, 183–184
PPAR-γ regulation, 178, 182–183
preadipocyte determination regulation, 178–181
studying, experimental systems for, 176
developing stages
determination/differentiation, 175
differentiation, genes in, 323–325
hypertrophy and lipogenesis, 326
lipolysis, 327
load, 7
number of, 174
types, 174
Adipocyte development and experimental obesity, 321–322
adipokines in SGA-associated obesity, 338–339
adipose tissue growth/function
adipocyte hypertrophy and lipogenesis, 326
adipocyte lipolysis, 327
hyperplasia *vs.* hypertrophy, 322–325
endocrinology of adipose tissue, 327–328
hormone signaling in SGA-associated obesity, 336–338
mechanisms in prenatal undernutrition, 339–340
prenatal development of adipose tissue depots
body fat distribution, 330–331
brown adipose tissue, 329–330
WAT *vs.* BAT, 330
white adipose tissue, 328–329
prenatal nutritional environment
role of accelerated postnatal growth, 332–334
undernutrition/LBW/adiposity, 331–332
prenatal undernutrition/LBW/adipocyte biology, 334
adipogenesis/lipogenesis/lipolysis in SGA humans/experimental models, 334–336
Adipogenesis, 116
appetite and, 220–221
and lipogenesis, 225–227
in white adipose tissue, 322
Adipose tissue
differentiation, 174, 390
endocrinology of, 327–328
growth and function, mechanisms of
adipocyte hypertrophy and lipogenesis, 326
adipocyte lipolysis, 327
hyperplasia *vs.* hypertrophy, 322–325
Adiposity, programming of, 225
enhanced adipogenesis and lipogenesis, 225–227
Adoption study
BMI, 43
Canadian study, 42
Danish group study, 42–43
design, 42
US study, 42

R.H. Lustig (ed.), *Obesity Before Birth*, Endocrine Updates 30,
DOI 10.1007/978-1-4419-7034-3, © Springer Science+Business Media, LLC 2011

Adult exposures to environmental agents and obesity, 362
  fructose, 362
  monosodium glutamate (MSG), 362–363
  phthalates, 363
Adult-onset obesity, HC intake during suckling, 261–262
  altered dietary experience in postnatal period, 263
  HC female rat (F0) in prepregnancy period, 266
  HC fetus (F1 generation), 268–269
  HC milk formula in rat pups (F0), 265
  HC offspring (F1) in postnatal period, 269–270
  HC pregnant rat (F0 generation), 266–267
  HC rat model, 263–265
  high-fat diet consumption and programming effects, 271–272
  long-term effects of HC dietary modification, 265–266
  metabolic programming of fetus, 262
  phenomenon of metabolic programming, 272
  reversal of transgenerational effect, 270–271
  transgenerational effect of HC dietary modification, 266
Agouti-related protein (AGRP), 11
AGRP, *see* Agouti-related protein (AGRP)
Albright hereditary osteodystrophy (AHO), 116, 137
ALMS, *see* Alström syndrome (ALMS)
Alström syndrome (ALMS), 72
  ALMS1 protein functions, 85
    siRNA-induced loss-of-cilia phenotype in, 86
  mouse models of, 85–86
  neurosensory problems, 85
Angelman syndrome, 115, 123
Animal models/species
  of hypothalamic maldevelopment
    neonatal leptin, role of, 11–12
  intrauterine growth restriction/SGA/experimental obesity, 218–220
  maternal diet in pregnancy on offspring, 242–243
  of maternal obesity/hypercaloric diet/high-fat feeding, 243–244
  prenatal glucocorticoid exposure in, 14
Appetite
  and adipogenesis, 220–221
  physiology, 221
  and satiety mechanisms, development of
    role of adipose tissue, 224–225
    role of leptin, 222–224

B

Bardet–Biedl syndrome (BBS), 72, 83
  in neuronal signaling and obesity, 81–82
  proteins and leptin signaling
    control of, 79–80
    mechanism, 81
    model, 80
  Roux-en-Y gastric bypass, 63–64
Bariatric surgery, 63
BBS, *see* Bardet–Biedl syndrome (BBS)
Bbs-induced aberrant Mchr1 signaling, 81
BBSome-like complex, 84–85
Beckwith–Weidemann syndrome, 116–117
Birth weight
  as biomarker, low, 332
  low and high, 332
Bisphenol A, 375–376
BMP, *see* Bone morphogenetic proteins (BMP)
Body composition
  genetic and environmental correlations, 36
  heritability of body fat distribution, 36
  somatotype, 35–36
  twin study, 37–38
Body fat distribution, 330–331
Body mass index (BMI), 26
  in adolescents
    genetic and environmental effects, 34
    longitudinal study, 34
    traits, 33
  in adults
    age-related weight gain, 34
    twin-pair studies, 34
  BMI–WHR correlation, 36
  in children
    DeFries–Fulker (DF) extremes analysis, 32–33
    heritability and, 33
    meta-analysis, 33
    model-fitting techniques, 32
    twin studies, 32
  genome-wide linkage study of, 44
Bone morphogenetic proteins (BMP), 177
Brain-derived neurotrophic factor (BDNF), 6
  expression in the VMH, 61
  food intake and
    MC4R downstream, 61

haploinsufficiency, obesity and, 61
WAGR syndrome, 61–62
Brown adipose tissue, 174, 329–330
vs. developmental origins of WAT, 330

C
CATCH and Pathways trials, 4
CCAAT-enhancer binding protein (C/EBP) family members
C/EBP® and C/EBP™, 82
CHARGE consortium, *see* Cohorts for Heart and Aging Research in Genomic Epidemiology (CHARGE) consortium
Childhood obesity, 53
Chromatin
and binding proteins intervention, 179
in adipogenesis, role of, 180
remodeling in
β-Cell of IUGR rats, 170–171
and C/EBP transcription factors, 181–182
Chronic hyperinsulinemia, 8
Chronic stress, 12
Cilia
and adipogenesis, 82–83
for cell types, 72
ciliary syndromes and obesity, 71
ciliogenesis, 82
in developmental signaling
Hh and Wnt signal transduction pathways, 75
in energy homeostasis, 79
function, 72
genes in adipocyte differentiation, 82
and Hedgehog signaling
Patched 1 (Ptc1) protein, 75
and IFT in vertebrates, 73
microtubules, 73
model, 73
primary vertebrate in, 73
roles of, 72
structure of, 73
types
motile and nonmotile, 73–74
and Wnt signaling, 76–77
Clinical obesity
body mass index (BMI), 26
defined, 26
diseases and, 147
skinfold thickness, 26
waist–hip ratio (WHR), 26
World Health Organization criteria, 26
CNV, *see* Copy number variants (CNV)
Cohorts for Heart and Aging Research in Genomic Epidemiology (CHARGE) consortium, 102
Copy number variants (CNV), 109
Corticotropin-releasing hormone (CRH), 12
Cotwin control study, 30
Cushing's syndrome, 13, 139
Cytoplasmic dynein 2, 74

D
DEBQ, *see* Dutch Eating Behavior Questionnaire (DEBQ)
Developmental exposure, 358, 360–362
"Developmental origins of health and disease" paradigm, 356
Developmental plasticity
canalization, 148
crowding species, 148
Darwinian fitness advantage, 148
and human metabolic disease, 149–151
Developmental programming, 6, 217, 241–242, 339, 358–359
of obesity related hypertension, 245
Dexfenfluramine obesity drugs, 5
Diabetic mothers and offspring
abnormal glucose tolerance and T2DM, 197
early life growth patterns and risk for obesity, 195
birthweight (BWT), 196
dose–response relationship between, 197
epidemiologic study, 196–197
long-term consequences, 200
SEARCH CC, 197
Diethylstilbestrol (DES), 370–375
body weight of control and DES-treated mice, 372
Diet-induced thermogenesis, 174
Discordant MZ twin study, 30
Dizygotic (DZ) twins pairs, 29
genetic linkage studies using, 31
genome-wide linkage scans, 32
meta-analysis, 32
DNA methylation, 168–169
DOHaD, 262, 274, 301–303, 356, 383–385, 392
Double-blind placebo-controlled trial, 9
Dutch Eating Behavior Questionnaire (DEBQ), 38

E

Early life programming, 279
  mechanisms, 290
Eating behavior
  DEBQ, 38
  external eating, 38–39
  heritability and, 38
  rate and styles, 39–40
  restraint and emotional eating, 38–39
  satiety and food responsiveness, 39
  Three-Factor Eating Questionnaire, 38–39
Emotional eating, 38–39
  See also Eating behavior
Endocrine disruptor, 362
Endocrine/endocrinology
  of adipose tissue, 327–328
  system disturbances, 139
Energy
  obesity
    intake and expenditure, 2
    physical activity and, 3
Environment(al)
  chemicals, 167, 291, 355, 357–359, 369
  defined, 26
  effects
    shared and nonshared, 31
  estrogens and obesity, 367–368
  obesogenic and rise in obesity, 26–27
    case–control studies, 27
  obesogens in obesity epidemic, role of, 383–384
    epigenetics: gene–environment connection, 390–392
    glucocorticoid metabolism, 387–389
    obesogens acting on estrogen/androgen metabolism, 385–387
    peroxisome proliferator-activated receptors, 389–390
    prenatal chemical exposure (obesogens): tributyltin, 384–385
  toxicants, 357–358
Environmental estrogens and obesity
  developmental origins of adult disease, 368–369
  environmental estrogens in obesity, 370
    bisphenol A, 375–376
    diethylstilbestrol (DES), 370–375
    EDC, 377–378
    phytoestrogens, 377
    proposed modes of action, 378
Epigenetic mechanisms
  adipocyte and, 173
    number of, 174
  chromatin remodeling in
    β-cell of IUGR rats, 170–171
    in muscle of IUGR rats, 172
  DNA methylation, 168–169
  gene–environment connection, 390–392
  and gene regulation, 155
    in animal model, 157–158
    in intrauterine growth retardation, 169–170
    mechanisms for induced changes in epigenome, 158–159
    prevention and reversal, 159–161
  histone modifications, 168
  in induced risk of obesity, 155
  noncoding RNA, 169
Estrogens
  and androgen metabolism, obesogens acting on, 385–387
  developmental origins of adult disease, 368–369
  environmental estrogens and obesity, 367–368, 370
    bisphenol A, 375–376
    diethylstilbestrol (DES), 370–375
    EDC, 377–378
    phytoestrogens, 377
    proposed modes of action, 378
  phytoestrogens, 377
Experimental models of maternal obesity, 241–242
  animal models, hypercaloric diet and high-fat feeding, 243–244
  animal models to study role of maternal diet, 242–243
  stimulus to developmental programming, 244–245
    appetite regulatory system, 250–252
    maternal diets, types of fatty acids, 246–247
    maternal hypercholesterolemia, 248–249
    maternal obesity and fat feeding, 245–246
    maternal obesity *vs.* maternal fat intake, 247–248
    postnatal period, altered appetite circuitry, 249–250
    SNS activity/obesity and hypertension, 252–253
External eating, 38–39
  See also Eating behavior

F
Family-based studies, 43–44
Fas apoptotic inhibitory molecule-2 *(FAIM2)*, 101
Fetal development
- effects of in utero environment, 217
- glucocorticoids and, 280–281

Fetal hyperinsulinemia
- association between
  - amniotic fluid insulin and symmetry index, 198
- fetal programming of future obesity, 198
- gestational age, 199

Fetal hypothalamic alterations
- in maternal overnutrition, 310–312
- in maternal undernutrition, 312–314

Fetal programming
- abnormal hypothalamic regulation
  - alterations in maternal overnutrition, 310–312
  - alterations in maternal undernutrition, 312–314
- central mechanisms for
  - perinatal hypothalamic controls of energy homeostasis, 306–308
  - perinatal leptin, 308–309
- glucocorticoids in, 283

Feto-placental glucocorticoid barrier, 281–283
Forced weight loss, 8
Fructose, 362

G
Gamma aminobutyric acid (GABA) receptor, 124
GDM, *see* Gestational diabetes mellitus (GDM)
GEF, *see* Guanine nucleotide exchange factor (GEF); Guanosyl exchange factor (GEF)
Gene expression in PWS, 128
- neurotransmitter serotonin receptor genes, 129
- regulatory mechanisms, 129
- whole-genome microarrays, 129

Generational effect, 264
Genetic effects, additive and dominant, 31
Gene transcription mechanisms of PPAR, 226
Genome-wide association (GWA) studies
- in children and adolescents, 106–107
- of copy number variants (CNV), 109
- established loci
  - follow-up and functional characterization, 104–105
- gene–lifestyle interaction, 108
- genotyping chips, 109
- GIANT consortium, 101
- HapMap Project, 96
- Human Genome Project, 96
- imputation, 98
- increased sample size, 106
- on intermediary traits of obesity, 107–108
- Manhattan plot, 99
- obesity loci
  - BMI and large-scale high-density, 103
  - impact and predictive value, 103
- obesity-related traits, 100
- presentation of, 98–99
- replication of variants, 108–109
- on risk of obesity, 107
- studies in populations, 106
- two-stage design
  - discovery, 97–98
  - replication, 98
- for type 2 diabetes mellitus (T2DM), 100
- "waves" of discoveries
  - fat mass and obesity-associated *(FTO)* gene, 99
  - first wave, 99–100
  - second wave, 100–101
  - third wave, 101–102

Genome-wide association studies (GWAS), 6, 76
- missing heritability problem, 44–45
- single nucleotide variation in genome, 45

Genomic imprinting, 116
Genomic Investigation of Anthropometric Traits (GIANT) consortium, 101
Gestational diabetes mellitus (GDM), 193
- community-based study, 194–195
- diagnosis
  - criteria for, 194
  - glucose tolerance test (OGTT), 194
- HAPO study, 195
- predictive of future diagnosis of T2DM, 199–200
- and pre-existing diabetes with insulin treatment, 196
- risk factors for, 194

Gestational diabetes mellitus (GDM), 249, 262, 306
Gestational weight gain (GWG)
- association between childhood obesity and, 208–210
- by BMI category and race/ethnicity, 208

GIANT consortium, *see* Genomic Investigation of Anthropometric Traits (GIANT) consortium
Gli family of proteins, 76
Glucocorticoids, 280
 administration, 13
  and food intake, 12
 and fetal development, 280–281
 in fetal programming, 283
 levels associated with chronic stress, 13
 metabolism, obesogens acting on, 387–389
 programming, 283–284
  in humans, evidence for, 288–290
 role of, 280
Glucocorticoid receptor (GR) expression, 151
Glucocorticoid replacement therapy, 59
Glucosamine-6-phosphate deaminase-2 *(GNPDA2)*, 101
GNPDA2, see Glucosamine-6-phosphate deaminase-2 *(GNPDA2)*
GPCR, *see* G Protein-coupled receptor (GPCR)
G protein-coupled receptor (GPCR), 54, 56, 81
Growth hormone treatment, 135
Guanine nucleotide exchange factor (GEF), 124
Guanosyl exchange factor (GEF), 84
GWAS, *see* Genome-wide association studies (GWAS)

H

HAPO study, *see* Hyperglycemia and Adverse Pregnancy Outcomes (HAPO) study
HC dietary modification in adulthood, long-term effects, 265–266
HC intake during suckling period, 261–262
 altered dietary experience in immediate postnatal period, 263
 HC female rat (F0) in prepregnancy period, 266
 HC fetus (F1 generation), 268–269
 HC milk formula in rat pups (F0), dietary modification, 265
 HC offspring (F1) in postnatal period, 269–270
 HC pregnant rat (F0 generation), 266–267
 HC rat model, 263–265
 high-fat diet consumption and programming effects, 271–272
 long-term effects of HC dietary modification, 265–266
 mechanisms, metabolic programming, 272
 metabolic programming of fetus for adult-onset disease, 262
 transgenerational effect
  of HC dietary modification, 266
  reversal of, 270–271
HC rat model, 263–265
 effects on HC offspring (F1), 273
 female rat (F0) in prepregnancy period, 266
 fetus (F1 generation), 268–269
 HC (F0) and age-matched MF control female rats on gestational day 21, 267
 HC (F1) and age-matched MF control term fetuses, 268
 HC milk formula in rat pups (F0) during dietary modification, 265
 intake during suckling period, 261–262
 offspring (F1) in postnatal period, 269–270
 pregnant rat (F0 generation), 266–267
Hedgehog (Hh) signaling pathway, 75
Heredity
 case–control studies, 44–45
 defined, 25
 law of independent assortment, 25
 law of segregation, 25
 and nongenetic traits in obesity, 45–46
 obesity-related phenotypes, 44
High carbohydrate milk formula, 264
High-resolution array comparative genomic hybridization (aCGH), 121
Histone modifications, 168
Hormone signaling in SGA-associated obesity, 336–338
Human ciliopathies and obesity, 83
Human data supporting, obesogen, 360
 persistent organic pollutants, 361–362
 smoking, 360–361
Human Genome Project, 96
11β-hydroxysteroid dehydrogenase type 2, 281–283
Hyperdynamic chromatin, 179
Hyperglycemia and Adverse Pregnancy Outcomes (HAPO) study, 195
Hyperinsulinemia, 7
Hyperphagia, 58–59
Hyperplasia *vs.* hypertrophy, 322–325
Hyperprolactinemia, 139
Hypothalamic fetal programming of energy homeostasis, 301
 abnormal hypothalamic regulation
  maternal overnutrition, 310–312
  maternal undernutrition, 312–314
 central mechanisms
  perinatal hypothalamic controls of energy homeostasis, 306–308

perinatal leptin, 308–309
prenatal maternal overnutrition, models
gestational diabetes mellitus (GDM), 306
high-fat diet, 304–306
prenatal maternal undernutrition, models
caloric restriction, 303–304
protein restriction, 304
prenatal programming
animal studies, 303
epidemiological studies, 302–303
Hypothalamic obesity, 9

I

IFT, *see* Intraflagellar transport (IFT)
IGF1R, see Insulin-like growth factor receptor 1 *(IGF1R)* gene
Immediate postnatal life, 264, 266
Imprinted genes, 117
Imputation software, 98
Institute of medicine guidelines for weight gain during pregnancy (2009), 207
Institute of Medicine (IOM) weight gain guidelines, 207
Insulin-like growth factor receptor 1 *(IGF1R)* gene, 118
Insulin receptor substrate 2 (IRS2), 8
Insulin suppression, 9
Intraflagellar transport (IFT)
discovery and characterization, 74
kinesin-2 and, 73
primary cilia structure, 73
Intrauterine growth restriction/SGA/experimental obesity, 215–216
animal models, 218–219
animal species, 219–220
appetite physiology, 221
development of appetite and satiety mechanisms
role of adipose tissue, 224–225
role of leptin, 222–224
effects of in utero environment on fetal development, 217
programmed obesity, mechanisms, 228
programming mechanisms, appetite/adipogenesis, 220–221
programming of adiposity, 225
enhanced adipogenesis and lipogenesis, 225–227
programming of obesity, 216–217
therapies and applications, 228–229
Intrauterine growth retardation (IUGR), 157, 169–170
Inversin (Inv) protein, 76
IRS, *see* Insulin receptor substrate 2 (IRS2)
IRS2/PI3K signaling cascade, 8
IUGR, *see* Intrauterine growth retardation (IUGR)

J

JATD, *see* Jeune asphyxiating thoracic dystrophy (JATD)
Jeune asphyxiating thoracic dystrophy (JATD), 72

K

KCTD15, see Potassium channel tetramerization domain containing-15 *(KCTD15)*
KLF, *see* Kruppel-like factors (KLF)
Kruppel-like factors (KLF), 178

L

Large-for-gestational age (LGA), 6
studies of, 10–11
LCA, *see* Leber congenital amaurosis (LCA)
Leber congenital amaurosis (LCA), 72
Leptin
administration, 6
deficiency
congenital, 57
treatment for, 62–63
gene mutation, 57
leptin receptor (LepR)
LepR gene mutations, 57–58
in vitro pull-down assay, 80
leptin-replete state, 5
resistance, 7–8
signaling in
BBS proteins, role for, 80–81
hypothalamus and body weight, 78
role of cilia, 79
Leptin–melanocortin system
of energy balance, 55
gene mutations and
BDNF, 61–62
LepR, 57–58
leptin, 57
MC4R, 54–56
monogenic obesity, 54
NTRK2, 62
PC1/3 and PC2, 59–60
POMC, 58–59
network of neurons, 54
LGA, *see* Large-for-gestational age (LGA)
Lipogenesis, 323
adipocyte hypertrophy and, 326

Lipolysis, 327
adipocyte, 327
Liver metabolism
induction of altered regulation, 160
Long-term peripheral energy homeostasis, 8
LYPLAL1, see Lysophospholipase-like 1 *(LYPLAL1)*
Lysophospholipase-like 1 *(LYPLAL1)*, 102

M

MAGE, *see* Melanoma-associated antigen gene (MAGE)
Mammals
predictive adaptive response
and future risk of disease, 149
Maternal hyperglycemia and fetal growth, 193
diabetic intrauterine environment, 194
glucose intolerance, 194
glycemia during pregnancy
and infant body size, 194–195
maternal fuel supply, 195
Maternal isodisomy, 118
Maternal obesity
due to high-fat diet consumption and programming effects, 271–272
vs. maternal fat intake, 247–248
Maternal overnutrition
fetal hypothalamic alterations in, 310–312
Maternal stress during pregnancy, 13
Maternal undernutrition
fetal hypothalamic alterations in, 312–314
Maternal weight gain and offspring obesity, 205
epidemiology and trends of pregnancy weight gain, 207–208
gestational weight gain (GWG) and childhood obesity, 208–210
Institute of Medicine (IOM) weight gain guidelines, 207
interventions to prevent weight gain, 211–212
optimal weight gain for obese women, 210–211
special diets for obese woman, 212–213
weight gain among obese and non-obese, 205–206
Mature Onset of Diabetes in Youth-4 (MODY4), 171
McCune–Albright syndrome (MAS), 116
bone thickening, 139
causes of, 139
cutaneous abnormalities, 139
MC4R, *see* Melanocortin-4 receptor (MC4R)
Meckel–Gruber syndrome (MKS), 72
Medullary reticular activating system, 4
Melanin-concentrating hormone receptor 1 (Mchr1), 81
Melanocortin-4 receptor (MC4R), 5, 54
deficiency, 56
bariatric surgery, 64
treatment for, 63
MC4R gene mutations
heterozygous and homozygous, 56
obesity and, 56
"MC4R syndrome," 56
regulation of
food intake, 56
long-term energy homeostasis, 56
α-Melanocyte stimulating hormone (α-MSH), 11
Melanoma-associated antigen gene (MAGE), 122
MAGEL2 gene, 123
Metabolic disease, 254, 263
Metabolic programming, 261
of fetus for adult-onset disease, 262
mechanisms supporting phenomenon of, 272
Methionine sulfoxide reductase A *(MSRA)*, 102
Missing heritability problem
case-control studies, 44–45
Mitochondrial carrier homologue-2 *(MTCH2)*, 101
MKS, *see* Meckel–Gruber syndrome (MKS)
MODY4, *see* Mature Onset of Diabetes in Youth-4 (MODY4)
Monogenic obesity, 54
Monosodium glutamate (MSG), 362–363
Monozygotic (MZ) twins pairs, 29
MSRA, see Methionine sulfoxide reductase A *(MSRA)*
MTCH2, see Mitochondrial carrier homologue-2 *(MTCH2)*
Myocyte enhancer factor 2 (MEF2), 172

N

National Diabetes Data Group (NDDG)
plasma glucose thresholds, 194
National Heart, Lung and Blood Institute Family Heart Study data, 44
"Nature" interpretation, 5–6
problem with, 7
NDDG, *see* National Diabetes Data Group (NDDG)
NDN, *see* Necdin (NDN)

Necdin (NDN), 85, 122–123
NEGR1, see Neuronal growth regulator-1 *(NEGR1)*
Nephrocystin in human cells, 75
Nephronophthisis (NPH), 72
Neurexin-3 *(NRXN3)*, 102
Neurodevelopment, gene mutations and
  SIM1 transcription factor
    deficiency in, 60
Neuronal growth regulator-1 *(NEGR1)*, 101
Niemann–Pick disease type C-1 *(NPC1)*, 102
Noncoding RNA, 169
NPC1, see Niemann–Pick disease type C-1 *(NPC1)*
NRXN3, see Neurexin-3 *(NRXN3)*
NTRK2 gene
  BDNF and, 62
  mutations
    early-onset obesity, 62
    heterozygous de novo, 62
    homozygous null, 62
    missense, 62
    post-developmental neuronal plasticity and, 62
Nutrition in early life and gene transcription, 151–154
Nutrition in first postnatal weeks of life, 201

O
Obesity
  bariatric surgery, 63
  epidemic, 1
    caloric intake and, 3
    PWS and, 140–141
  frequency and severity in global, 1
  genetic and environmental effects
    balance of, 46
    distinguish between, 31
  hyperinsulinemic pregnancy, 264, 273
  obese and non-obese women, physiology of weight gain, 205–206
  obese women during pregnancy
    optimal weight gain for, 210–211
    special diets for, 212–213
  paradigms
    "nature" and "nurture," 2
  population shift due to programming, 216
  prevention and risk reduction strategies, 201, 210
  problems with, 3–5
  programming of, 216–217, 228
  related hypertension, 245, 252
  risk factors, 3, 331
Obesogen hypothesis of obesity, 252–253, 355–356, 358–360
  adult exposures to environmental agents and obesity, 362
    fructose, 362
    monosodium glutamate (MSG), 362–363
    phthalates, 363
  "developmental origins of health and disease" paradigm, 356
  environmental toxicants, 357–358
  human data supporting, 360
    persistent organic pollutants, 361–362
    smoking, 360–361
Offspring and diabetic mothers
  abnormal glucose tolerance and T2DM, 197
  early life growth patterns and risk for obesity
    dose–response relationship between, 197
    epidemiologic study, 196–197
  long-term consequences, 200
  SEARCH CC, 197
Open-label trial, 9
Orlistat obesity drugs, 5

P
Pancreatic beta cells, 376
Paraventricular nucleus (PVN) of hypothalamus, 54
Patched 1 (Ptc1) protein, 75–76
Pdx-1, homeodomain-containing transcription factor, 170
  targeted homozygous disruption of, 171
PEPCK, *see* Phosphoenolpyruvate carboxykinase (PEPCK)
Peroxisome proliferator-activated receptor- (PPAR), 82
  α expression, 152
Peroxisome proliferator-activated receptors, obesogens acting on, 389–390
Persistent organic pollutants, 361–362
Phosphatidyl inositol-3-kinase (PI3K), 8
Phosphoenolpyruvate carboxykinase (PEPCK), 151–152
Phosphotriesterase related *(PTER)*, 102
PHP, *see* Pseudohypoparathyroidism (PHP)
Phthalates, 363
Physical activity, 40–42
Phytoestrogens, 377
PI3K, *see* Phosphatidyl inositol-3-kinase (PI3K)

Plasma insulin levels in HC (F1), 269
Polycystin-2, 75
Polydactyly, 83–84
POMC, *see* Proopiomelanocortin (POMC)
Postnatal environment and intrauterine exposure, 199–200
Postnatal hyperinsulinemia, 8
Postnatal period
altered dietary experience in, immediate, 263
importance of, 249–250
Postnatal stress, 13
Potassium channel tetramerization domain containing-15 *(KCTD15)*, 101
PPARgamma, 225–226
PPAR, gene transcription mechanisms of, 226
PPHP, *see* Pseudopseudohypoparathyroidism (PPHP)
Prader–Willi syndrome (PWS), 6, 60, 115
with atypical 15q11–q13 Deletions, 127–128
behavioral problems, 120
clinical stages and natural history, 129–132
compulsive symptoms, 120
deletion *vs.* maternal disomy 15, 119–120
fatness patterns and body composition measures in, 132–133
genetic subtypes, 117
GNAS locus
genetic defects affecting, 137
heterozygous mutations within, 137
NESP55 transcript, 136–137
somatic mutations of, 139
XLAS transcript, 136
molecular genetics and deletion types, 120
aCGH, 121–122
breakpoints, 121
clinical findings associated with, 124–125
expression of, 126–127
genes/transcripts, 122–123
high-resolution chromosome, 121
larger Type I (TI) deletion, 121
smaller Type II (TII) deletion, 121
nutritional management
energy expenditure, 136
growth hormone treatment, 135
metabolic rates, 135
strategies for, 135
obesity and
energy expenditure components, 134
food exchange programs, 134
food monitoring program, 135
ghrelin and peptide YY, 134
pharmacological agents, 134
physical activity, 134
restricted caloric intake, 134–135
weight control and dietary restrictions, 134
obsessive–compulsive behavior, 124–125
seizures in, 120
self-injurious behavior, 120
translocations and causative genes, 127–128
treatment
exercise program, 63
types
heterodisomy and isodisomy, 118
X chromosome inactivation ratio, 119
X-linked disorders, 119
Pregnancy weight gain
epidemiology and trends of, 207–208
interventions to prevent excessive, 211–212
Prenatal chemical exposure (obesogens), tributyltin, 384–385
Prenatal development of adipose tissue depots
body fat distribution, 330–331
brown adipose tissue, 329–330
developmental origins of WAT *vs.* BAT, 330
white adipose tissue, 328–329
Prenatal maternal overnutrition, models
gestational diabetes mellitus (GDM), 306
high-fat diet, 304–306
Prenatal maternal undernutrition, models
caloric restriction, 303–304
protein restriction, 304
Prenatal nutritional environment
prenatal undernutrition, low birth weight, and adiposity, 331–332
role of accelerated postnatal growth, 332–334
Prenatal programming
conditions of, 218
and obesity, animal studies, 303
and obesity, epidemiological studies, 302–303
Prenatal stress, glucocorticoids, and metabolic syndrome, 279
11β-hydroxysteroid dehydrogenase type 2 and feto-placental glucocorticoid barrier, 281–283
glucocorticoids
and fetal development, 280–281

programming, 283–284
programming in humans, 288–290
role of, 280
mechanisms of early life programming, 290
programming of cardiovascular and metabolic systems
blood pressure and vascular function, 284–285
fatty liver, 287–288
glucose and insulin homeostasis, 285–287
muscle and fat, 288
pancreas, 287
Prenatal undernutrition
adipocyte hypertrophy, 336
adipogenesis/lipogenesis/lipolysis
in experimental models, 335–336
in SGA humans, 334
associated obesity
epigenetic and developmental mechanisms in, 339–340
Pre-pregnancy BMI category, gestational weight gain by, 209
Primary cilia in appetite control, 77
leptin signaling in
BBS proteins and control, 79–81
hypothalamus and body weight, 78
IFT requirement for, 78–79
Prohormone convertase 1/3 (PC1/3), 54
mutations in
and obesity, 59
proinsulin processing and, 60
Promelanocortin-expressing cells of hypothalamus, 72
Proopiomelanocortin (POMC), 54
coding region of, 58
deficiency
glucocorticoid replacement therapy, 59
POMC gene mutations, 58
hyperphagia and obesity, 58–59
loss-of-function, 58
processing, 58
tissue-specific cleavage of, 58
Protein-restricted (PR) diet, 151–154
Pseudohypoparathyroidism (PHP), 137–138
Pseudopseudohypoparathyroidism (PPHP), 137–138
Psychosocial stresses, 13
PTER, *see* Phosphotriesterase related *(PTER)*
Public health consequences, 200
Putative causative mechanisms, 228

R
Rab family of GTPases, 84
Rabin8, 84
REE, *see* Resting energy expenditure (REE)
Resting energy expenditure (REE), 5
REE:leptin ratio, 9
Rett syndrome, 119
RXR, 226, 389–390

S
Satiety, 221
SEARCH Case–Control Study (SEARCH CC), 197
Self-propagating epigenetic cycle, 171
Serotonin receptor 6, 81
Sexual precocity, 139
SGA, *see* Small-for-gestational age (SGA)
SGA-associated obesity and experimental models
adipokines in, 338–339
hormone signaling in, 336–338
SH2B adaptor protein-1 *(SH2B1)*, 101
Sibutramine obesity drugs, 5
Silver–Russell syndrome, 116–117
Single-copy snoRNA genes *(SNORD)*, 123
SIRT1 regulation of PPARγ, 227
Small-for-gestational age (SGA), 6
studies of, 10
Small nuclear ribonucleoprotein N (SNRPN), 122
Smoking, 360–361
Smoothened (Smo), 75
SNS, *see* Sympathetic nervous system (SNS)
SNS activity, obesity, and hypertension, programming of, 252–253
SNURF–SNRPN transcript, 123
Somatostatin 3 (Sstr3), 81
Somatotype, 35
categories of
ectomorph, 36
endomorph, 36
mesomorph, 36
SSTR, *see* Subscapular/triceps skin thickness ratio (SSTR)
Stem cell, 322, 325
Stimulus to developmental programming, 244–245
appetite regulatory system, 250–252
effect of maternal hypercholesterolemia, 248–249

Stimulus to developmental (*cont.*)
  effects of maternal obesity and fat feeding, 245–246
Stress, *see* Prenatal stress, glucocorticoids, and metabolic syndrome
Stress and glucocorticoids, 12
Subscapular/triceps skin thickness ratio (SSTR), 36
Sympathetic nervous system (SNS), 5
  tone drops, 5

T
Tachyphylaxis obesity drugs, 5
TFAP2B, see Transcription factor AP-2 beta *(TFAP2B)*
Three-Factor Eating Questionnaire, 38–39
TMEM18, see Transmembrane protein 18 *(TMEM18)*
Total energy expenditure, 5
Transcription factor AP-2 beta *(TFAP2B)*, 102
Transgenerational effect
  of HC dietary modification, 266
  reversal of, 270–271
Transmembrane protein 18 *(TMEM18)*, 101
Tributyltin (TBT), 384–385
  prenatal exposure to, 386
Trichostatin A (TSA) treatment, 171
TRKB, *see* Tropomyosin-related kinase B (TRKB)
Tropomyosin-related kinase B (TRKB), 62
Tubby gene role in obesity, 81
Twin studies
  analysis of variance (ANOVA), 29
  designs, 28
  genetic and environmental effects, distinguish between, 31
  intraclass correlations analysis, 29
  and obesity
    BMI, 31
    skinfold thickness, 31
  of obesity-related traits
    anthropometric measures, 35
    BMI in adolescents, 33–34
    BMI in adults, 34
    BMI in children, 32–33
    body composition, 35–38
    eating behavior, 38–40
    physical activity, 40–42
  structural equation modeling (SEM), 29
  types
    classical, 29
    Cotwin control study, 30
    discordant MZ twin study, 30
    twins reared apart, 30–31

U
UCP-1, *see* Uncoupling protein-1 (UCP-1)
UCP levels, *see* Uncoupling protein (UCP) levels
Uncoupling protein-1 (UCP-1), 174
Uncoupling protein (UCP) levels, 5

V
Ventromedial hypothalamus (VMH), 11
  as starvation, 5
Visceral adiposity, 13–14
V-maf musculoaponeurotic fibrosarcoma oncogene homologue *(MAF)*, 102
VMH, *see* Ventromedial hypothalamus (VMH)

W
WAGR syndrome, *see* Wilms' tumor, aniridia, genitourinary anomalies, and mental retardation (WAGR syndrome)
Waist circumference (WC), 13, 30, 35, 39, 44
Waist–hip ratio (WHR), 26, 35
Weight gain in pregnancy and offspring obesity, 205
  epidemiology and trends, 207–208
  gestational weight gain (GWG) and childhood obesity, 208–210
  Institute of Medicine (IOM) weight gain guidelines, 207
  interventions to prevent excessive pregnancy weight gain, 211–212
  optimal weight gain for obese women, 210–211
  special diets during pregnancy, 212–213
  weight gain in obese/non-obese women, physiology, 205–206
White adipose tissue, 174, 328–329
  adipogenesis in, 322
  developmental origins of BAT *vs.*, 330
Willi syndrome, 85
Wilms' tumor, aniridia, genitourinary anomalies, and mental retardation (WAGR syndrome), 61
Wnt signaling, 76
  and adiposity, 77

Made in the USA
Las Vegas, NV
22 October 2026

07bc9f6c-2aa9-44c8-b5c9-63ab9bf891eaR01